"十三五"国家重点出版物出版规划项目

总 主 编　刘树伟
副总主编　赵　斌　柳　澄　李振平　徐以发

Color Atlas of Digital Human Cross Sectional Anatomy
Pelvis and Perineum

数字人连续横断层解剖学彩色图谱
盆部与会阴分册

主编　林祥涛　王　青　吴凤霞

山东科学技术出版社

图书在版编目（CIP）数据

数字人连续横断层解剖学彩色图谱. 盆部与会阴分册/林祥涛, 王青, 吴凤霞主编. -- 济南：山东科学技术出版社, 2020.12
ISBN 978-7-5723-0678-5

Ⅰ.①数… Ⅱ.①林… ②王… ③吴… Ⅲ.①骨盆—计算机X线扫描体层摄影—断面解剖学—图谱②会阴—计算机X线扫描体层摄影—断面解剖学—图谱 Ⅳ.①R814.42-64

中国版本图书馆CIP数据核字(2020)第166493号

数字人连续横断层解剖学彩色图谱·盆部与会阴分册

SHUZIREN LIANXU HENGDUANCENG JIEPOUXUE CAISE TUPU · PENBUYUHUIYIN FENCE

责任编辑：王　涛　徐日强
装帧设计：侯　宇　李晨溪

主管单位：山东出版传媒股份有限公司
出 版 者：山东科学技术出版社
　　　　　地址：济南市市中区英雄山路189号
　　　　　邮编：250002　电话：（0531）82098088
　　　　　网址：www.lkj.com.cn
　　　　　电子邮件：sdkj@sdcbcm.com
发 行 者：山东科学技术出版社
　　　　　地址：济南市市中区英雄山路189号
　　　　　邮编：250002　电话：（0531）82098071
印 刷 者：济南新先锋彩印有限公司
　　　　　地址：济南市工业北路188-6号
　　　　　邮编：250101　电话：（0531）88615699

规格：8开（285mm×420mm）
印张：40.75　　字数：252千　　印数：1~2000
版次：2020年12月第1版　2020年12月第1次印刷
定价：490.00元

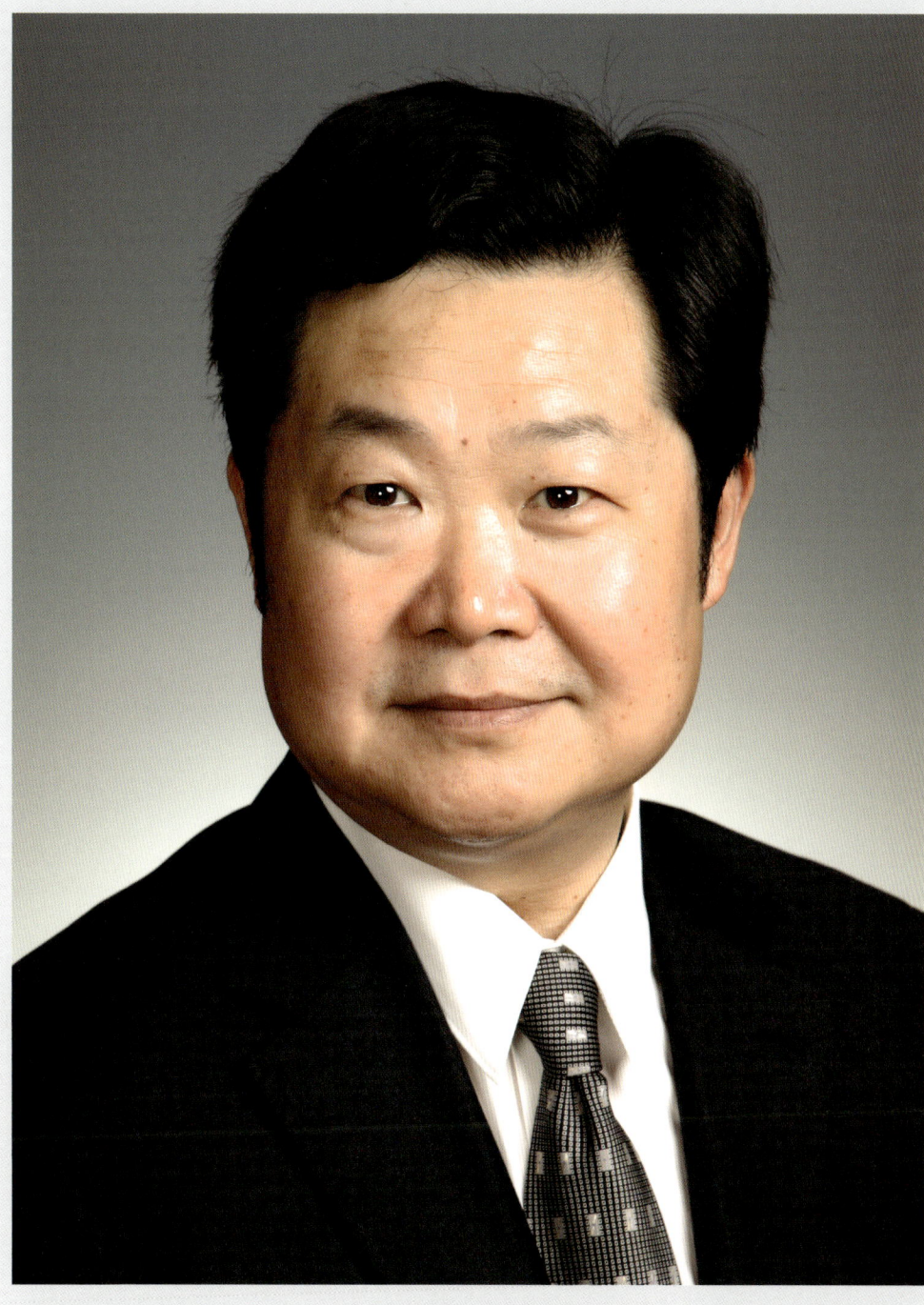

总主编　刘树伟

刘树伟，医学博士，山东大学基础医学院解剖学与神经生物学系教授、博士生导师，山东大学断层影像解剖学研究中心主任，山东大学数字人研究院院长，山东大学脑与类脑科学研究院副院长。曾任山东大学研究生院常务副院长、医学院副院长、人体解剖与组织胚胎学系主任等职，兼任亚洲临床解剖学会副主席、中国解剖学会副理事长和断层影像解剖学分会主任委员、中华医学会数字医学分会常务委员等职。获"卫生部有突出贡献的中青年专家"和"山东省教学名师"称号，享受国务院政府特殊津贴。潜心断层影像解剖学、数字人体和计算神经科学研究，承担国家及省部级课题20余项，在 Radiology、NeuroImage 和 Cerebral Cortex 等杂志发表论文320余篇（其中SCI收录70余篇），主编《人体断层解剖学》《临床中枢神经解剖学》和《功能神经影像学》等著作40余部，获省部级科技进步奖4项（其中一等奖1项）。长期从事人体解剖学教学，主持的"顺应现代影像学发展，创建断层解剖学课程"教学改革项目于1997年获山东省教学成果奖一等奖和国家级教学成果奖二等奖，主持完成的"我国数字解剖学教学体系创建与推广"教学研究项目于2018年获山东省教学成果奖特等奖和国家级教学成果奖二等奖。

主要学术著作、论文如下：

1. 刘树伟. 断层解剖学. 北京：人民卫生出版社，1998.
2. 刘树伟. 人体断层解剖学图谱. 济南：山东科学技术出版社，2003.
3. 刘树伟. 人体断层解剖学. 北京：高等教育出版社，2006.
4. 刘树伟，柳澄，胡三元. 腹部外科临床解剖学图谱. 济南：山东科学技术出版社，2006.
5. 刘树伟，王怀经. 应用解剖学（全六册）. 北京：高等教育出版社，2007.
6. 刘树伟，尹岭，唐一源. 功能神经影像学. 济南：山东科学技术出版社，2011.
7. 刘树伟，李瑞锡. 局部解剖学. 8版. 北京：人民卫生出版社，2013.
8. 刘树伟，杨晓飞，邓雪飞. 临床解剖学·腹盆部分册. 2版. 北京：人民卫生出版社，2014.
9. 刘树伟. 断层解剖学. 3版. 北京：高等教育出版社，2017.
10. 刘树伟，林祥涛. 影像解剖学系列图谱（全六册）. 济南：山东科学技术出版社，2020.
11. Tang Y, Hojatkashani C, Dinov ID, Sun B, Fan L, Lin X, Qi H, Hua X, Liu S*, Toga AW*. The construction of a Chinese MRI brain atlas: a morphometric comparison study between Chinese and Caucasian cohorts. NeuroImage, 2010, 51(1): 33-41.
12. Liu F, Zhang Z, Lin X, Teng G, Meng H, Yu T, Fang F, Zang F, Li Z, Liu S*. Development of the human fetal cerebellum in the second trimester: a post mortem magnetic resonance imaging evaluation. J Anat, 2011, 219: 582–588.
13. Zuo Y, Liu C, Liu S*. Pulmonary intersegmental planes: imaging appearance and possible reasons leading to their visualization. Radiology, 2013, 267(1): 267-275.
14. Yin X, Han Y, Ge H, Xu W, Huang R, Zhang D, Xu J, Fan L, Pang Z, Liu S*. Inferior frontal white matter asymmetry correlates with executive control of attention. Hum Brain Mapp, 2013, 34(4): 796-813.
15. Zhan J, Dinov ID, Li J, Zhang Z, Hobel S, Shi Y, Lin X, Zamanyan A, Lei F, Teng G, Fang F, Tang Y, Zang F, Toga AW*, Liu S*. Spatial-temporal atlas of fetal brain development during the early second trimester. NeuroImage, 2013, 82:115-126.
16. Ge X, Shi Y, Li J, Zhang Z, Lin X, Zhan J, Ge H, Xu J, Yu Q, Leng Y, Teng G, Feng L, Meng H, Tang Y, Zang F, Toga AW*, Liu S*. Development of the human fetal hippocampal formation during early second trimester. NeuroImage, 2015, 119: 33-43.
17. Xu J, Yin X, Ge H, Han Y, Pang Z, Liu B*, Liu S*, Friston K. Heritability of the effective connectivity in the resting-state default mode network. Cerebral Cortex，2017, 27(12): 5626-5634.
18. Tang Y, Zhao L, Lou Y, Shi Y, Fang R, Lin X, Liu S*, Toga AW. Brain structure differences between Chinese and Caucasian cohorts: A comprehensive morphometry study. Hum Brain Mapp, 2018, 39(5): 2147-2155.
19. Li Z, Xu F, Zhang Z, Lin X, Teng G, Zang F, Liu S*. Morphologic evolution and coordinated development of the fetal lateral ventricles in the second and third trimesters. Am J Neuroradiol, 2019, 40(4): 718-725.
20. Xu F, Ge X, Shi Y, Zhang Z, Tang Y, Lin X, Teng G, Zang F, Gao N, Liu H, Toga AW*, Liu S*. Morphometric development of the human fetal cerebellum during the early second trimester. NeuroImage, 2020, 207: 116372.

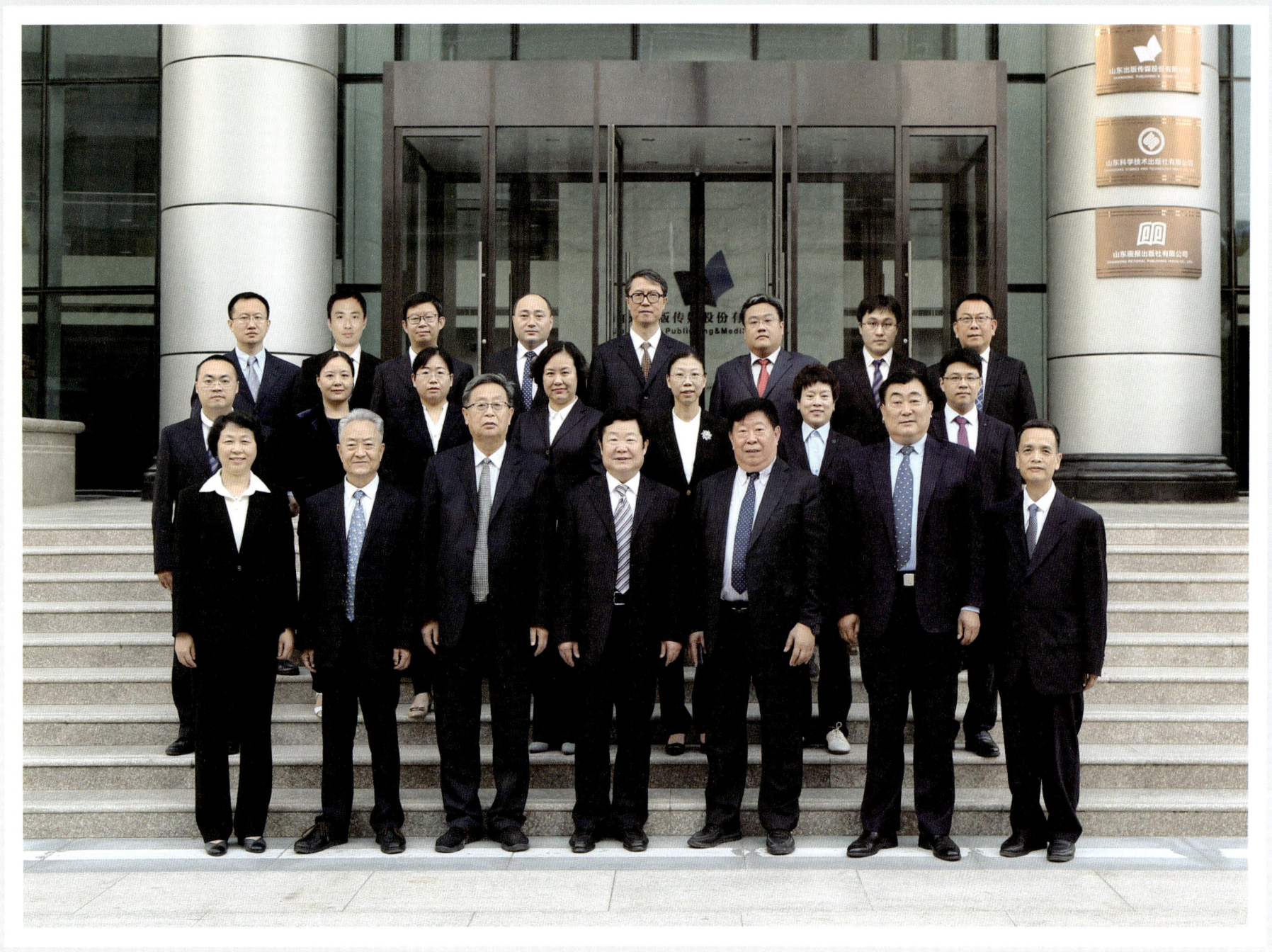

编委会全体人员合影

前排（从左至右）：王 青　李振平　柳 澄　刘树伟　赵 斌　徐以发　林祥涛
中排（从左至右）：孙 博　孟海伟　冯 蕾　张 杨　吴凤霞　王韶玉　任福欣
后排（从左至右）：侯中煜　左一智　于德新　汤煜春　于台飞　张忠和　于乔文　王增涛

《数字人连续横断层解剖学彩色图谱》编委会

总 主 编 刘树伟

副总主编 赵 斌　柳 澄　李振平　徐以发

编　　委（以姓氏笔画为序）

于台飞（山东省医学影像学研究所）　　　　汤煜春（山东大学齐鲁医学院）

于乔文（山东省立医院）　　　　　　　　　吴凤霞（山东大学齐鲁医学院）

于德新（山东大学齐鲁医院）　　　　　　　张　杨（山东大学齐鲁医院）

王　青（山东大学齐鲁医院）　　　　　　　张忠和（山东省立医院）

王韶玉（山东大学齐鲁医院）　　　　　　　李振平（山东大学齐鲁医学院）

王增涛（山东大学齐鲁医学院，山东省立医院）　孟海伟（山东大学齐鲁医学院）

刘树伟（山东大学齐鲁医学院）　　　　　　林祥涛（山东大学齐鲁医学院，山东省立医院）

冯　蕾（山东大学齐鲁医学院）　　　　　　赵　斌（山东省医学影像学研究所）

左一智（南京医科大学）　　　　　　　　　柳　澄（山东省医学影像学研究所）

孙　博（山东省医学影像学研究所）　　　　侯中煜（山东省立医院）

任福欣（山东省医学影像学研究所）　　　　徐以发（山东省数字人工程技术研究中心）

盆部与会阴分册

主　　编　林祥涛　王　青　吴凤霞

编　　者　（以姓氏笔画为序）

　　　　　王　青（山东大学齐鲁医院）　　　　　　　吴　锋（皖南医学院）

　　　　　田迷迷（山东大学齐鲁医学院）　　　　　　林祥涛（山东大学齐鲁医学院，山东省立医院）

　　　　　刘　冰（山东大学齐鲁医学院）　　　　　　徐兴华（山东大学齐鲁医院）

　　　　　李小莉（山东大学齐鲁医学院）　　　　　　夏　青（山东大学齐鲁医学院）

　　　　　吴凤霞（山东大学齐鲁医学院）　　　　　　韩晓宇（山东大学齐鲁医院）

标本图像处理

　　　　　魏　昱（山东省数字人工程技术研究中心）

　　　　　蒋　瑜（山东省数字人工程技术研究中心）

　　　　　韩　冰（山东省数字人工程技术研究中心）

序 一

我在人体解剖学园地里已耕耘七十余年了，对这个园地里新出现的每一朵鲜花和每一颗小草，都备感欣慰和鼓舞。今天，当看到山东大学刘树伟教授寄来的《数字人连续横断层解剖学彩色图谱》的书稿时，我眼前一亮，心情十分振奋。这将是一部巨著，是人体解剖学园地里一朵引人注目的鲜花。第一，它的人体标本数字断层彩色图像国际领先。"剖开顽石方知玉，淘尽泥沙始见金。"外形适中、结构正常、色泽鲜艳的人体断层标本相当难得。刘树伟教授团队历时 5 年，共铣削了 6 具人体标本，选择其中 2 具的断层图像来制成这部图谱，十分难能可贵。这套断层图像的分辨率高达 16 000 像素 ×26 000 像素，为当今国际上人体标本断层图像的最高分辨率。更令人感到欣喜的是，动脉和静脉均灌注颜料，使小血管得以展示，更有益于疾病的影像诊断和微创外科手术参考，大大增加了这套图谱的临床适用性。第二，书中标本断层与活体薄层 CT、MR 图像匹配得当。"天机云锦用在我，裁剪妙处非刀尺。"由于非同一个体，人体标本断层与活体 CT、MR 图像的匹配十分困难，在毫米级的层厚上二者间的匹配更是难上加难。同时，在国内外同类图谱中往往不配 CT、MR 图像。刘树伟教授团队"明知山有虎，偏向虎山行"，动员了十几名志愿者参与 CT、MR 配图，终获成功，使这部图谱的科学性、临床实用价值大为提高。第三，这部图谱是"医工结合""解剖与影像结合"的典范。"几番磨砺方成器，十载耕耘自见功。"刘树伟教授在山东大学先后创建了山东大学断层影像解剖学研究中心、数字人研究院，形成了一支"医工结合""解剖与影像结合"的科研团队，承担了一批国家级科研项目，在国内外杂志上发表了 400 余篇论文，获得 10 余项省部级科技进步奖和国家级教学成果奖，开发了教学软件"中国数字人解剖系统"，为我国断层影像解剖学和数字医学的发展做出了突出贡献。这部图谱是这种合作的杰出代表，我十分赞赏。

总之，刘树伟教授总主编的这部《数字人连续横断层解剖学彩色图谱》具有极强的创新性、科学性和实用性，出版价值重大。我真诚地希望不远的将来有数字人连续矢状断层和冠状断层的解剖学图谱出版。若如斯，解剖与影像皆幸莫大焉！

中国工程院院士 钟世镇

2020 年 10 月

序 二

进入 21 世纪以来，医学影像技术发展迅速，扫描层厚越来越薄，图像分辨率不断提高，所显示的解剖细节也越来越丰富，亟需与之相适应的断层解剖学图谱为其提供形态学基础。正值此时，山东大学刘树伟教授团队利用数控冷冻铣削技术获得了 0.1 mm 层厚的人体标本连续断层数据集，并编写成《数字人连续横断层解剖学彩色图谱》。我有幸先于广大读者看到书稿，感到此部图谱有以下特色：

特色之一，断层薄，精度高。人体连续断层标本彩色图像 0.1 mm 层厚，每隔 20 层选 1 层，分辨率高达 16 000 像素 ×26 000 像素，达到了同类图谱的国际领先水平。CT、MR 图像均为 2 mm 层厚，能做到与断层标本较好地契合。

特色之二，标注细，结构全。全书对 5 000 多个解剖结构进行了中英文标注，脑部结构标注到了大脑沟回、神经核团，肺、肝等均标注到了亚段级结构，对心包腔、胸膜腔、腹膜腔等均进行了连续追踪观察。

特色之三，注重将具体知识总结提升为解剖学理论。每一断层均有概要性文字，不仅描述了断层结构的整体配布规律，还讨论了关键结构的断面形态变化类型、大小、变异及其影像学特征等。

特色之四，努力做到理论联系实际。关键结构的选择以临床需要为原则，具体内容强调结合临床诊疗技术进展讨论解剖结构在疾病影像学诊断、介入治疗和外科手术中的应用。

总之，这是一部优秀的大型人体断层解剖学专著。它的公开出版，不仅在解剖学上有着重要的意义，而且对疾病影像诊断水平的提高也将大有裨益。因之为序，并郑重地向广大临床工作者推荐。

中国工程院院士 张运

2020 年 10 月

序 三

山东大学刘树伟教授是我国著名的断层影像解剖学专家,目前担任中国解剖学会副理事长兼断层影像解剖学分会主任委员。他不仅在 Radiology 和 NeuroImage 等国际著名杂志上发表了一系列研究论文,而且在断层解剖学和数字解剖学教学方面 2 次获得国家级教学成果奖。最近,刘树伟教授团队用数控冷冻铣削技术获取了 6 套中国人连续横断层解剖数据,计划出版一部《数字人连续横断层解剖学彩色图谱》。我仔细阅读了他寄来的书稿,感到这是一部人体断层解剖学的巨著,拥有以下创新:

(1)人体标本连续断层彩色图像来源于数字人研究,分辨率高,达到了同类图谱的国际领先水平。刘树伟教授团队改进了数控冷冻铣削技术,使用了大型龙门刨床,革新了切削刀具和切削工艺,使用 LED 光源和线阵扫描式相机摄影,获得了 0.1 mm 层厚的真彩色人体标本断层图像,分辨率达到了 16 000 像素 × 26 000 像素,而且较好地保留了标本原始色彩。

(2)使用 2 mm 间距选择标本和活体 CT、MR 图像制作图谱,8 开本印刷,是国内外同类图谱中绝无仅有的。使用数字人断面制作断层解剖学图谱在美国和中国已有先例,但断面间距均在 10 mm 以上,且无活体 CT、MR 图像相匹配,因此已不能满足当今数字人研究和疾病 CT、MR 图像诊断的需求,亟需薄层断层解剖学图谱的出版。

(3)标注细致和断面特点总结是该部图谱的又一显著特点。该部图谱使用《中国解剖学名词》对 5 000 多个解剖结构进行了中英文标注,每幅图像的标注结构大多超过 40 个,每隔 10 mm 增加了重要结构断层解剖的特点总结、断面数值和临床应用意义介绍,使这部图谱不仅科学理论价值巨增,也提高了其临床实用性,受众面大大增加。

我相信这部图谱代表了当今断层影像解剖学的发展前沿,将使该学科又上了一个新台阶,不仅将促进我国断层解剖学学科水平的整体提高,也将推动疾病 CT、MR 诊断水平的进一步改善,从而产生巨大的社会效益。因此,我很高兴为之作序,并向广大读者推荐。

中国工程院院士

2020 年 11 月

总前言

"图谱是表达断层解剖的最好形式。"这是我的导师四川大学王永贵教授34年前的谆谆教诲，当时只是一名硕士研究生的我并未完全理解。随着岁月的磨炼，我逐渐认识到这真是一句至理名言。时间进入21世纪，尤其是近10年间，人体断层解剖学发展迅速。在断层数据的获取方面，数控冷冻铣削技术使标本断层层厚达到了亚毫米水平，以CT和MRI为代表的医学影像设备的扫描速度更快、层厚更薄、分辨力更高；在断层图像的处理方面，多平面重组、三维重建、多模态影像融合、虚拟现实、增强现实和生物学计量等技术的发展更加深入、应用更趋广泛；在研究内容方面，对人体局部断层解剖信息的要求更加精细，形态与功能的结合更加密切，临床应用的针对性更强。在这种学术背景下，无论是人体解剖学工作者，还是临床医师，均呼唤着层厚在毫米级的薄层连续人体断层解剖学彩色图谱的出版。"好雨知时节，当春乃发生。"这部《数字人连续横断层解剖学彩色图谱》应运而生，既是人体解剖学领域最重要的前沿进展之一，又迎合了临床医师尤其是医学影像学医师的祈盼，还实现了本人的终生夙愿。

《数字人连续横断层解剖学彩色图谱》共包括头颈部、胸部、腹部、盆部与会阴、上肢和下肢6个分册，图像共4 519幅（含断层标本彩色图像917幅、螺旋CT图像1 753幅、3T MR图像1 841幅、其他图像8幅），文字约170万字。从图像采集到全书定稿，主要由山东大学数字人研究院完成。我们的目标是把本套图谱打造成断层解剖学的传世经典、解剖学工作者案头必备的工具书、临床工作者爱不释手的阅片指南。努力追求做到以下四个突出。第一，突出薄层断层解剖。以往的厚片断层解剖切片多在厘米级，许多解剖结构难以显示。本图谱标本断层层厚为0.1 mm，每隔20层选用1层，因此可充分展示一些细小的解剖结构。在标注和文字描述中，重点突出那些以往厚片无法展示的解剖细节，使断层解剖学为之一新。第二，突出解剖与影像的融合。标本断层和影像断层是断层解剖学两大支柱内容，在以往的研究中往往强调相互对照，而融合不够。本图谱不但强调二者之间的相互匹配，而且更强调二者的融合，旨在给出关键结构影像学表现的精准解剖学阐释。第三，突出断层解剖学规律的总结。以往的许多图谱，只注重断层结构的标注，而忽略了解剖结构在连续断层中的变化规律。本图谱每一断层均有300～500字的总结性短文，以讨论关键结构的断层形态变化规律、类型、大小、位置、毗邻、分区、发育、变异、影像学特征、生理功能、诊断和治疗意义等，以期将具体知识总结升华为断层解剖学理论。第四，突出基础理论与临床应用的结合。伟大导师恩格斯说过："没有解剖学就没有医学。"因此，解剖学知识只有应用于临床才能显示出其巨大实用意义和社会价值。书中关键结构的选择以临床需要为标准，在写作中强调精选内容，重点讨论关键结构在疾病诊断、介入治疗和外科手术中的应用价值。

"雄关漫道真如铁，而今迈步从头越。"在全书即将付梓之际，心中百感交集，思绪万千。我要衷心感谢国家自然科学基金委员会和山东省科技厅，是其立项的科研项目使本图谱使用的原始数据得以成功获取；我要衷心感谢我的同事们和研究生们，是大家齐心协力、忘我无私的工作，才使本书得以完成；我要衷心感谢中国工程院钟世镇院士、张运院士、顾晓松院士及西安交通大学刘军教授，是他们的推荐意见和序，照亮了我前进的道路；我要衷心感谢我的解剖学、影像学和外科学同仁，他们富有建设性的意见和建议使得本书内容在解剖学与临床的结合上更加紧密；我要衷心感谢山东科学技术出版社，是其领导和编辑们的视野、耐心和意志使得本图谱历尽千辛万苦而得以出版并入选"十三五"国家重点出版物出版规划项目。书是在使用中日臻完善的。最后，我衷心希望和感谢广大读者，不断提出您的意见和需求，以使本书更具理论价值和临床适用性。

2020年是中国解剖学会成立100周年。特将本部图谱献给中国解剖学会，以隆重纪念其百年华诞。

总主编 刘树伟

2020年10月15日

前 言

《数字人连续横断层解剖学彩色图谱·盆部与会阴分册》包括女性和男性两部分。前者从 L5-S1 椎间盘开始至外阴消失结束，共有标本断层图像 93 幅，CT 图像 93 幅，MR T1WI 图像 93 幅、T2WI 图像 95 幅；后者从股骨头中份开始至外阴消失结束，共有标本断层图像 57 幅，CT 图像 58 幅，MR T1WI 图像 57 幅、T2WI 图像 59 幅。标本断层图像由山东大学数字人研究院制作，CT 及 MR 图像采集自山东省立医院影像科。CT 扫描由 Siemens Force 双源 CT 扫描仪完成，MR 图像由 Siemens Prisma 3.0T MR 扫描仪制作。为体现本书的前沿性、思想性和学术性，在女性盆部，引用了作者完成的国家自然科学基金委员会资助的关于胎儿脊柱发育的最新研究成果，增加了子宫的正中矢状位及冠状位 T2WI 各 1 幅图像，以显示子宫壁的层次结构；在男性盆部，增加了目前临床最新应用的前列腺 T2WI 高分辨成像，清晰地显示了前列腺不同分区及相应信号改变。

以盆腔器官的变化为依据，自上而下大致可分女性盆部与会阴为五段。第 1 段（断层 1～26），从第 5 腰椎间盘平面至第 3 骶椎平面，主要为腹部带有系膜的肠道，如回肠、阑尾、乙状结肠。可重点观察髂骨翼、骶骨、骶髂关节、腹直肌、腹外斜肌及其腱膜、腹内斜肌与腹横肌、髂腰肌、梨状肌、臀大中小肌、回肠、盲肠、阑尾、降结肠和乙状结肠、输尿管、肠系膜、阑尾系膜、乙状结肠系膜、髂外动静脉、髂内动静脉、髂内外淋巴结、腰丛和骶丛等。第 2 段（断层 27～44），从骶髂关节消失平面到髋臼上缘平面，此段腹腔、盆腔器官共存，前部为消化道（回肠、乙状结肠），中部为内生殖器（卵巢、子宫底和体），后部为直肠。可观察的结构还有尾骨、梨状肌、闭孔内肌、腹前外侧壁肌、臀肌、输尿管、子宫阔韧带、乙状结肠系膜、髂外动静脉、髂内动静脉、髂内外淋巴结、腰丛及骶丛等。第 3 段（断层 45～62），从髋臼上缘平面至耻骨联合上缘平面，由前向后为膀胱、子宫颈或阴道上部、直肠。可观察的结构还有尾骨、耻骨、坐骨、闭膜管、闭孔内外肌、输尿管、子宫主韧带、股动静脉、腹股沟淋巴结、阴道静脉丛、直肠系膜、肛提肌及坐骨肛门窝等。第 4 段（断层 63～82），从耻骨联合上缘平面至耻骨弓下缘平面，由前向后依次为尿道、前庭球、阴道及肛管。除上述外，还有耻骨联合、坐骨结节、坐骨支、闭孔、闭孔内外肌、肛提肌、耻骨后间隙、坐骨肛门窝、阴部管、前庭球、阴蒂、阴蒂海绵体肌及肛门外括约肌等。第 5 段（断层 83～93），从耻骨弓下缘平面至女阴消失平面，主要为女阴，包括大阴唇、小阴唇、阴蒂、阴道前庭和会阴中心腱等。

男性盆腔器官自上而下大致可分为三段。第 1 段（断层 1～16），从髋臼上份平面至耻骨联合上缘平面。盆腔内的结构主要为膀胱、输尿管、输精管、精囊及直肠，盆壁结构主要观察精索。第 2 段（断层 17～27），耻骨联合上下缘层面，盆腔内的结构主要为前列腺、尿道、射精管及直肠，其他结构可观察会阴深横肌、会阴深隙、精索及男性外阴。第 3 段（断层 28～57），从耻骨联合下缘平面至阴囊消失平面，主要为男性会阴部的结构，包括会阴肌、男性外生殖器（阴茎、阴囊）、睾丸、附睾、精索、男性尿道、肛管及肛门外括约肌等。

在本册图谱图像采集及文字整理过程中，山东大学硕士研究生单德娟、杨咏青及山东第一医科大学硕士研究生马文静等同学做了大量具体工作，同时也得到了山东省立医院影像科王锡明主任、袁宪顺技师等同志们的大力帮助。在此，主编对所有为本图谱做出贡献的同仁们表示衷心的感谢！

编撰层厚 2 mm 标本及影像学图像匹配图谱尚属首次。尽管我们刻苦工作，反复校对，由于结构繁多、精细及作者水平所限，难免会有错误和不足之处。愿读者多多批评和提出合理建议，以便本图谱在应用中不断得以改进和完善。

林祥涛　王　青　吴凤霞
2020 年 11 月 5 日

目 录

女性盆部与会阴连续横断层解剖

女性盆部与会阴连续横断层 1（FH.9370）..................2
女性盆部与会阴连续横断层 2（FH.9350）..................4
女性盆部与会阴连续横断层 3（FH.9330）..................6
女性盆部与会阴连续横断层 4（FH.9310）..................8
女性盆部与会阴连续横断层 5（FH.9290）..................10
女性盆部与会阴连续横断层 6（FH.9270）..................12
女性盆部与会阴连续横断层 7（FH.9250）..................14
女性盆部与会阴连续横断层 8（FH.9230）..................16
女性盆部与会阴连续横断层 9（FH.9210）..................18
女性盆部与会阴连续横断层 10（FH.9190）..................20
女性盆部与会阴连续横断层 11（FH.9170）..................22
女性盆部与会阴连续横断层 12（FH.9150）..................24
女性盆部与会阴连续横断层 13（FH.9130）..................26
女性盆部与会阴连续横断层 14（FH.9110）..................28
女性盆部与会阴连续横断层 15（FH.9090）..................30
女性盆部与会阴连续横断层 16（FH.9070）..................32
女性盆部与会阴连续横断层 17（FH.9050）..................34
女性盆部与会阴连续横断层 18（FH.9030）..................36
女性盆部与会阴连续横断层 19（FH.9010）..................38
女性盆部与会阴连续横断层 20（FH.8990）..................40
女性盆部与会阴连续横断层 21（FH.8970）..................42
女性盆部与会阴连续横断层 22（FH.8950）..................44
女性盆部与会阴连续横断层 23（FH.8930）..................46
女性盆部与会阴连续横断层 24（FH.8910）..................48
女性盆部与会阴连续横断层 25（FH.8890）..................50
女性盆部与会阴连续横断层 26（FH.8870）..................52
女性盆部与会阴连续横断层 27（FH.8850）..................54
女性盆部与会阴连续横断层 28（FH.8830）..................56
女性盆部与会阴连续横断层 29（FH.8810）..................58
女性盆部与会阴连续横断层 30（FH.8790）..................60
女性盆部与会阴连续横断层 31（FH.8770）..................62
女性盆部与会阴连续横断层 32（FH.8750）..................64
女性盆部与会阴连续横断层 33（FH.8730）..................66
女性盆部与会阴连续横断层 34（FH.8710）..................68
女性盆部与会阴连续横断层 35（FH.8690）..................70
女性盆部与会阴连续横断层 36（FH.8670）..................72
女性盆部与会阴连续横断层 37（FH.8650）..................74
女性盆部与会阴连续横断层 38（FH.8630）..................76
女性盆部与会阴连续横断层 39（FH.8610）..................78
女性盆部与会阴连续横断层 40（FH.8590）..................80
女性盆部与会阴连续横断层 41（FH.8570）..................82
女性盆部与会阴连续横断层 42（FH.8550）..................84

女性盆部与会阴连续横断层 43（FH.8530）..........86
女性盆部与会阴连续横断层 44（FH.8510）..........88
女性盆部与会阴连续横断层 45（FH.8490）..........90
女性盆部与会阴连续横断层 46（FH.8470）..........92
女性盆部与会阴连续横断层 47（FH.8450）..........94
女性盆部与会阴连续横断层 48（FH.8430）..........96
女性盆部与会阴连续横断层 49（FH.8410）..........98
女性盆部与会阴连续横断层 50（FH.8390）..........100
女性盆部与会阴连续横断层 51（FH.8370）..........102
女性盆部与会阴连续横断层 52（FH.8350）..........104
女性盆部与会阴连续横断层 53（FH.8330）..........106
女性盆部与会阴连续横断层 54（FH.8310）..........108
女性盆部与会阴连续横断层 55（FH.8290）..........110
女性盆部与会阴连续横断层 56（FH.8270）..........112
女性盆部与会阴连续横断层 57（FH.8250）..........114
女性盆部与会阴连续横断层 58（FH.8230）..........116
女性盆部与会阴连续横断层 59（FH.8210）..........118
女性盆部与会阴连续横断层 60（FH.8190）..........120
女性盆部与会阴连续横断层 61（FH.8170）..........122
女性盆部与会阴连续横断层 62（FH.8150）..........124
女性盆部与会阴连续横断层 63（FH.8130）..........126
女性盆部与会阴连续横断层 64（FH.8110）..........128
女性盆部与会阴连续横断层 65（FH.8090）..........130
女性盆部与会阴连续横断层 66（FH.8070）..........132
女性盆部与会阴连续横断层 67（FH.8050）..........134
女性盆部与会阴连续横断层 68（FH.8030）..........136
女性盆部与会阴连续横断层 69（FH.8010）..........138
女性盆部与会阴连续横断层 70（FH.7990）..........140
女性盆部与会阴连续横断层 71（FH.7970）..........142
女性盆部与会阴连续横断层 72（FH.7950）..........144
女性盆部与会阴连续横断层 73（FH.7930）..........146
女性盆部与会阴连续横断层 74（FH.7910）..........148
女性盆部与会阴连续横断层 75（FH.7890）..........150
女性盆部与会阴连续横断层 76（FH.7870）..........152
女性盆部与会阴连续横断层 77（FH.7850）..........154
女性盆部与会阴连续横断层 78（FH.7830）..........156
女性盆部与会阴连续横断层 79（FH.7810）..........158
女性盆部与会阴连续横断层 80（FH.7790）..........160
女性盆部与会阴连续横断层 81（FH.7770）..........162
女性盆部与会阴连续横断层 82（FH.7750）..........164
女性盆部与会阴连续横断层 83（FH.7730）..........166
女性盆部与会阴连续横断层 84（FH.7710）..........168
女性盆部与会阴连续横断层 85（FH.7690）..........170
女性盆部与会阴连续横断层 86（FH.7670）..........172
女性盆部与会阴连续横断层 87（FH.7650）..........174
女性盆部与会阴连续横断层 88（FH.7630）..........176
女性盆部与会阴连续横断层 89（FH.7610）..........178
女性盆部与会阴连续横断层 90（FH.7590）..........180
女性盆部与会阴连续横断层 91（FH.7570）..........182
女性盆部与会阴连续横断层 92（FH.7550）..........184
女性盆部与会阴连续横断层 93（FH.7530）..........186

男性盆部与会阴连续横断层解剖

男性盆部连续横断层 1（MH.6580）..........190
男性盆部连续横断层 2（MH.6570）..........192
男性盆部连续横断层 3（MH.6560）..........194
男性盆部连续横断层 4（MH.6550）..........196

男性盆部连续横断层 5（MH.6540）	198
男性盆部连续横断层 6（MH.6530）	200
男性盆部连续横断层 7（MH.6520）	202
男性盆部连续横断层 8（MH.6510）	204
男性盆部连续横断层 9（MH.6500）	206
男性盆部连续横断层 10（MH.6490）	208
男性盆部连续横断层 11（MH.6480）	210
男性盆部连续横断层 12（MH.6470）	212
男性盆部连续横断层 13（MH.6460）	214
男性盆部连续横断层 14（MH.6450）	216
男性盆部连续横断层 15（MH.6440）	218
男性盆部连续横断层 16（MH.6430）	220
男性盆部连续横断层 17（MH.6420）	222
男性盆部连续横断层 18（MH.6410）	224
男性盆部连续横断层 19（MH.6400）	226
男性盆部连续横断层 20（MH.6390）	228
男性盆部连续横断层 21（MH.6380）	230
男性盆部连续横断层 22（MH.6370）	232
男性盆部连续横断层 23（MH.6360）	234
男性盆部连续横断层 24（MH.6350）	236
男性盆部连续横断层 25（MH.6340）	238
男性盆部连续横断层 26（MH.6330）	240
男性盆部连续横断层 27（MH.6320）	242
男性盆部连续横断层 28（MH.6310）	244
男性盆部连续横断层 29（MH.6300）	246
男性盆部连续横断层 30（MH.6290）	248
男性盆部连续横断层 31（MH.6280）	250
男性盆部连续横断层 32（MH.6270）	252
男性盆部连续横断层 33（MH.6260）	254
男性盆部连续横断层 34（MH.6250）	256
男性盆部连续横断层 35（MH.6240）	258
男性盆部连续横断层 36（MH.6230）	260
男性盆部连续横断层 37（MH.6220）	262
男性盆部连续横断层 38（MH.6210）	264
男性盆部连续横断层 39（MH.6200）	266
男性盆部连续横断层 40（MH.6190）	268
男性盆部连续横断层 41（MH.6180）	270
男性盆部连续横断层 42（MH.6170）	272
男性盆部连续横断层 43（MH.6160）	274
男性盆部连续横断层 44（MH.6150）	276
男性盆部连续横断层 45（MH.6140）	278
男性盆部连续横断层 46（MH.6130）	280
男性盆部连续横断层 47（MH.6120）	282
男性盆部连续横断层 48（MH.6110）	284
男性盆部连续横断层 49（MH.6100）	286
男性盆部连续横断层 50（MH.6090）	288
男性盆部连续横断层 51（MH.6080）	290
男性盆部连续横断层 52（MH.6070）	292
男性盆部连续横断层 53（MH.6060）	294
男性盆部连续横断层 54（MH.6050）	296
男性盆部连续横断层 55（MH.6040）	298
男性盆部连续横断层 56（MH.6030）	300
男性盆部连续横断层 57（MH.6020）	302

参考文献 ... 304

索　引 ... 306

女性盆部与会阴连续横断层解剖

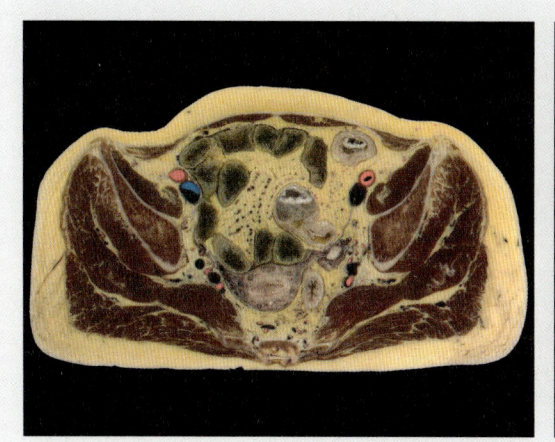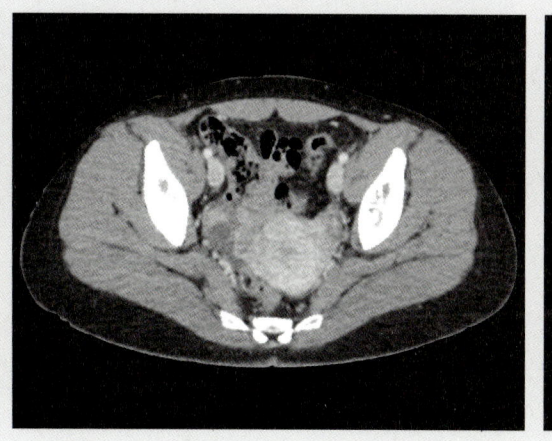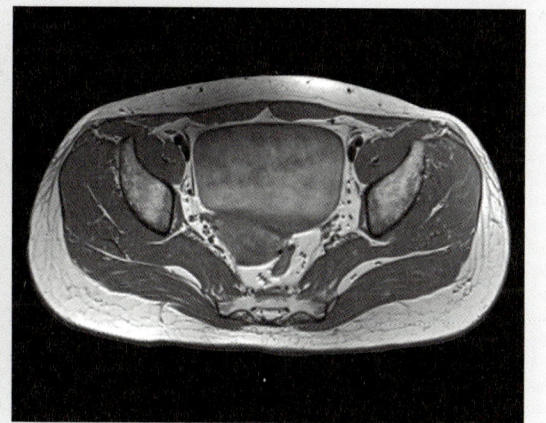

女性盆部与会阴连续横断层 1（FH.9370）

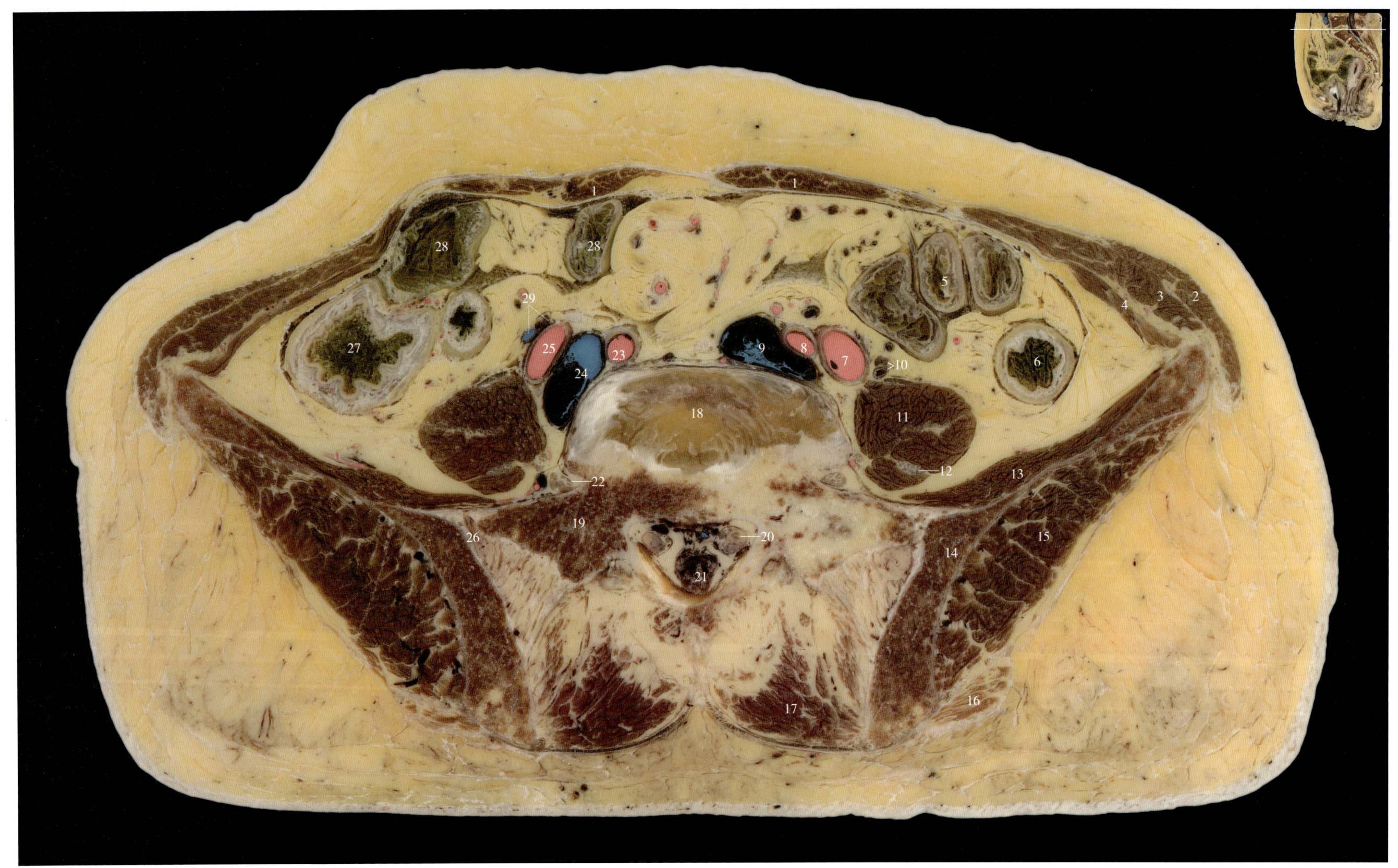

A. 断层标本图像

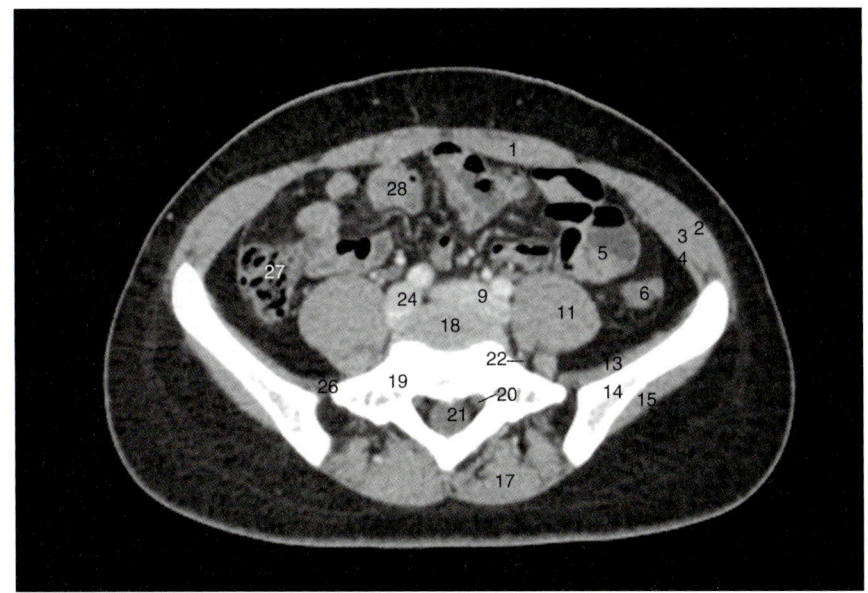
B. CT 增强图像

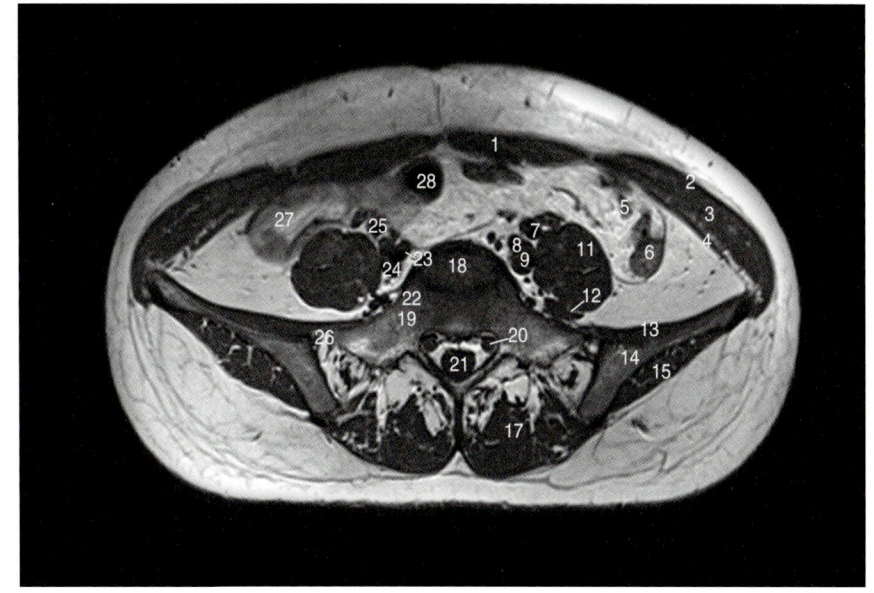
C. MR T1WI

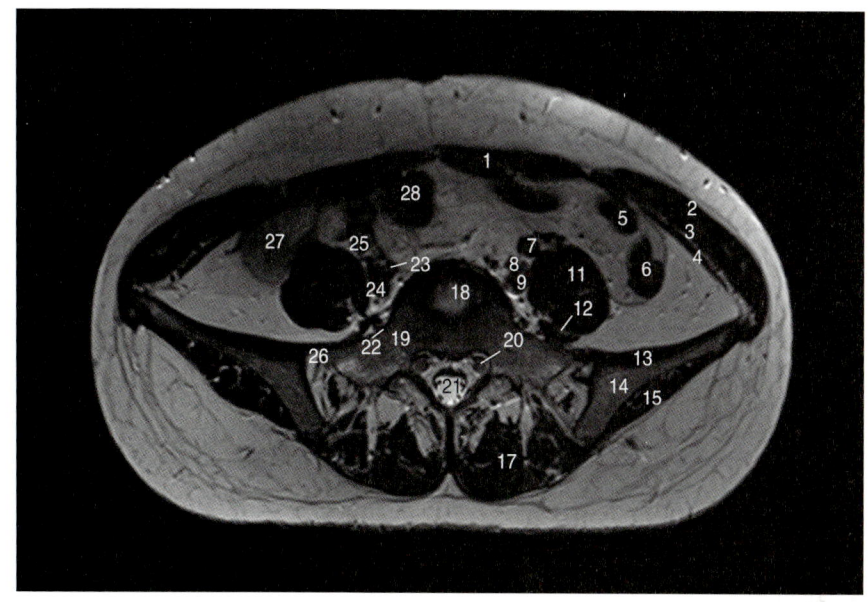
D. MR T2WI

1. 腹直肌 rectus abdominis
2. 腹外斜肌 obliquus externus abdominis
3. 腹内斜肌 obliquus internus abdominis
4. 腹横肌 transversus abdominis
5. 空肠 jejunum
6. 降结肠 descending colon
7. 左髂外动脉 left external iliac artery
8. 左髂内动脉 left internal iliac artery
9. 左髂总静脉 left common iliac vein
10. 左卵巢动、静脉 left ovarian artery and vein
11. 腰大肌 psoas major
12. 股神经 femoral nerve
13. 髂肌 iliacus
14. 髂骨翼 ala of ilium
15. 臀中肌 gluteus medius
16. 臀大肌 gluteus maximus
17. 竖脊肌 erector spinae
18. L5-S1 椎间盘 L5-S1 intervertebral disc
19. 骶骨侧部 lateral part of sacrum
20. 第 1 骶神经 1st sacral nerve
21. 马尾 cauda equina
22. 腰骶干 lumbosacral trunk
23. 右髂内动脉 right internal iliac artery
24. 右髂总静脉 right common iliac vein
25. 右髂外动脉 right external iliac artery
26. 骶髂骨间韧带 interosseous sacroiliac ligaments
27. 盲肠 cecum
28. 回肠 ileum
29. 右卵巢动、静脉 right ovarian artery and vein

关键结构：L5-S1 椎间盘，髂血管，肠管。

此断面经过 L5-S1 椎间盘（临床上常写作 L5-S1 椎间盘）。

L5-S1 椎间盘居于盆部后壁中央，连接第 5 腰椎椎体和第 1 骶椎椎体的上下面。椎间盘由髓核、纤维环、Sharpey 纤维和透明软骨终板组成。纤维环围绕髓核周围，由纤维板层构成，其后部相对薄弱，故髓核易向后外侧和后方突出，突入椎间孔和椎管，压迫脊神经根或脊髓而出现相应症状，称椎间盘突出症。在 CT 图像上，椎间盘的密度低于椎体，髓核和纤维环难以区分。在 MR T1WI 上，外纤维环与 Sharpey 纤维呈低信号，而内纤维环和髓核呈略高信号；在 MR T2WI 上，髓核呈明显的高信号[1]。椎间盘后方及两侧分别是第 1 骶椎椎体及髂骨，L5-S1 椎间盘外侧为腰大肌，二者之间形成的夹角内见粗大的髂血管。髂外动脉外侧、腰大肌前方见细小的卵巢动、静脉断面。肠管集中于断面的前半部，左髂窝处为降结肠，右髂窝处为盲肠，降结肠内侧是空肠，空肠黏膜皱襞丰富。盲肠内侧是回肠，回肠黏膜皱襞较空肠少。两侧髂骨翼呈浅"S"形，髂骨翼前面微微凹陷形成髂窝，窝内为髂肌。髂骨翼后外侧见臀中肌，其后方是臀大肌。腹前壁为白线及两侧的腹直肌，前外侧壁从外侧向内侧分别是腹外斜肌、腹内斜肌、腹横肌。骶骨侧部与髂骨间见骶髂骨间韧带，骶骨正中嵴两侧为竖脊肌。

女性盆部与会阴连续横断层 2（FH.9350）

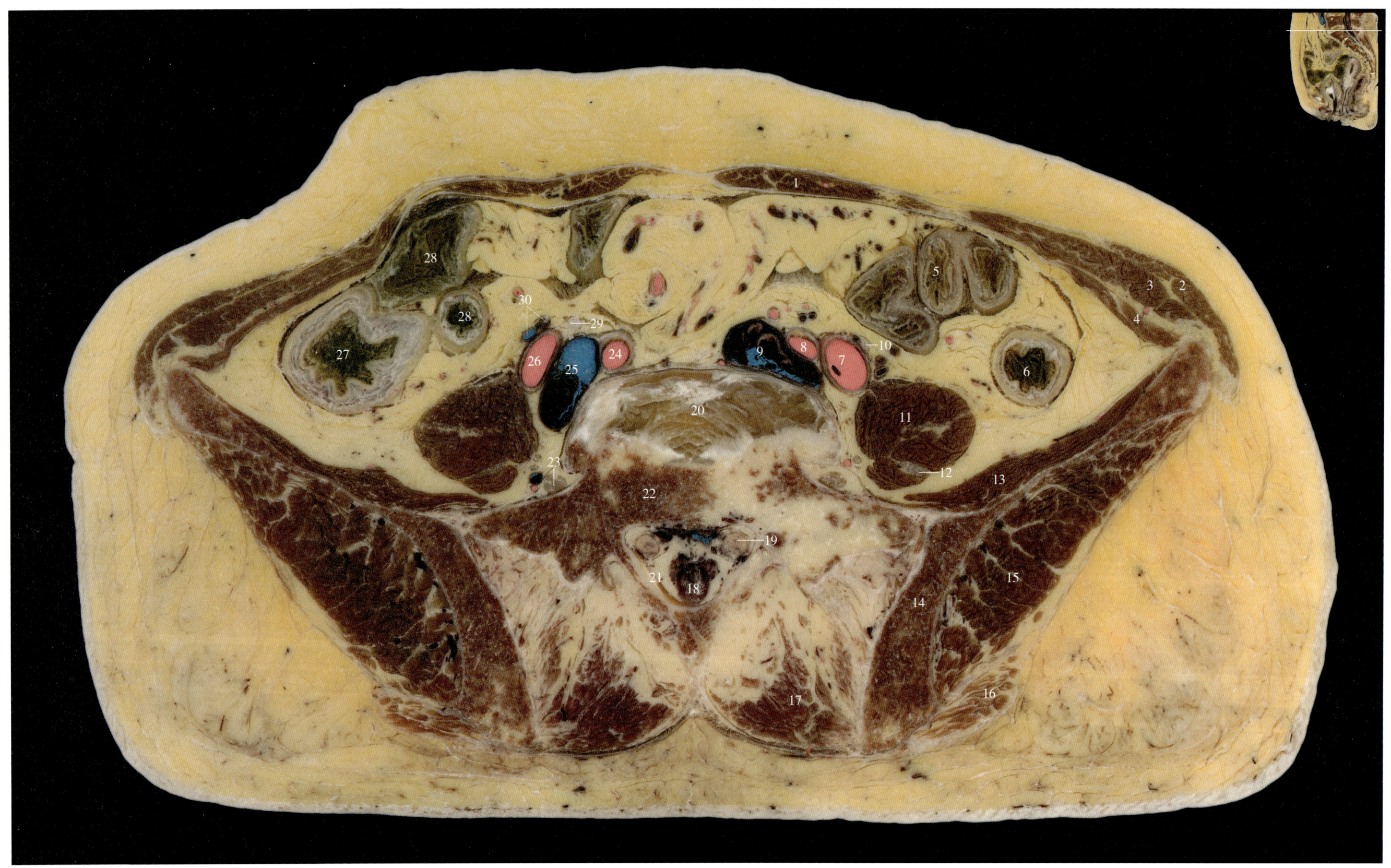

A. 断层标本图像

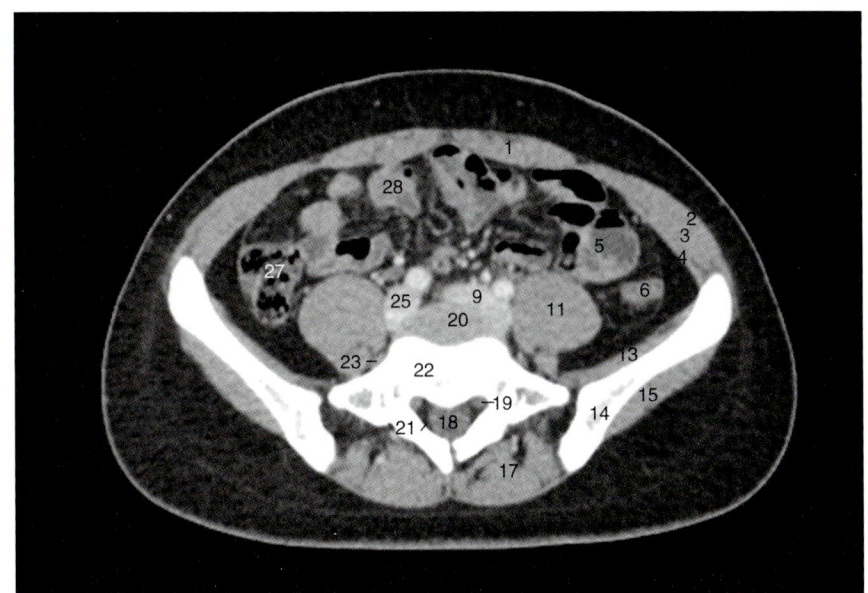

B. CT 增强图像

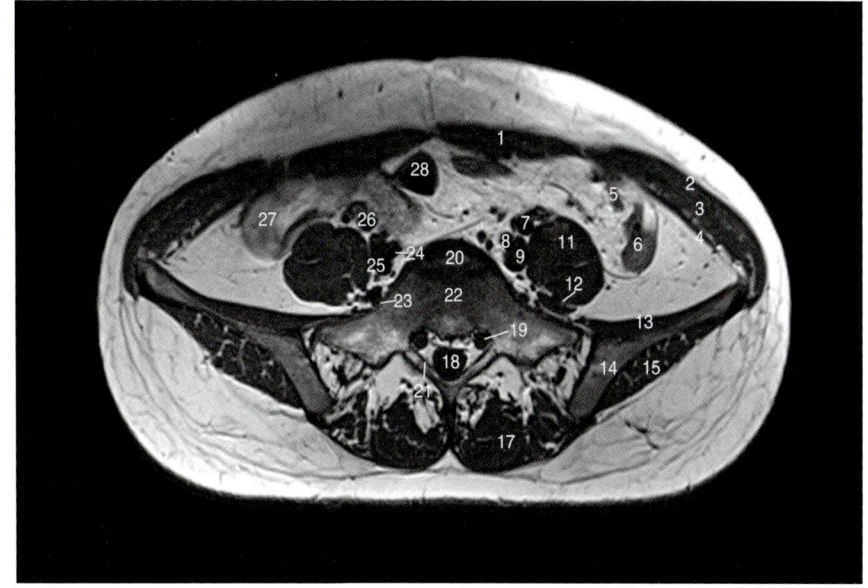

C. MR T1WI

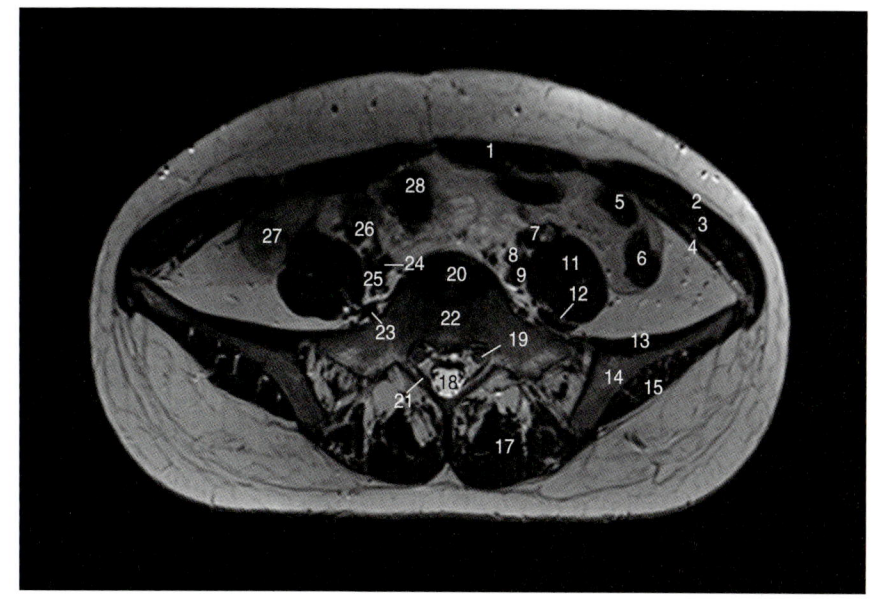

D. MR T2WI

1. 腹直肌 rectus abdominis
2. 腹外斜肌 obliquus externus abdominis
3. 腹内斜肌 obliquus internus abdominis
4. 腹横肌 transversus abdominis
5. 空肠 jejunum
6. 降结肠 descending colon
7. 左髂外动脉 left external iliac artery
8. 左髂内动脉 left internal iliac artery
9. 左髂总静脉 left common iliac vein
10. 左输尿管 left ureter
11. 腰大肌 psoas major
12. 股神经 femoral nerve
13. 髂肌 iliacus
14. 髂骨翼 ala of ilium
15. 臀中肌 gluteus medius
16. 臀大肌 gluteus maximus
17. 竖脊肌 erector spinae
18. 马尾 cauda equina
19. 第 1 骶神经 1st sacral nerve
20. L5-S1 椎间盘 L5-S1 intervertebral disc
21. 硬脊膜 spinal dura mater
22. 第 1 骶椎 1st sacral vertebra
23. 腰骶干 lumbosacral trunk
24. 右髂内动脉 right internal iliac artery
25. 右髂总静脉 right common iliac vein
26. 右髂外动脉 right external iliac artery
27. 盲肠 cecum
28. 回肠 ileum
29. 右输尿管 right ureter
30. 右卵巢动、静脉 right ovarian artery and vein

关键结构：骶髂骨间韧带，髂血管，肠管。

此断面经过 L5-S1 椎间盘。

其后方为第 1 骶椎椎体及骶管，骶管内容纳骶、尾神经根。L5-S1 椎间盘外侧与腰大肌形成的夹角内见髂血管：左侧自内向前外为髂总静脉、髂内动脉、髂外动脉，右侧自内侧向外侧为髂内动脉、髂总静脉、髂外动脉。髂外动脉外侧、腰大肌前方见卵巢动、静脉断面。左输尿管位于髂外动脉的前外侧，右输尿管位于髂外动脉与髂总静脉间前方。骶骨侧部与髂骨间为骶髂骨间韧带。骶髂骨间韧带是人体最坚强的韧带，位于关节后方的骨间隙中，韧带纤维较短，连接髂骨和骶骨，起自髂骨翼内侧面，横跨骶髂关节后方，止于骶骨背侧面，维持后方骶髂关节复合体的稳定性。男、女骶髂骨间韧带的高度分别为 32.1 mm ± 8.0 mm、27.1 mm ± 8.1 mm，长度和宽度由近端至远端不一，但长度基本约为 10 mm，而宽度约为 25 mm[2]。在 CT 图像上，韧带呈软组织密度，与周围软组织难以区分。MR T1WI 及 T2WI 图像上，韧带表现为低信号，轴位图像可显示骶髂骨间韧带全长[3]。

女性盆部与会阴连续横断层 3（FH.9330）

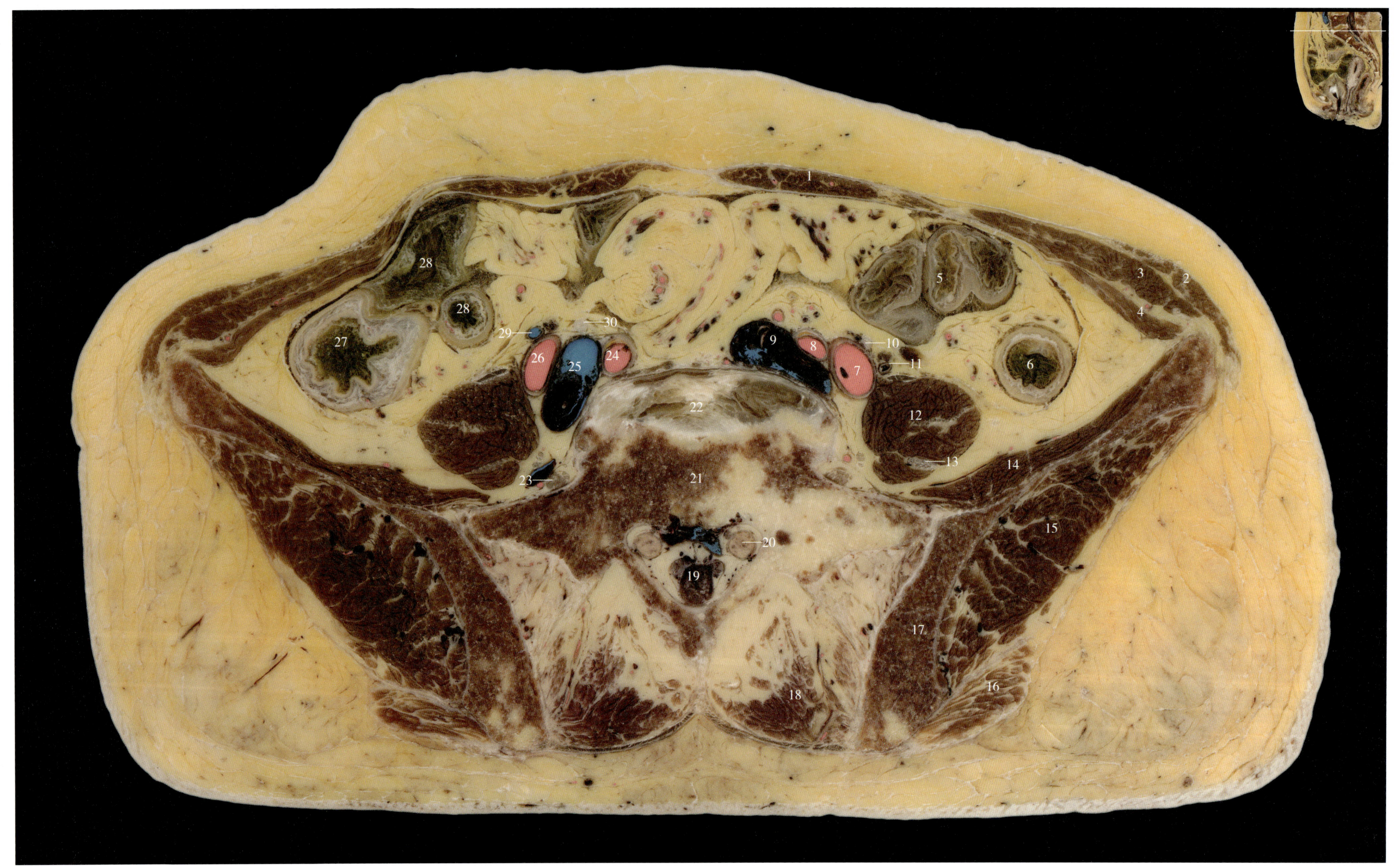

A. 断层标本图像

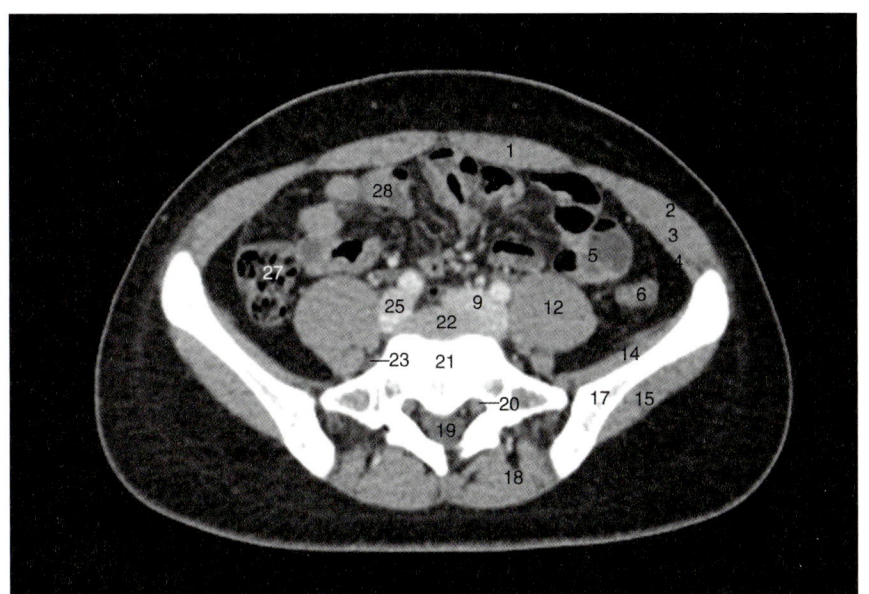
B. CT 增强图像

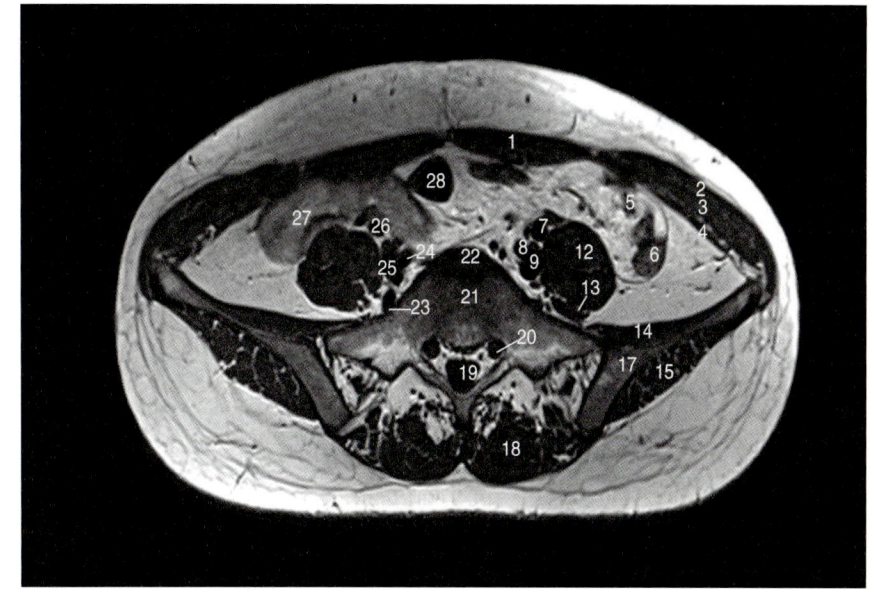
C. MR T1WI

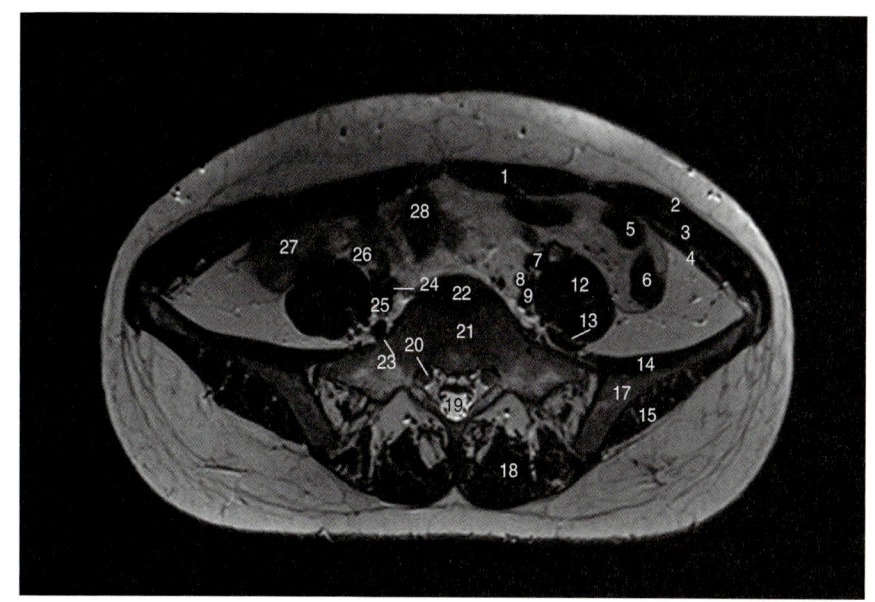
D. MR T2WI

1. 腹直肌 rectus abdominis
2. 腹外斜肌 obliquus externus abdominis
3. 腹内斜肌 obliquus internus abdominis
4. 腹横肌 transversus abdominis
5. 空肠 jejunum
6. 降结肠 descending colon
7. 左髂外动脉 left external iliac artery
8. 左髂内动脉 left internal iliac artery
9. 左髂总静脉 left common iliac vein
10. 左输尿管 left ureter
11. 左卵巢动、静脉 left ovarian artery and vein
12. 腰大肌 psoas major
13. 股神经 femoral nerve
14. 髂肌 iliacus
15. 臀中肌 gluteus medius
16. 臀大肌 gluteus maximus
17. 髂骨翼 ala of ilium
18. 竖脊肌 erector spinae
19. 马尾 cauda equina
20. 第 1 骶神经 1st sacral nerve
21. 第 1 骶椎 1st sacral vertebra
22. L5-S1 椎间盘 L5-S1 intervertebral disc
23. 腰骶干 lumbosacral trunk
24. 右髂内动脉 right internal iliac artery
25. 右髂总静脉 right common iliac vein
26. 右髂外动脉 right external iliac artery
27. 盲肠 cecum
28. 回肠 ileum
29. 右卵巢动、静脉 right ovarian artery and vein
30. 右输尿管 right ureter

关键结构：空肠，回肠，髂血管，输尿管。

此断面经过第 1 骶椎椎体上份。

其后方为骶管，骶管内容纳骶、尾神经根。臀大肌位于 L5-S1 椎间盘外侧，二者之间的夹角内见髂血管。左侧腰大肌前方、右侧髂外动脉前方分别见左侧卵巢动、静脉断面。左右输尿管位于髂血管前方。腰大肌后份内见股神经。肠管集中于断面的前半部，左髂窝处有降结肠，右髂窝处有盲肠，盲肠内侧是回肠，降结肠内侧是空肠。空回肠间没有绝对界线，通常空肠位于左上腹，约占 2/5，管径稍大，黏膜皱襞密而高，管壁稍厚；而回肠以右下腹为主，约占空回肠总长的 3/5，管径较细，管壁略薄，黏膜皱襞少。钡餐透视时空肠黏膜多为环状皱襞，蠕动活跃，常显示为羽毛状影像，钡剂通过迅速；回肠黏膜平坦，运动明显不及空肠活跃，常显示为充盈像，轮廓光滑。在 CT 图像上，充盈良好的小肠壁厚约 3 mm，回肠末端肠壁厚约 5 mm。在 MR 图像上，肠管壁在肠腔内气体低信号或高信号口服对比剂的衬托下能够显示清楚[4]。

女性盆部与会阴连续横断层 4（FH.9310）

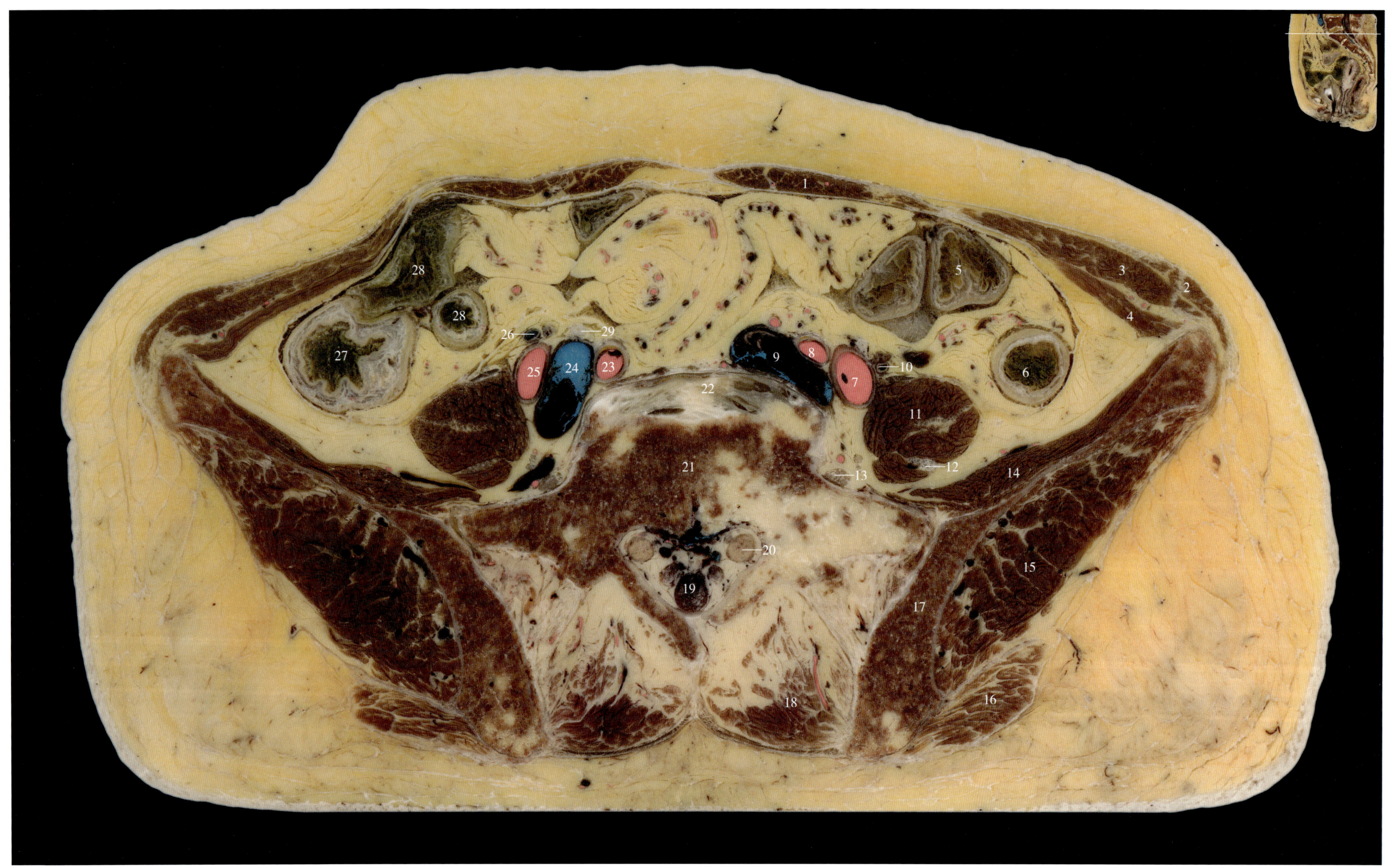

A. 断层标本图像

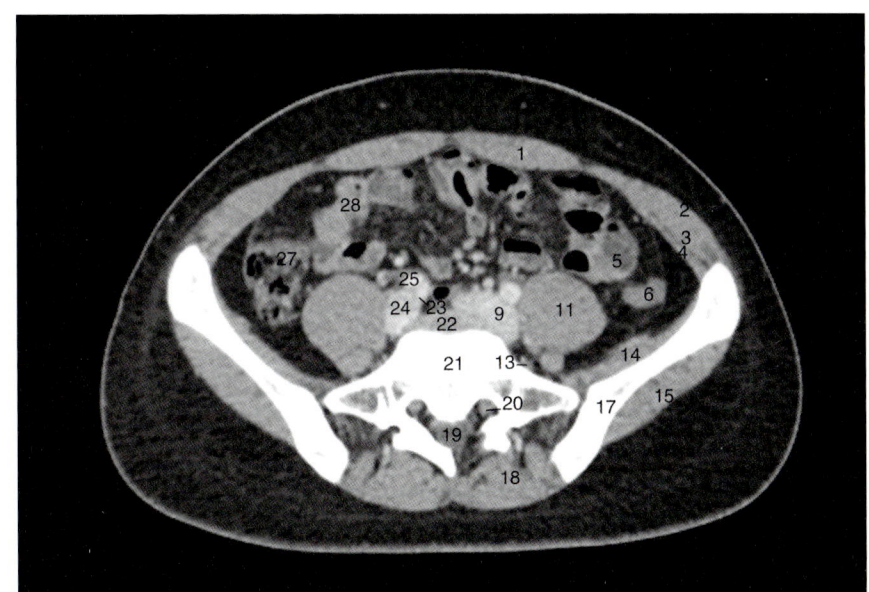

B. CT 增强图像

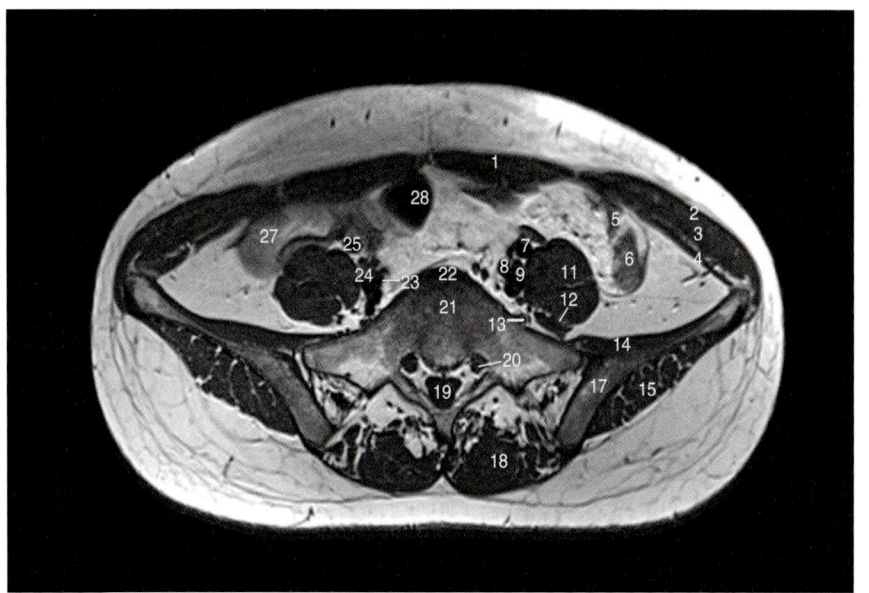

C. MR T1WI

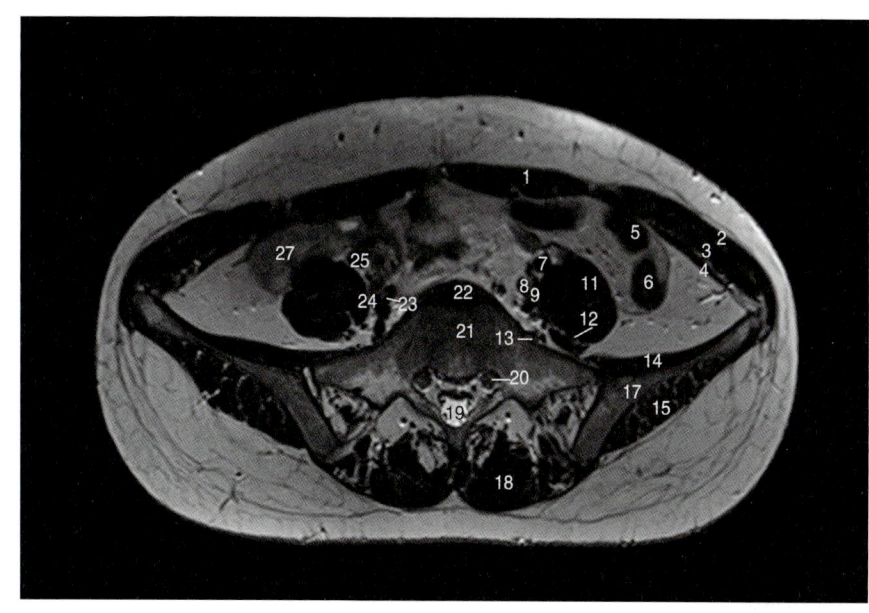

D. MR T2WI

1. 腹直肌 rectus abdominis
2. 腹外斜肌 obliquus externus abdominis
3. 腹内斜肌 obliquus internus abdominis
4. 腹横肌 transversus abdominis
5. 空肠 jejunum
6. 降结肠 descending colon
7. 左髂外动脉 left external iliac artery
8. 左髂内动脉 left internal iliac artery
9. 左髂总静脉 left common iliac vein
10. 左卵巢动、静脉 left ovarian artery and vein
11. 腰大肌 psoas major
12. 股神经 femoral nerve
13. 腰骶干 lumbosacral trunk
14. 髂肌 iliacus
15. 臀中肌 gluteus medius
16. 臀大肌 gluteus maximus
17. 髂骨翼 ala of ilium
18. 竖脊肌 erector spinae
19. 马尾 cauda equina
20. 第 1 骶神经 1st sacral nerve
21. 第 1 骶椎 1st sacral vertebra
22. L5-S1 椎间盘 L5-S1 intervertebral disc
23. 右髂内动脉 right internal iliac artery
24. 右髂总静脉 right common iliac vein
25. 右髂外动脉 right external iliac artery
26. 右卵巢动、静脉 right ovarian artery and vein
27. 盲肠 cecum
28. 回肠 ileum
29. 右输尿管 right ureter

关键结构：空肠，回肠，髂血管，输尿管。

此断面经过第 1 骶椎椎体上份。

其后方为骶管，骶管内容纳骶、尾神经根。腰大肌位于椎体外侧，腰大肌内侧为输尿管、髂血管和腰骶干，呈前后方向排列，腰大肌后份内见股神经。肠管集中于断面的前半部，左髂窝处有降结肠，降结肠内侧是空肠。右髂窝处有盲肠，盲肠为大肠的起始部，下端为盲端，形似口袋，长约 6 cm，位于回肠与结肠的交界处之下，通常盲肠靠近腹前壁，但有时大网膜或小肠袢可插入二者之间。腹膜常将盲肠表面完全覆盖，并向后下方的右髂窝底发生返折，从而起自盲肠后壁的腹膜皱襞在盲肠周围形成多个隐窝：回盲上隐窝、回盲下隐窝、盲肠后隐窝和结肠旁隐窝。这些隐窝是发生内疝的可能部位。盲肠具有可膨大的口袋样结构因而可容纳来自小肠的大量半流质食糜。盲肠相对较粗，故而在结肠内压升高时容易扩张，结肠膨胀（因梗阻或其他病理因素）导致的大肠继发性穿孔也最易发生于盲肠[5]。

女性盆部与会阴连续横断层 5（FH.9290）

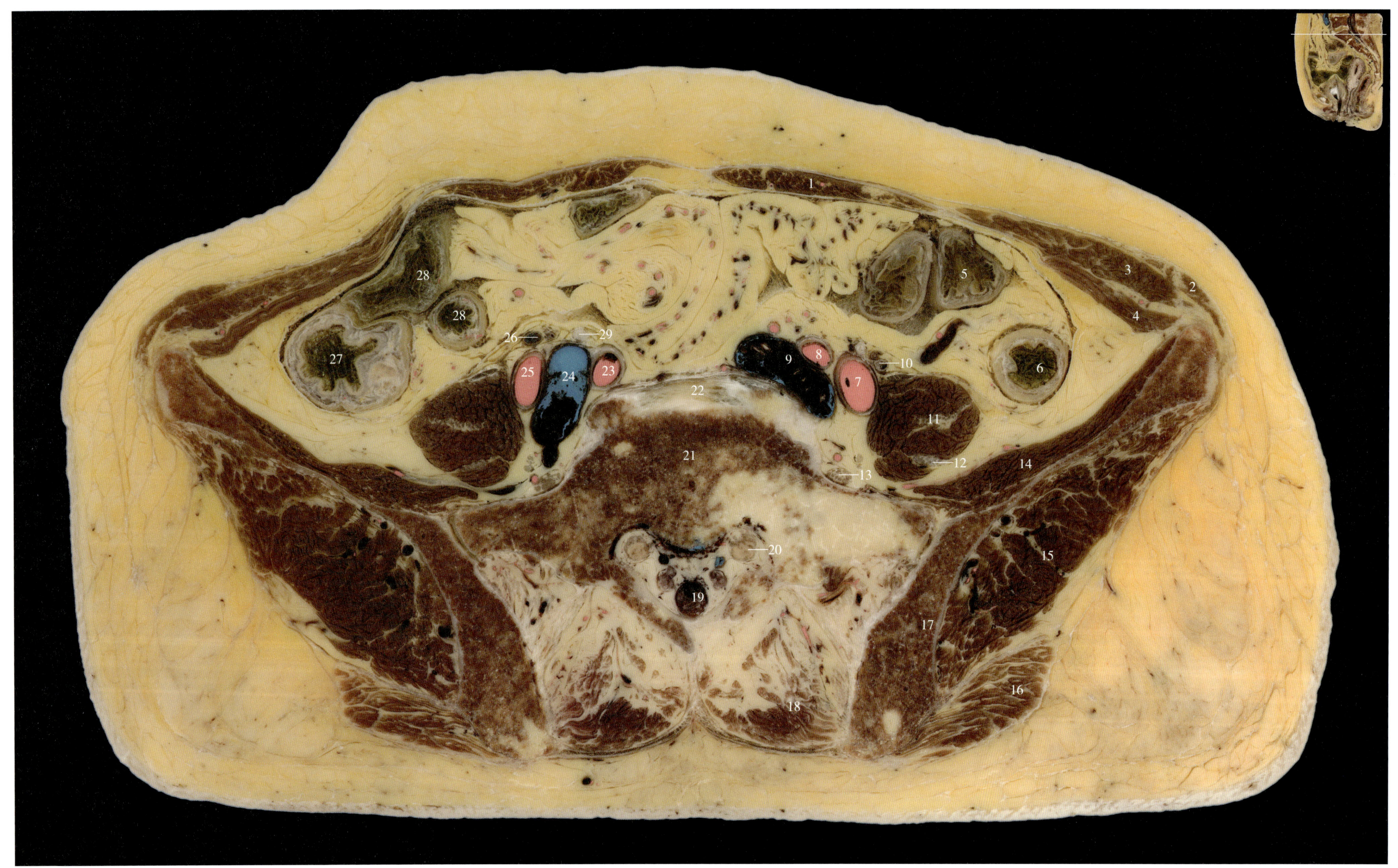

A. 断层标本图像

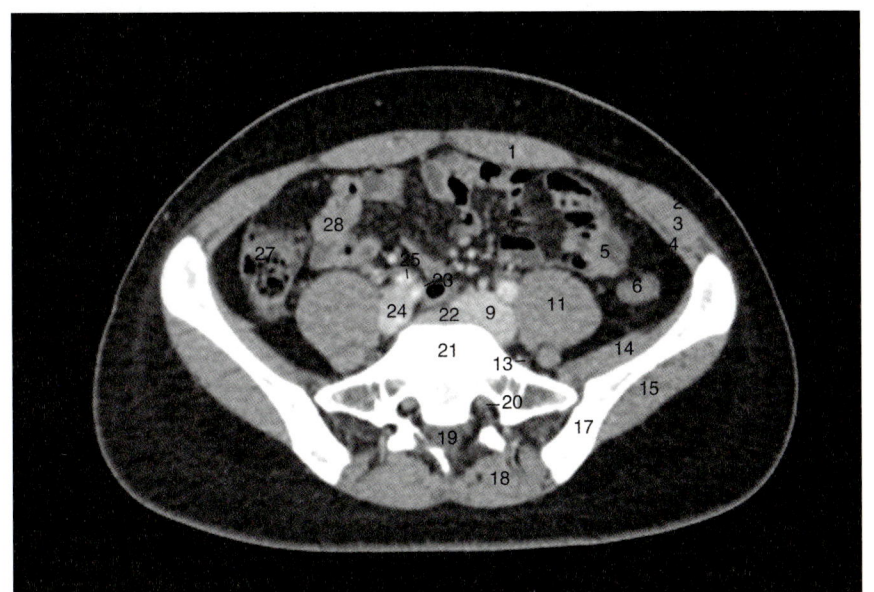

B. CT 增强图像

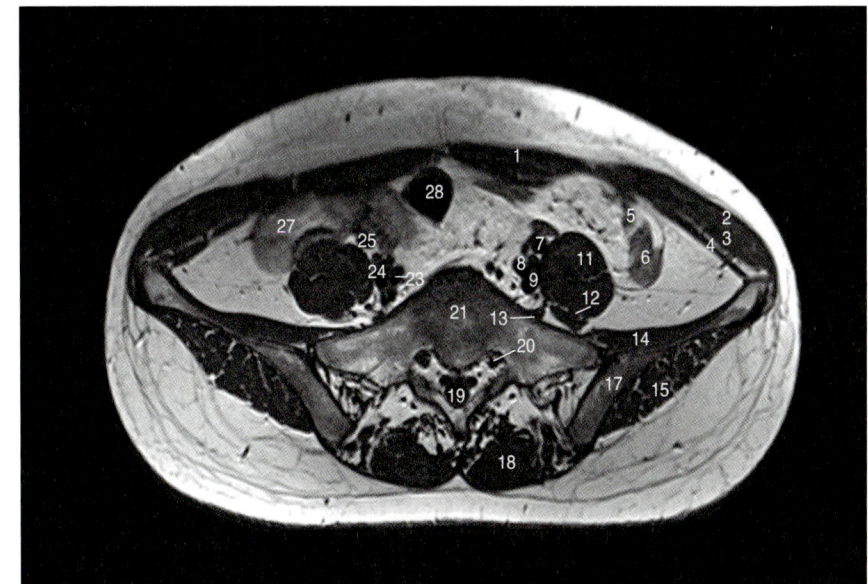

C. MR T1WI

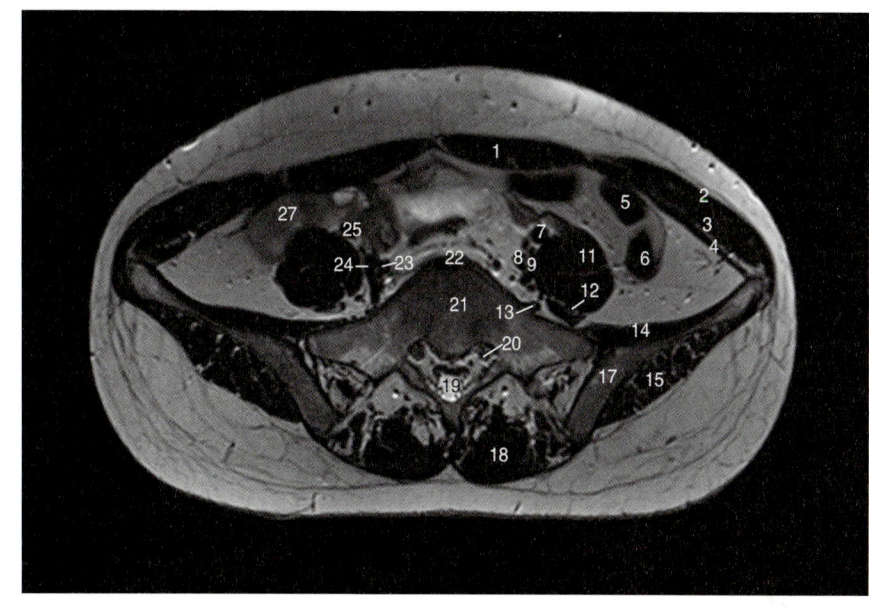

D. MR T2WI

1. 腹直肌 rectus abdominis
2. 腹外斜肌 obliquus externus abdominis
3. 腹内斜肌 obliquus internus abdominis
4. 腹横肌 transversus abdominis
5. 空肠 jejunum
6. 降结肠 descending colon
7. 左髂外动脉 left external iliac artery
8. 左髂内动脉 left internal iliac artery
9. 左髂总静脉 left common iliac vein
10. 左卵巢动、静脉 left ovarian artery and vein
11. 腰大肌 psoas major
12. 股神经 femoral nerve
13. 腰骶干 lumbosacral trunk
14. 髂肌 iliacus
15. 臀中肌 gluteus medius
16. 臀大肌 gluteus maximus
17. 髂骨翼 ala of ilium
18. 竖脊肌 erector spinae
19. 马尾 cauda equina
20. 第 1 骶神经 1st sacral nerve
21. 第 1 骶椎 1st sacral vertebra
22. L5-S1 椎间盘 L5-S1 intervertebral disc
23. 右髂内动脉 right internal iliac artery
24. 右髂总静脉 right common iliac vein
25. 右髂外动脉 right external iliac artery
26. 右卵巢动、静脉 right ovarian artery and vein
27. 盲肠 cecum
28. 回肠 ileum
29. 右输尿管 right ureter

关键结构：小肠系膜，骶髂关节，肠管。

此断面经过第 1 骶椎椎体中份，后方为骶管。

骶翼宽大，其前外侧与髂骨翼之间出现骶髂关节上部。腰大肌位于椎体外侧，腰大肌内侧由前向后依次为输尿管、髂血管和腰骶干，腰大肌后份内见股神经。肠管集中于断面的前半部两侧，右髂窝处为盲肠，盲肠内侧是回肠，左髂窝处为降结肠，盆腔前部被肠系膜脂肪充填。小肠系膜是将空肠和回肠固定于腹后壁的双层腹膜结构，面积较大，呈扇形，其附于腹后壁的部分称为肠系膜根，长约 15 cm，起自第 2 腰椎左侧，斜向右下跨过脊柱及其前方结构，止于右骶髂关节前方。肠系膜的两层腹膜间含有肠系膜上血管及其分支、淋巴管、淋巴结、神经丛和脂肪等[1]。在 CT 横断面图像上系膜脂肪组织呈低密度，系膜内的血管多为点状、细条状，增强扫描动、静脉期可以区分伴行的动脉、静脉。如果发生栓塞或血栓形成时，增强的血管管腔内见低密度充盈缺损。当发现肠系膜上动、静脉走行存在异常时，要考虑是否存在肠管排列异常或肠扭转。肠系膜动脉发生夹层时，增强的血管管腔分为真、假两个腔，两腔中间见纤细的低密度内膜片。

女性盆部与会阴连续横断层 6（FH.9270）

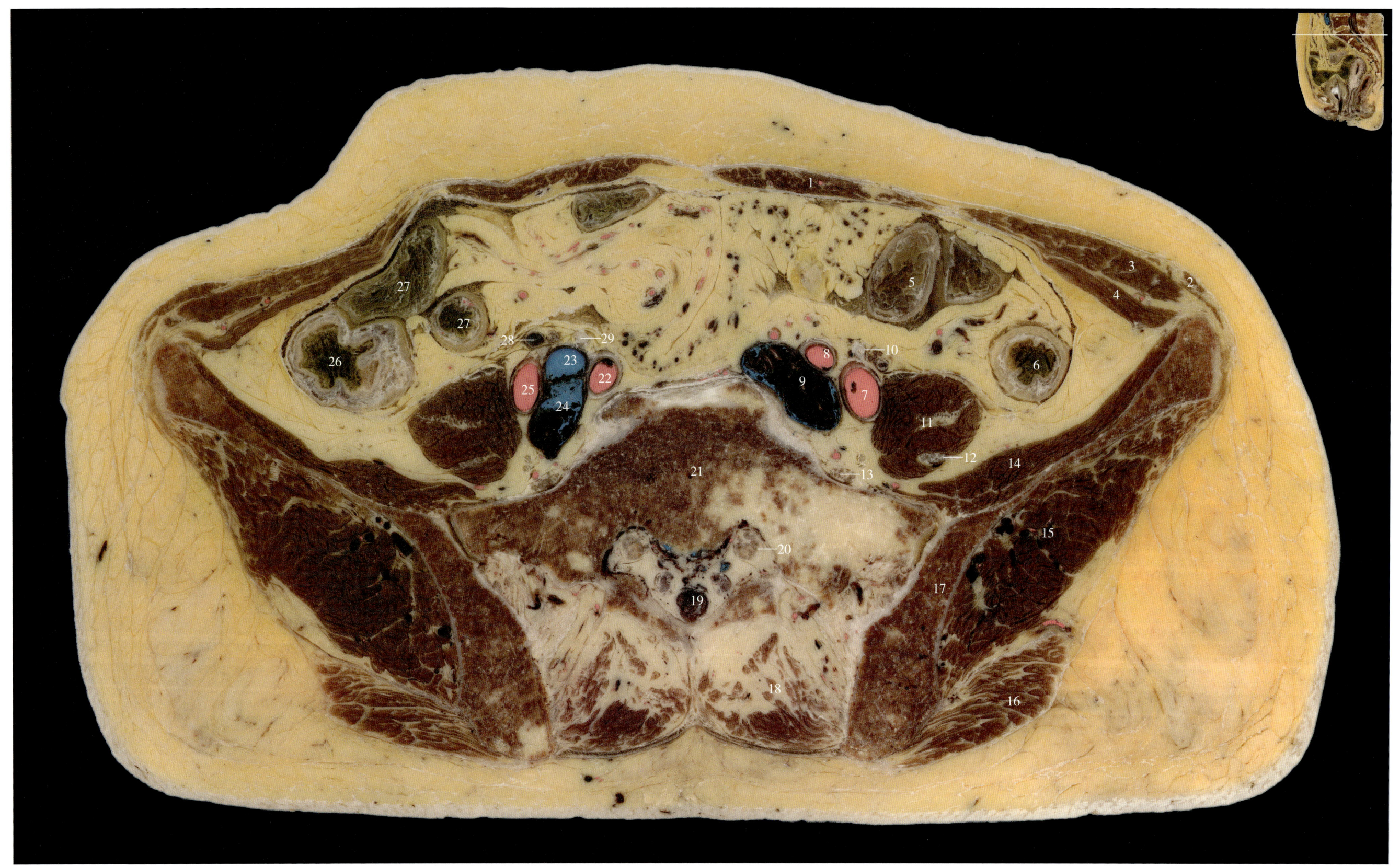

A. 断层标本图像

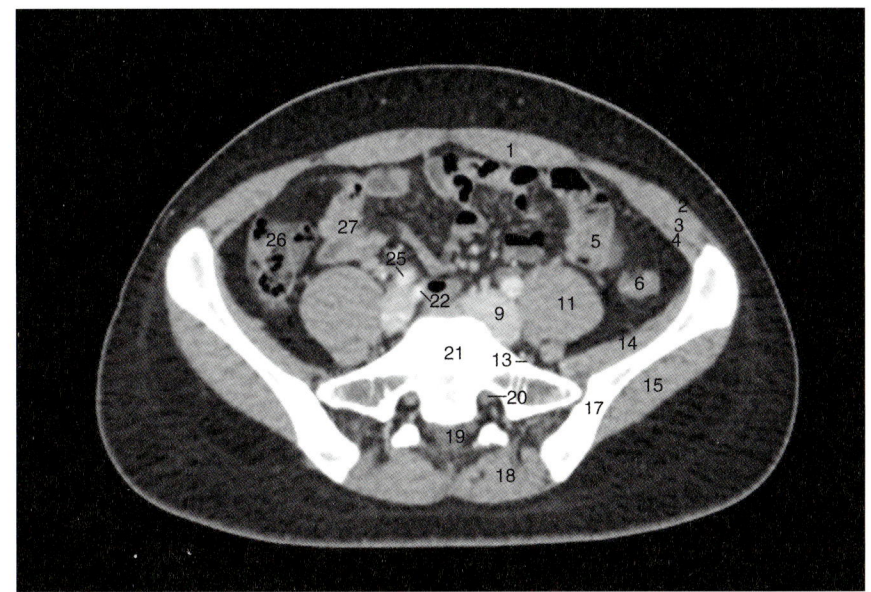
B. CT 增强图像

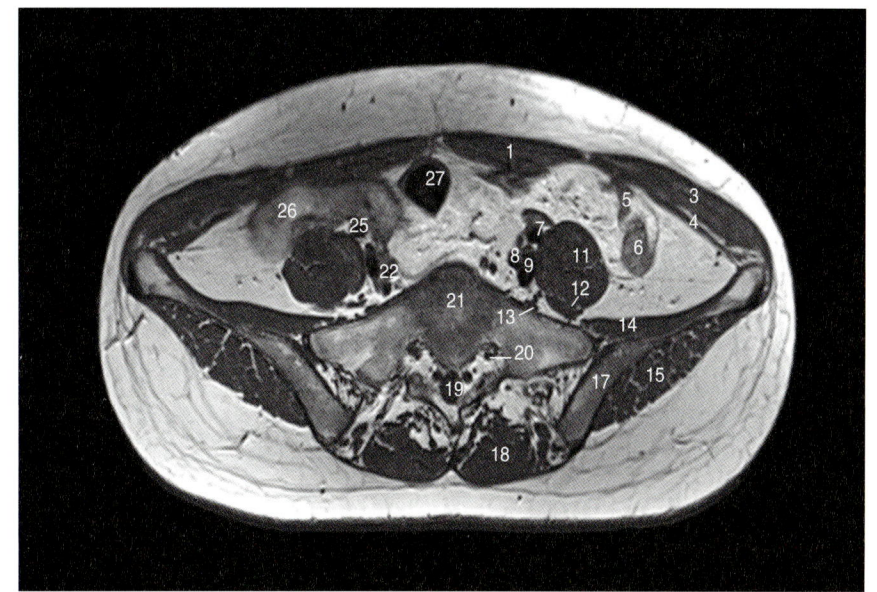
C. MR T1WI

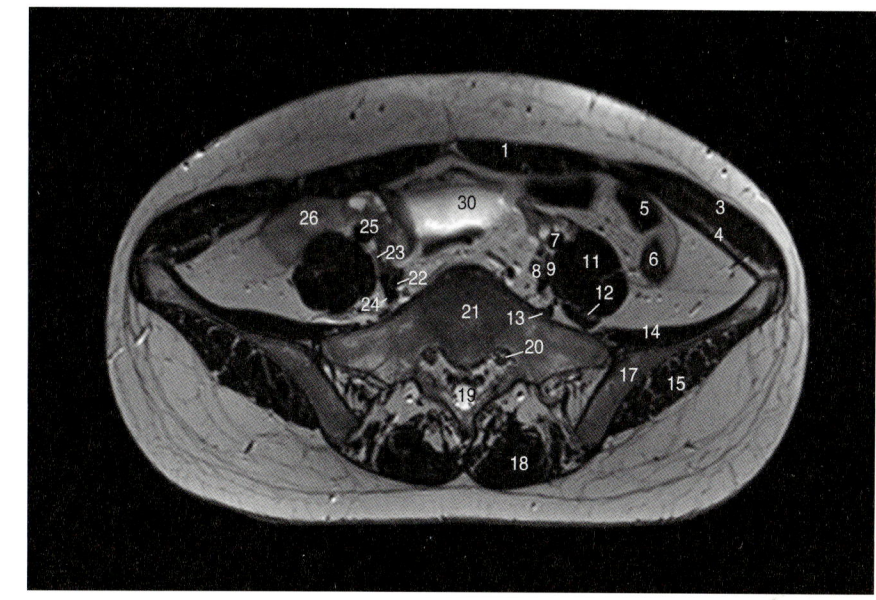
D. MR T2WI

1. 腹直肌 rectus abdominis
2. 腹外斜肌 obliquus externus abdominis
3. 腹内斜肌 obliquus internus abdominis
4. 腹横肌 transversus abdominis
5. 空肠 jejunum
6. 降结肠 descending colon
7. 左髂外动脉 left external iliac artery
8. 左髂内动脉 left internal iliac artery
9. 左髂总静脉 left common iliac vein
10. 左输尿管 left ureter
11. 腰大肌 psoas major
12. 股神经 femoral nerve
13. 腰骶干 lumbosacral trunk
14. 髂肌 iliacus
15. 臀中肌 gluteus medius

16. 臀大肌 gluteus maximus
17. 髂骨翼 ala of ilium
18. 竖脊肌 erector spinae
19. 马尾 cauda equina
20. 第 1 骶神经 1st sacral nerve
21. 第 1 骶椎 1st sacral vertebra
22. 右髂内动脉 right internal iliac artery
23. 右髂外静脉 right external iliac vein
24. 右髂内静脉 right internal iliac vein
25. 右髂外动脉 right external iliac artery
26. 盲肠 cecum
27. 回肠 ileum
28. 右卵巢动、静脉 right ovarian artery and vein
29. 右输尿管 right ureter
30. 膀胱 urinary bladder

关键结构：髂静脉，输尿管，肠管。

此断面经过第 1 骶椎椎体中份。

其前方向前突为骶骨岬，L5-S1 椎间盘几乎消失；后方为骶管及骶管内的骶、尾神经根。腰大肌位于椎体外侧，略向外侧移行，腰大肌与椎体之间见输尿管、髂血管及腰骶干。右侧髂总静脉在此断面分为前方的髂外静脉及后方的髂内静脉，左侧髂总静脉长而倾斜，先沿左髂总动脉内侧，后沿左髂总动脉后方上行。右侧髂总静脉短而垂直，先行于右髂总动脉后方，后行于髂总动脉外侧。双侧髂总静脉的汇合位置，多在髂总动脉分叉点下方（左侧 92.31% ± 2.61%，右侧为 97.12% ± 1.64%）。左、右髂总静脉一般于第 5 腰椎体右侧汇入下腔静脉，该处位于伴行的髂总动脉及腰骶椎之间。临床上左髂总静脉有时受到右侧髂总动脉及腰骶椎的压迫，合并静脉内粘连结构形成，引起下肢和盆腔的静脉回流障碍，从而产生一系列的临床症状和体征称为髂静脉压迫综合征[6]。

女性盆部与会阴连续横断层 7（FH.9250）

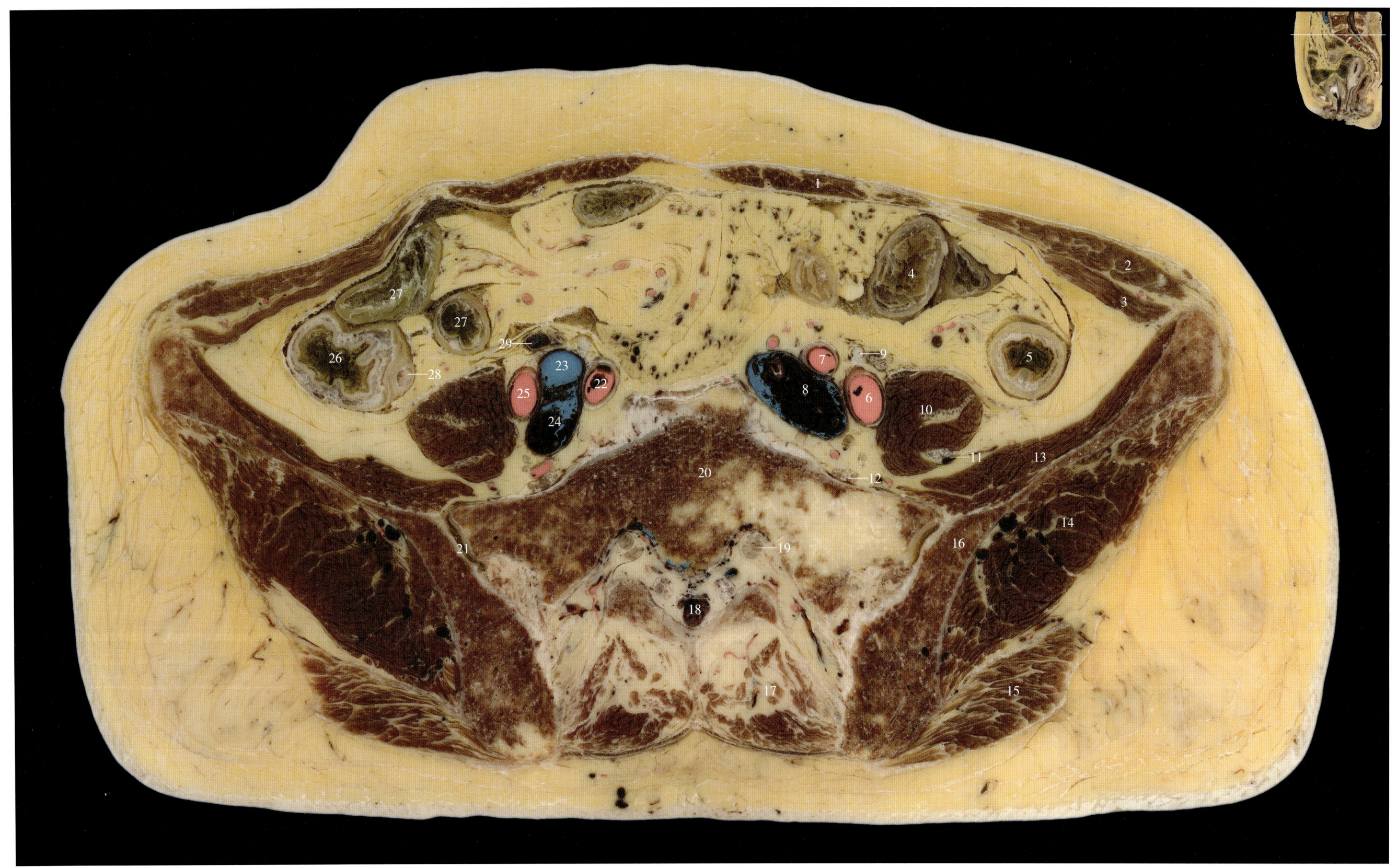

A. 断层标本图像

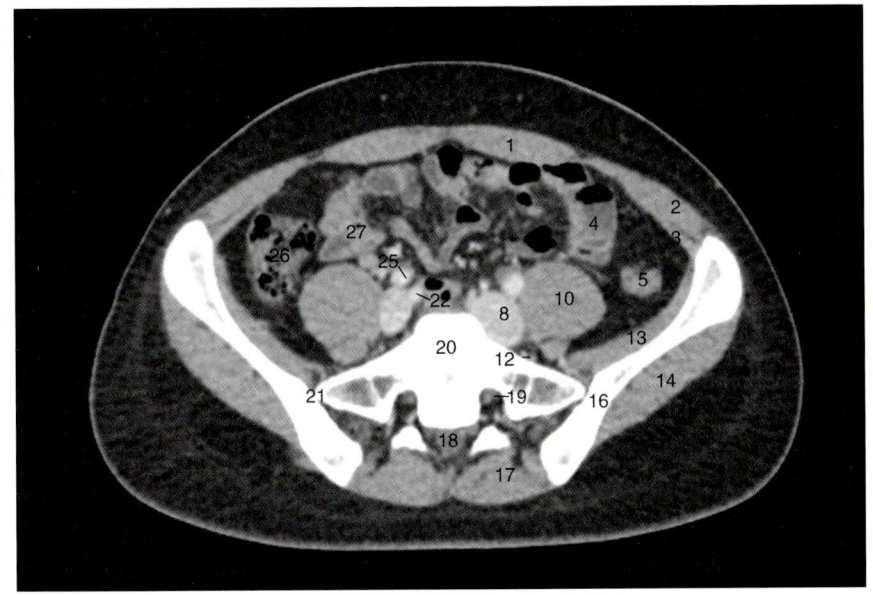
B. CT 增强图像

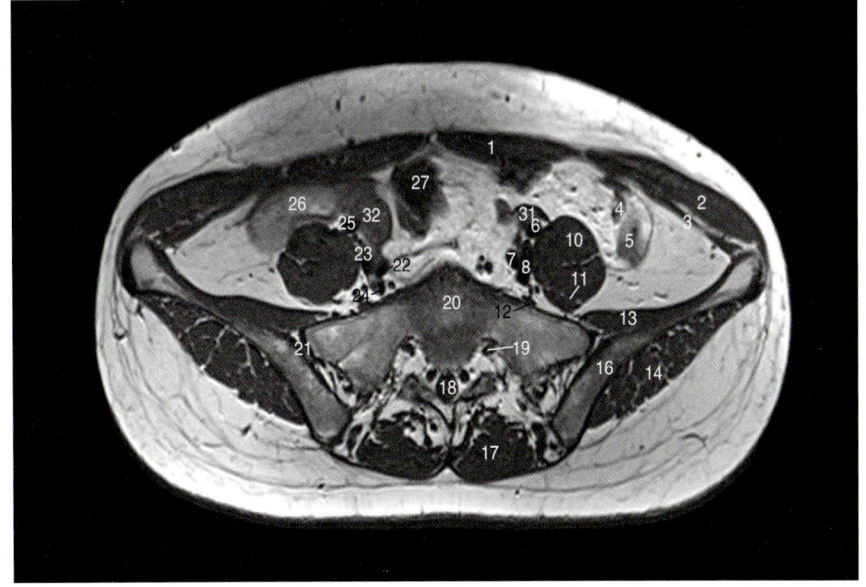
C. MR T1WI

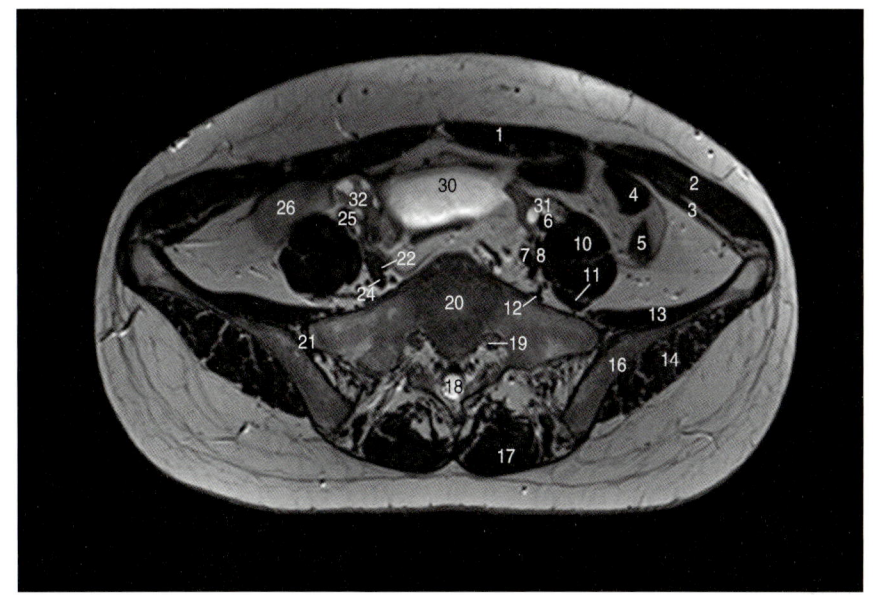
D. MR T2WI

关键结构：卵巢血管，骶髂关节，输尿管。

此断面经过第 1 骶椎椎体中份，后方为骶管。

髂骨翼略增大，其内、外侧面分别为髂肌和臀中肌所附着。腰大肌位于骶髂关节前方，腰大肌内侧见输尿管、髂血管及腰骶干，呈前后顺序排列。腰大肌内前方见细小的卵巢动、静脉断面，卵巢动脉十分纤细，管径为 0.5~0.8 mm，育龄期管径可达 1.1 mm，妊娠期卵巢动脉管径可代偿性增粗，绝经期管径可小于 0.5 mm[7]。卵巢动脉血管造影显示 95.8% 发自腹主动脉，96.7% 开口于 L2 椎体上缘至 L3 椎体下缘间，右侧直径约为 0.9 mm，左侧约为 0.8 mm，呈螺旋状在腰椎旁外下走行，分布于卵巢和输卵管壶腹[8]。卵巢静脉起自卵巢静脉丛，在卵巢悬韧带内上行，合成卵巢静脉，与同名动脉伴行。同时，部分静脉丛与同侧或对侧子宫静脉丛相通，部分子宫和输卵管血液回流其中。右侧卵巢静脉在右肾静脉下方直接汇入下腔静脉（IVC），左侧卵巢静脉行程长，呈直角汇入左肾静脉。左侧卵巢静脉管径比右侧粗。此断面右侧髂窝内盲肠已近盲端，其内侧阑尾开始出现。

1. 腹直肌 rectus abdominis
2. 腹内斜肌 obliquus internus abdominis
3. 腹横肌 transversus abdominis
4. 空肠 jejunum
5. 降结肠 descending colon
6. 左髂外动脉 left external iliac artery
7. 左髂内动脉 left internal iliac artery
8. 左髂总静脉 left common iliac vein
9. 左输尿管 left ureter
10. 腰大肌 psoas major
11. 股神经 femoral nerve
12. 腰骶干 lumbosacral trunk
13. 髂肌 iliacus
14. 臀中肌 gluteus medius
15. 臀大肌 gluteus maximus
16. 髂骨翼 ala of ilium
17. 竖脊肌 erector spinae
18. 马尾 cauda equina
19. 第 1 骶神经 1st sacral nerve
20. 第 1 骶椎 1st sacral vertebra
21. 骶髂关节 sacroiliac joint
22. 右髂内动脉 right internal iliac artery
23. 右髂外静脉 right external iliac vein
24. 右髂内静脉 right internal iliac vein
25. 右髂外动脉 right external iliac artery
26. 盲肠 cecum
27. 回肠 ileum
28. 阑尾 vermiform appendix
29. 右卵巢动、静脉 right ovarian artery and vein
30. 膀胱 urinary bladder
31. 左卵巢 left ovary
32. 右卵巢 right ovary

女性盆部与会阴连续横断层 8（FH.9230）

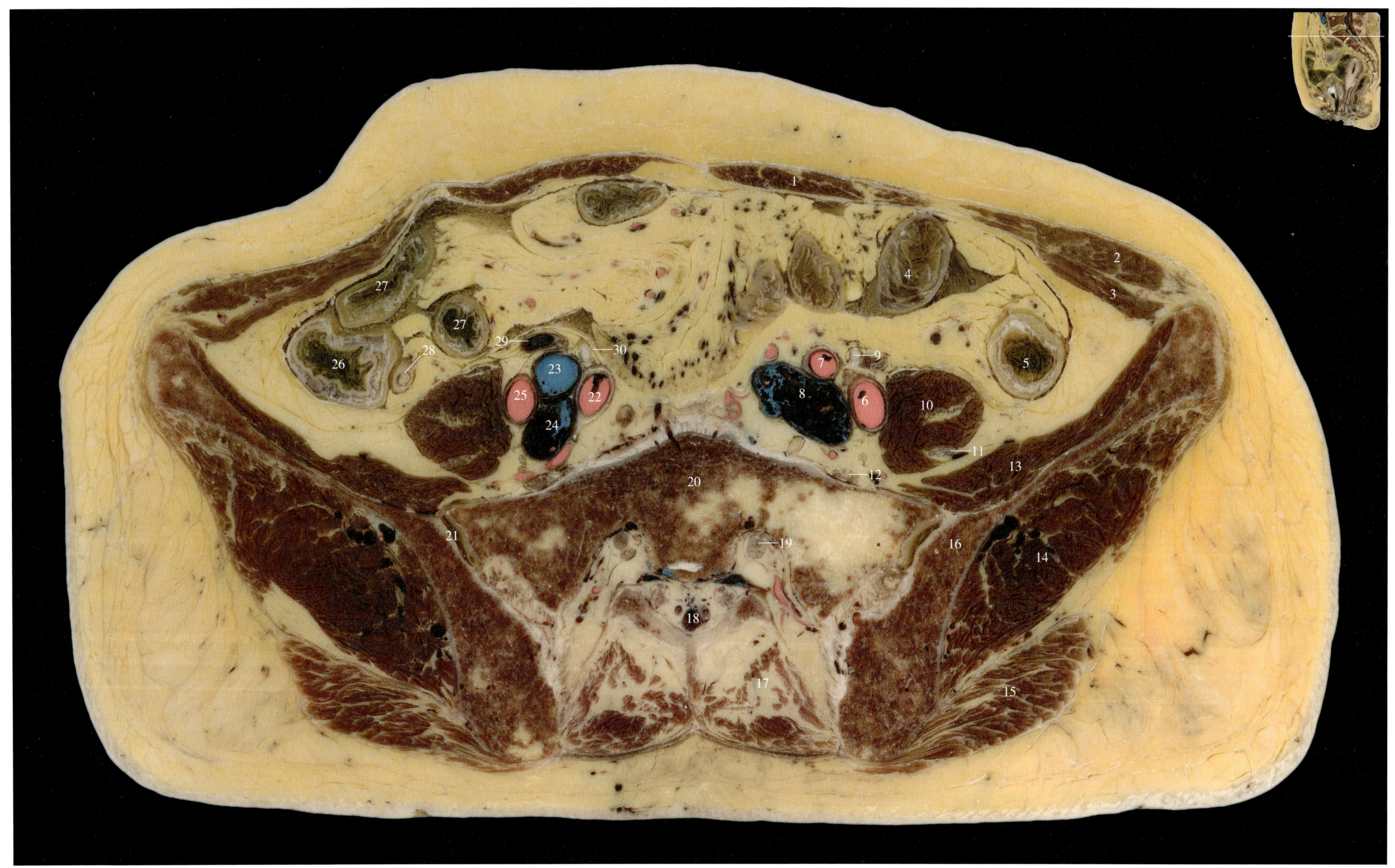

A. 断层标本图像

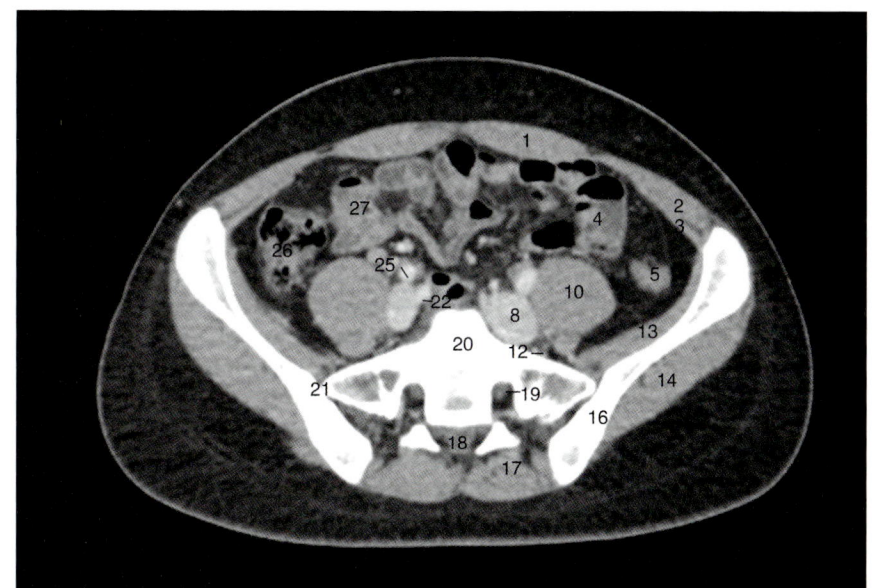

B. CT 增强图像

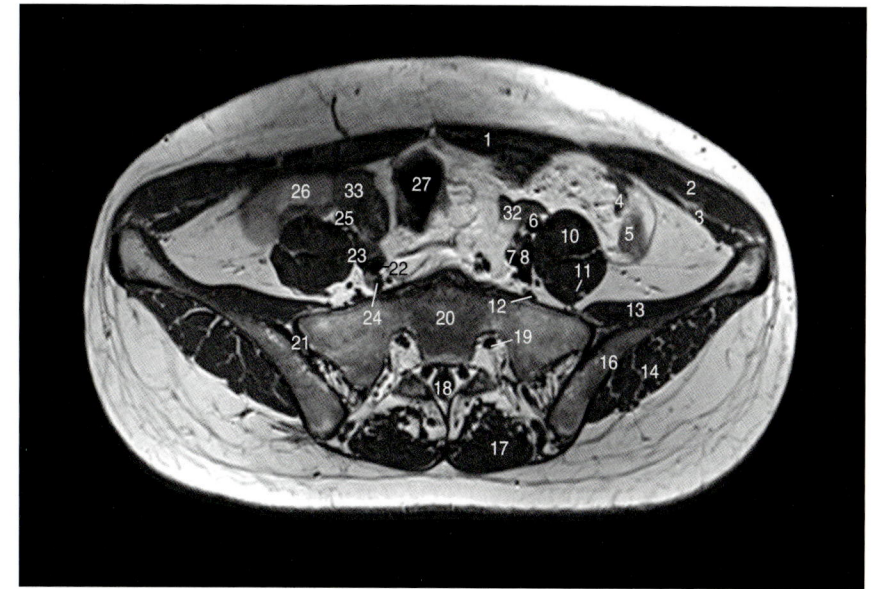

C. MR T1WI

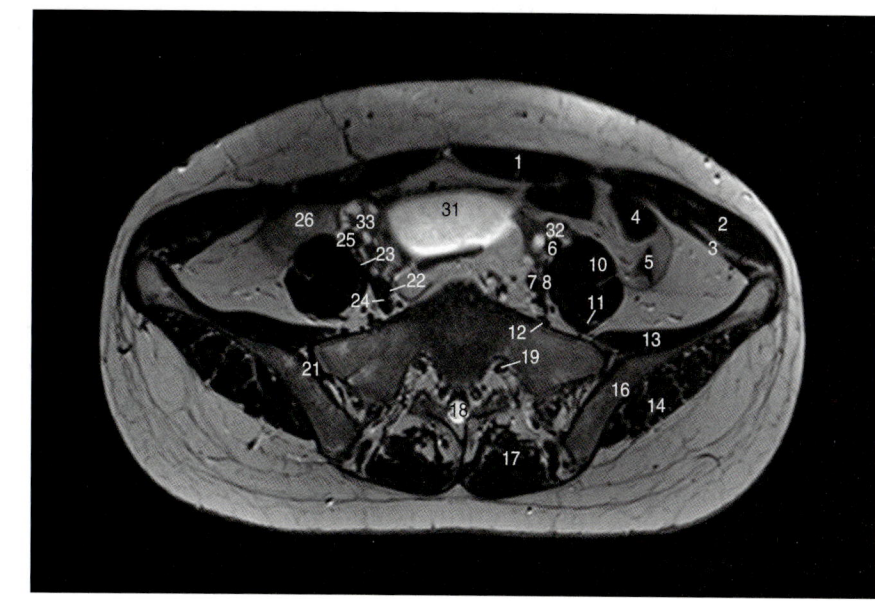

D. MR T2WI

1. 腹直肌 rectus abdominis
2. 腹内斜肌 obliquus internus abdominis
3. 腹横肌 transversus abdominis
4. 空肠 jejunum
5. 降结肠 descending colon
6. 左髂外动脉 left external iliac artery
7. 左髂内动脉 left internal iliac artery
8. 左髂总静脉 left common iliac vein
9. 左输尿管 left ureter
10. 腰大肌 psoas major
11. 股神经 femoral nerve
12. 腰骶干 lumbosacral trunk
13. 髂肌 iliacus
14. 臀中肌 gluteus medius
15. 臀大肌 gluteus maximus
16. 髂骨翼 ala of ilium
17. 竖脊肌 erector spinae
18. 马尾 cauda equina
19. 第1骶神经 1st sacral nerve
20. 第1骶椎 1st sacral vertebra
21. 骶髂关节 sacroiliac joint
22. 右髂内动脉 right internal iliac artery
23. 右髂外静脉 right external iliac vein
24. 右髂内静脉 right internal iliac vein
25. 右髂外动脉 right external iliac artery
26. 盲肠 cecum
27. 回肠 ileum
28. 阑尾 vermiform appendix
29. 右卵巢动、静脉 right ovarian artery and vein
30. 右输尿管 right ureter
31. 膀胱 urinary bladder
32. 左卵巢 left ovary
33. 右卵巢 right ovary

关键结构：骶髂关节，输尿管，髂血管。

此断面经过第1骶椎椎体下份，后方为骶管。

骶管内容纳骶、尾神经根，第1骶神经进入骶前孔内。盆后壁两侧骶髂关节面增大。骶髂关节具有明显的年龄变化。在儿童期，骶髂关节具有滑膜关节的所有特征，具有相对活动性；在青少年期和成年早期中，骶髂关节逐渐从运动性（滑膜）关节转化为不动关节，其中最显著的变化特征是关节面由光滑变得粗糙；随年龄增长，关节间隙逐渐增宽，皮质边缘光滑度降低，关节面出现小囊变、骨质硬化及骨质增生的发生率逐渐增多，并且这种变化在关节的髂骨侧明显多于骶骨侧，增生的部位也以关节的髂骨前上缘多见。当发生强直性脊柱炎时，几乎骶髂关节全部受累，常导致脊柱韧带广泛骨化而致骨性强直，其主要的病变特征是骶髂关节炎[9]。腰大肌位于骶髂关节前方，腰大肌内侧见输尿管、髂血管及腰骶干，呈前后顺序排列。腰大肌后份内见股神经。

17

女性盆部与会阴连续横断层 9（FH.9210）

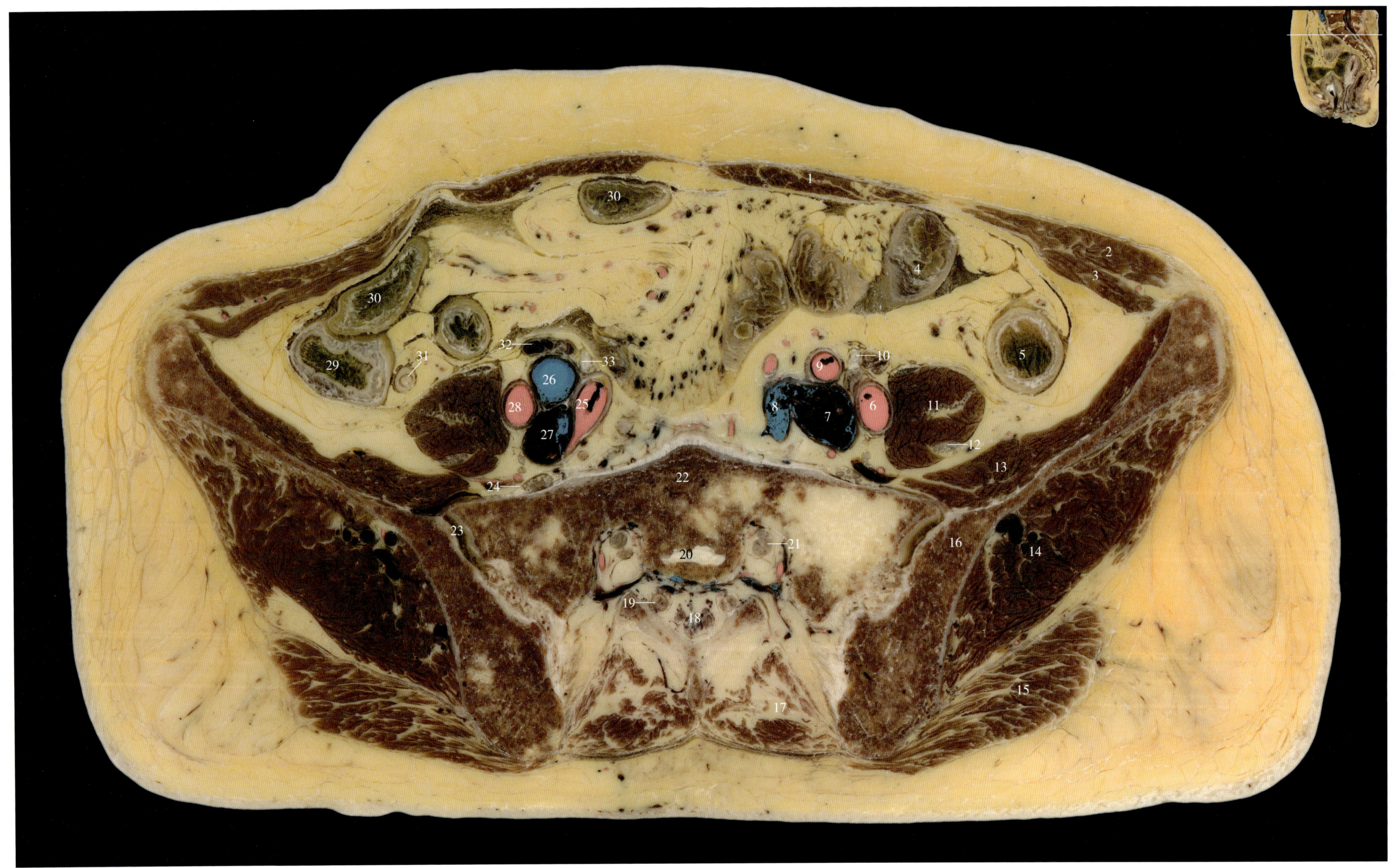

A. 断层标本图像

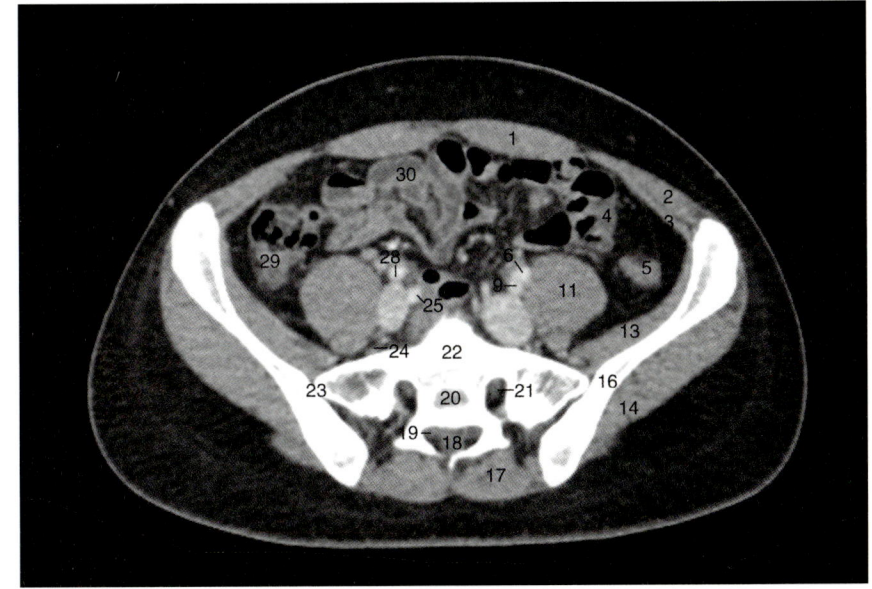
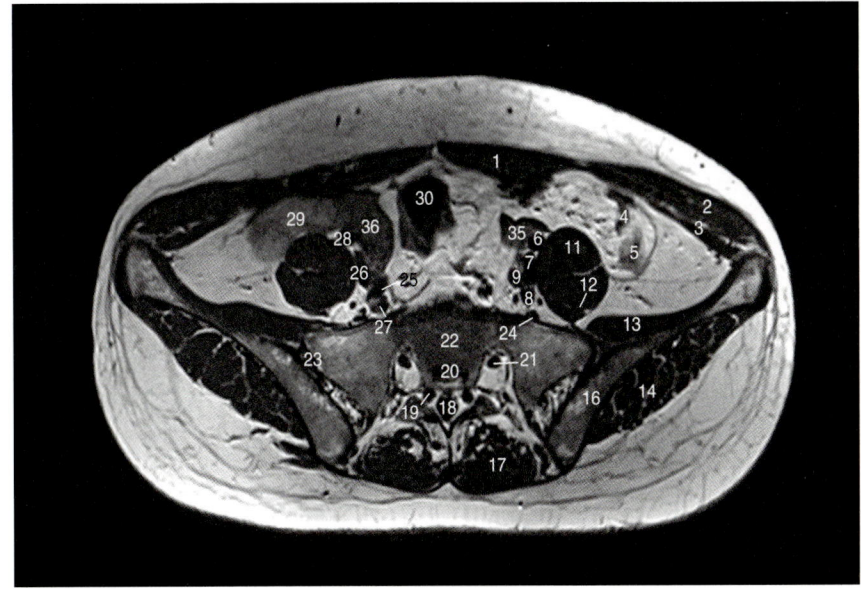
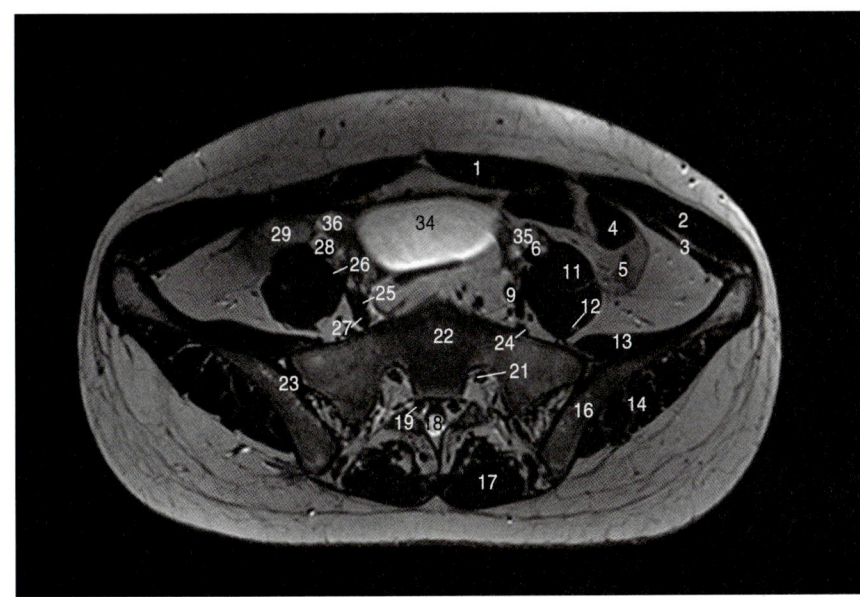

B. CT 增强图像　　　　　　C. MR T1WI　　　　　　D. MR T2WI

1. 腹直肌 rectus abdominis
2. 腹内斜肌 obliquus internus abdominis
3. 腹横肌 transversus abdominis
4. 空肠 jejunum
5. 降结肠 descending colon
6. 左髂外动脉 left external iliac artery
7. 左髂外静脉 left external iliac vein
8. 左髂内静脉 left internal iliac vein
9. 左髂内动脉 left internal iliac artery
10. 左输尿管 left ureter
11. 腰大肌 psoas major
12. 股神经 femoral nerve
13. 髂肌 iliacus
14. 臀中肌 gluteus medius
15. 臀大肌 gluteus maximus
16. 髂骨翼 ala of ilium
17. 竖脊肌 erector spinae
18. 骶管 sacral canal
19. 第 2 骶神经 2nd sacral nerve
20. S1-2 骶椎间盘 S1-2 intervertebral disc
21. 第 1 骶神经 1st sacral nerve
22. 第 1 骶椎 1st sacral vertebra
23. 骶髂关节 sacroiliac joint
24. 腰骶干 lumbosacral trunk
25. 右髂内动脉 right internal iliac artery
26. 右髂外静脉 right external iliac vein
27. 右髂内静脉 right internal iliac vein
28. 右髂外动脉 right external iliac artery
29. 盲肠 cecum
30. 回肠 ileum
31. 阑尾 vermiform appendix
32. 右卵巢动、静脉 right ovarian artery and vein
33. 右输尿管 right ureter
34. 膀胱 urinary bladder
35. 左卵巢 left ovary
36. 右卵巢 right ovary

关键结构：马尾，髂血管，股神经。

此断面经过第 1 骶椎椎体下份，后方为骶管，骶管内见马尾。

马尾由腰骶神经根在脊髓圆锥下方聚集而成，由于腰骶神经根束在椎管内的走行顺序排列，并不相互交叉或编织，从而表现出排列的规律性。整体上，脊髓末端到第 3 腰椎椎弓根的下缘，脊神经前后根分别占据马尾的前半部和后半部，且各节段的前后根排列基本一致；第 3 腰椎椎弓根以下，马尾呈弓背向后的半弧形，呈马蹄形排列，脊神经前根位居弧形马尾的前内侧半，后根则居于弧形的外后侧半[10, 11]。临床上由于各种先天或后天的原因致腰椎椎管绝对或相对狭窄，压迫马尾而产生一系列神经功能障碍，称为马尾综合征。在 MR 图像上能够辨别腰骶椎管内的脊神经节，从而辨别脊神经后根和前根。盆腔内各器官与上一断面变化不大。腰大肌内侧自前向后依次排列输尿管、髂血管及腰骶干，股神经位于腰大肌后份内。

女性盆部与会阴连续横断层 10（FH.9190）

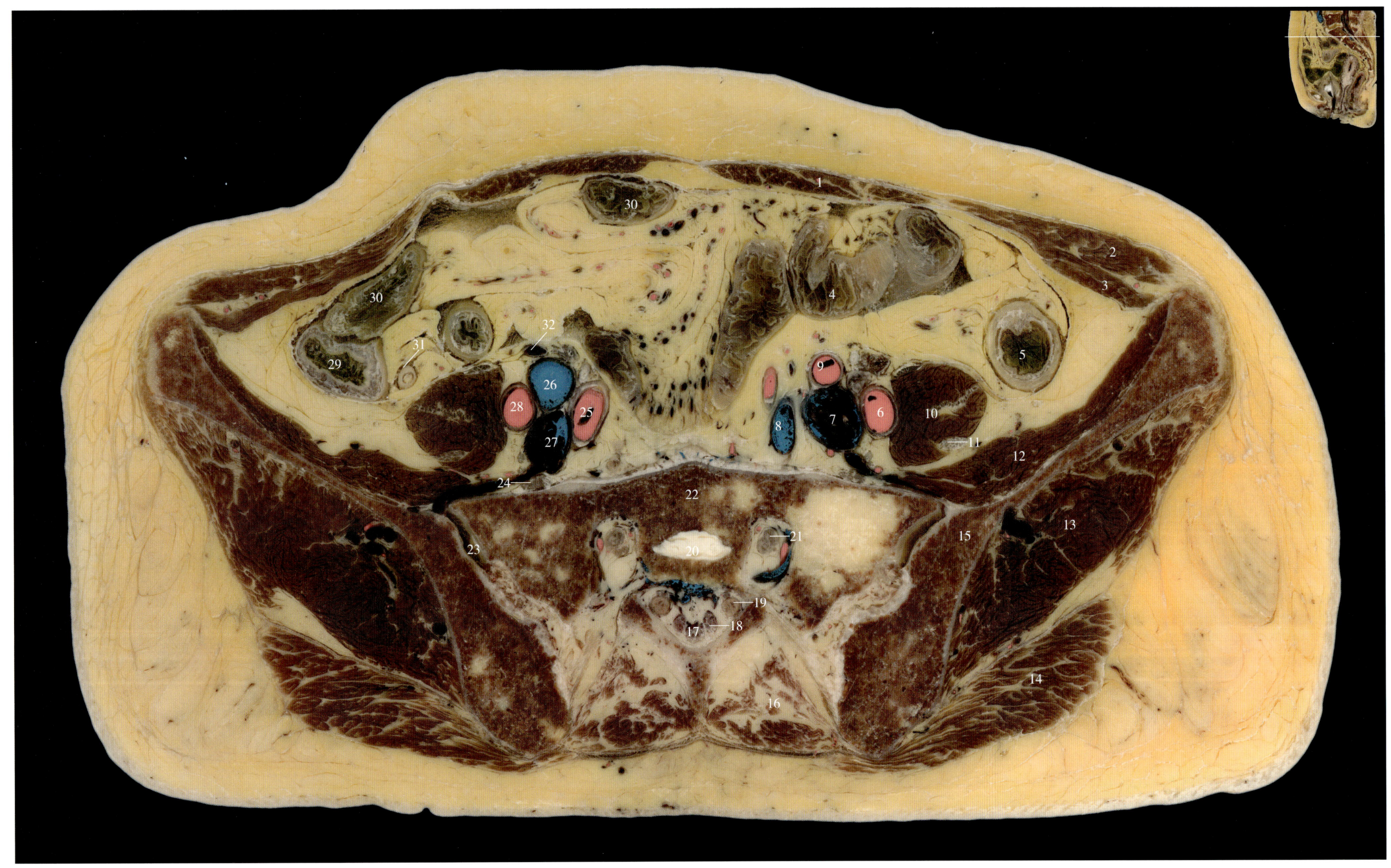

A. 断层标本图像

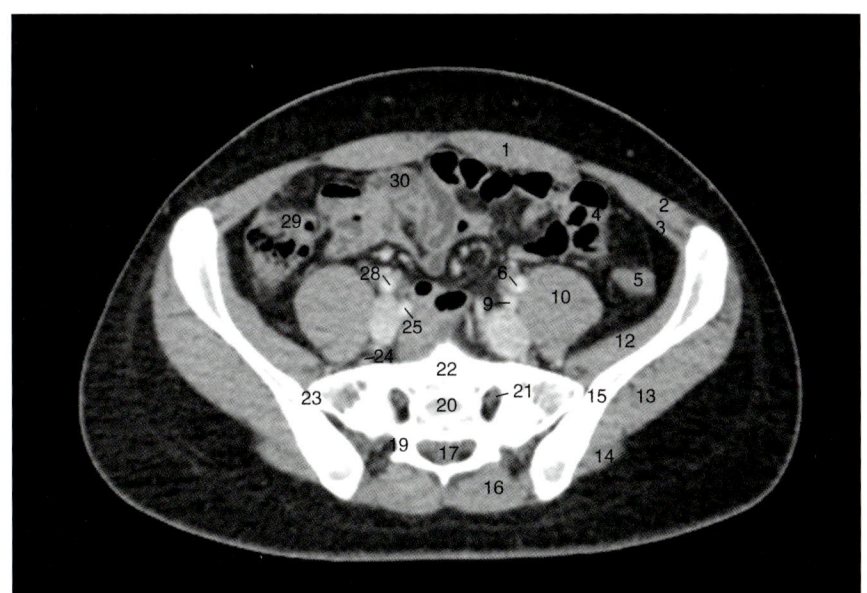

B. CT 增强图像

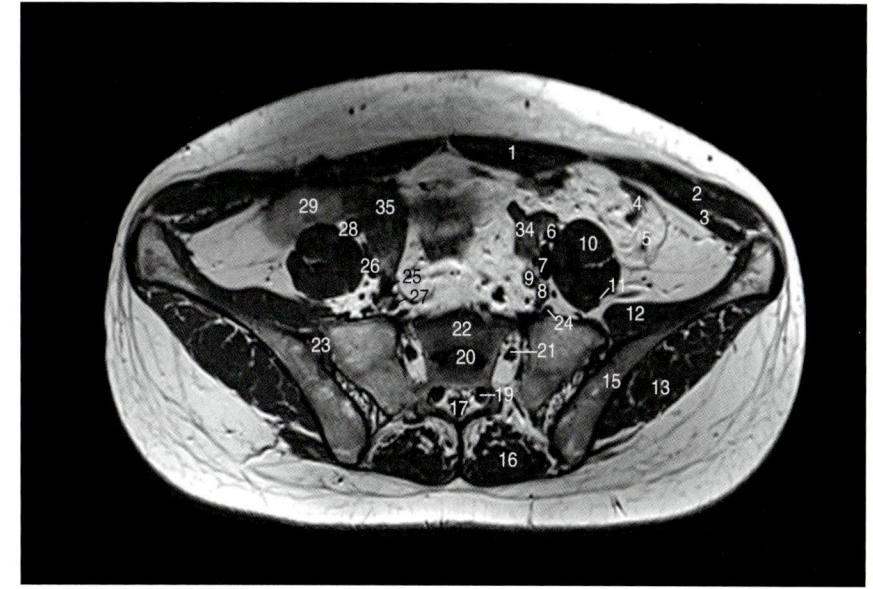

C. MR T1WI

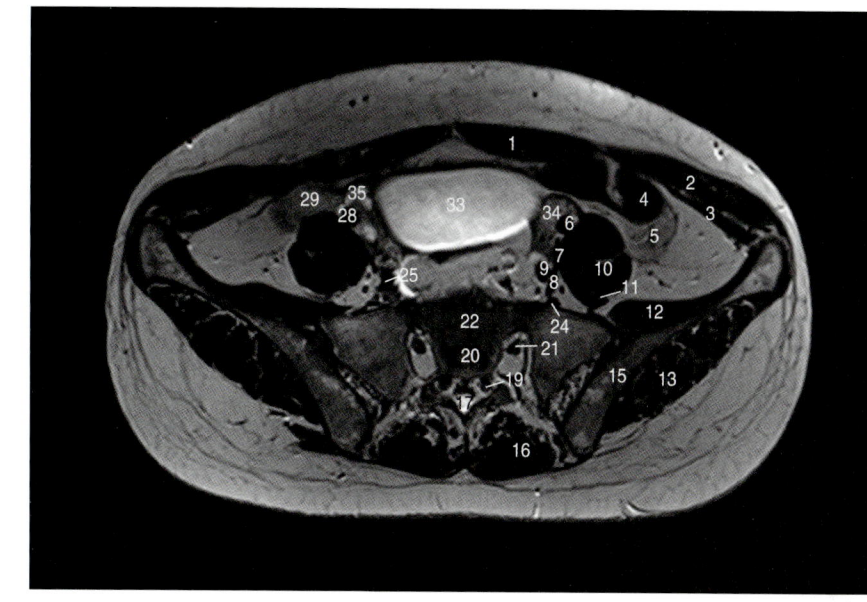

D. MR T2WI

1. 腹直肌 rectus abdominis
2. 腹内斜肌 obliquus internus abdominis
3. 腹横肌 transversus abdominis
4. 空肠 jejunum
5. 降结肠 descending colon
6. 左髂外动脉 left external iliac artery
7. 左髂外静脉 left external iliac vein
8. 左髂内静脉 left internal iliac vein
9. 左髂内动脉 left internal iliac artery
10. 腰大肌 psoas major
11. 股神经 femoral nerve
12. 髂肌 iliacus
13. 臀中肌 gluteus medius
14. 臀大肌 gluteus maximus
15. 髂骨翼 ala of ilium
16. 竖脊肌 erector spinae
17. 骶管 sacral canal
18. 第 3 骶神经 3rd sacral nerve
19. 第 2 骶神经 2nd sacral nerve
20. S1-2 椎间盘 S1-2 intervertebral disc
21. 第 1 骶神经 lst sacral nerve
22. 第 1 骶椎 1st sacral vertebra
23. 骶髂关节 sacroiliac joint
24. 腰骶干 lumbosacral trunk
25. 右髂内动脉 right internal iliac artery
26. 右髂外静脉 right external iliac vein
27. 右髂内静脉 right internal iliac vein
28. 右髂外动脉 right external iliac artery
29. 盲肠 cecum
30. 回肠 ileum
31. 阑尾 vermiform appendix
32. 右卵巢动、静脉 right ovarian artery and vein
33. 膀胱 urinary bladder
34. 左卵巢 left ovary
35. 右卵巢 right ovary

关键结构：骶管，骶髂关节，股神经。

此断面经过 S1-2 椎间盘（临床上常写作 S1/2 椎间盘），后方为骶管。

骶管上部与腰椎椎管相连，下部开口于骶管裂孔，两侧借椎间孔、骶前孔和骶后孔与外界相通。骶管断面的形态上段呈三角形逐渐变为下段的长椭圆形。硬膜囊的下界大多位于第 2 骶椎或第 3 骶椎椎体水平，因此该水平上、下骶管内的结构有一定的差异，在该水平以上，骶管内的结构包含硬膜外隙、硬膜囊及硬膜囊内的终池、马尾和终丝等结构；该水平以下骶管已无硬膜囊及蛛网膜下隙等结构，主要为下位骶神经根、尾神经根、终丝、椎内静脉丛和脂肪组织等。腰大肌位于骶髂关节前方，其内侧见前后排列的输尿管、髂血管和腰骶干，两侧的髂内静脉与髂外静脉已经完全分离，腰骶干向外移行。腰大肌后外侧份内见股神经。

女性盆部与会阴连续横断层 11（FH.9170）

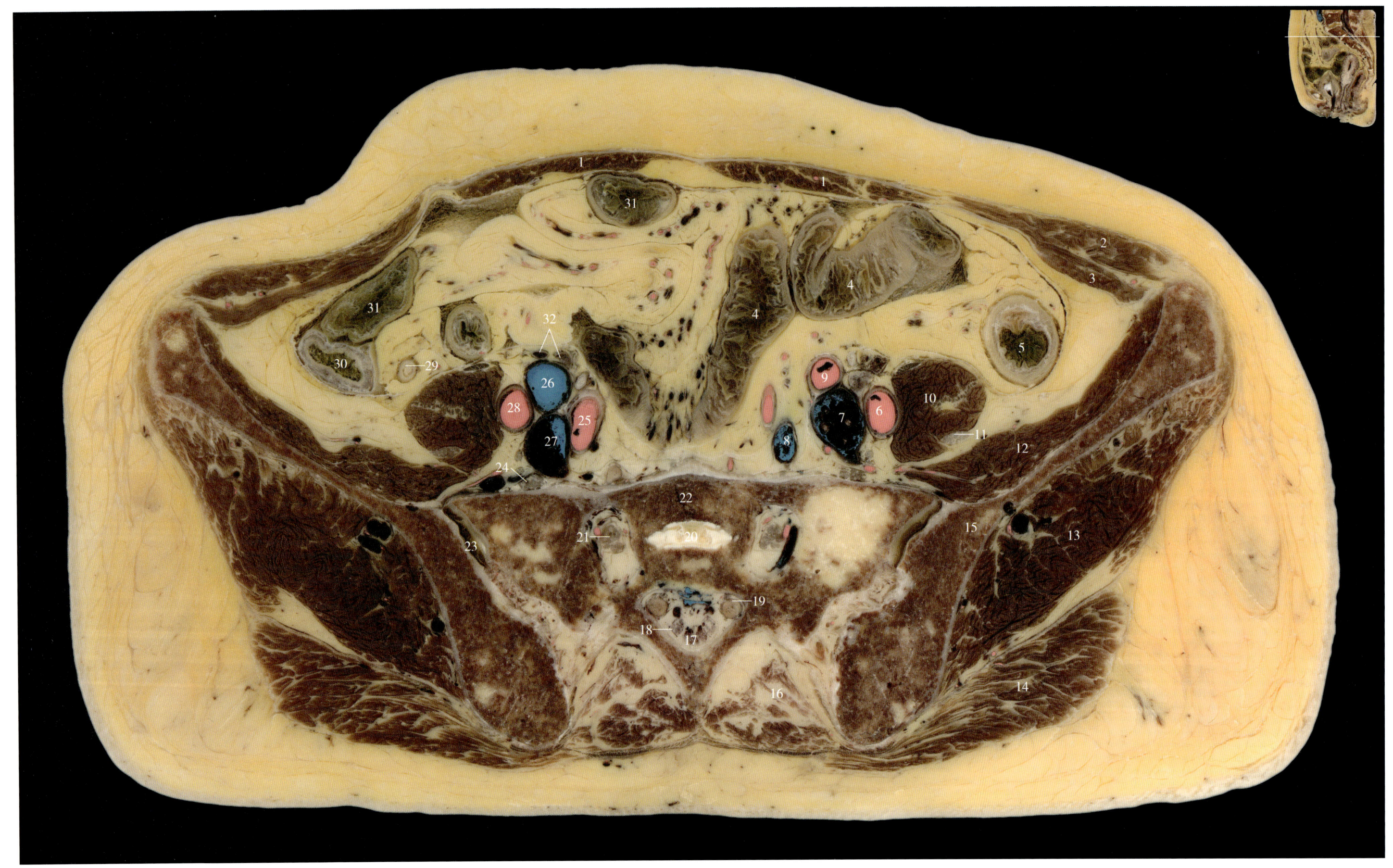

A. 断层标本图像

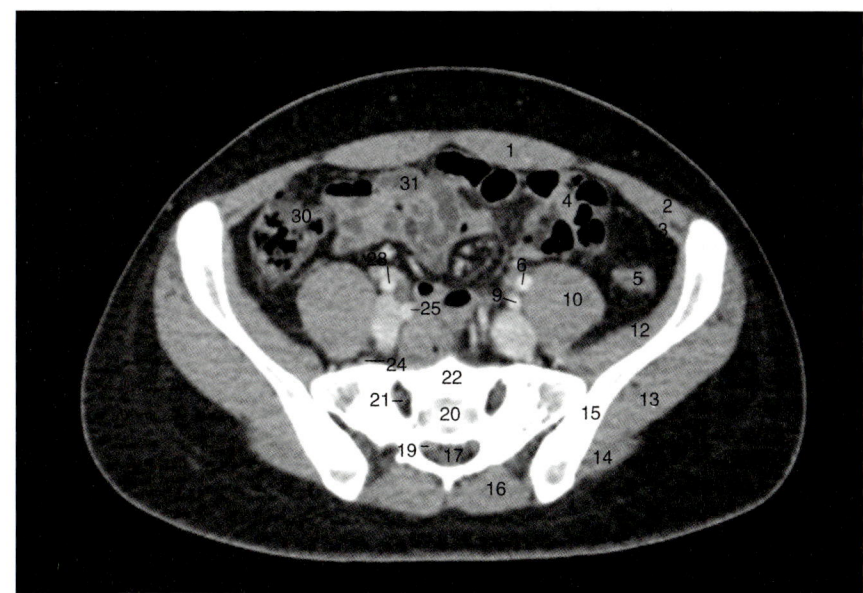
B. CT 增强图像

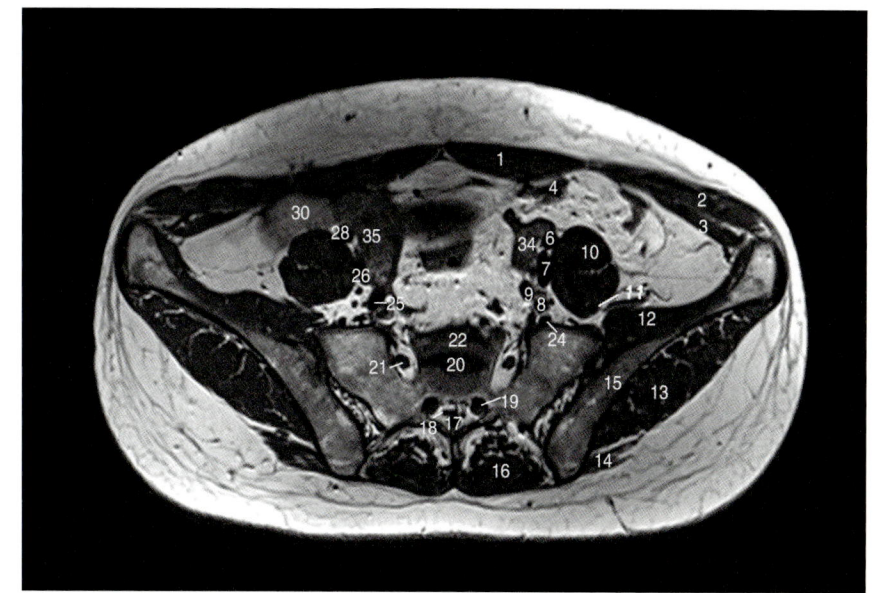
C. MR T1WI

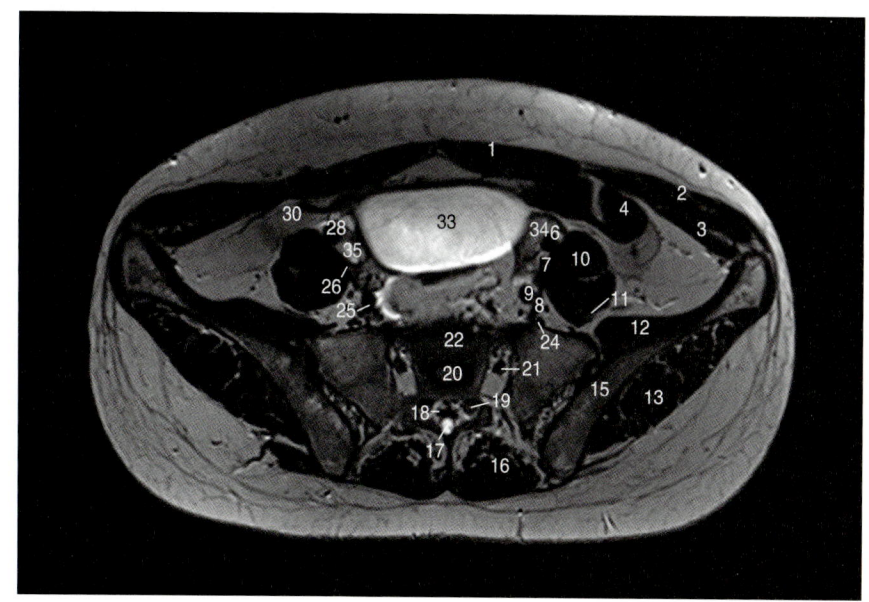
D. MR T2WI

1. 腹直肌 rectus abdominis
2. 腹内斜肌 obliquus internus abdominis
3. 腹横肌 transversus abdominis
4. 空肠 jejunum
5. 降结肠 descending colon
6. 左髂外动脉 left external iliac artery
7. 左髂外静脉 left external iliac vein
8. 左髂内静脉 left internal iliac vein
9. 左髂内动脉 left internal iliac artery
10. 腰大肌 psoas major
11. 股神经 femoral nerve
12. 髂肌 iliacus
13. 臀中肌 gluteus medius
14. 臀大肌 gluteus maximus
15. 髂骨翼 ala of ilium
16. 竖脊肌 erector spinae
17. 骶管 sacral canal
18. 第 3 骶神经 3rd sacral nerve
19. 第 2 骶神经 2nd sacral nerve
20. S1-2 椎间盘 S1-2 intervertebral disc
21. 第 1 骶神经 1st sacral nerve
22. 第 1 骶椎 1st sacral vertebra
23. 骶髂关节 sacroiliac joint
24. 腰骶干 lumbosacral trunk
25. 右髂内动脉 right internal iliac artery
26. 右髂外静脉 right external iliac vein
27. 右髂内静脉 right internal iliac vein
28. 右髂外动脉 right external iliac artery
29. 阑尾 vermiform appendix
30. 盲肠 cecum
31. 回肠 ileum
32. 右卵巢动、静脉 right ovarian artery and vein
33. 膀胱 urinary bladder
34. 左卵巢 left ovary
35. 右卵巢 right ovary

关键结构：骨盆，髂血管，股神经。

此断面经过 S1-2 椎间盘。

椎间盘后方为骶管，骶管内含骶、尾神经根。腰大肌位于骶髂关节前方，腰大肌内侧见输尿管、髂血管及腰骶干，呈前后方向排列。腰大肌后外侧份内见股神经。男女骨盆存在差异，主要表现在：①男性骨盆外形窄而长，骨盆上口接近心形，较小，骨盆下口较窄；女性骨盆宽而短，上口接近圆形，骨盆下口较宽；②第 1 骶椎椎体最大宽度女性大于男性，女性平均为 11.34 cm ± 0.48 cm，男性平均为 10.84 cm ± 1.09 cm；③髂骨翼形态，男性髂骨翼前份呈弓形伸向前外，女性髂骨翼前份呈平直斜向前外；④男性耻骨下角较小，角度明显，为 50°~60°；而女性耻骨下角圆润，不易测量，为 80°~85°；⑤男性的坐骨棘间的距离比较近，且弯向内侧。女性的坐骨大切迹较男性宽，男、女平均值分别为 50.4°、74.4°[5]。

女性盆部与会阴连续横断层 12（FH.9150）

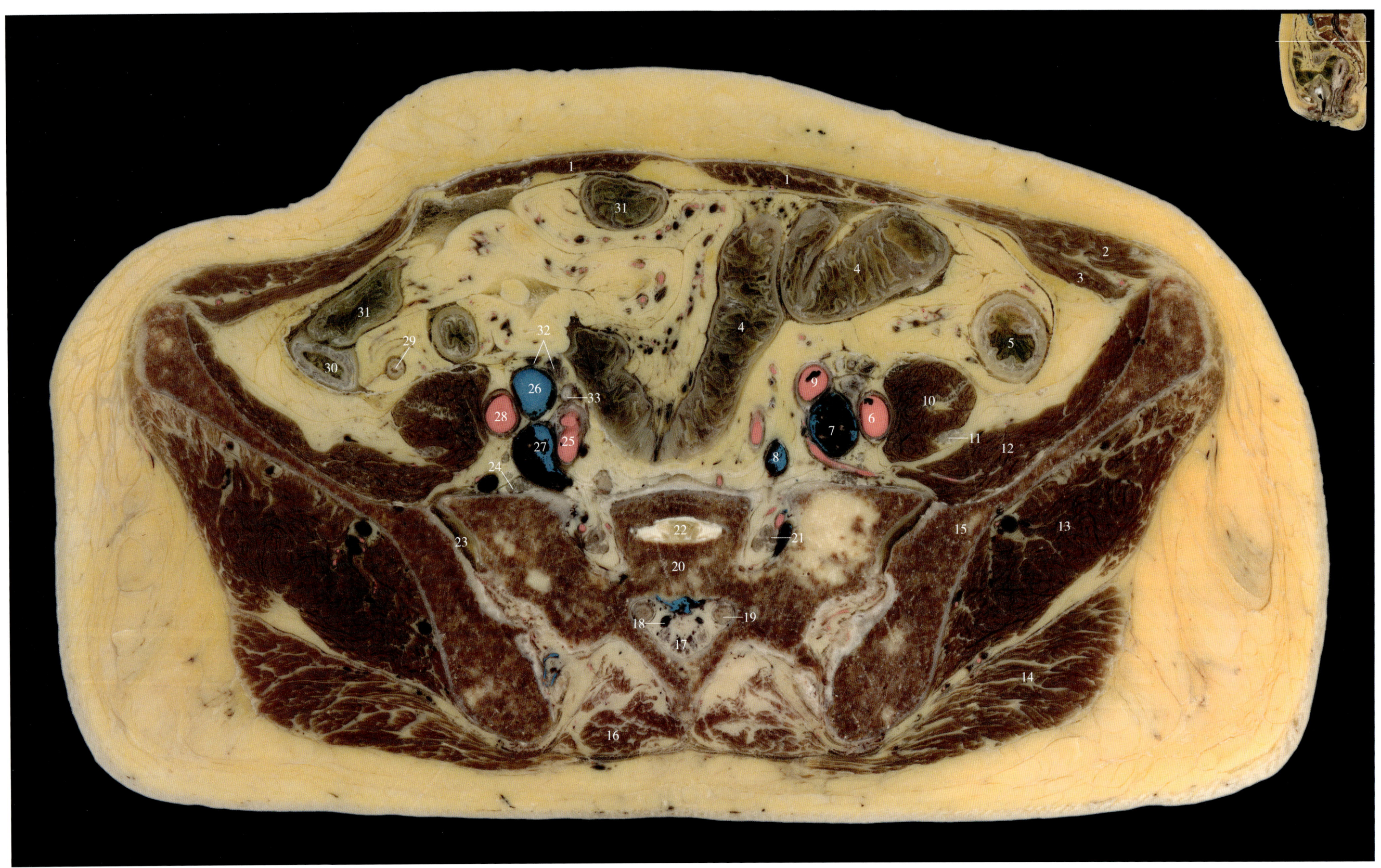

A. 断层标本图像

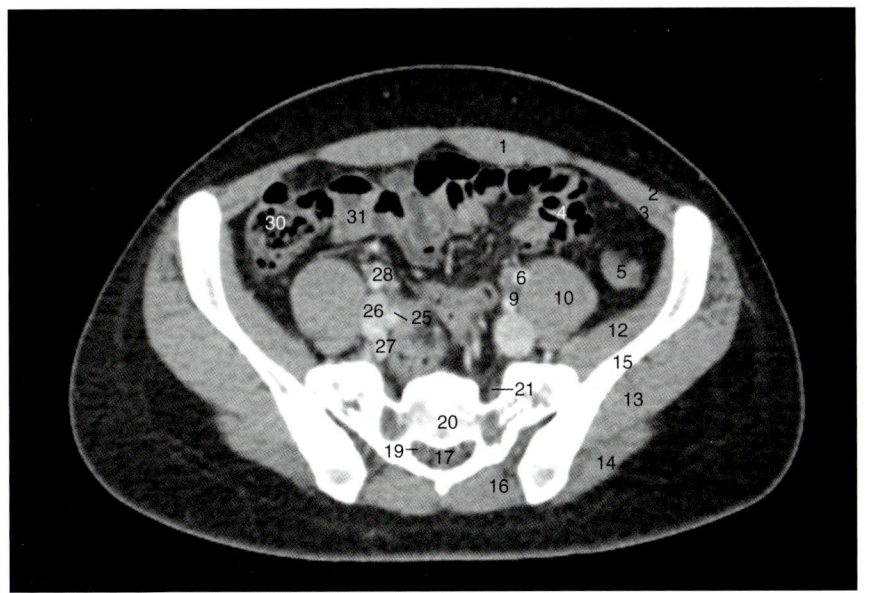

B. CT 增强图像

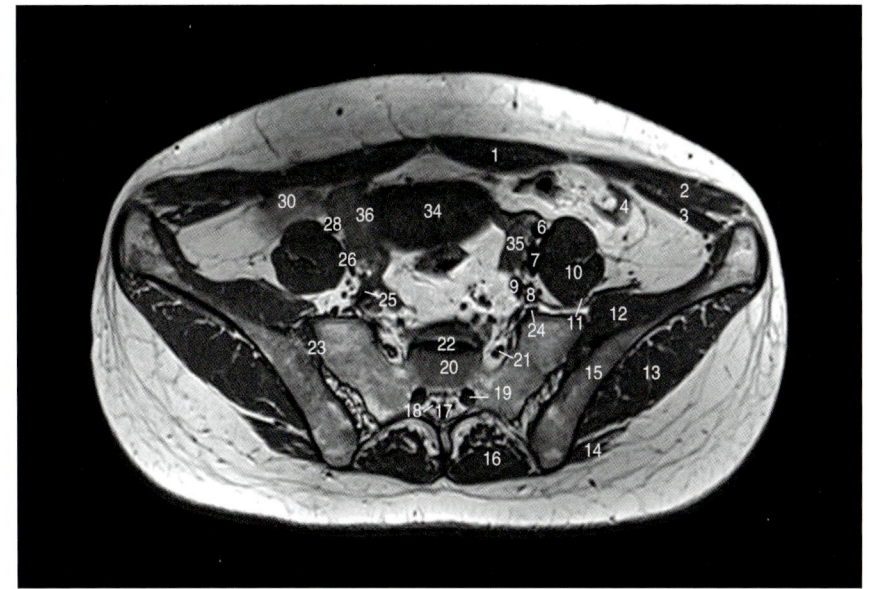

C. MR T1WI

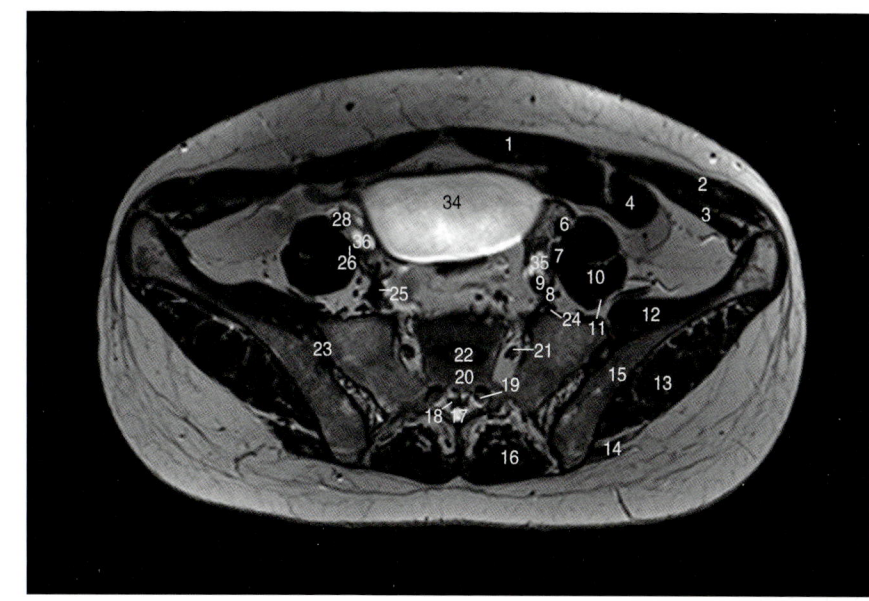

D. MR T2WI

1. 腹直肌 rectus abdominis
2. 腹内斜肌 obliquus internus abdominis
3. 腹横肌 transversus abdominis
4. 空肠 jejunum
5. 降结肠 descending colon
6. 左髂外动脉 left external iliac artery
7. 左髂外静脉 left external iliac vein
8. 左髂内静脉 left internal iliac vein
9. 左髂内动脉 left internal iliac artery
10. 腰大肌 psoas major
11. 股神经 femoral nerve
12. 髂肌 iliacus
13. 臀中肌 gluteus medius
14. 臀大肌 gluteus maximus
15. 髂骨翼 ala of ilium
16. 竖脊肌 erector spinae
17. 骶管 sacral canal
18. 第 3 骶神经 3rd sacral nerve
19. 第 2 骶神经 2nd sacral nerve
20. 第 2 骶椎 2nd sacral vertebra
21. 第 1 骶神经 lst sacral nerve
22. S1-2 椎间盘 S1-2 intervertebral disc
23. 骶髂关节 sacroiliac joint
24. 腰骶干 lumbosacral trunk
25. 右髂内动脉 right internal iliac artery
26. 右髂外静脉 right external iliac vein
27. 右髂内静脉 right internal iliac vein
28. 右髂外动脉 right external iliac artery
29. 阑尾 vermiform appendix
30. 盲肠 cecum
31. 回肠 ileum
32. 右卵巢动、静脉 right ovarian artery and vein
33. 右输尿管 right ureter
34. 膀胱 urinary bladder
35. 左卵巢 left ovary
36. 右卵巢 right ovary

关键结构：阑尾，髂骨翼骶髂关节，股神经。

此断面经过 S1-2 椎间盘。

骶椎间盘后方为骶管，骶管内容纳骶、尾神经根。髂骨为骨盆重要组成结构之一，前部宽大的为髂骨翼，后部窄小为髂骨体。髂骨翼内面光滑稍凹，称髂窝，内见髂腰肌断面，窝的下界为突出的弓状线。髂骨翼的外面称臀面，有臀肌附着，从内侧向外侧依次为臀小肌、臀中肌、臀大肌。在骶翼与髂骨翼（中部）之间为骶髂关节，关节面较上一断层增大。腰大肌位于骶髂关节前方。腰大肌内侧见输尿管、髂血管及腰骶干，呈前后方向排列。股神经向外移行，位于腰大肌与髂肌之间。盆腔内右侧髂窝内盲端已近盲端，阑尾位于盲肠内侧，从盲肠下端后内侧壁向外延伸的一条细管样器官，长度因人而异，成人一般长 5~7 cm。幼儿时期阑尾长而粗，至 3 岁左右即接近成年人大小。阑尾最常见于盲肠后位或结肠后位，也可出现在其他位置，包括盲肠下位、回肠前位或回肠后位，尤其是阑尾系膜较长、阑尾活动度较大时[5]。在 CT 图像上，正常阑尾不易找到，当发生阑尾炎时，可表现为阑尾增粗，周围系膜密度增高、邻近腹膜增厚和少量腹膜腔积液。

女性盆部与会阴连续横断层 13（FH.9130）

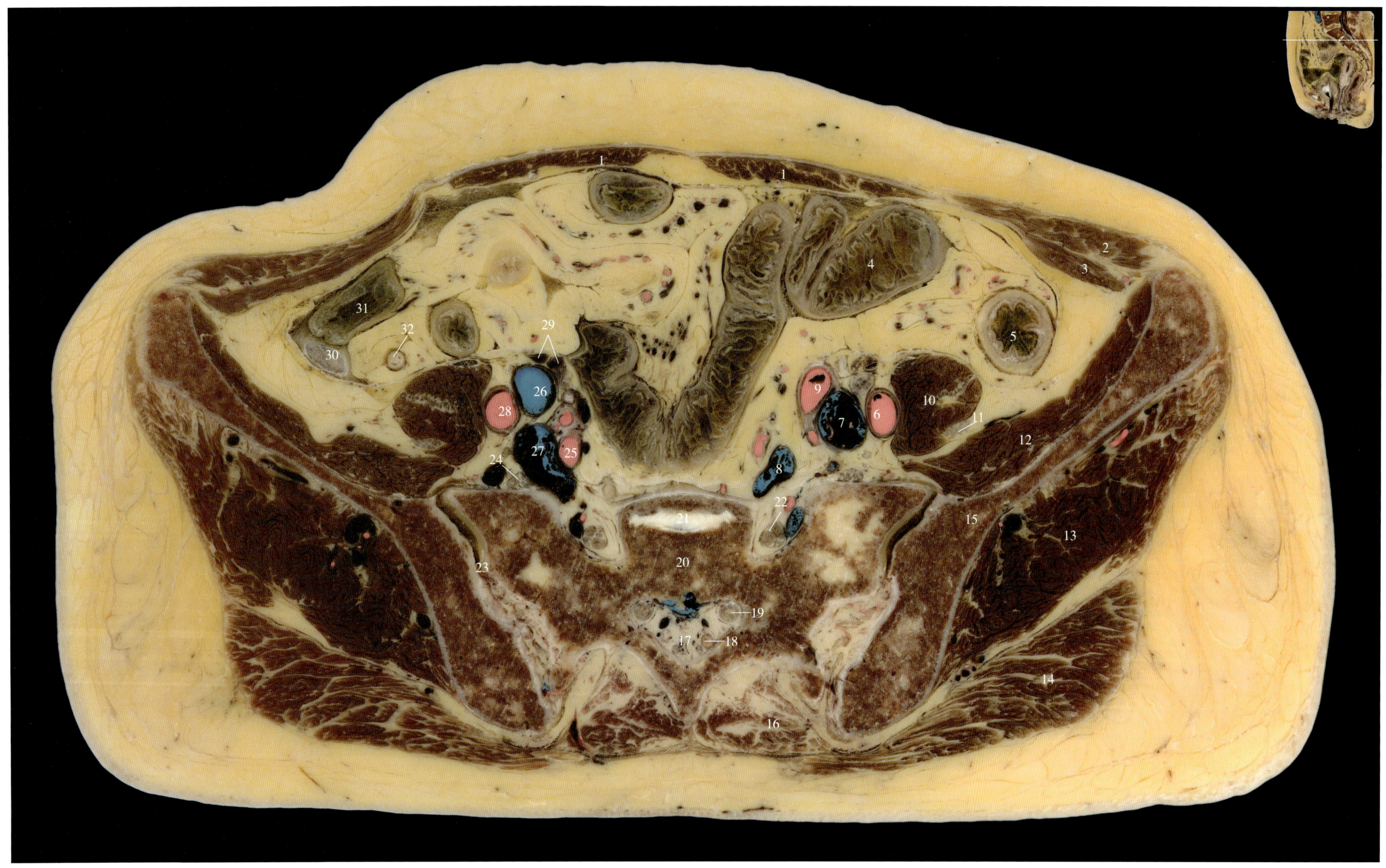

A. 断层标本图像

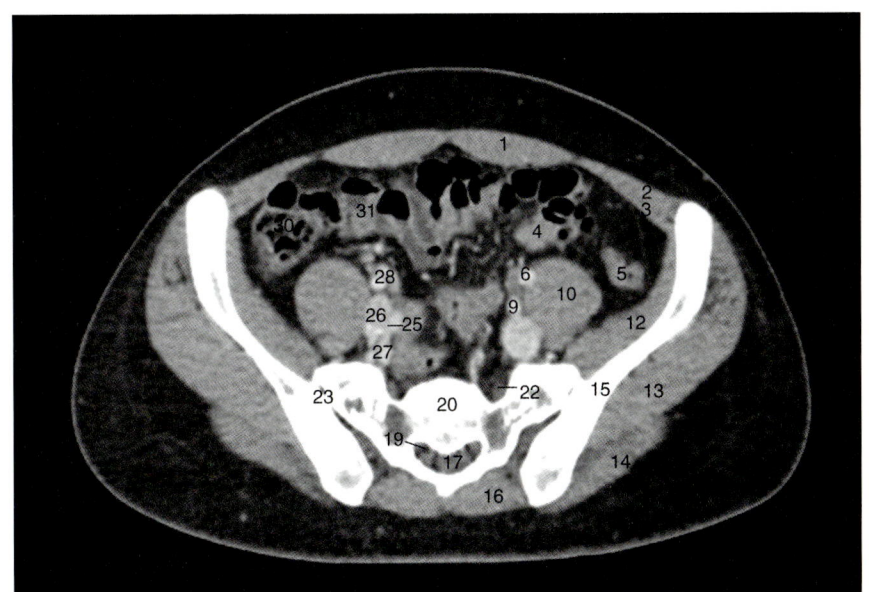

B. CT 增强图像

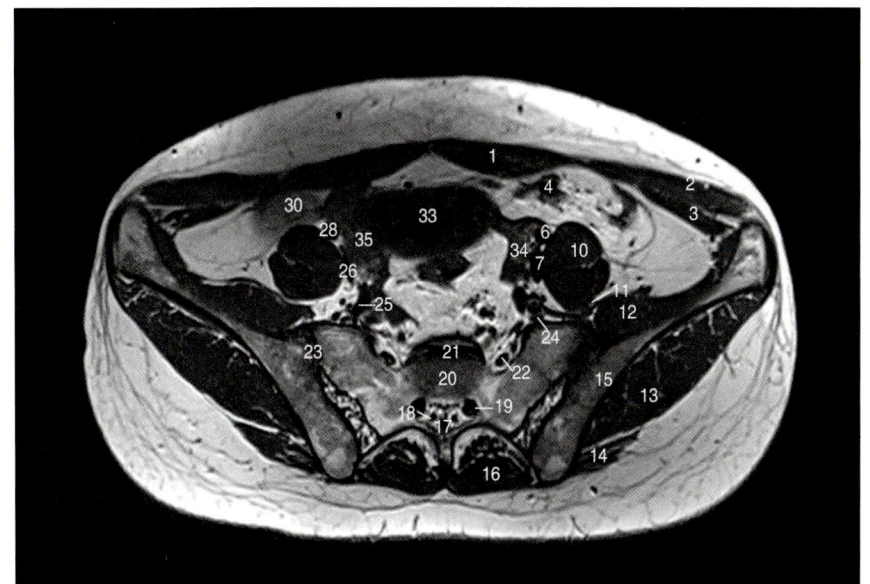

C. MR T1WI

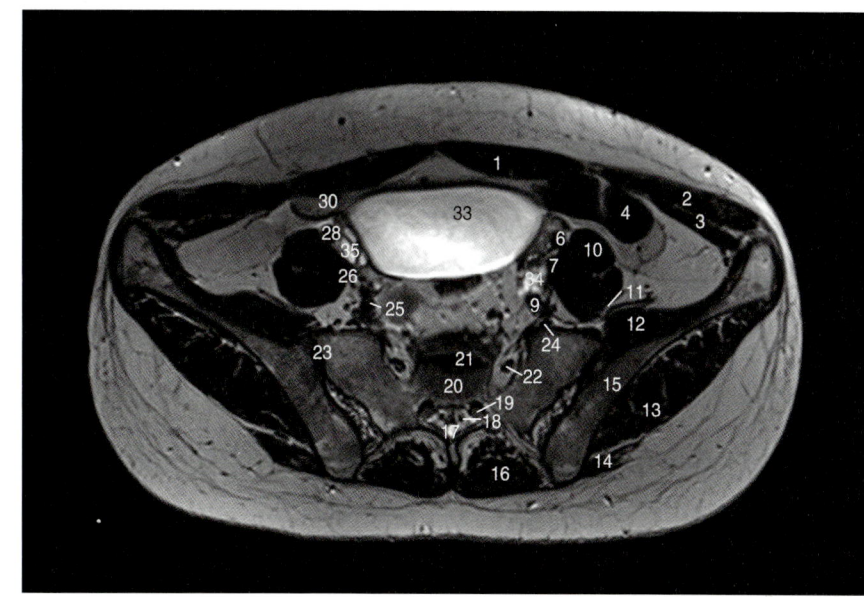

D. MR T2WI

1. 腹直肌 rectus abdominis
2. 腹内斜肌 obliquus internus abdominis
3. 腹横肌 transversus abdominis
4. 空肠 jejunum
5. 降结肠 descending colon
6. 左髂外动脉 left external iliac artery
7. 左髂外静脉 left external iliac vein
8. 左髂内静脉 left internal iliac vein
9. 左髂内动脉 left internal iliac artery
10. 腰大肌 psoas major
11. 股神经 femoral nerve
12. 髂肌 iliacus
13. 臀中肌 gluteus medius
14. 臀大肌 gluteus maximus
15. 髂骨翼 ala of ilium
16. 竖脊肌 erector spinae
17. 骶管 sacral canal
18. 第 3 骶神经 3rd sacral nerve
19. 第 2 骶神经 2nd sacral nerve
20. 第 2 骶椎 2nd sacral vertebra
21. S1-2 椎间盘 S1-2 intervertebral disc
22. 第 1 骶神经 1st sacral nerve
23. 骶髂关节 sacroiliac joint
24. 腰骶干 lumbosacral trunk
25. 右髂内动脉 right internal iliac artery
26. 右髂外静脉 right external iliac vein
27. 右髂内静脉 right internal iliac vein
28. 右髂外动脉 right external iliac artery
29. 右卵巢动、静脉 right ovarian artery and vein
30. 盲肠 cecum
31. 回肠 ileum
32. 阑尾 vermiform appendix
33. 膀胱 urinary bladder
34. 左卵巢 left ovary
35. 右卵巢 right ovary

关键结构：骶骨，输尿管，股神经。

此断面经过第 2 骶椎椎体上份。

第 2 骶椎椎体位于盆部后壁中央，第 2 骶椎椎体较第 1 骶椎椎体缩小，骶椎融合形成骶骨。骶骨呈三角形，底朝上与第 5 腰椎椎体相连结，尖向下连于尾骨；其前面平滑凹向前，有四对骶前孔；后面由后凸且高低不平，正中线上有骶正中嵴，嵴两侧有四对骶后孔。骶前、后孔通过相应的椎间孔与骶管相通。骶 1~4 脊神经根经相应的椎间孔并发出前、后支分别穿过骶前、后孔出骶骨。椎间孔和骶前、后孔内有血管、淋巴管、脂肪组织等通过。椎骨在胚胎发育过程中数目可发生变异，如第 1 骶椎椎体不与其他骶椎融合而成第 6 腰椎，则称骶椎腰化；反之，如第 5 腰椎与骶骨融合，则称腰椎骶化。由于骶椎发育过程复杂，变异及畸形多见。检测胎儿骨化中心的出现时间和形态，对于评估脊柱发育及发现椎体畸形有重要意义。胎儿在 17 孕周时，第 1~3 骶椎椎体的骨化中心全部出现，第 4 骶椎骨化中心出现于第 19 孕周，第 5 骶椎体骨化中心出现于第 28 孕周。腰大肌位于骶髂关节前方，内侧见输尿管、髂血管及腰骶干。股神经位于腰大肌与髂肌之间[13]。

女性盆部与会阴连续横断层 14（FH.9110）

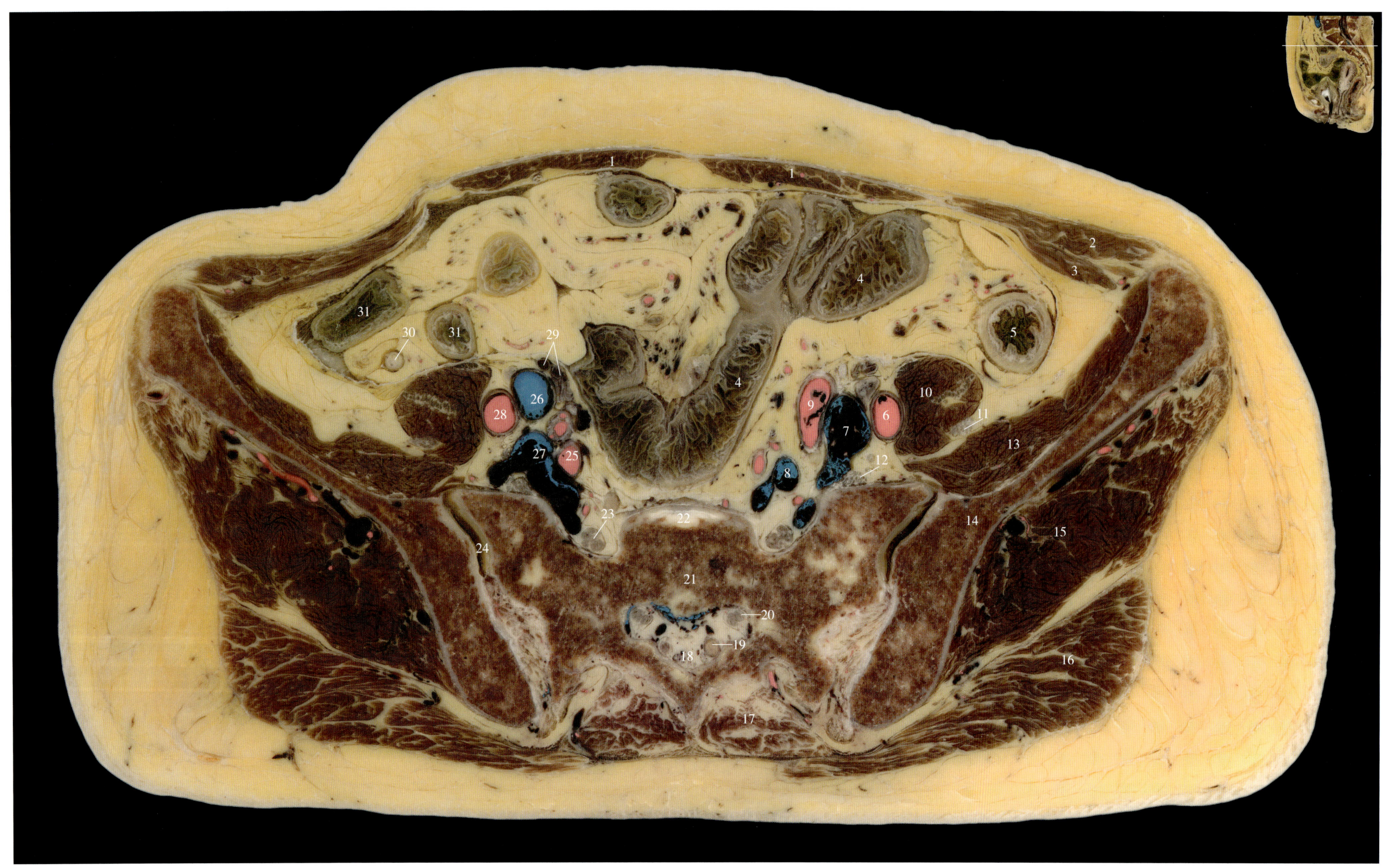

A. 断层标本图像

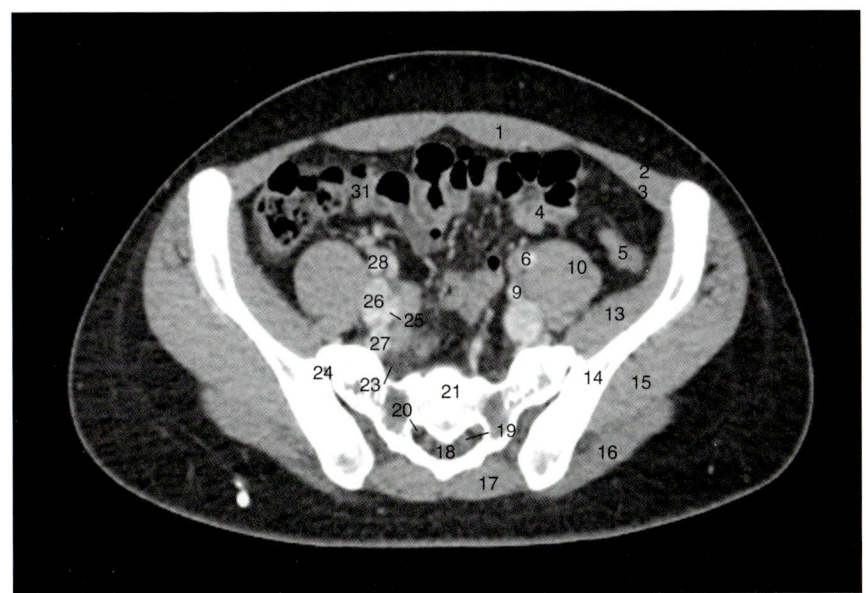
B. CT 增强图像

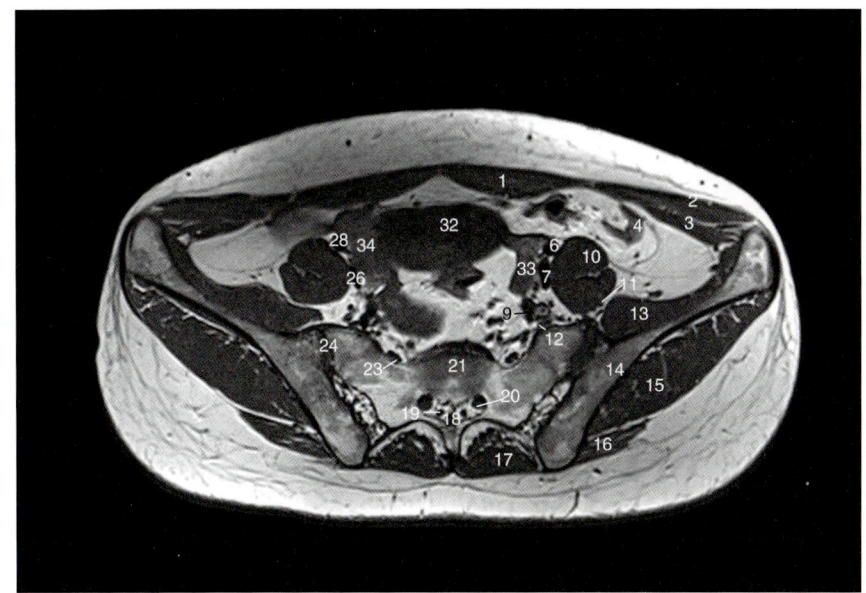
C. MR T1WI

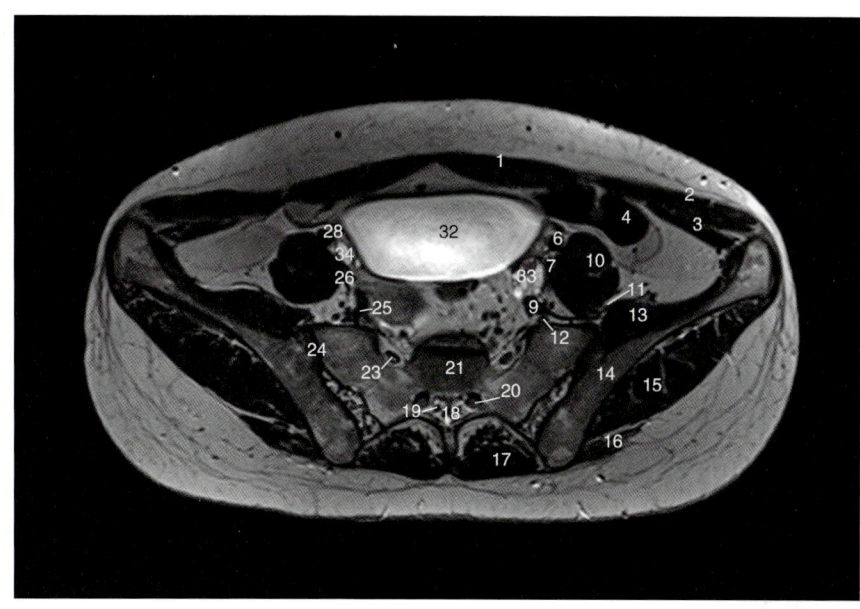
D. MR T2WI

1. 腹直肌 rectus abdominis
2. 腹内斜肌 obliquus internus abdominis
3. 腹横肌 transversus abdominis
4. 空肠 jejunum
5. 降结肠 descending colon
6. 左髂外动脉 left external iliac artery
7. 左髂外静脉 left external iliac vein
8. 左髂内静脉 left internal iliac vein
9. 左髂内动脉 left internal iliac artery
10. 腰大肌 psoas major
11. 股神经 femoral nerve
12. 腰骶干 lumbosacral trunk
13. 髂肌 iliacus
14. 髂骨翼 ala of ilium
15. 臀中肌 gluteus medius
16. 臀大肌 gluteus maximus
17. 竖脊肌 erector spinae
18. 骶管 sacral canal
19. 第 3 骶神经 3rd sacral nerve
20. 第 2 骶神经 2nd sacral nerve
21. 第 2 骶椎 2nd sacral vertebra
22. S1-2 椎间盘 S1-2 intervertebral disc
23. 第 1 骶神经 1st sacral nerve
24. 骶髂关节 sacroiliac joint
25. 右髂内动脉 right internal iliac artery
26. 右髂外静脉 right external iliac vein
27. 右髂内静脉 right internal iliac vein
28. 右髂外动脉 right external iliac artery
29. 右卵巢动、静脉 right ovarian artery and vein
30. 阑尾 vermiform appendix
31. 回肠 ileum
32. 膀胱 urinary bladder
33. 左卵巢 left ovary
34. 右卵巢 right ovary

关键结构：臀大肌，输尿管，髂血管。

此断面经过第 2 骶椎椎体上份。

椎体后方为骶管，骶管内容纳骶、尾神经根。腰大肌位于骶髂关节前方，内侧见输尿管，输尿管在从盆腔边缘到子宫动脉下交叉后，进入宫旁组织并在"输尿管通道"内行走，大致沿主韧带的前纤维和子宫骶韧带的后纤维的分界走行。在这一区域，输尿管沿子宫颈前外侧和阴道上方走行，然后在阴道前壁上方走行而后下入膀胱，止于膀胱壁内输尿管开口处[14]。股神经位于腰大肌与髂肌之间。两侧髂骨翼为盆后外侧壁，其内、外侧面分别为髂肌与臀中肌所附着，臀中肌后份是臀大肌。臀大肌起止面广泛，自上而下起于髂骨翼外面和骶骨背面，止于髂胫束和股骨的臀肌粗隆。臀大肌纤维非常粗大，平行向外向下。臀大肌呈菱形，上缘长为 9.1 cm ± 0.2 cm，下缘长为 10.3 cm ± 0.1 cm，止点宽为 9.8 cm ± 0.5 cm。臀大肌覆盖臀中肌的后部、臀小肌及出入盆腔的血管、神经。臀大肌收缩时，使髋关节伸和旋外，下肢固定时，能伸直躯干，防止躯干前倾。此肌受臀下神经支配。臀大肌的滋养血管和神经入肌点多在其上下 1/4 交界处，血管和神经分支在上部较多而下部较少，手术时，应在臀大肌中部沿肌纤维走行方向钝性牵拉以显露深层组织[15, 16]。

29

女性盆部与会阴连续横断层 15（FH.9090）

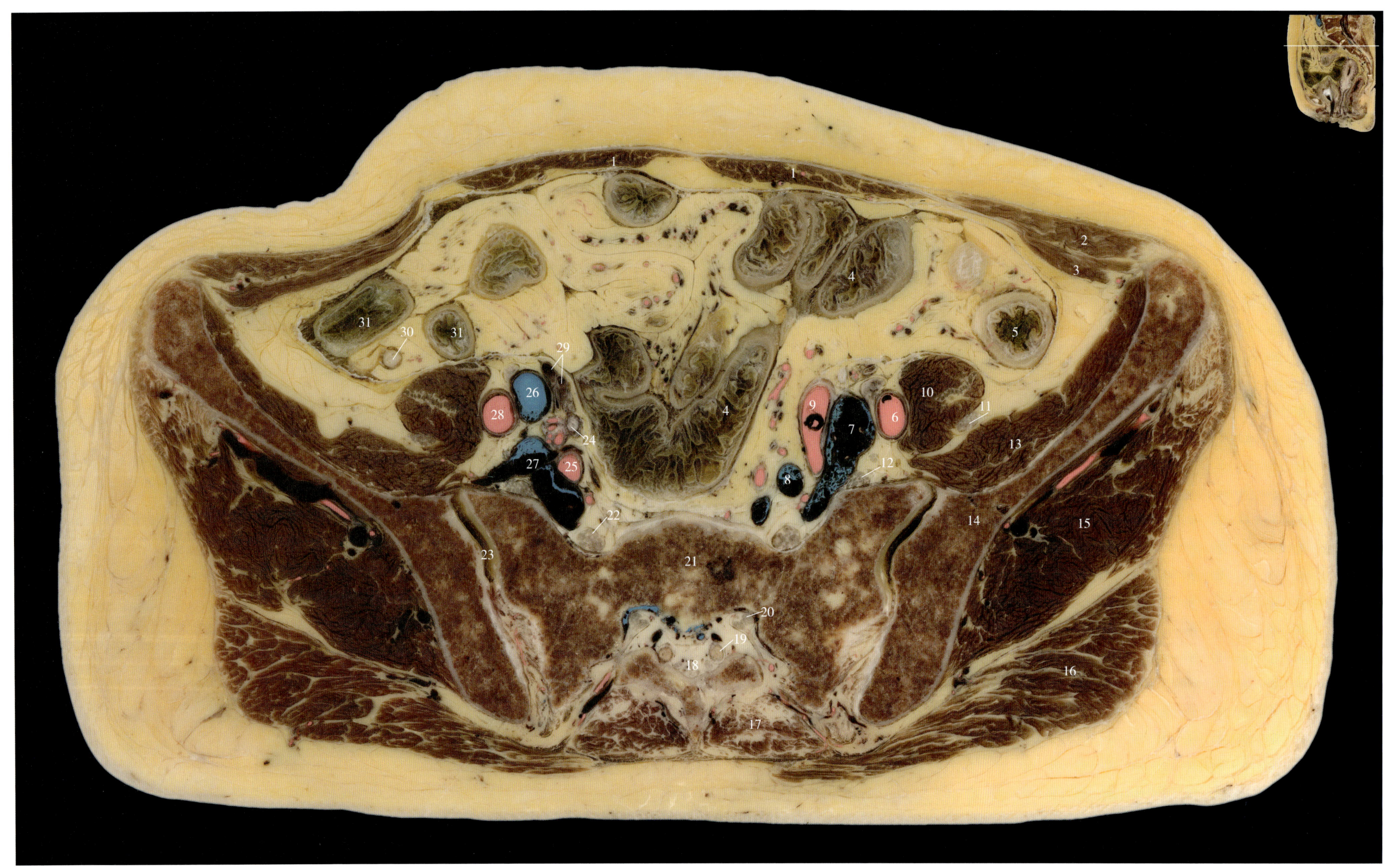

A. 断层标本图像

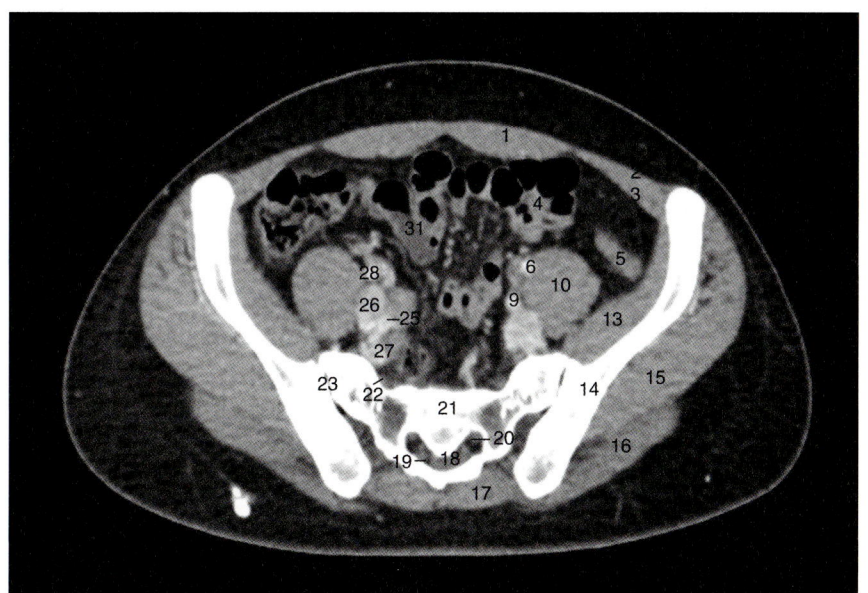

B. CT 增强图像

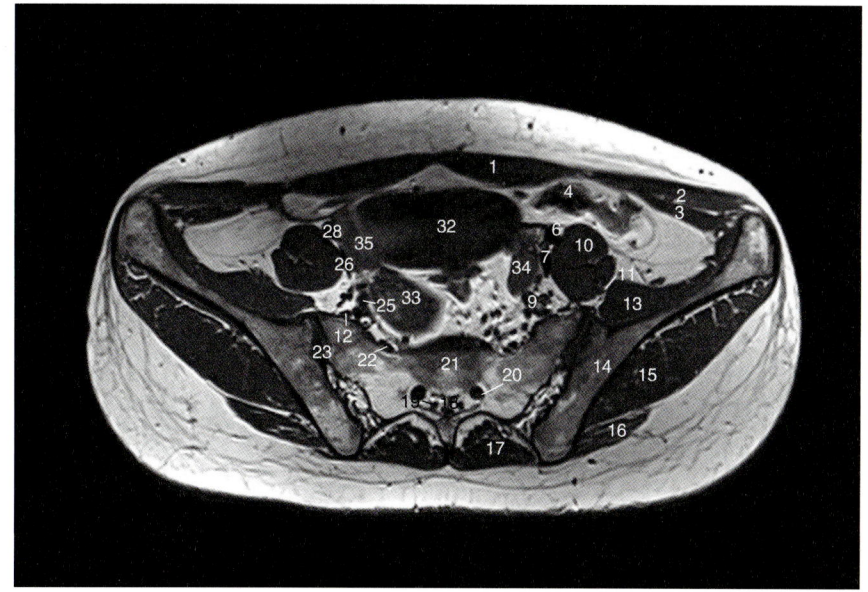

C. MR T1WI

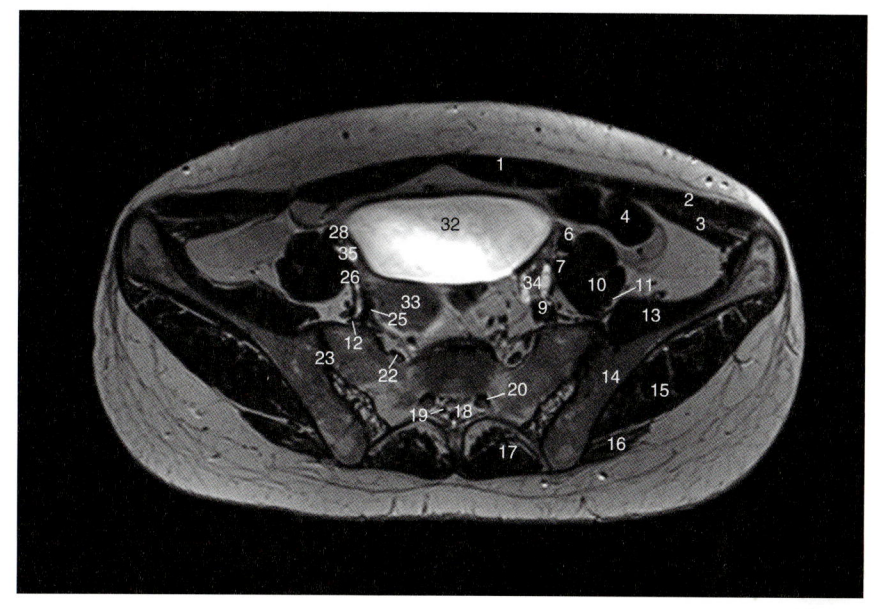

D. MR T2WI

1. 腹直肌 rectus abdominis
2. 腹内斜肌 obliquus internus abdominis
3. 腹横肌 transversus abdominis
4. 空肠 jejunum
5. 降结肠 descending colon
6. 左髂外动脉 left external iliac artery
7. 左髂外静脉 left external iliac vein
8. 左髂内静脉属支 tributary of left internal iliac vein
9. 左髂内动脉分支 branch of left internal iliac artery
10. 腰大肌 psoas major
11. 股神经 femoral nerve
12. 腰骶干 lumbosacral trunk
13. 髂肌 iliacus
14. 髂骨翼 ala of ilium
15. 臀中肌 gluteus medius
16. 臀大肌 gluteus maximus
17. 竖脊肌 erector spinae
18. 骶管 sacral canal
19. 第3骶神经 3rd sacral nerve
20. 第2骶神经 2nd sacral nerve
21. 第2骶椎 2nd sacral vertebra
22. 第1骶神经 1st sacral nerve
23. 骶髂关节 sacroiliac joint
24. 右输尿管 right ureter
25. 右髂内动脉 right internal iliac artery
26. 右髂外静脉 right external iliac vein
27. 右髂内静脉属支 tributary of right internal iliac vein
28. 右髂外动脉 right external iliac artery
29. 右卵巢动、静脉 right ovarian artery and vein
30. 阑尾 vermiform appendix
31. 回肠 ileum
32. 膀胱 urinary bladder
33. 子宫底 fundus of uterus
34. 左卵巢 left ovary
35. 右卵巢 right ovary

关键结构：肠管，阑尾，股神经。

此断面经过第2骶椎椎体中份。

椎体后方为骶管，骶管内容纳骶、尾神经根。腰大肌位于骶髂关节前方，内侧见输尿管、髂血管及腰骶干呈前后方向排列。腰骶干向外侧移行，左侧腰骶干位于左髂外静脉外侧，右侧腰骶干位于右髂内静脉外侧。股神经位于腰大肌与髂肌之间。盆腔内盲肠已消失，左髂窝处有降结肠，降结肠内侧及右侧髂血管之间是空肠，右侧髂窝内见回肠，回肠断面之间见类圆形阑尾。阑尾表面通常会覆盖阑尾系膜，系膜的形态通常以扇形为主。阑尾系膜是一含有脂肪组织的角形腹膜襞，通过回肠末端系膜的后面、紧邻回盲肠连接处和阑尾。阑尾尖端有时很短，为一薄的、含有脂肪的腹膜，包裹阑尾的血管、神经和淋巴管，常含有淋巴结[1]。系膜内的阑尾动脉起源于回结肠动脉，或其分支盲肠前动脉、盲肠后动脉或回肠支。阑尾静脉与动脉伴行，经回结肠静脉、肠系膜上静脉汇入肝门静脉。

女性盆部与会阴连续横断层 16（FH.9070）

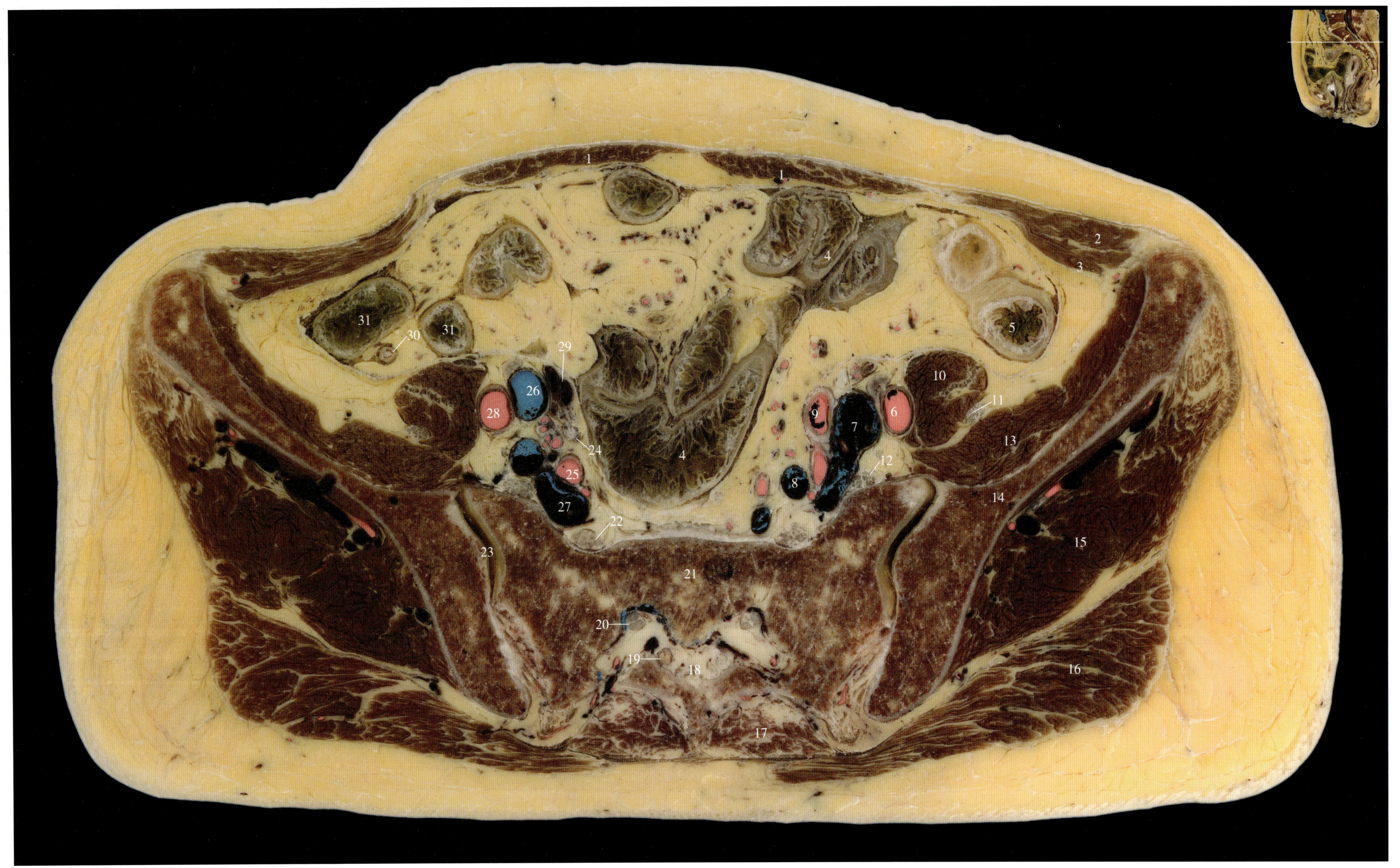

A. 断层标本图像

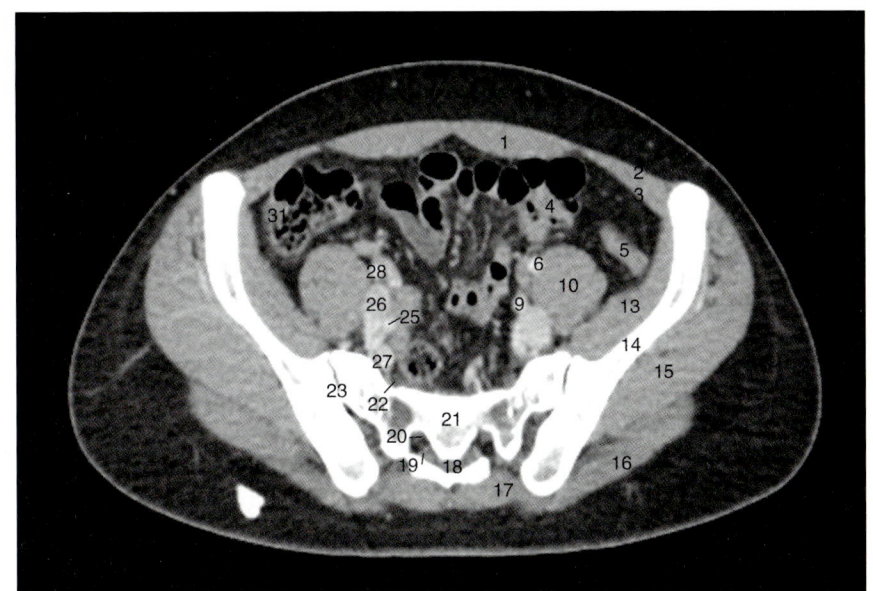
B. CT 增强图像

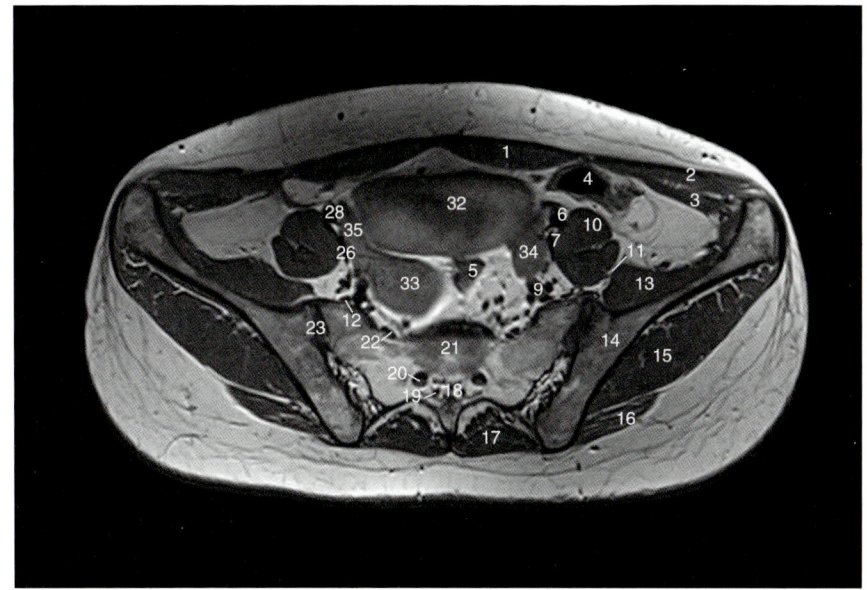
C. MR T1WI

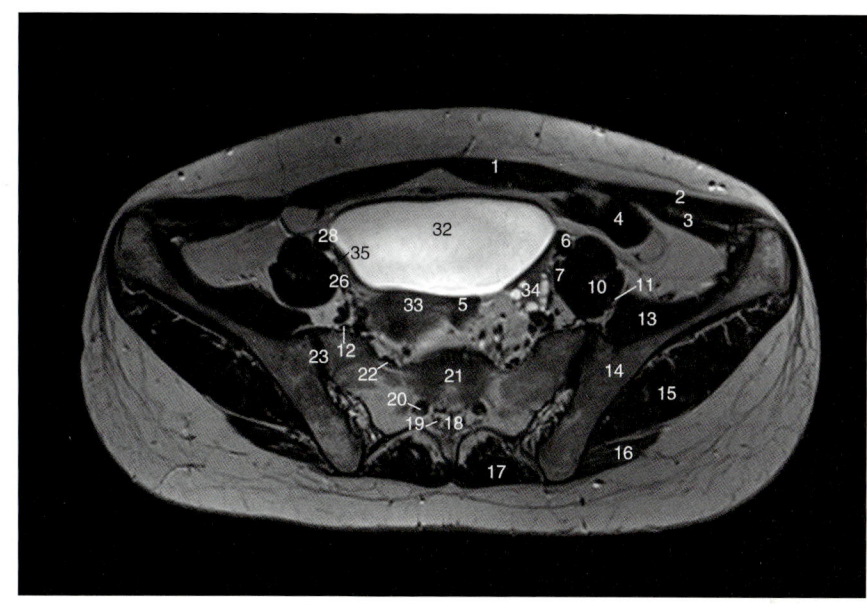
D. MR T2WI

1. 腹直肌 rectus abdominis
2. 腹内斜肌 obliquus internus abdominis
3. 腹横肌 transversus abdominis
4. 空肠 jejunum
5. 乙状结肠 sigmoid colon
6. 左髂外动脉 left external iliac artery
7. 左髂外静脉 left external iliac vein
8. 左髂内静脉 left internal iliac vein
9. 左髂内动脉 left internal iliac artery
10. 腰大肌 psoas major
11. 股神经 femoral nerve
12. 腰骶干 lumbosacral trunk
13. 髂肌 iliacus
14. 髂骨翼 ala of ilium
15. 臀中肌 gluteus medius
16. 臀大肌 gluteus maximus
17. 竖脊肌 erector spinae
18. 骶管 sacral canal
19. 第3骶神经 3rd sacral nerve
20. 第2骶神经 2nd sacral nerve
21. 第2骶椎 2nd sacral vertebra
22. 第1骶神经 1st sacral nerve
23. 骶髂关节 sacroiliac joint
24. 右输尿管 right ureter
25. 右髂内动脉 right internal iliac artery
26. 右髂外静脉 right external iliac vein
27. 右髂内静脉 right internal iliac vein
28. 右髂外动脉 right external iliac artery
29. 右卵巢动、静脉 right ovarian artery and vein
30. 阑尾 vermiform appendix
31. 回肠 ileum
32. 膀胱 urinary bladder
33. 子宫底 fundus of uterus
34. 左卵巢 left ovary
35. 右卵巢 right ovary

关键结构：股神经，腰大肌，髂血管。

此断面经过第2骶椎椎体中份。

椎体后方为骶管，骶管内容纳骶、尾神经根。腰大肌位于骶髂关节前方，其内侧与骶骨翼前方见输尿管、髂血管、腰骶干及第1骶神经。股神经位于腰大肌与髂肌之间，自腰大肌外侧缘发出后，在腰大肌与髂肌之间下行，经肌腔隙于股动脉的外侧进入股三角，并分为肌支、皮支和关节支。股神经肌支分布到股四头肌、缝匠肌和耻骨肌，关节支分布到膝关节，皮支分布到股前内侧区皮肤。皮支中最长的皮神经为隐神经，分布于髌骨下方、小腿内侧和足内侧的皮肤。股神经受损后主要表现为屈髋无力、坐位时不能伸膝、行走困难、膝跳反射消失、大腿前面和小腿内侧面皮肤感觉障碍等。在CT图像上，股神经呈小圆形的软组织密度。在MR轴位图像上，正常的股神经神经束呈排列整齐的圆形结构，在T1WI及T2WI上呈等或略高信号，其轮廓由神经外膜间的脂肪层勾勒。神经束的宽度通常与邻近脂肪组织的宽度相似或略宽。神经束膜层通常不能辨别，除非异常增厚。正常的神经外膜层不太明显，在T1WI和T2WI图像上显示为包绕神经的低信号层，此层增厚≥2 mm通常视为异常，提示先前有神经损伤或炎症。此断面降结肠在髂肌前方转而向内，延续成为乙状结肠，乙状结肠内侧是空肠。右侧髂窝内见回肠，回肠断面之间见类圆形阑尾。

女性盆部与会阴连续横断层 17（FH.9050）

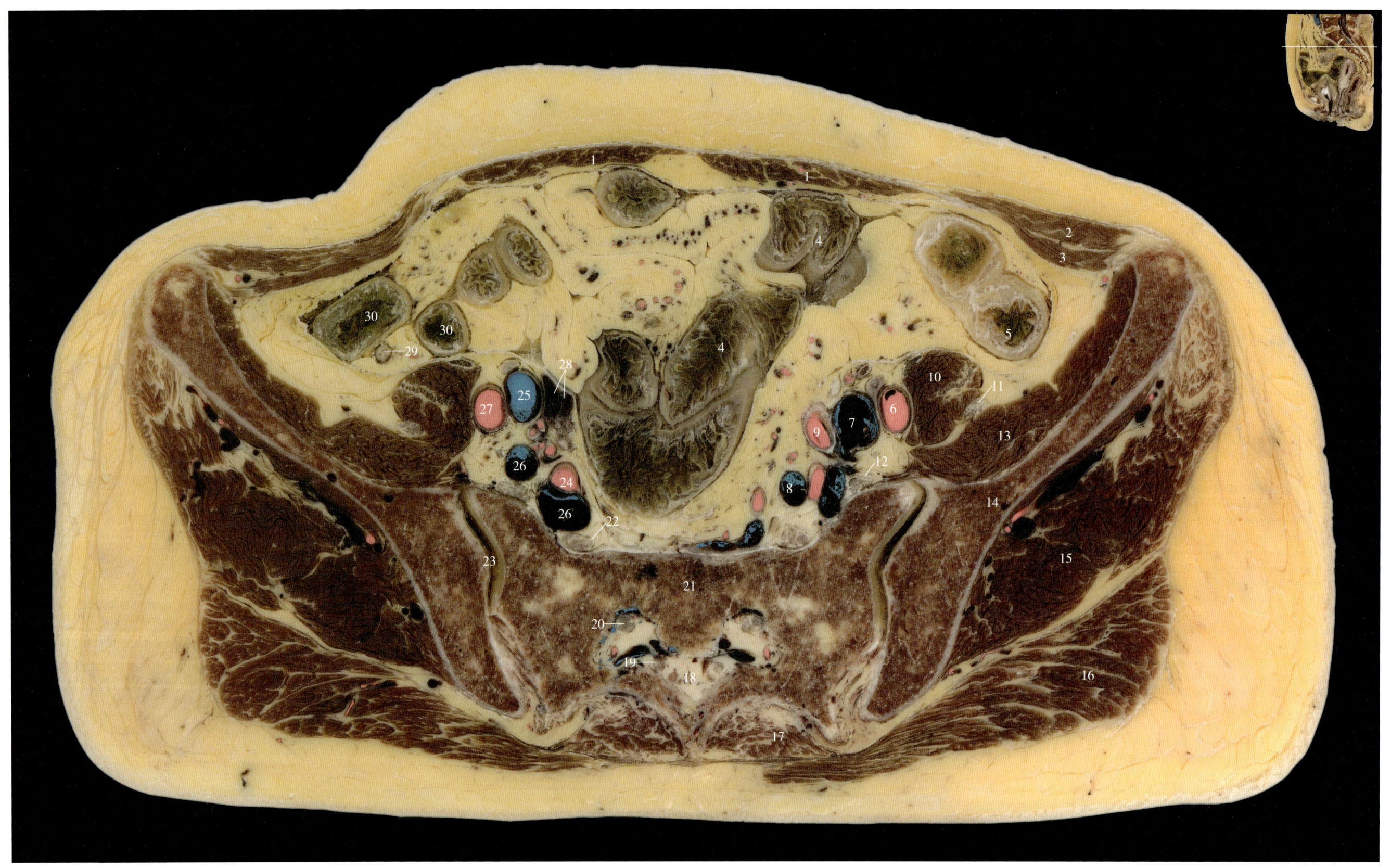

A. 断层标本图像

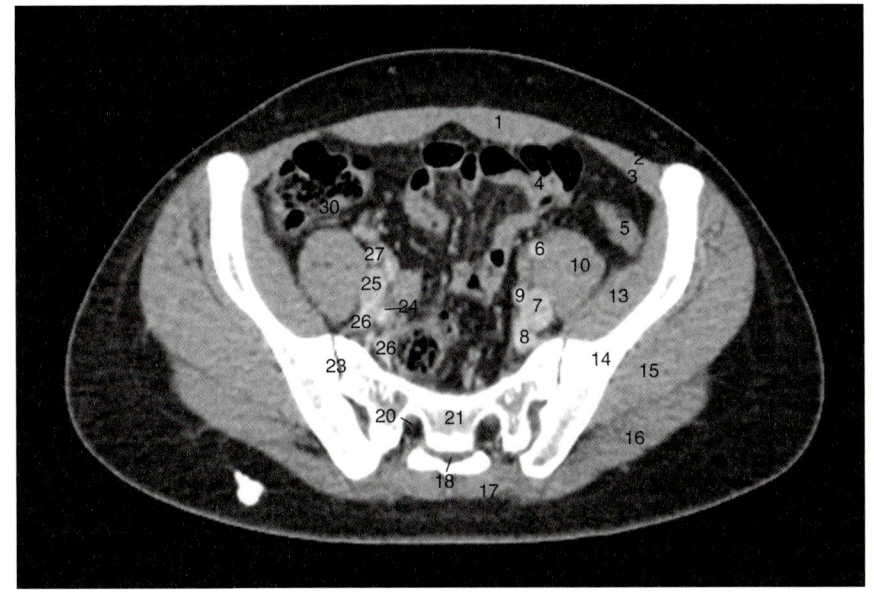

B. CT 增强图像

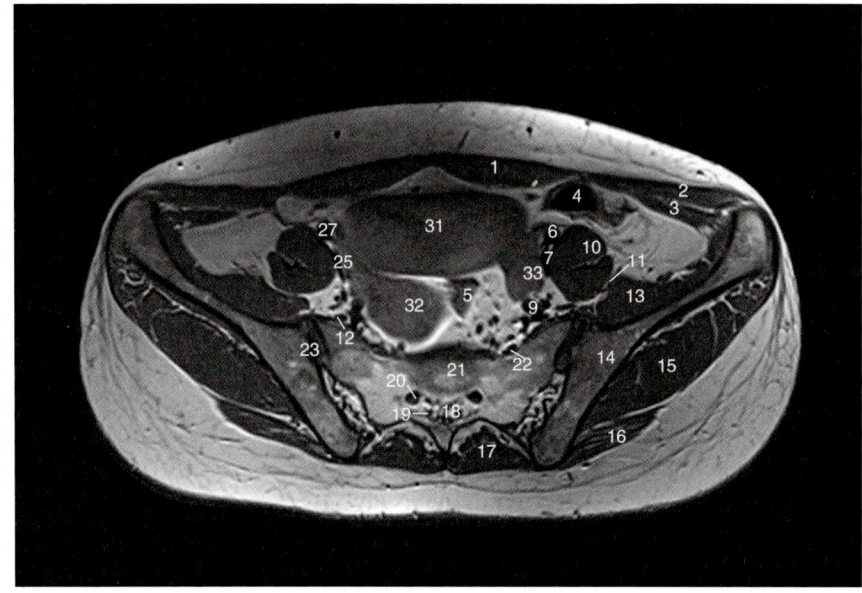

C. MR T1WI

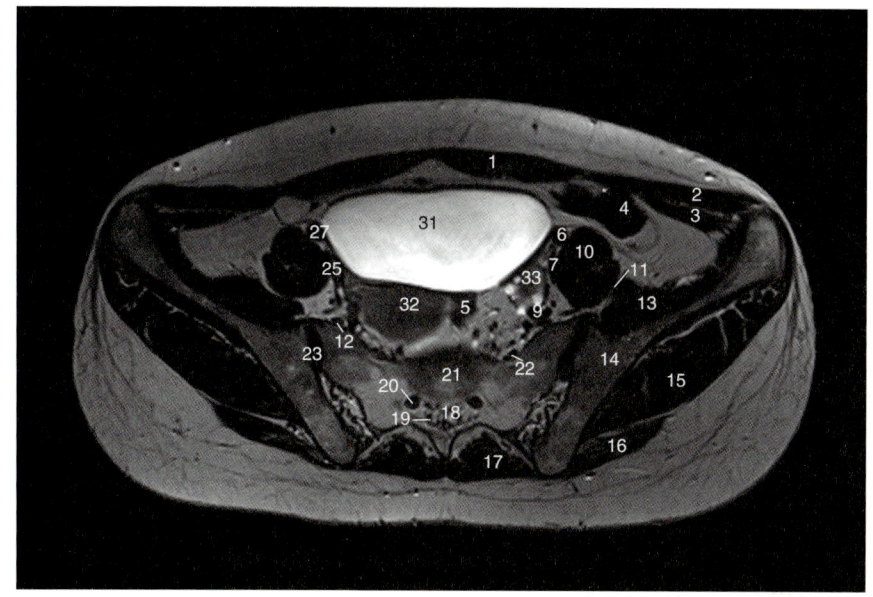

D. MR T2WI

1. 腹直肌 rectus abdominis
2. 腹内斜肌 obliquus internus abdominis
3. 腹横肌 transversus abdominis
4. 空肠 jejunum
5. 乙状结肠 sigmoid colon
6. 左髂外动脉 left external iliac artery
7. 左髂外静脉 left external iliac vein
8. 左髂内静脉 left internal iliac vein
9. 左髂内动脉 left internal iliac artery
10. 腰大肌 psoas major
11. 股神经 femoral nerve
12. 腰骶干 lumbosacral trunk
13. 髂肌 iliacus
14. 髂骨翼 ala of ilium
15. 臀中肌 gluteus medius
16. 臀大肌 gluteus maximus
17. 竖脊肌 erector spinae
18. 骶管 sacral canal
19. 第3骶神经 3rd sacral nerve
20. 第2骶神经 2nd sacral nerve
21. 第2骶椎 2nd sacral vertebra
22. 第1骶神经 1st sacral nerve
23. 骶髂关节 sacroiliac joint
24. 右髂内动脉 right internal iliac artery
25. 右髂外静脉 right external iliac vein
26. 右髂内静脉 right internal iliac vein
27. 右髂外动脉 right external iliac artery
28. 右卵巢动、静脉 right ovarian artery and vein
29. 阑尾 vermiform appendix
30. 回肠 ileum
31. 膀胱 urinary bladder
32. 子宫底 fundus of uterus
33. 左卵巢 left ovary

关键结构：髂内静脉，盆静脉丛，输尿管，股神经。

此断面经过第2骶椎椎体中份。

椎体后方为骶管，骶管内容纳马尾。腰大肌位于骶髂关节前方，腰大肌内侧与骶骨翼前方见输尿管、髂血管、腰骶干及第1骶神经，双侧髂内静脉在此断面分为两个断面，左侧髂内静脉两个断面呈左右方向排列，右侧髂内静脉两个断面呈前后方向排列，髂内静脉长为 3.21 cm ± 0.28 cm，左侧外径为 11.08 cm ± 0.22 mm，右侧外径为 11.99 cm ± 0.23 mm[16]。髂内静脉沿髂内动脉后内侧上行，与髂外静脉汇合成髂总静脉。髂内静脉的属支与同名动脉伴行。盆腔内静脉在器官壁内或表面形成丰富的静脉丛，男性有膀胱静脉丛和直肠静脉丛，女性此外还有子宫静脉丛和阴道静脉丛。这些静脉丛在盆腔器官扩张或受压迫时有助于血液回流，但是如果在外科手术时受损，可能会影响静脉引流而导致单侧或双侧下肢水肿[5]。股神经向外移行，位于腰大肌与髂肌之间。

女性盆部与会阴连续横断层 18（FH.9030）

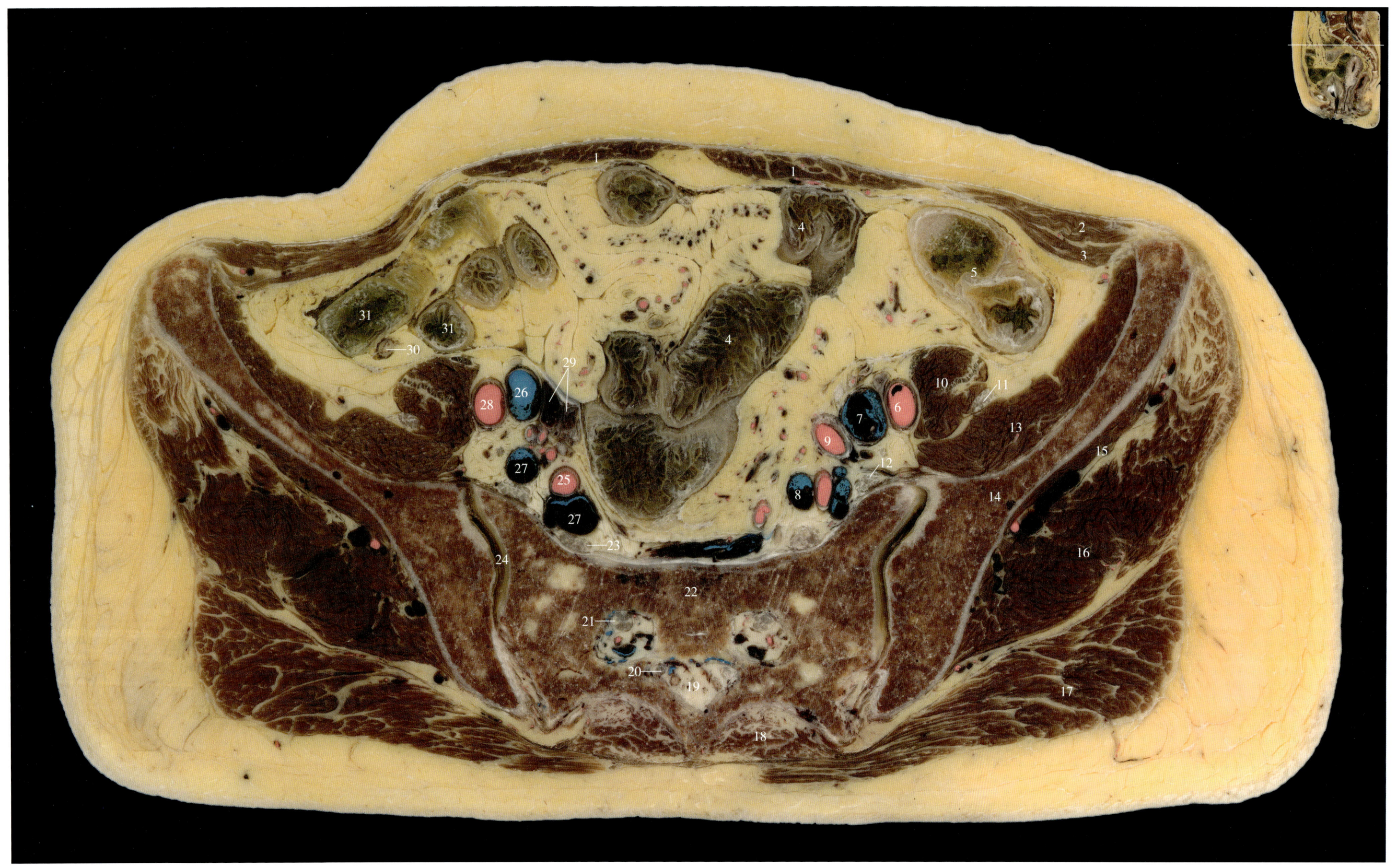

A. 断层标本图像

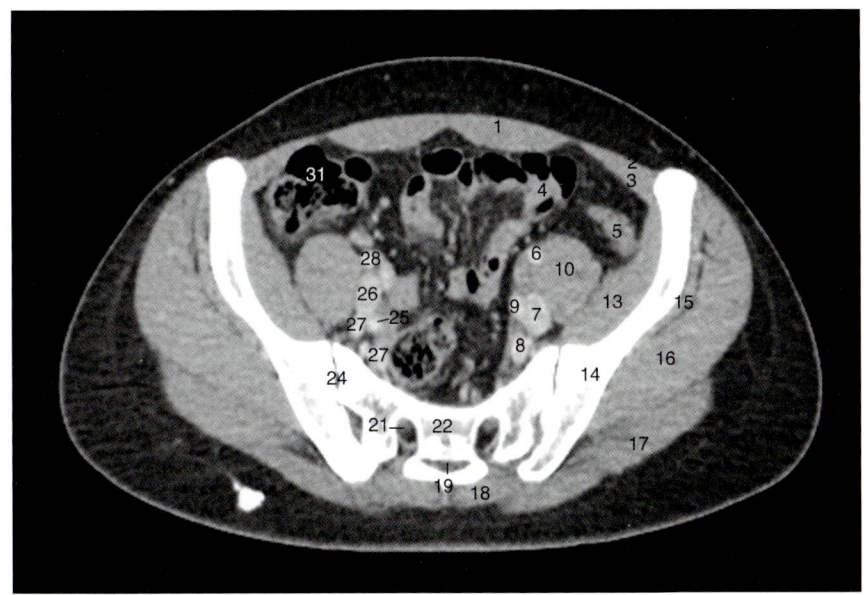
B. CT 增强图像

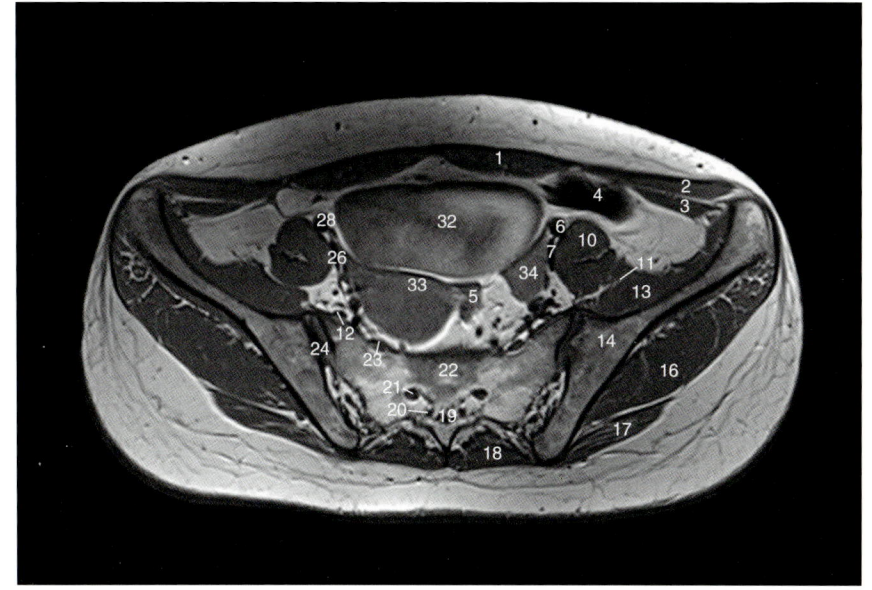
C. MR T1WI

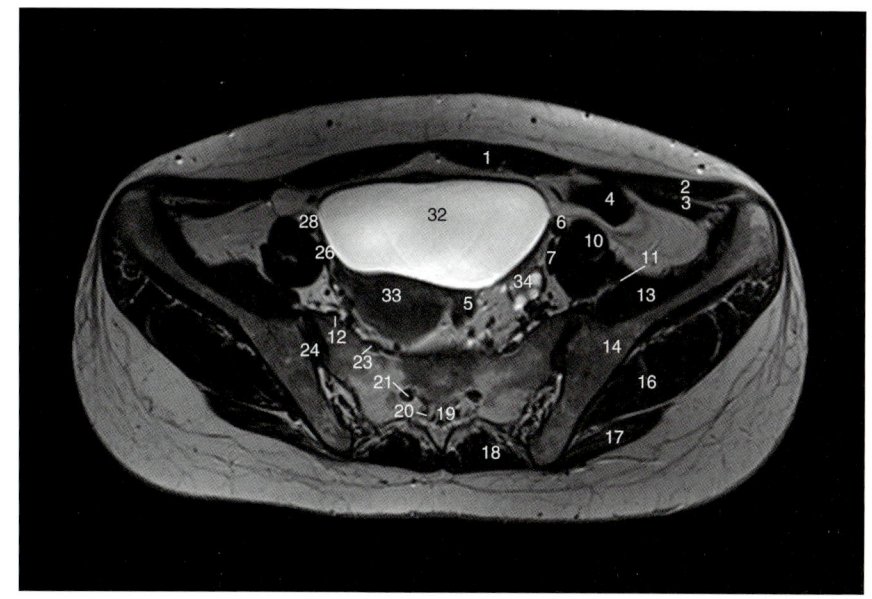
D. MR T2WI

1. 腹直肌 rectus abdominis
2. 腹内斜肌 obliquus internus abdominis
3. 腹横肌 transversus abdominis
4. 空肠 jejunum
5. 乙状结肠 sigmoid colon
6. 左髂外动脉 left external iliac artery
7. 左髂外静脉 left external iliac vein
8. 左髂内静脉 left internal iliac vein
9. 左髂内动脉 left internal iliac artery
10. 腰大肌 psoas major
11. 股神经 femoral nerve
12. 腰骶干 lumbosacral trunk
13. 髂肌 iliacus
14. 髂骨翼 ala of ilium
15. 臀小肌 gluteus minimuss
16. 臀中肌 gluteus medius
17. 臀大肌 gluteus maximus
18. 竖脊肌 erector spinae
19. 骶管 sacral canal
20. 第 3 骶神经 3rd sacral nerve
21. 第 2 骶神经 2nd sacral nerve
22. 第 2 骶椎 2nd sacral vertebra
23. 第 1 骶神经 1st sacral nerve
24. 骶髂关节 sacroiliac joint
25. 右髂内动脉 right internal iliac artery
26. 右髂外静脉 right external iliac vein
27. 右髂内静脉 right internal iliac vein
28. 右髂外动脉 right external iliac artery
29. 右卵巢动、静脉 right ovarian artery and vein
30. 阑尾 vermiform appendix
31. 回肠 ileum
32. 膀胱 urinary bladder
33. 子宫底 fundus of uterus
34. 左卵巢 left ovary

关键结构：骶髂关节，股神经，髂血管。

此断面经过第 2 骶椎椎体下份。

椎体后方为骶管，骶管内容纳马尾。骶翼与髂骨翼之间为骶髂关节，由骶骨耳状关节面和髂骨耳状关节面构成，位于第 1~2 骶椎平面，男性可至第 3 骶椎平面。骶髂关节形态男女差别较大，男性以直线型为主，女性以"S"形为主，正常关节间隙宽为 2.28 cm ± 0.81 mm，髂骨侧皮质厚度为 1.42 cm ± 0.49 mm，骶骨侧皮质厚度为 1.34 cm ± 0.37 mm。约 14% 的人在髂后上棘内面与第 2 骶后孔外侧未退化的横结节之间可出现副骶髂关节，部分为出生时就存在，系可以活动的关节，但更多为负重所致的获得性纤维软骨关节。腰大肌位于骶髂关节前方，腰大肌与髂肌位置相对前移并相互靠近，构成小骨盆的盆缘。腰大肌内侧与骶骨翼前方见输尿管、髂血管、腰骶干及第 1 骶神经，股神经向外移行，位于腰大肌与髂肌之间。此断面臀小肌开始出现，髂骨翼后方从前向后依次为臀小肌、臀中肌、臀大肌，其余肌肉骨骼分布较上一断面无明显变化。

女性盆部与会阴连续横断层 19（FH.9010）

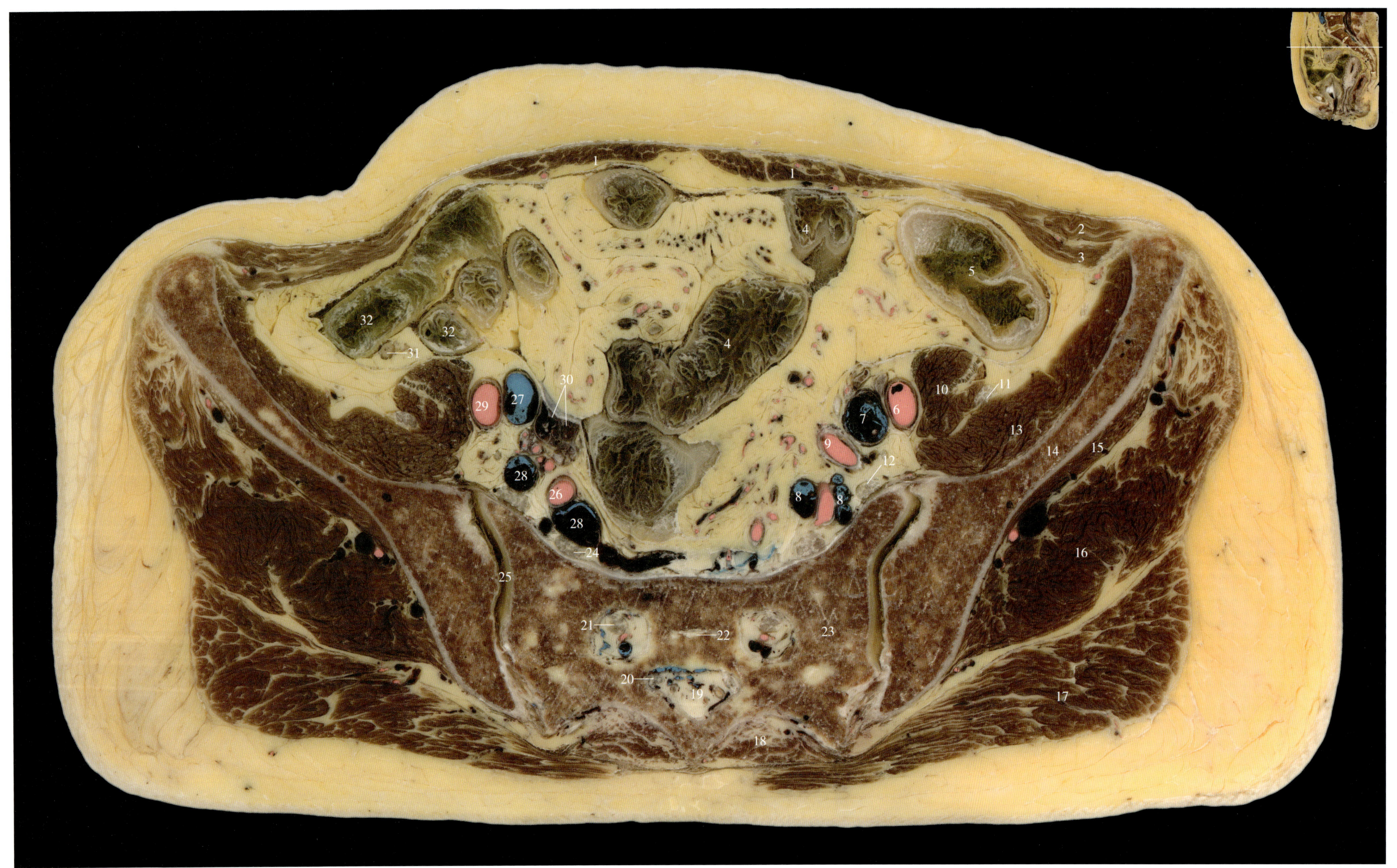

A. 断层标本图像

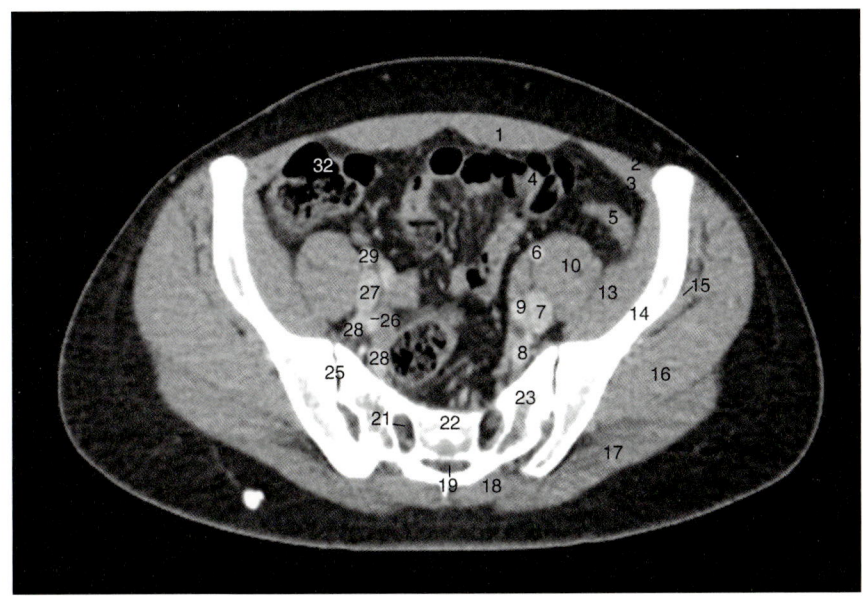
B. CT 增强图像

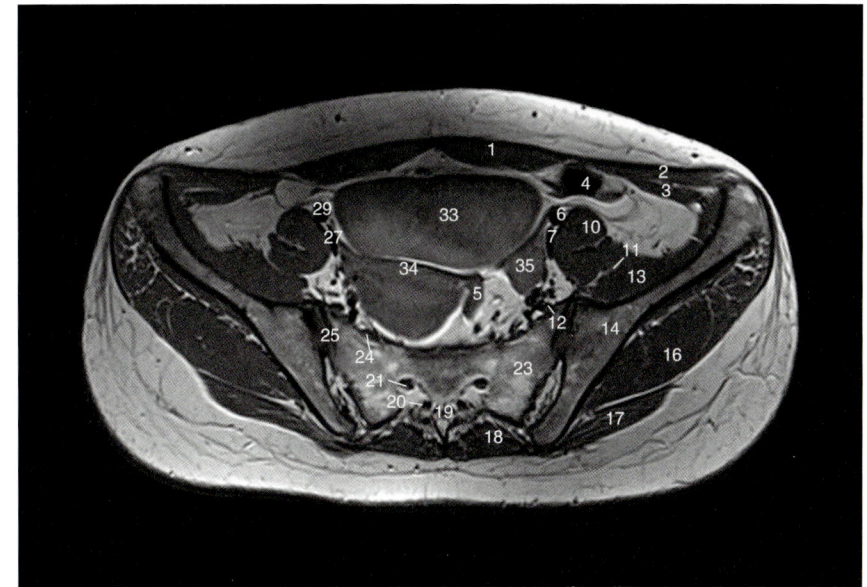
C. MR T1WI

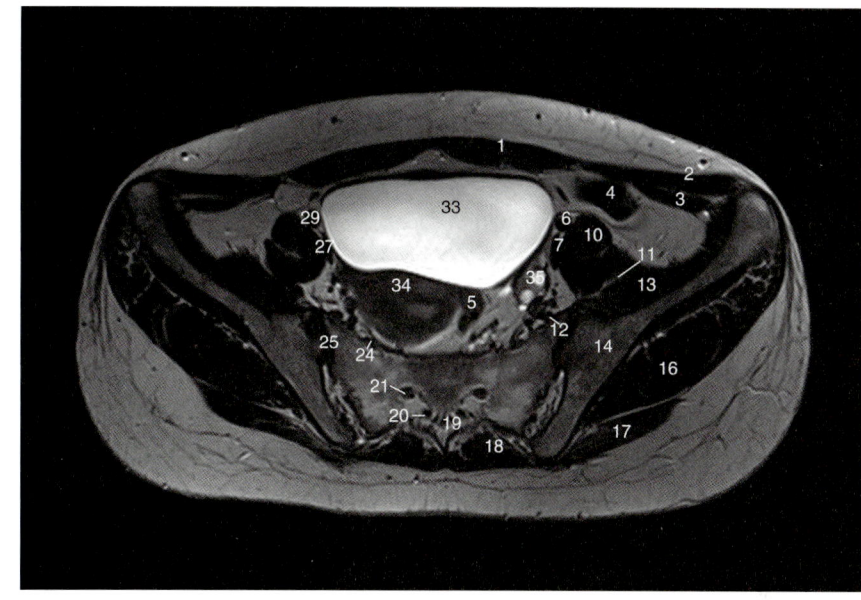
D. MR T2WI

1. 腹直肌 rectus abdominis
2. 腹内斜肌 obliquus internus abdominis
3. 腹横肌 transversus abdominis
4. 空肠 jejunum
5. 乙状结肠 sigmoid colon
6. 左髂外动脉 left external iliac artery
7. 左髂外静脉 left external iliac vein
8. 左髂内静脉 left internal iliac vein
9. 左髂内动脉 left internal iliac artery
10. 腰大肌 psoas major
11. 股神经 femoral nerve
12. 腰骶干 lumbosacral trunk
13. 髂肌 iliacus
14. 髂骨翼 ala of ilium
15. 臀小肌 gluteus minimuss
16. 臀中肌 gluteus medius
17. 臀大肌 gluteus maximus
18. 竖脊肌 erector spinae
19. 骶管 sacral canal
20. 第3骶神经 3rd sacral nerve
21. 第2骶神经 2nd sacral nerve
22. S2-3 椎间盘 S2-3 intervertebral disc
23. 第2骶椎 2nd sacral vertebra
24. 第1骶神经 lst sacral nerve
25. 骶髂关节 sacroiliac joint
26. 右髂内动脉 right internal iliac artery
27. 右髂外静脉 right external iliac vein
28. 右髂内静脉 right internal iliac vein
29. 右髂外动脉 right external iliac artery
30. 右卵巢动、静脉 right ovarian artery and vein
31. 阑尾 vermiform appendix
32. 回肠 ileum
33. 膀胱 urinary bladder
34. 子宫体 body of uterus
35. 左卵巢 left ovary

关键结构：髂骨，输尿管，髂血管。

此断面经过第2骶椎椎体下份。

椎体后方为骶管，骶管内容纳马尾。腰大肌位于骶髂关节前方，腰大肌与髂肌位置继续相对前移并相互靠近。两侧的输尿管、髂血管、腰骶干及第1骶神经呈"U"形排列于腰大肌内侧和第2骶椎前方。盆侧壁髂骨翼的前端为髂前上棘，突至皮下，为髂嵴末端向上的突起，髂嵴的后端为髂后上棘。髂前上棘在腹股沟褶皱外侧端可以触诊到，腹股沟韧带外侧端附着在髂前上棘上。髂后上棘不能触到，但通常位于骶骨第2棘突外侧4cm。两侧髂嵴最高点的连线平对第4腰椎棘突。男性第5腰椎多位于髂嵴最高点水平线以下，而女性整个第5腰椎或其上半部位于髂嵴最高点水平线以上。两侧髂后上棘的连线平对第2骶椎棘突及硬膜囊和终池的下端[1]。髂骨翼后方从前向后依次为臀小肌、臀中肌、臀大肌。

女性盆部与会阴连续横断层 20（FH.8990）

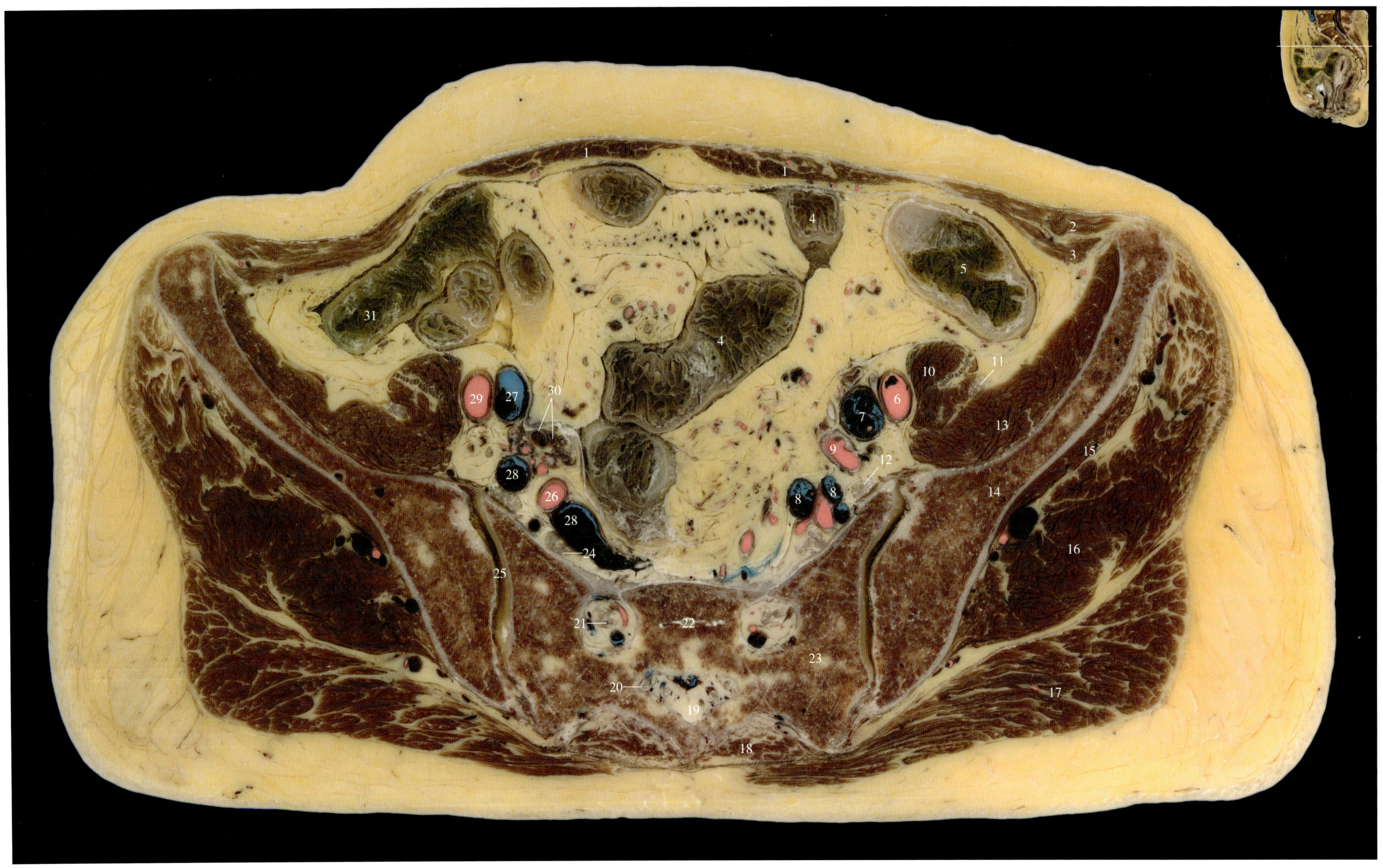

A. 断层标本图像

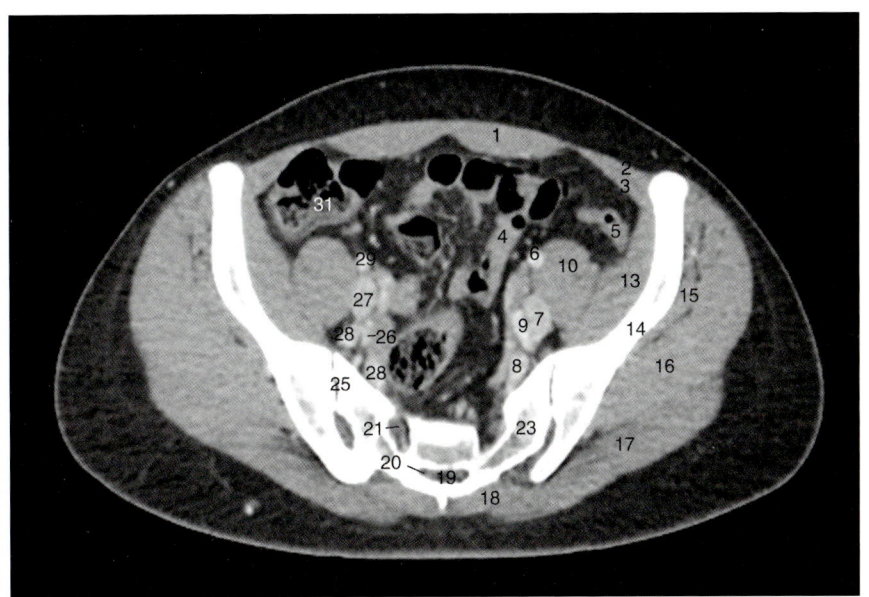

B. CT 增强图像

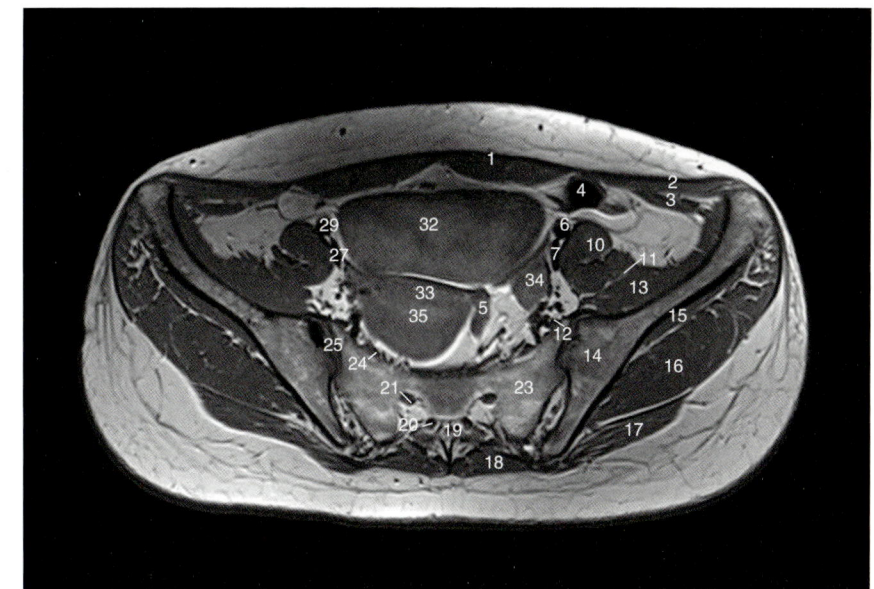

C. MR T1WI

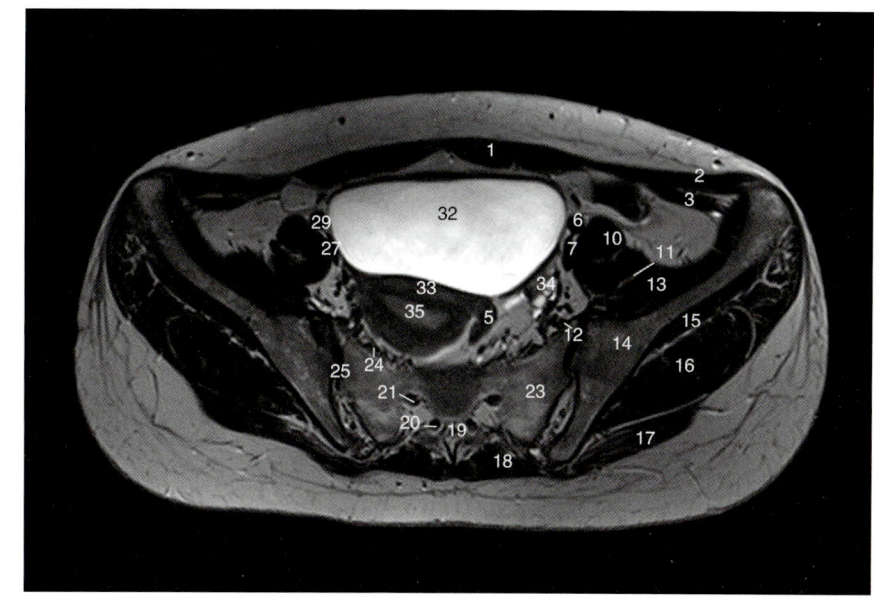

D. MR T2WI

关键结构：臀中肌，臀小肌，髂骨，髂血管。

此断面经过第 2 骶椎椎体下份。

腰大肌与髂肌位置相对前移并相互融合。两侧的输尿管、髂血管、腰骶干及第 1 骶神经呈 "U" 形排列于腰大肌内侧和第 2 骶椎椎体前方，双侧髂外动、静脉位置随着腰大肌前移，腰骶干及第 1 骶神经向外侧移行。股神经继续向前外侧移行，位于腰大肌与髂肌之间。两侧髂骨翼为盆后外侧壁，其内、外侧面分别为髂肌与臀中肌所附着，髂骨翼后方从前向后依次为臀小肌、臀中肌、臀大肌，臀中肌前上部位于皮下、后下部位于臀大肌的深面，臀小肌位于臀中肌的深面。臀中肌和臀小肌都呈扇形，皆起自髂骨翼外面，肌束向下集中形成短腱，止于股骨大转子。二肌的作用是使髋关节外展，前部肌束可使髋关节旋内，后部肌束使髋关节旋外。此二肌受臀上神经支配。在 CT 及 MR 图像上，由于肌肉与肌肉之间通常会有少量脂肪的相隔，T1WI 及 T2WI 上高信号的脂肪与低信号肌肉形成自然对比，CT 显示的低密度脂肪与软组织密度肌肉形成对比，可以辨别不同的肌肉轮廓。

1. 腹直肌 rectus abdominis
2. 腹内斜肌 obliquus internus abdominis
3. 腹横肌 transversus abdominis
4. 空肠 jejunum
5. 乙状结肠 sigmoid colon
6. 左髂外动脉 left external iliac artery
7. 左髂外静脉 left external iliac vein
8. 左髂内静脉 left internal iliac vein
9. 左髂内动脉 left internal iliac artery
10. 腰大肌 psoas major
11. 股神经 femoral nerve
12. 腰骶干 lumbosacral trunk
13. 髂肌 iliacus
14. 髂骨翼 ala of ilium
15. 臀小肌 gluteus minimuss
16. 臀中肌 gluteus medius
17. 臀大肌 gluteus maximus
18. 竖脊肌 erector spinae
19. 骶管 sacral canal
20. 第 3 骶神经 3rd sacral nerve
21. 第 2 骶神经 2nd sacral nerve
22. S2-3 椎间盘 S2-3 intervertebral disc
23. 第 3 骶椎 3rd sacral vertebra
24. 第 1 骶神经 lst sacral nerve
25. 骶髂关节 sacroiliac joint
26. 右髂内动脉 right internal iliac artery
27. 右髂外静脉 right external iliac vein
28. 右髂内静脉 right internal iliac vein
29. 右髂外动脉 right external iliac artery
30. 右卵巢动、静脉 right ovarian artery and vein
31. 回肠 ileum
32. 膀胱 urinary bladder
33. 子宫体 body of uterus
34. 左卵巢 left ovary
35. 子宫内膜 endometrium

女性盆部与会阴连续横断层 21（FH.8970）

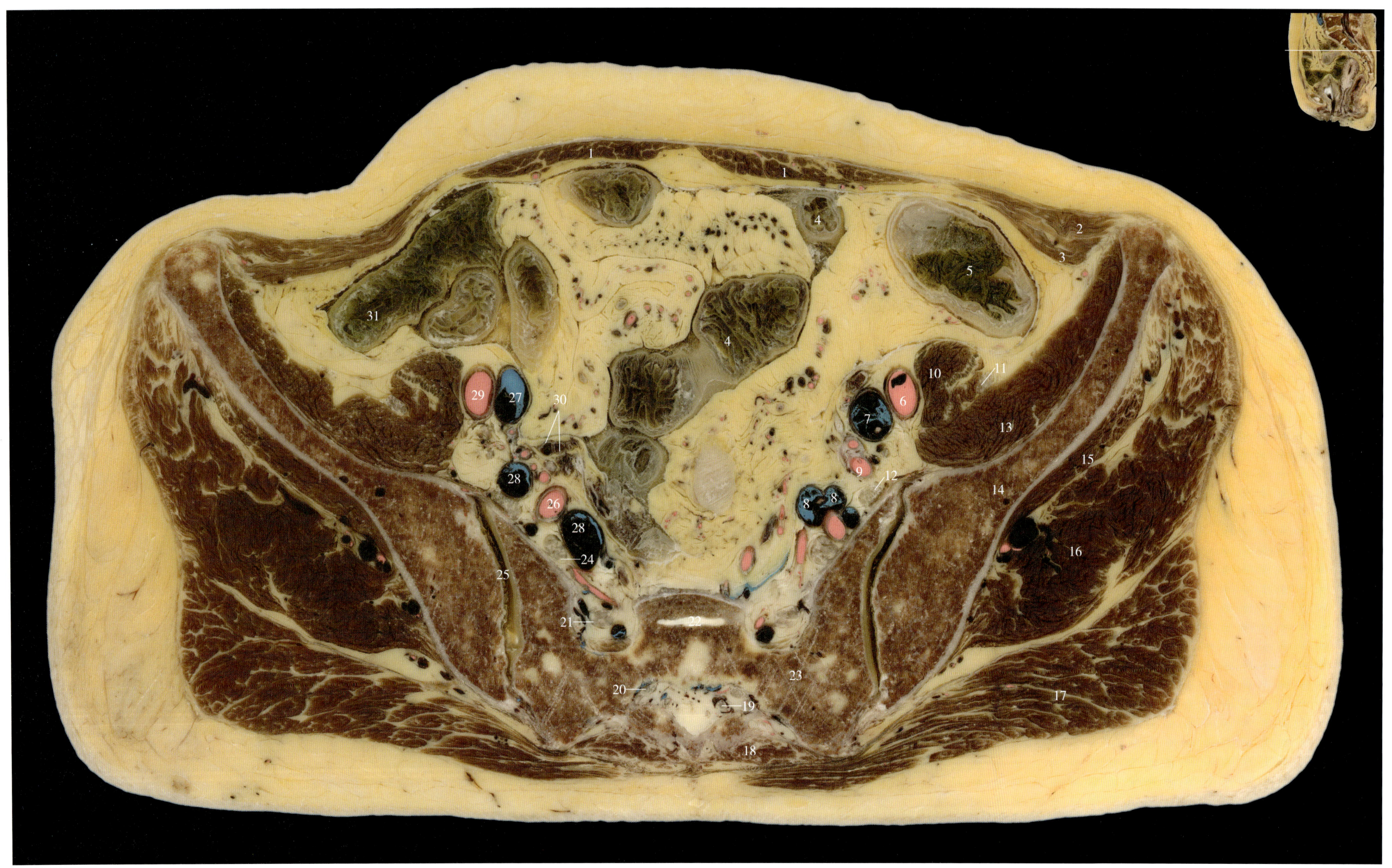

A. 断层标本图像

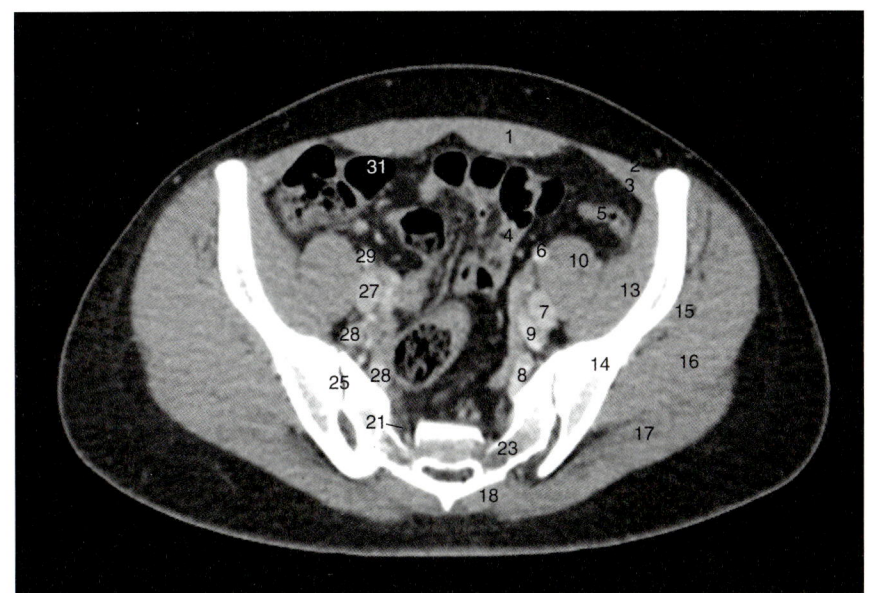
B. CT 增强图像

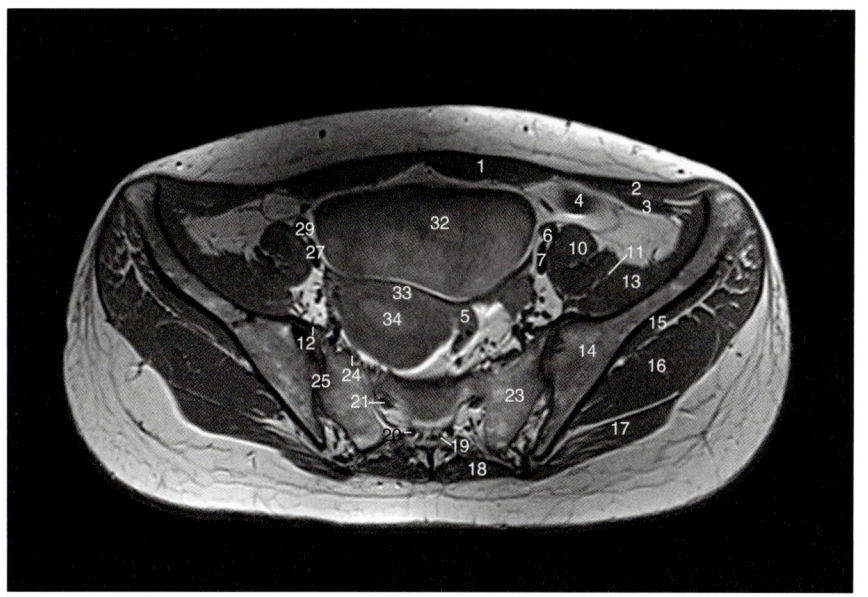
C. MR T1WI

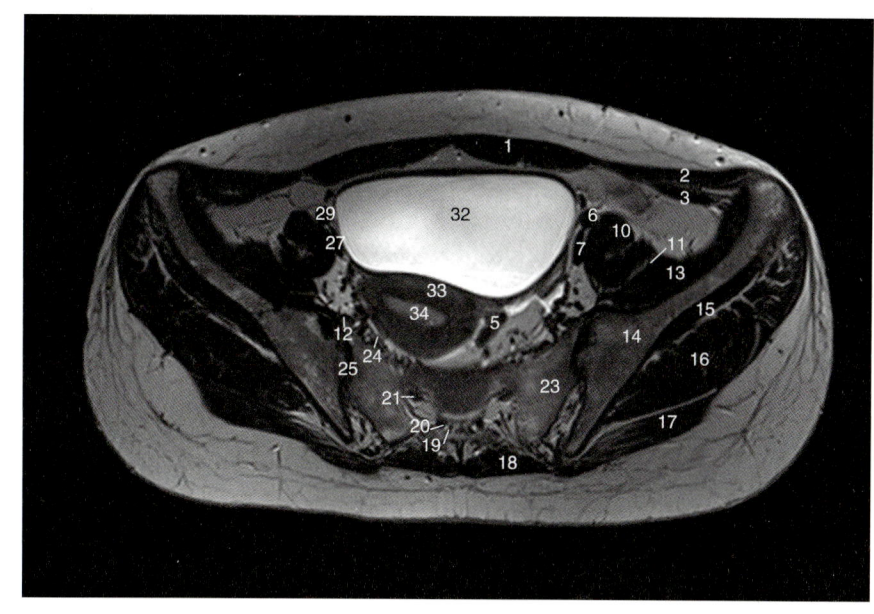
D. MR T2WI

1. 腹直肌 rectus abdominis
2. 腹内斜肌 obliquus internus abdominis
3. 腹横肌 transversus abdominis
4. 空肠 jejunum
5. 乙状结肠 sigmoid colon
6. 左髂外动脉 left external iliac artery
7. 左髂外静脉 left external iliac vein
8. 左髂内静脉 left internal iliac vein
9. 左髂内动脉 left internal iliac artery
10. 腰大肌 psoas major
11. 股神经 femoral nerve
12. 腰骶干 lumbosacral trunk
13. 髂肌 iliacus
14. 髂骨翼 ala of ilium
15. 臀小肌 gluteus minimuss
16. 臀中肌 gluteus medius
17. 臀大肌 gluteus maximus
18. 竖脊肌 erector spinae
19. 第 4 骶神经 4th sacral nerve
20. 第 3 骶神经 3rd sacral nerve
21. 第 2 骶神经 2nd sacral nerve
22. S2-3 椎间盘 S2-3 intervertebral disc
23. 第 3 骶椎 3rd sacral vertebra
24. 第 1 骶神经 1st sacral nerve
25. 骶髂关节 sacroiliac joint
26. 右髂内动脉 right internal iliac artery
27. 右髂外静脉 right external iliac vein
28. 右髂内静脉 right internal iliac vein
29. 右髂外动脉 right external iliac artery
30. 右卵巢动、静脉 right ovarian artery and vein
31. 回肠 ileum
32. 膀胱 urinary bladder
33. 子宫体 body of uterus
34. 子宫内膜 endometrium

关键结构：髂动脉，股神经，肠管。

此断面经过 S2-3 椎间盘（临床上常写作 S2/3 椎间盘），椎间盘后方为骶管。

髂窝由外侧向内侧为髂肌及腰大肌，两肌已大部分融合，两肌之间其交界处的稍前方见股神经。髂外动、静脉位于髂腰肌内侧，髂内动、静脉位于骶椎前方，右侧的髂内动脉位于髂内静脉两个断面之间，左侧髂内动脉位于髂内、外静脉之间。髂内动脉起源于髂总动脉分叉，沿骨盆壁在腹膜后脂肪组织中下行，57%~77% 的人至坐骨大孔上缘分为前干和后干，前干的分支供应膀胱、子宫、直肠、阴道，并通过闭孔动脉供应骨盆和骨盆内、外的肌肉，后干的分支供应骨、肌肉和神经，包括形成坐骨神经的腰、骶神经的近段[17]。髂内动脉阙如的情况极少见。肠管集中于断面的前半部。CT 图像显示乙状结肠在此断面被切成两个断面，一个位于左髂窝内，一个位于骶骨前方，右髂窝处有回肠，中间为空肠。

女性盆部与会阴连续横断层 22（FH.8950）

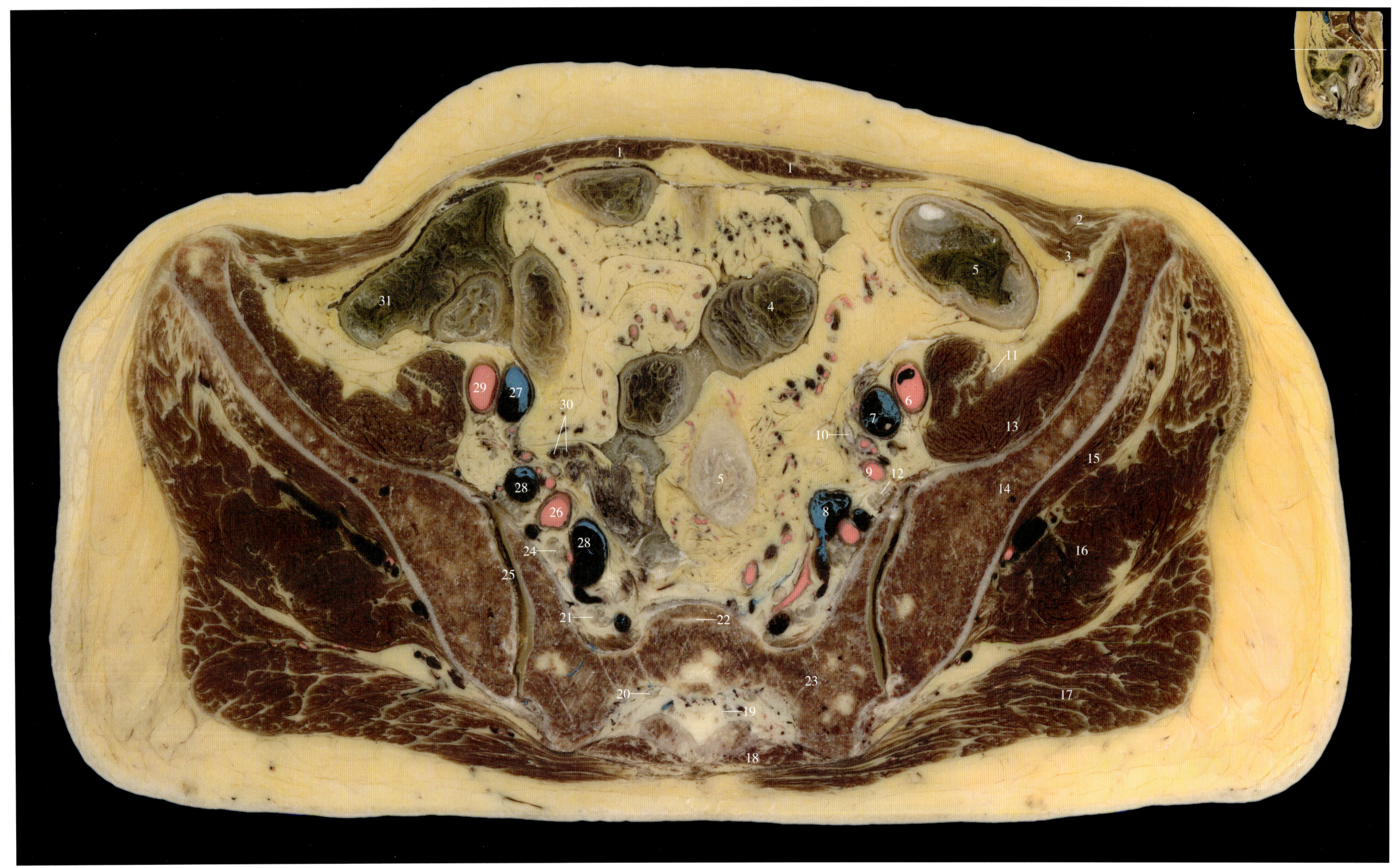

A. 断层标本图像

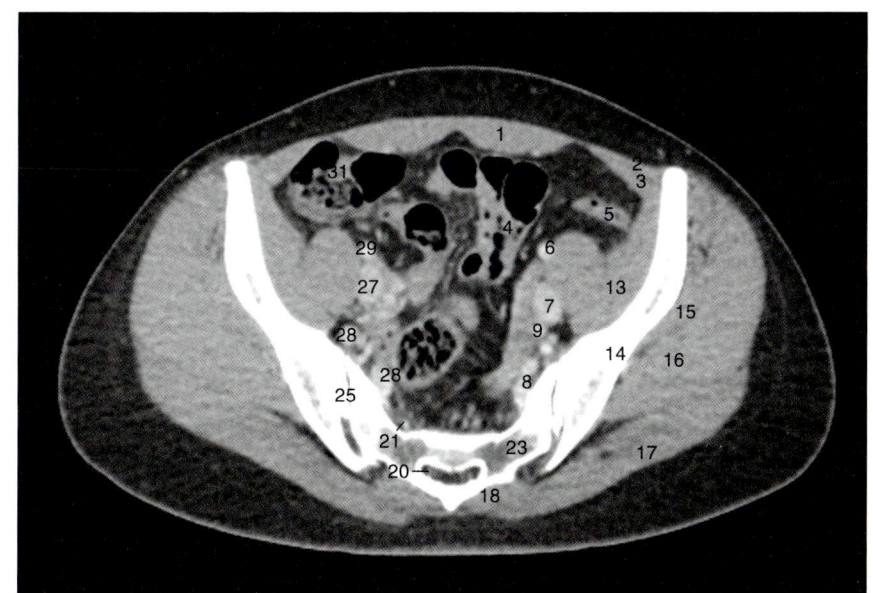
B. CT 增强图像

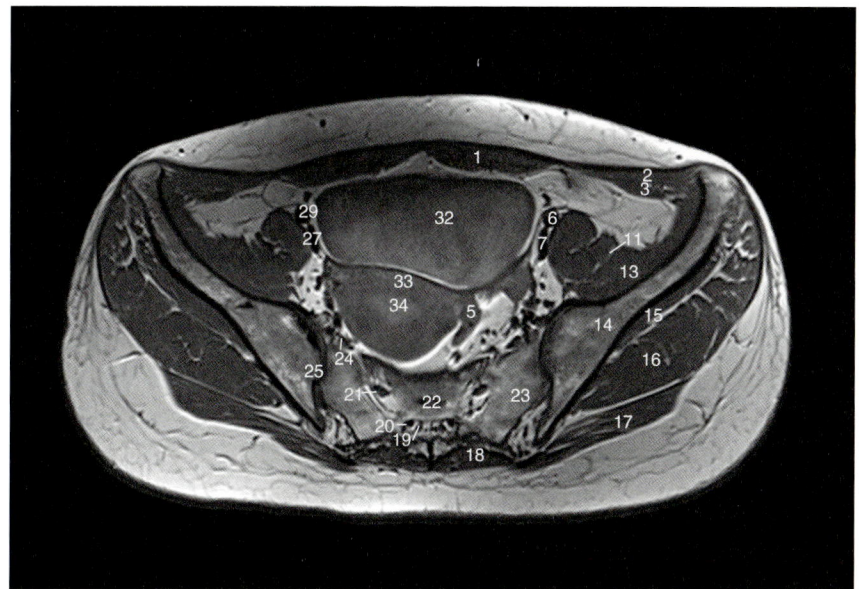
C. MR T1WI

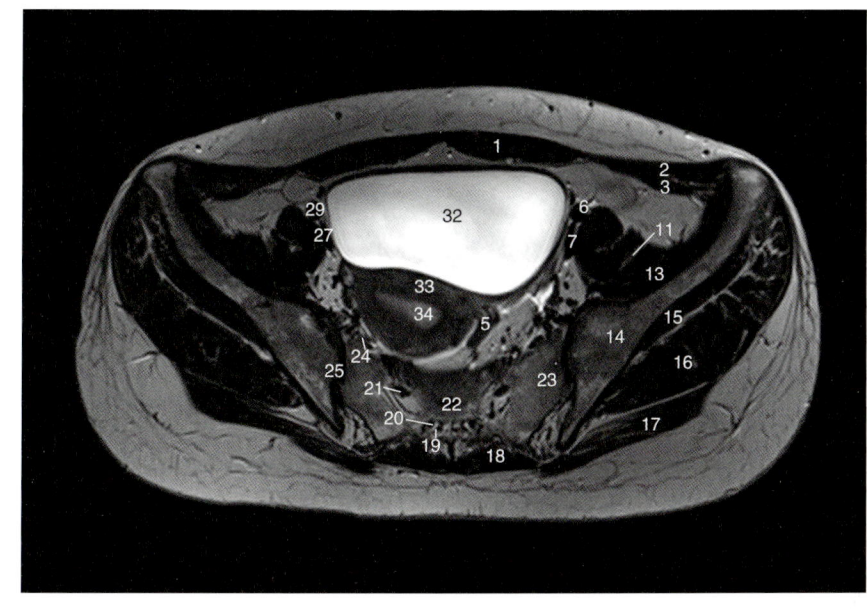
D. MR T2WI

关键结构：肠管，髂腰肌，骶骨。

此断面经过 S2-3 椎间盘。

髂窝内腰大肌与髂肌完全融合形成髂腰肌，股神经沿髂腰肌向下延伸。髂腰肌内侧和骶椎前方见髂血管，神经及输尿管沿盆壁肌内侧下行。标本图像显示肠管集中于断面的前中部，右髂窝处有回肠，中间为空肠，左髂窝内见乙状结肠，骶骨前方断面较上一断面增大，乙状结肠周围有乙状结肠系膜。乙状结肠系膜是将乙状结肠固定于左下腹的双层腹膜结构，其根部附于左髂窝和骨盆左后壁，呈倒"V"形，其尖部近于左髂总动脉分叉处，左侧沿腰大肌内侧下行，右侧进入骨盆，于中线处止于第 3 骶椎平面，系膜根尖后方常可见左输尿管进入盆腔；该系膜较长，故乙状结肠活动度较大，易发生肠扭转。系膜内含有乙状结肠血管、直肠上血管、淋巴管、淋巴结和神经丛等。在 CT 图像上，乙状结肠系膜脂肪组织呈低密度，当炎症及恶性肿瘤累及时，可表现为系膜密度增高及结节；另外，系膜内可出现淋巴结转移[18]。

1. 腹直肌 rectus abdominis
2. 腹内斜肌 obliquus internus abdominis
3. 腹横肌 transversus abdominis
4. 空肠 jejunum
5. 乙状结肠 sigmoid colon
6. 左髂外动脉 left external iliac artery
7. 左髂外静脉 left external iliac vein
8. 左髂内静脉 left internal iliac vein
9. 左髂内动脉 left internal iliac artery
10. 左输尿管 left ureter
11. 股神经 femoral nerve
12. 腰骶干 lumbosacral trunk
13. 髂腰肌 iliopsoas
14. 髂骨翼 ala of ilium
15. 臀小肌 gluteus minimuss
16. 臀中肌 gluteus medius
17. 臀大肌 gluteus maximus
18. 竖脊肌 erector spinae
19. 第 4 骶神经 4th sacral nerve
20. 第 3 骶神经 3rd sacral nerve
21. 第 2 骶神经 2nd sacral nerve
22. S2-3 椎间盘 S2-3 intervertebral disc
23. 第 3 骶椎 3rd sacral vertebra
24. 第 1 骶神经 lst sacral nerve
25. 骶髂关节 sacroiliac joint
26. 右髂内动脉 right internal iliac artery
27. 右髂外静脉 right external iliac vein
28. 右髂内静脉 right internal iliac vein
29. 右髂外动脉 right external iliac artery
30. 右卵巢动、静脉 right ovarian artery and vein
31. 回肠 ileum
32. 膀胱 urinary bladder
33. 子宫体 body of uterus
34. 子宫内膜 endometrium

女性盆部与会阴连续横断层 23（FH.8930）

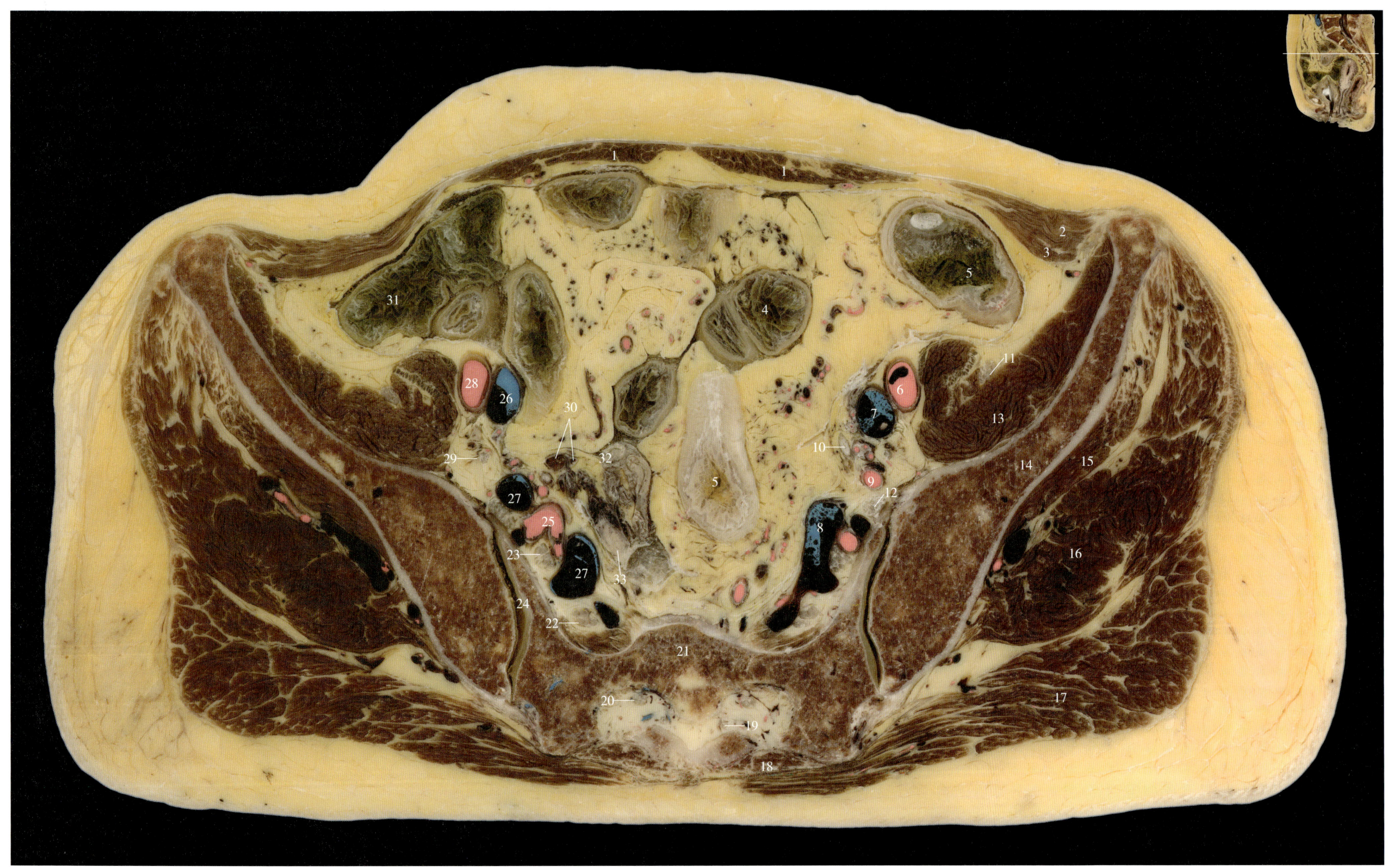

A. 断层标本图像

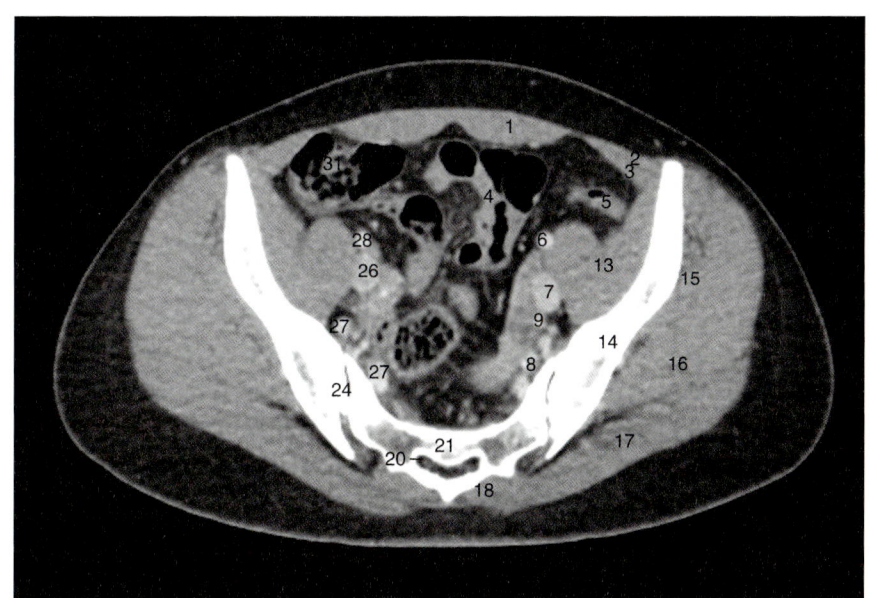

B. CT 增强图像

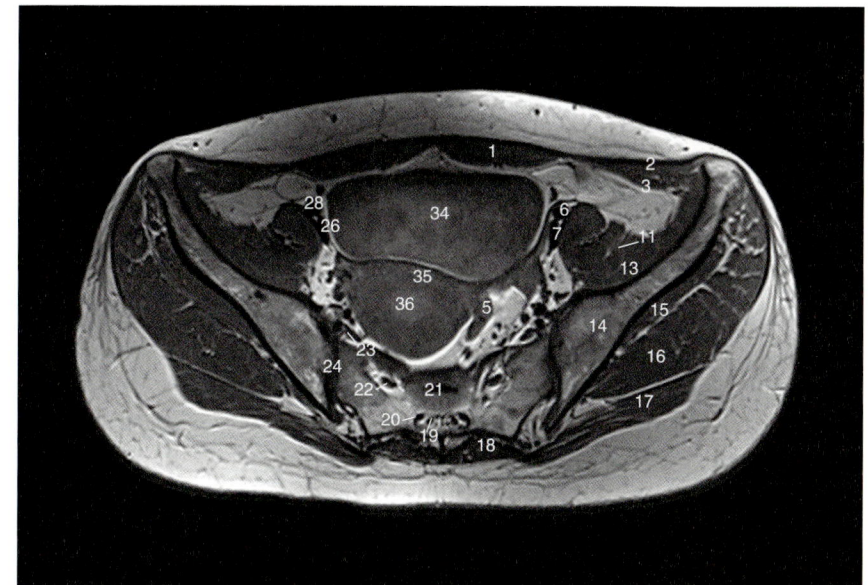

C. MR T1WI

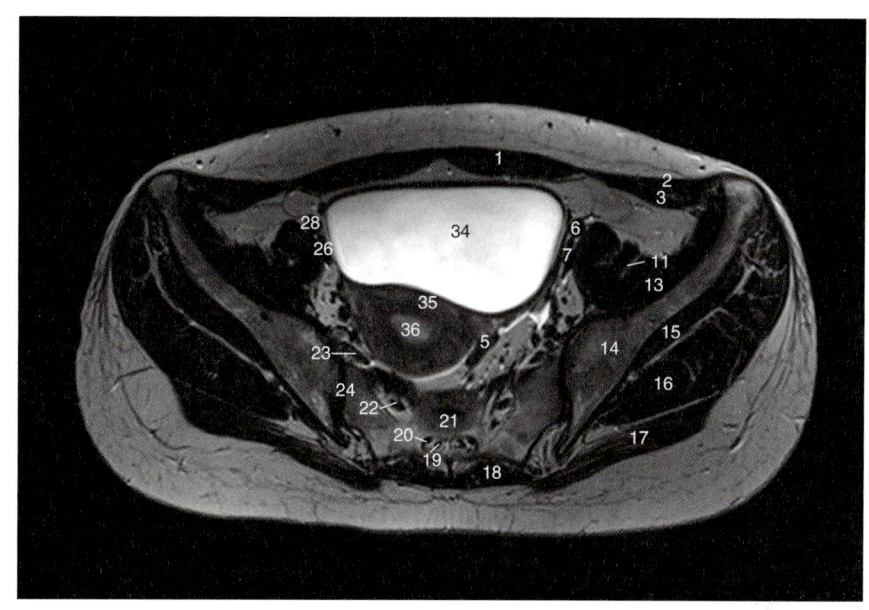

D. MR T2WI

关键结构：髂腰肌，股神经，卵巢。

此断面经过第3骶椎体上份。

髂窝内见髂腰肌，髂腰肌由腰大肌和髂肌组成。腰大肌位于脊柱腰部两侧，起自腰椎体侧面和横突；髂肌位于腰大肌外侧，呈扇形，起自髂窝。两肌向下汇合，经腹股沟韧带深面，止于股骨小转子。髂腰肌收缩时，使髋关节前屈和旋外；下肢固定时，可使躯干前屈。此肌肉受腰神经丛支配。脊柱来源的脓肿（如结核脓肿）可沿腰大肌向下流至股部形成肿块[19]。髂筋膜内血肿或感染可形成小包块或使髋关节屈曲畸形。在仰卧位屈髋屈膝时，可通过对抗阻力屈髋关节进行临床检测。股神经沿髂腰肌向下延伸。髂腰肌内侧和骶椎前方见髂血管、神经及输尿管沿盆壁肌内缘下行。此标本断面右侧输卵管及右侧卵巢开始出现，位于髂内动、静脉及空肠之间。左髂窝内见乙状结肠，右髂窝处有回肠，中间为空肠。

1. 腹直肌 rectus abdominis
2. 腹内斜肌 obliquus internus abdominis
3. 腹横肌 transversus abdominis
4. 空肠 jejunum
5. 乙状结肠 sigmoid colon
6. 左髂外动脉 left external iliac artery
7. 左髂外静脉 left external iliac vein
8. 左髂内静脉 left internal iliac vein
9. 左髂内动脉 left internal iliac artery
10. 左输尿管 left ureter
11. 股神经 femoral nerve
12. 腰骶干 lumbosacral trunk
13. 髂腰肌 iliopsoas
14. 髂骨翼 ala of ilium
15. 臀小肌 gluteus minimuss
16. 臀中肌 gluteus medius
17. 臀大肌 gluteus maximus
18. 竖脊肌 erector spinae
19. 第4骶神经 4th sacral nerve
20. 第3骶神经 3rd sacral nerve
21. 第3骶椎 3rd sacral vertebra
22. 第2骶神经 2nd sacral nerve
23. 第1骶神经 1st sacral nerve
24. 骶髂关节 sacroiliac joint
25. 右髂内动脉 right internal iliac artery
26. 右髂外静脉 right external iliac vein
27. 右髂内静脉 right internal iliac vein
28. 右髂外动脉 right external iliac artery
29. 闭孔神经 obturator nerve
30. 右卵巢动、静脉 right ovarian artery and vein
31. 回肠 ileum
32. 右输卵管 right uterine tube
33. 右卵巢 right ovary
34. 膀胱 urinary bladder
35. 子宫体 body of uterus
36. 子宫内膜 endometrium

女性盆部与会阴连续横断层 24（FH.8910）

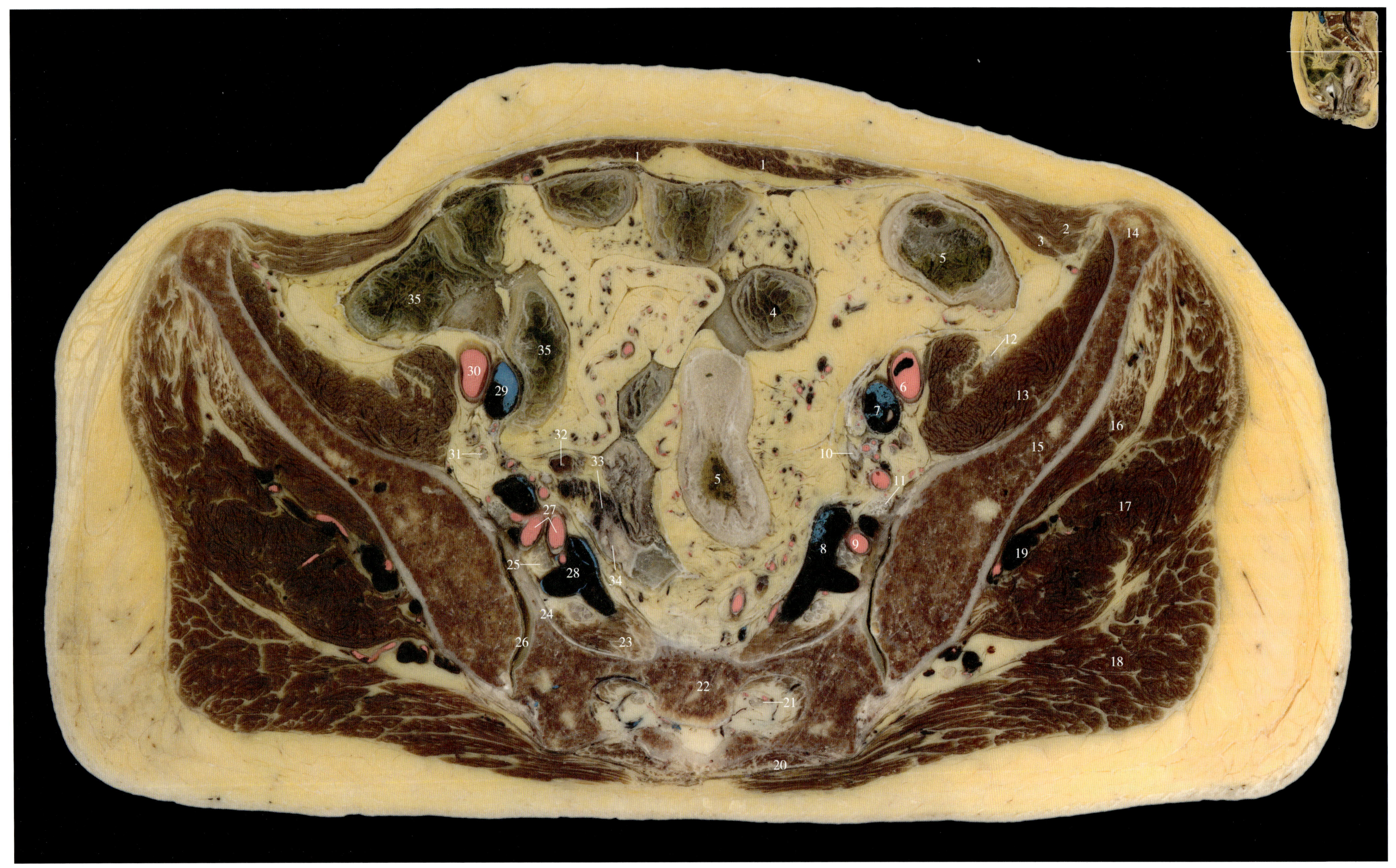

A. 断层标本图像

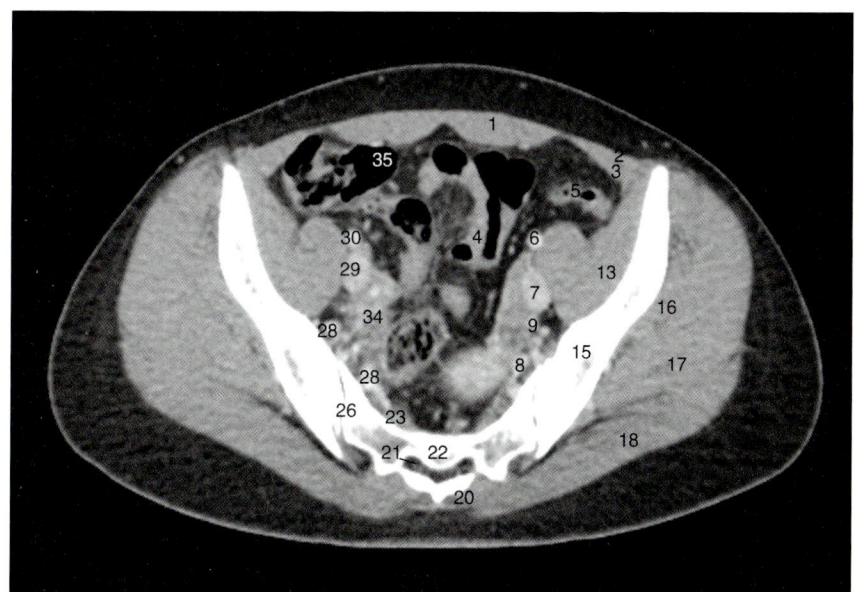

B. CT 增强图像

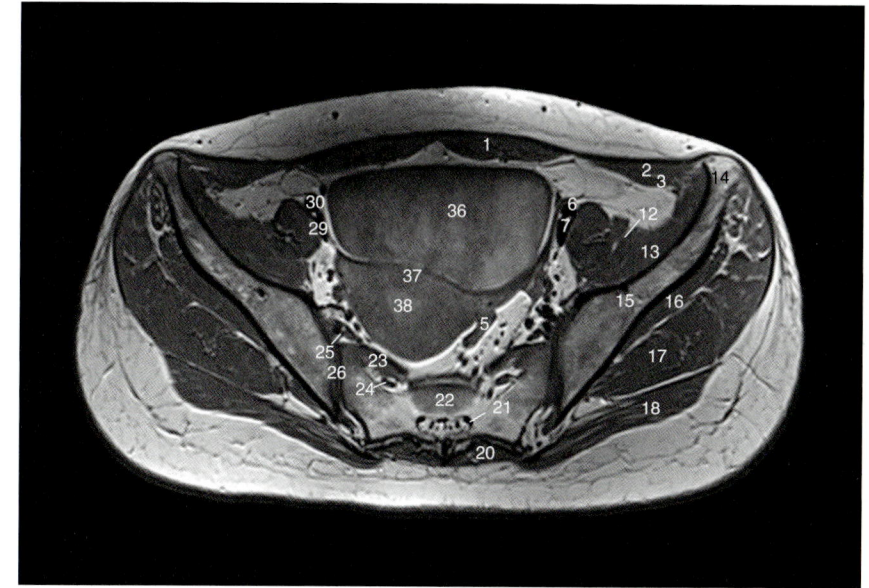

C. MR T1WI

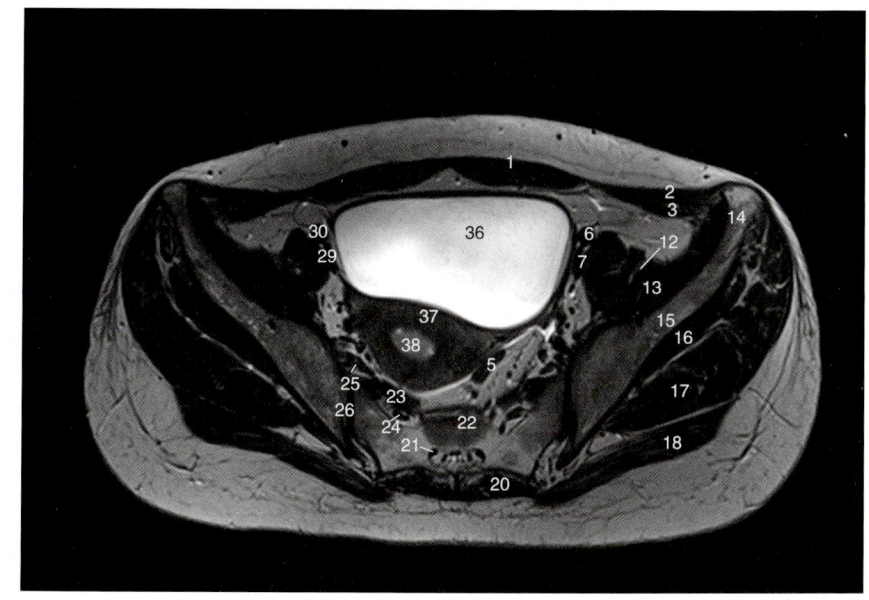

D. MR T2WI

关键结构：骶骨，梨状肌，卵巢。

此断面经过第 3 骶椎椎体中份。

梨状肌开始出现，附着在第 3 骶椎椎体凹面前方。骶髂关节骶骨面内侧从前向后见腰骶干、第 1 骶神经、第 2 骶神经。此断面的骶髂关节断面较中份断面变小。参与构成小骨盆边界的髂腰肌进一步前移，股神经沿髂腰肌向下延伸，髂内、外动、静脉和输尿管分别位于髂腰肌和髂骨翼内侧的腹膜壁层深面。骶骨形态有性别差异。女性骶骨较为平坦，曲度主要存在于第 1、2 段之间及第 3、4 段之间，而二者之间较为平坦。男性的骶骨较为弯曲且狭长。第一骶椎上缘与水平线夹角称骶骨角，立位照片平均为 40°，此角越大，脊柱越不稳定。在骶骨角水平，髂总动脉分叉为髂外动脉和髂内动脉，输尿管由外侧向内侧穿过髂总动脉骶骨前宽长比（宽：耳状面最前点之间；长：骶骨前缘峡部和尖中点的连线）男性为 105%，女性为 115%。女性的耳状面相对较小且更倾斜，男性和女性的耳状面都延伸至上 3 个骶椎。女性耳状面的背侧缘更加凹陷。总之，男性的骨盆腔长，呈圆锥形；女性的短，呈圆柱形，二者的轴线都是弯曲的[5]。右侧输卵管及右侧卵巢位于髂内动、静脉及空肠之间，卵巢断面较上一断面更大。

1. 腹直肌 rectus abdominis
2. 腹内斜肌 obliquus internus abdominis
3. 腹横肌 transversus abdominis
4. 空肠 jejunum
5. 乙状结肠 sigmoid colon
6. 左髂外动脉 left external iliac artery
7. 左髂外静脉 left external iliac vein
8. 左髂内静脉 left internal iliac vein
9. 左髂内动脉 left internal iliac artery
10. 左输尿管 left ureter
11. 腰骶干 lumbosacral trunk
12. 股神经 femoral nerve
13. 髂腰肌 iliopsoas
14. 髂前上棘 anterior superior iliac spine
15. 髂骨翼 ala of ilium
16. 臀小肌 gluteus minimus
17. 臀中肌 gluteus medius
18. 臀大肌 gluteus maximus
19. 臀上静脉 superior gluteal vein
20. 竖脊肌 erector spinae
21. 第 3 骶神经 3rd sacral nerve
22. 第 3 骶椎 3rd sacral vertebra
23. 梨状肌 piriformis
24. 第 2 骶神经 2nd sacral nerve
25. 第 1 骶神经 1st sacral nerve
26. 骶髂关节 sacroiliac joint
27. 右髂内动脉分支 branches of right internal iliac artery
28. 右髂内静脉 right internal iliac vein
29. 右髂外静脉 right external iliac vein
30. 右髂外动脉 right external iliac artery
31. 闭孔神经 obturator nerve
32. 右卵巢动、静脉 right ovarian artery and vein
33. 右输卵管 right uterine tube
34. 右卵巢 right ovary
35. 回肠 ileum
36. 膀胱 urinary bladder
37. 子宫体 body of uterus
38. 子宫内膜 endometrium

女性盆部与会阴连续横断层 25（FH.8890）

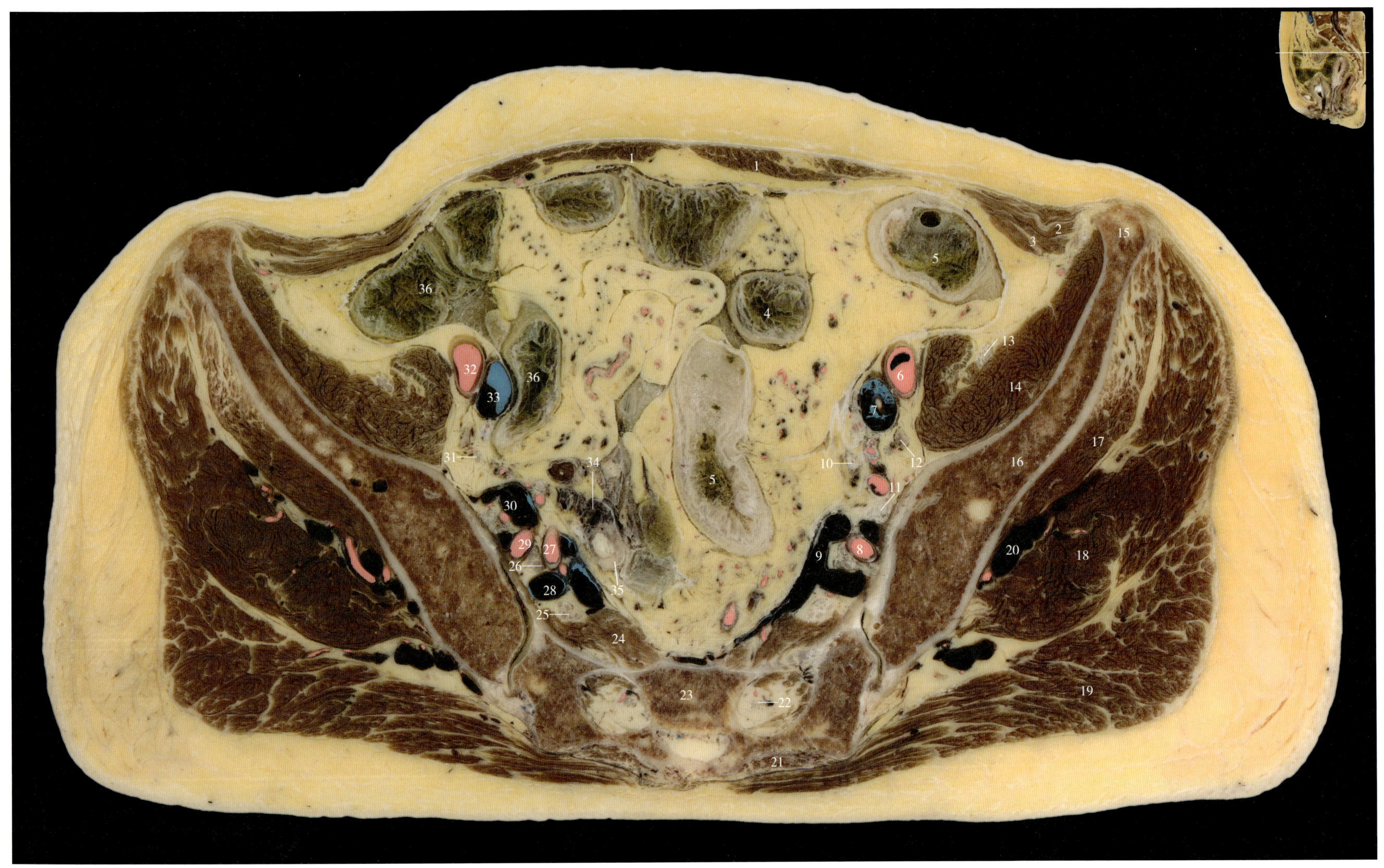

A. 断层标本图像

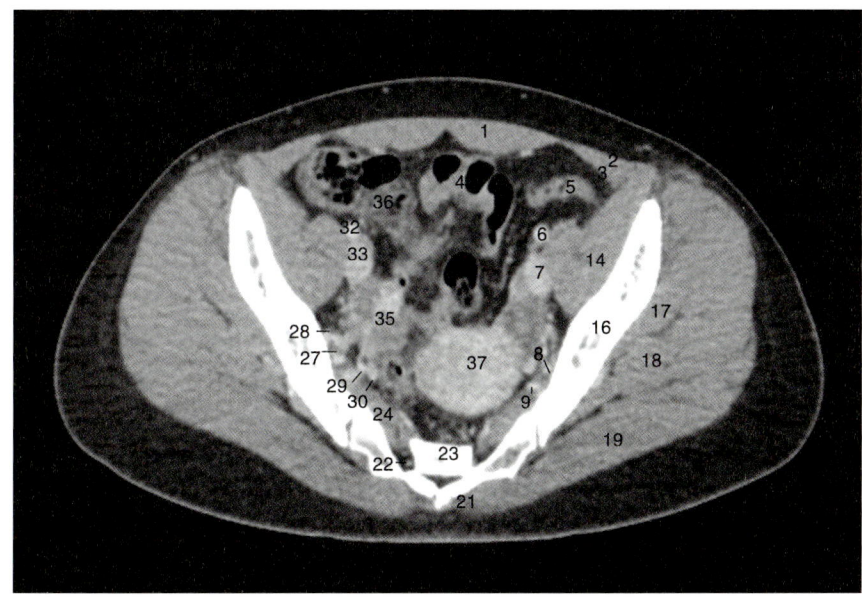
B. CT 增强图像

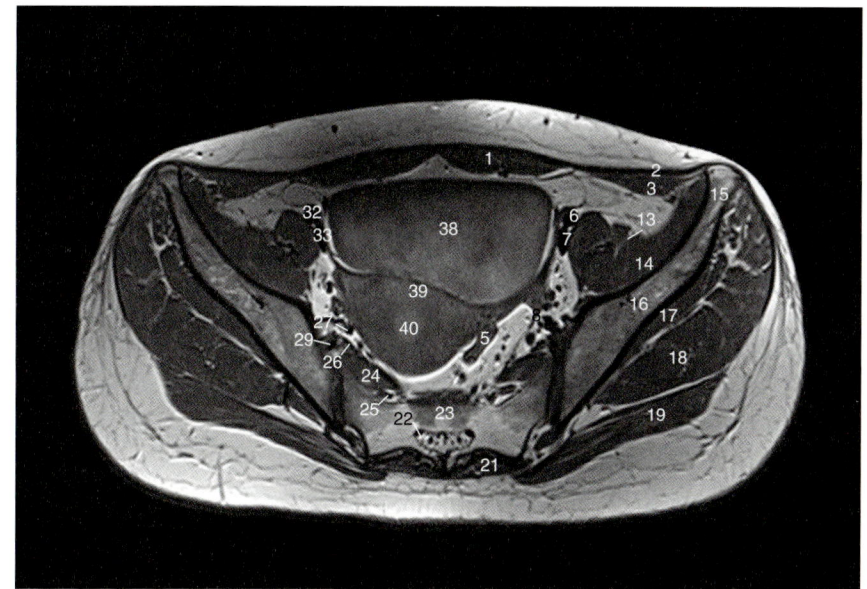
C. MR T1WI

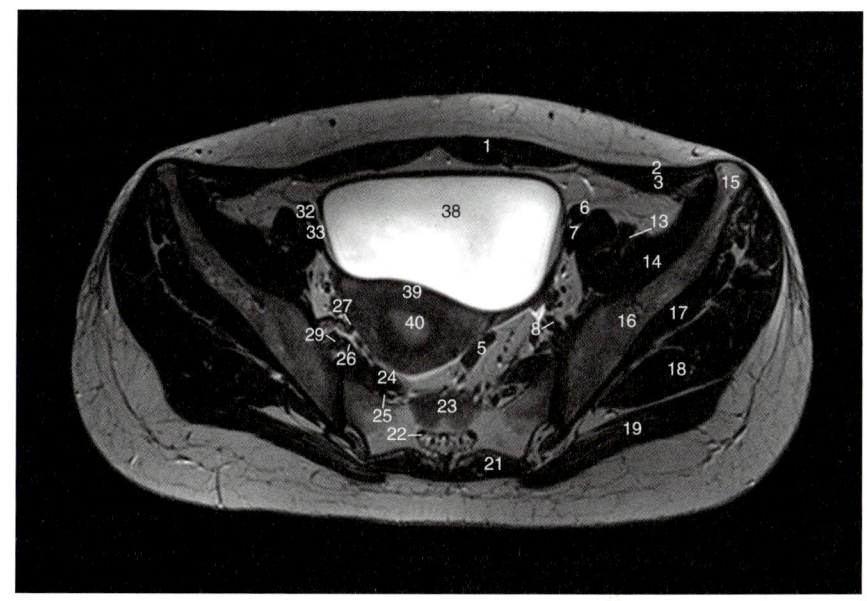
D. MR T2WI

1. 腹直肌 rectus abdominis
2. 腹内斜肌 obliquus internus abdominis
3. 腹横肌 transversus abdominis
4. 空肠 jejunum
5. 乙状结肠 sigmoid colon
6. 左髂外动脉 left external iliac artery
7. 左髂外静脉 left external iliac vein
8. 左臀上动脉 left superior gluteal artery
9. 髂内静脉属支 tributary of internal iliac vein
10. 左输尿管 left ureter
11. 腰骶干 lumbosacral trunk
12. 髂外淋巴结 external iliac lymph nodes
13. 股神经 femoral nerve
14. 髂腰肌 iliopsoas
15. 髂前上棘 anterior superior iliac spine
16. 髂骨翼 ala of ilium
17. 臀小肌 gluteus minimuss
18. 臀中肌 gluteus medius
19. 臀大肌 gluteus maximus
20. 左臀上静脉 left superior gluteal vein
21. 竖脊肌 erector spinae
22. 第 3 骶神经 3rd sacral nerve
23. 第 3 骶椎 3rd sacral vertebra
24. 梨状肌 piriformis
25. 第 2 骶神经 2nd sacral nerve
26. 第 1 骶神经 1st sacral nerve
27. 右臀下动脉 right inferior gluteal artery
28. 右臀上静脉 right superior gluteal vein
29. 右臀上动脉 right superior gluteal artery
30. 右臀下静脉 right inferior gluteal vein
31. 闭孔神经 obturator nerve
32. 右髂外动脉 right external iliac artery
33. 右髂外静脉 right external iliac vein
34. 右输卵管 right uterine tube
35. 右卵巢 right ovary
36. 回肠 ileum
37. 子宫底 fundus of uterus
38. 膀胱 urinary bladder
39. 子宫体 body of uterus
40. 子宫内膜 endometrium

关键结构：髂血管，臀上动、静脉，卵巢。

此断面经过第 3 骶椎椎体中份。

第 3 骶椎椎体凹面前方见梨状肌，髂骨翼内侧从前向后见腰骶干、第 1 骶神经、第 2 骶神经。两侧髂内动、静脉随着髂腰肌前移，仍然位于髂腰肌内侧，股神经沿髂腰肌向下延伸。在此断面，右髂内动脉分为外侧的臀上动脉及内侧的臀下动脉，右侧髂内静脉移行为前方的臀上静脉及后方的臀下静脉。左髂内动脉分为前方的臀上动脉及后方的臀下动脉。左侧髂内静脉分为前方的臀上静脉及后方的臀下静脉。臀上动脉是髂内动脉的最大分支，它是后干的直接延续。臀上动脉走行于腰骶干和第 1 骶神经或第 1~2 骶神经之间，随后稍向下行穿过梨状肌上方的坐骨大孔离开骨盆并分为浅、深两支：浅支供应臀大肌，并与臀下动脉及骶外侧动脉的后支相吻合；深支分为上、下两支，上支与旋髂深动脉及旋股外侧动脉升支相吻合，下支与旋股外侧动脉、臀下动脉及旋骨内侧动脉升支相吻合。臀上静脉的各属支，经梨状肌上方的坐骨大孔并行进入骨盆，并作为单干加入髂内静脉[5]。右侧输卵管及右侧卵巢位于臀下动、静脉内侧。

女性盆部与会阴连续横断层 26（FH.8870）

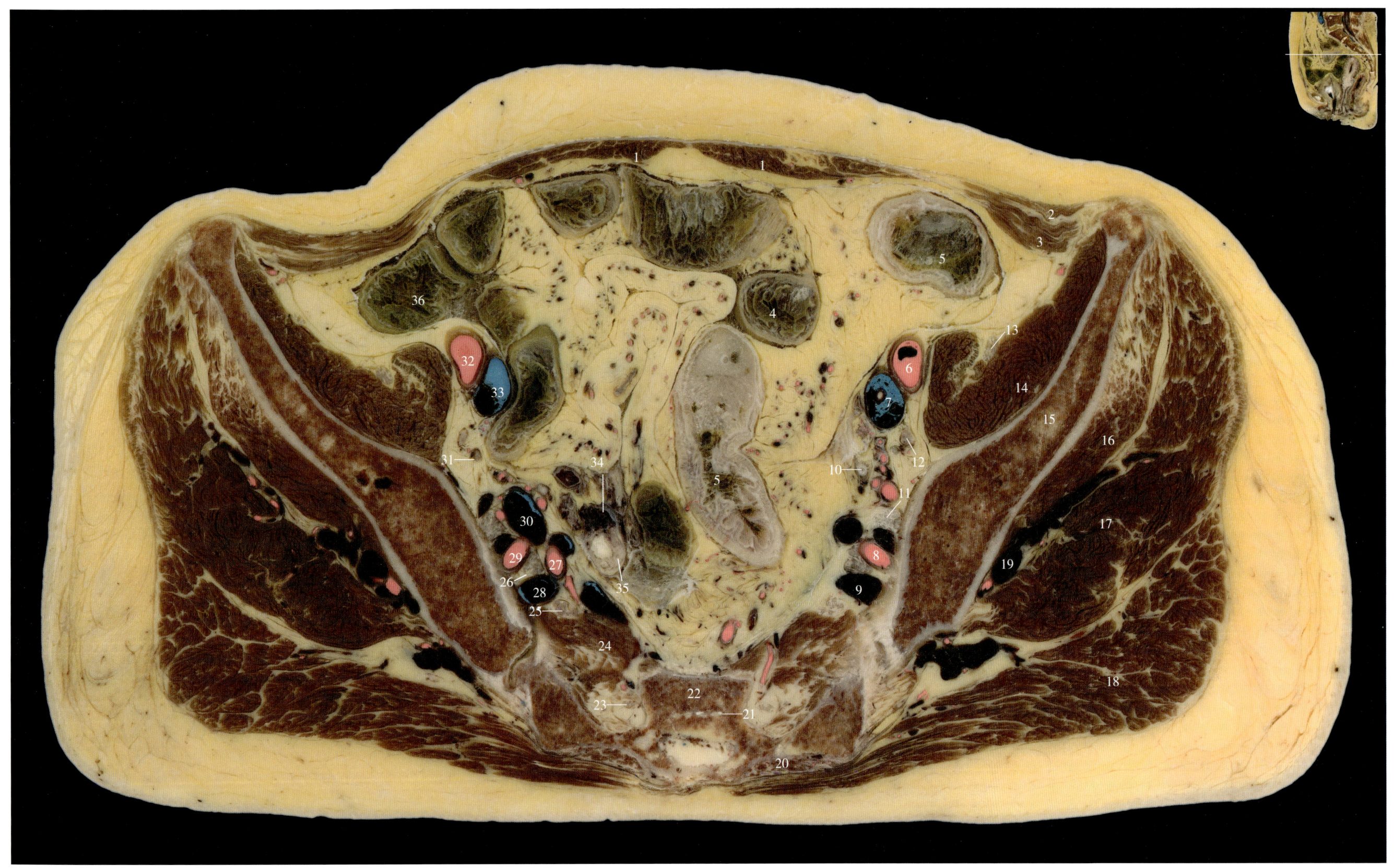

A. 断层标本图像

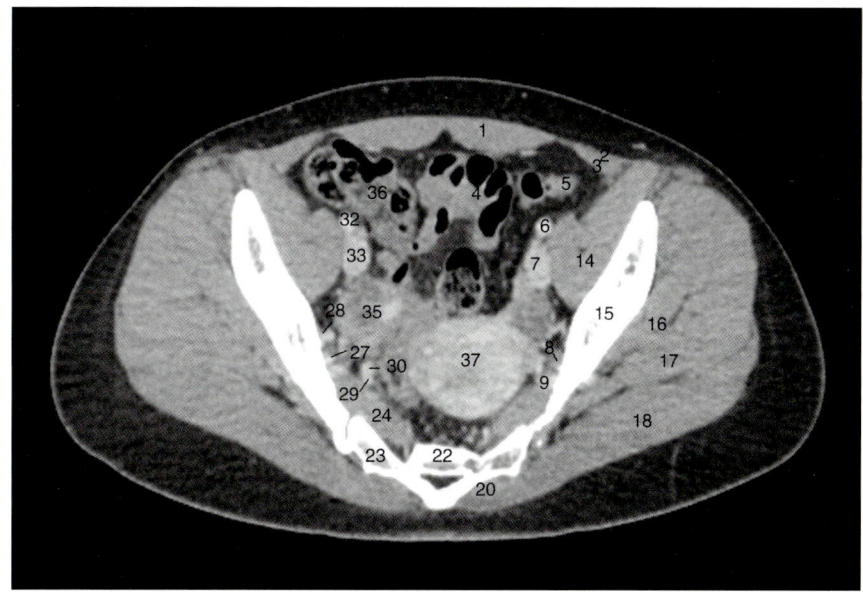

B. CT 增强图像

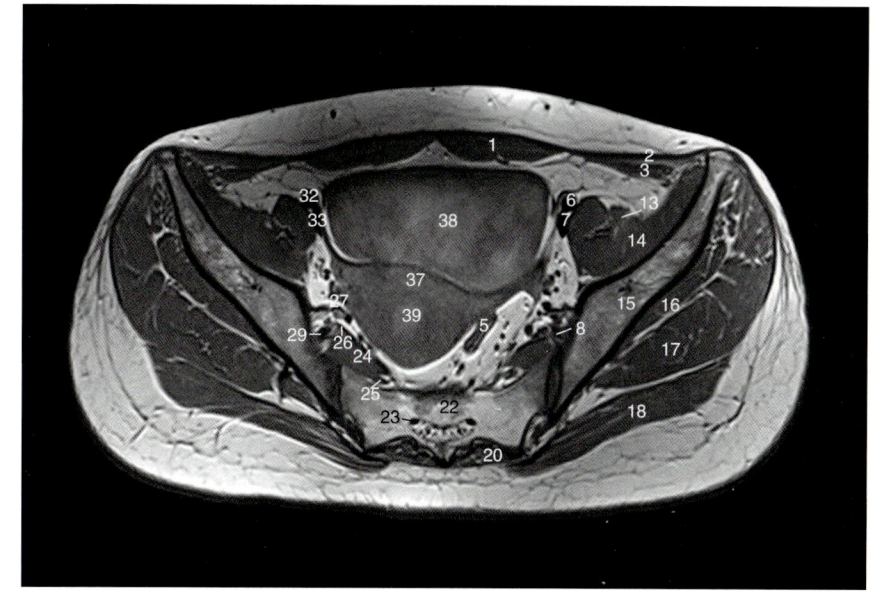

C. MR T1WI

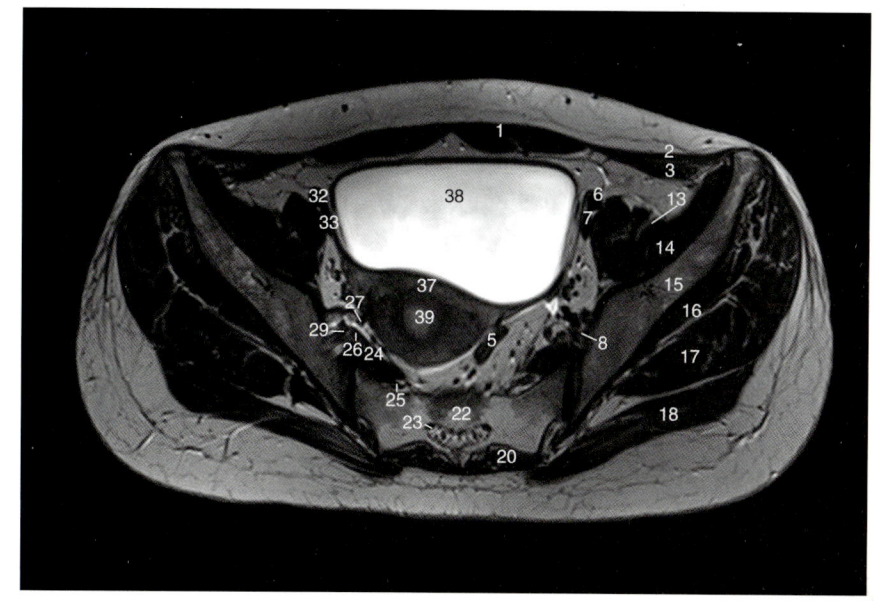

D. MR T2WI

1. 腹直肌 rectus abdominis
2. 腹内斜肌 obliquus internus abdominis
3. 腹横肌 transversus abdominis
4. 空肠 jejunum
5. 乙状结肠 sigmoid colon
6. 左髂外动脉 left external iliac artery
7. 左髂外静脉 left external iliac vein
8. 左臀上动脉 left superior gluteal artery
9. 左臀上静脉 left superior gluteal vein
10. 左输尿管 left ureter
11. 腰骶干 lumbosacral trunk
12. 髂外淋巴结 external iliac lymph nodes
13. 股神经 femoral nerve
14. 髂腰肌 iliopsoas
15. 髂骨翼 ala of ilium
16. 臀小肌 gluteus minimuss
17. 臀中肌 gluteus medius
18. 臀大肌 gluteus maximus
19. 臀上静脉属支 tributary of superior gluteal vein
20. 竖脊肌 erector spinae

21. S3-4 椎间盘 S3-4 intervertebral disc
22. 第 3 骶椎 3rd sacral vertebra
23. 第 3 骶神经 3rd sacral nerve
24. 梨状肌 piriformis
25. 第 2 骶神经 2nd sacral nerve
26. 第 1 骶神经 1st sacral nerve
27. 右臀下动脉 right inferior gluteal artery
28. 右臀上静脉 right superior gluteal vein
29. 右臀上动脉 right superior gluteal artery
30. 右臀下静脉 right inferior gluteal vein
31. 闭孔神经 obturator nerve
32. 右髂外动脉 right external iliac artery
33. 右髂外静脉 right external iliac vein
34. 右输卵管 right uterine tube
35. 右卵巢 right ovary
36. 回肠 ileum
37. 子宫体 body of uterus
38. 膀胱 urinary bladder
39. 子宫内膜 endometrium

关键结构：骶丛，梨状肌，股神经。

此断面经过第 3 骶椎椎体下份。

盆后壁骶骨及骶髂关节明显变小，骶管内容纳骶、尾神经根。第 3 骶椎椎体凹面前方见梨状肌。髂骨翼内侧从前向后见腰骶干、第 1 骶神经、第 2 骶神经，上述神经汇聚形成骶丛，骶丛由来自腰丛的腰骶干和所有骶、尾神经前支组成。腰骶干由第 4 腰神经前支的部分纤维和第 5 腰神经前支的所有纤维在腰丛下方合成，随后下行越过盆腔上口进入小骨盆，加入骶丛。骶丛位于梨状肌的前面，向远端走行分出坐骨神经。在 MR 轴位和冠状位 T1WI 图像上，细长的神经纤维束信号与腰大肌信号相近，在周围脂肪层的衬托下神经轮廓清晰可见。在冠状位 3D 高分辨 T2WI 图像上，双侧骶丛神经表现为对称的高信号，且粗细相近。两侧髂腰肌位于髂骨翼内侧面，股神经沿髂腰肌向下延伸，髂腰肌与骶髂关节之间为输尿管、髂血管及其分支。右侧输卵管及右侧卵巢位于臀下动、静脉内侧。盆腔内，左髂窝及骶骨前方见乙状结肠，右髂窝处有回肠，中间为空肠，空肠所占范围缩小。

53

女性盆部与会阴连续横断层 27（FH.8850）

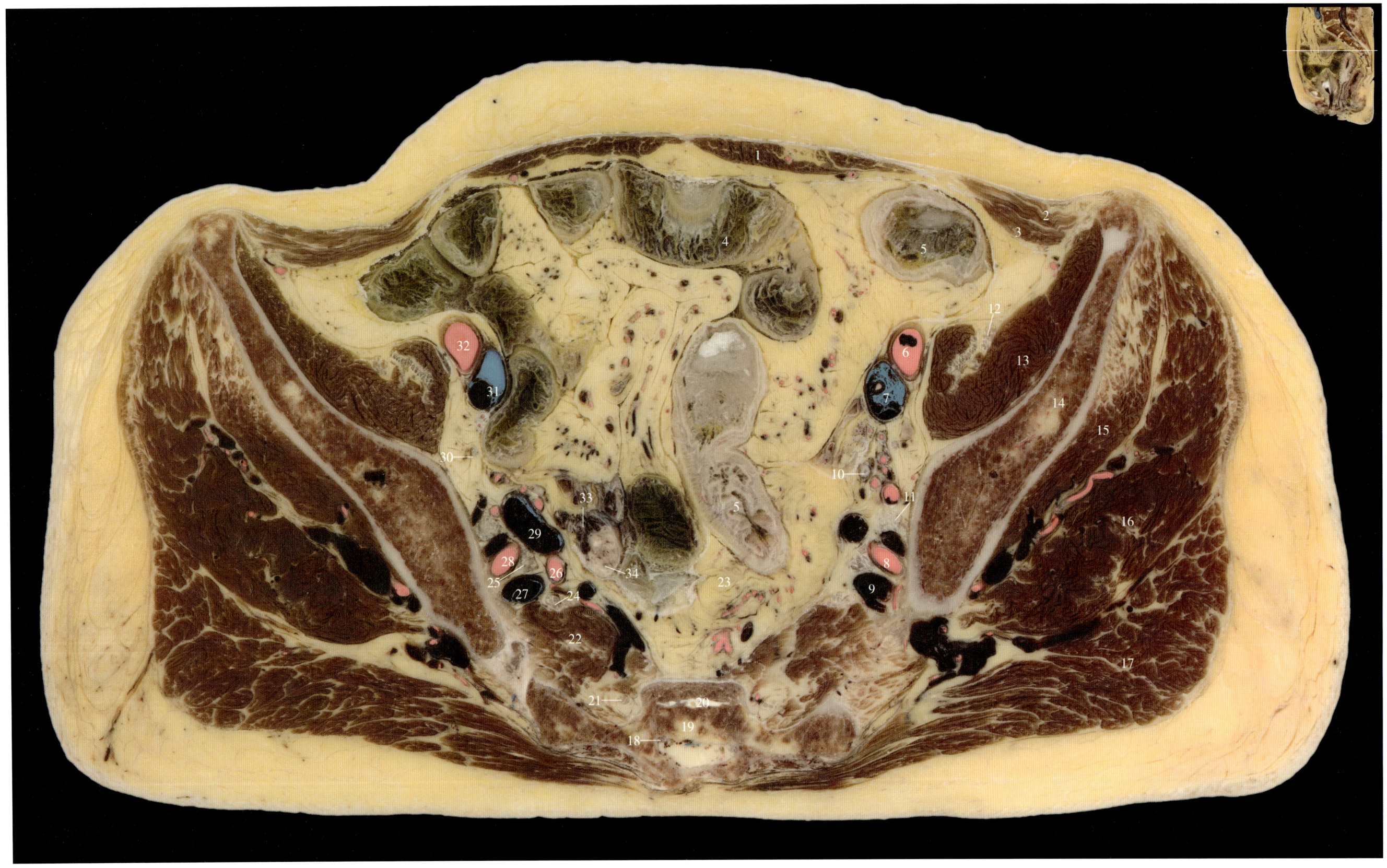

A. 断层标本图像

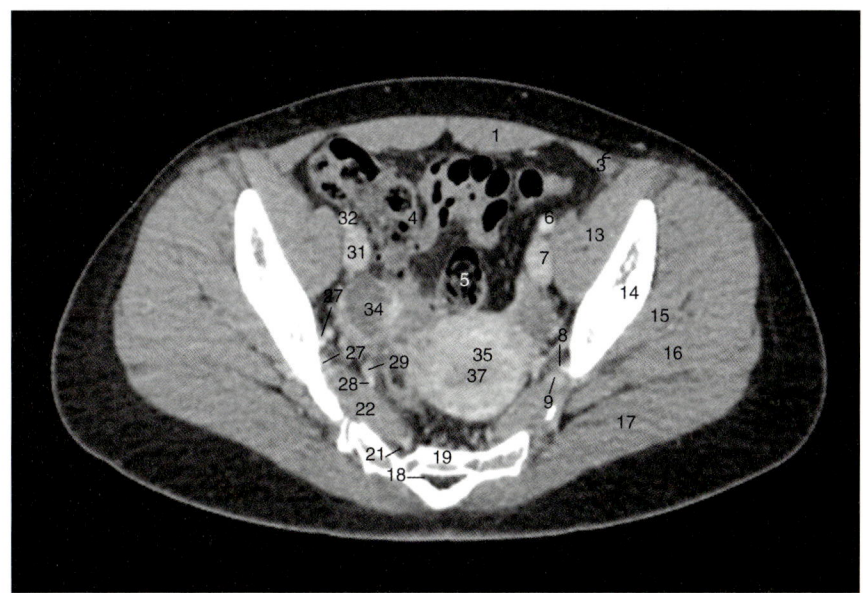

B. CT 增强图像

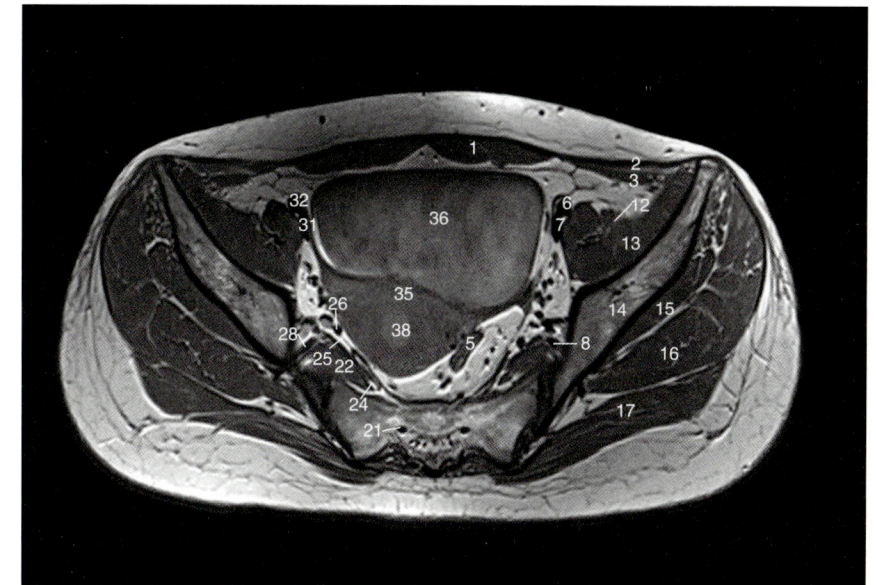

C. MR T1WI

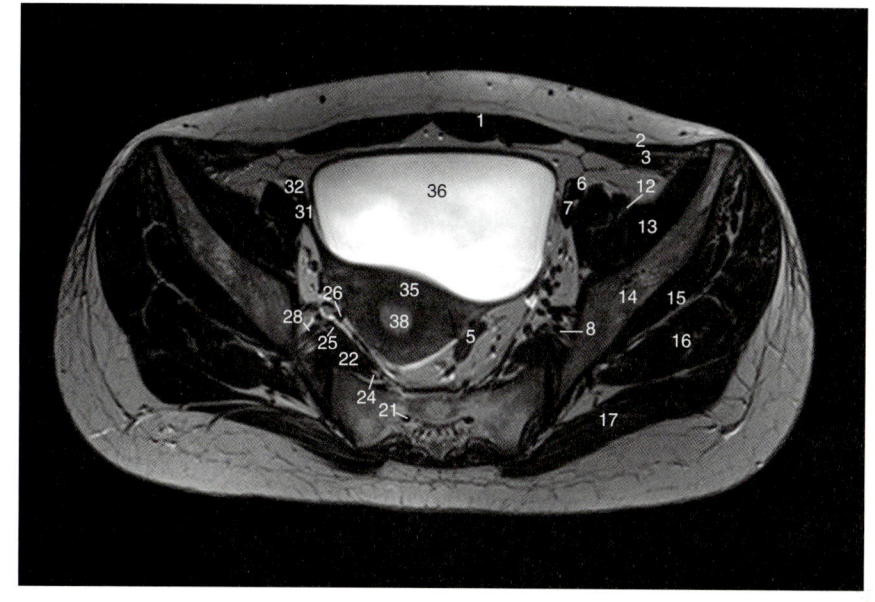

D. MR T2WI

1. 腹直肌 rectus abdominis
2. 腹内斜肌 obliquus internus abdominis
3. 腹横肌 transversus abdominis
4. 回肠 ileum
5. 乙状结肠 sigmoid colon
6. 左髂外动脉 left external iliac artery
7. 左髂外静脉 left external iliac vein
8. 左臀上动脉 left superior gluteal artery
9. 左臀上静脉 left superior gluteal vein
10. 左输尿管 left ureter
11. 腰骶干 lumbosacral trunk
12. 股神经 femoral nerve
13. 髂腰肌 iliopsoas
14. 髂骨翼 ala of ilium
15. 臀小肌 gluteus minimuss
16. 臀中肌 gluteus medius
17. 臀大肌 gluteus maximus
18. 第 4 骶神经 4th sacral nerve
19. 第 4 骶椎 4th sacral vertebra
20. S3-4 椎间盘 S3-4 intervertebral disc
21. 第 3 骶神经 3rd sacral nerve
22. 梨状肌 piriformis
23. 乙状结肠系膜 sigmoid mesocolon
24. 第 2 骶神经 2nd sacral nerve
25. 第 1 骶神经 1st sacral nerve
26. 右臀下动脉 right inferior gluteal artery
27. 右臀上静脉 right superior gluteal vein
28. 右臀上动脉 right superior gluteal artery
29. 右臀下静脉 right inferior gluteal vein
30. 闭孔神经 obturator nerve
31. 右髂外静脉 right external iliac vein
32. 右髂外动脉 right external iliac artery
33. 右输卵管 right uterine tube
34. 右卵巢 right ovary
35. 子宫体 body of uterus
36. 膀胱 urinary bladder
37. 子宫腔 cavity of uterus
38. 子宫内膜 endometrium

关键结构：髂血管，臀下动、静脉，梨状肌。

此断面经过 S3-4 椎间盘（临床上常写作 S3/4 椎间盘）。

第 4 骶椎体前方见梨状肌，腰骶干、第 1 骶神经、第 2 骶神经由前外侧向后内侧依次位于梨状肌前方并相互靠近。此断面骶髂关节已完全消失，髂骨翼位于盆壁两侧，髂骨翼与骶骨分离。两侧髂腰肌位于髂骨翼内侧面，股神经沿髂腰肌向下延伸。髂腰肌与骶骨之间为髂血管及其分支，臀下动脉是髂内动脉前干最大的终末支，供应臀部及大腿的肌肉。臀下动脉位于骶丛和梨状肌的前方、阴部内动脉的后方，穿过骶前脊神经的第 1~2 或第 2~3 分支之间，随后位于梨状肌和坐骨耻骨肌之间，穿过坐骨大孔下部至臀区。髂内动脉和臀下动脉的栓塞可能导致神经缺血和下肢麻木。在骨盆外臀下动脉可与臀上动脉、阴部内动脉、闭孔动脉和旋股内侧动脉相互吻合。臀下静脉的各属支并行上升至大腿根近端后部与旋股内侧静脉、第一穿静脉汇合，经坐骨大孔的下部进入骨盆，汇入髂内静脉，并通过臀部的穿静脉与臀浅静脉相联系[5]。右侧输卵管及右侧卵巢位于臀下动、静脉内侧。

女性盆部与会阴连续横断层 28（FH.8830）

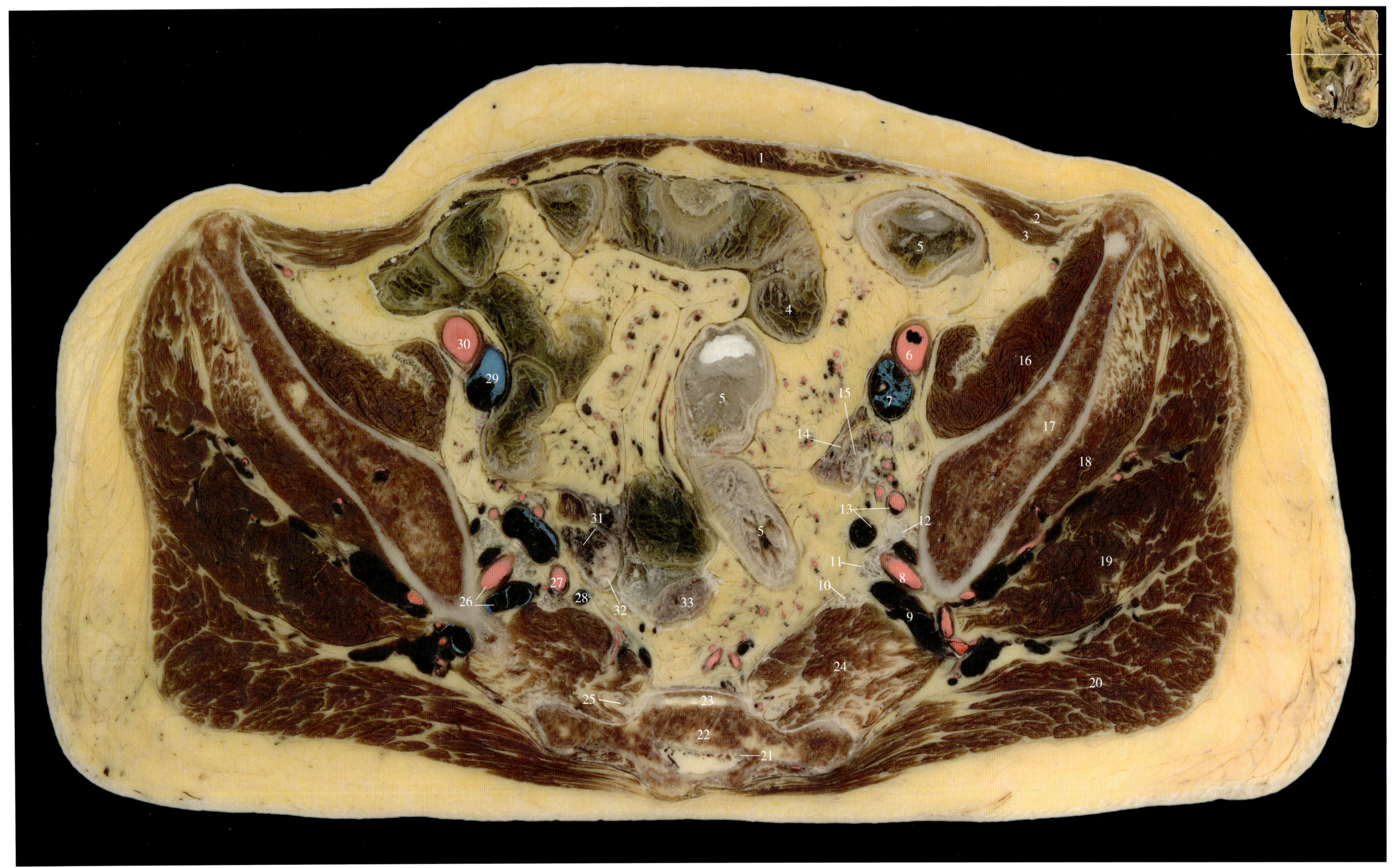

A. 断层标本图像

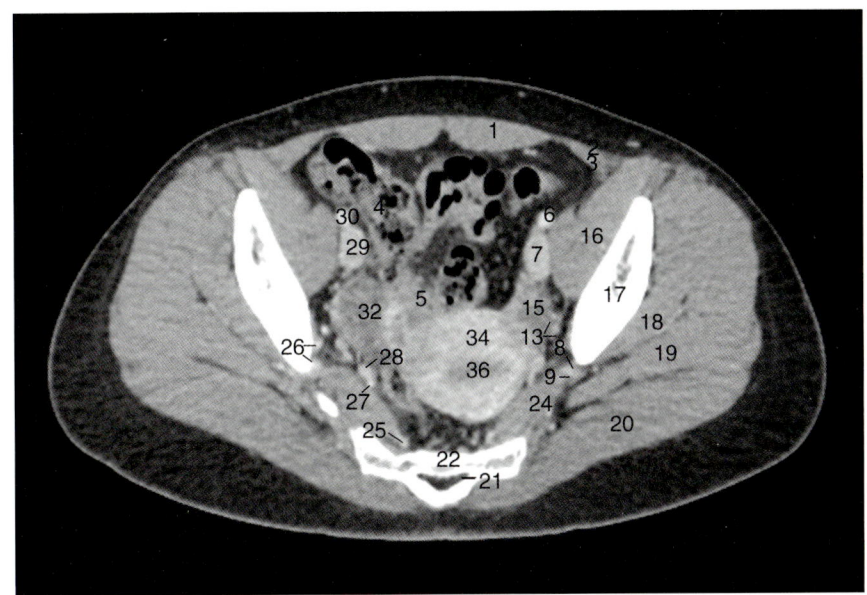
B. CT 增强图像

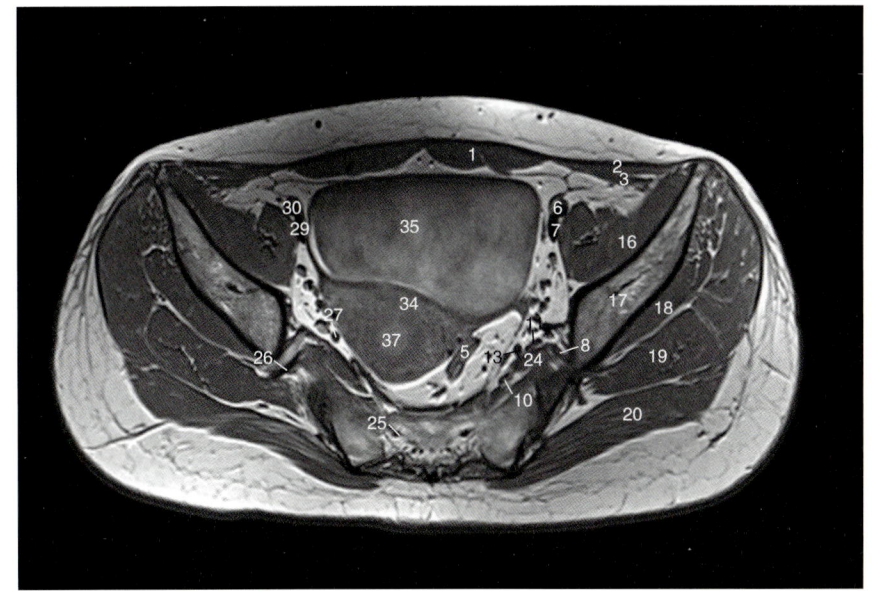
C. MR T1WI

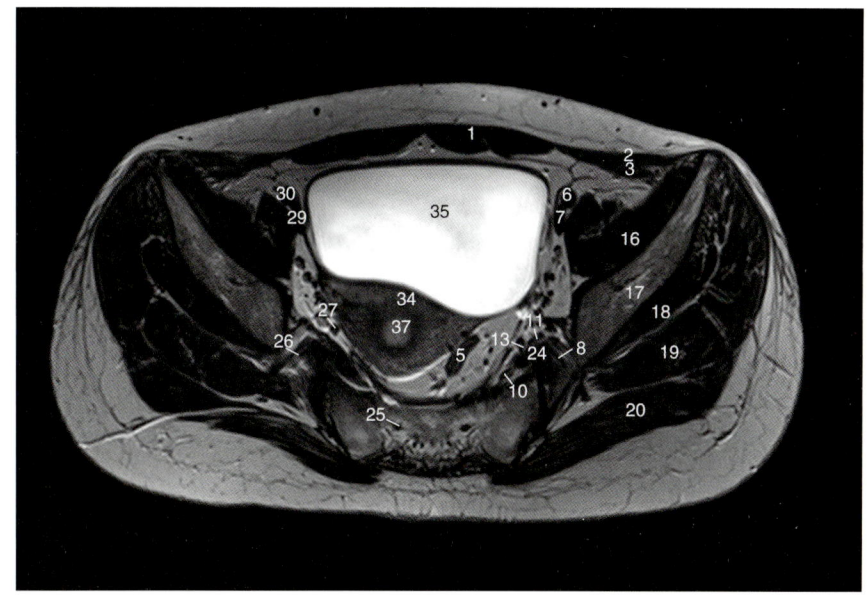
D. MR T2WI

1. 腹直肌 rectus abdominis
2. 腹内斜肌 obliquus internus abdominis
3. 腹横肌 transversus abdominis
4. 回肠 ileum
5. 乙状结肠 sigmoid colon
6. 左髂外动脉 left external iliac artery
7. 左髂外静脉 left external iliac vein
8. 左臀上动脉 left superior gluteal artery
9. 左臀上静脉 left superior gluteal vein
10. 第 2 骶神经 2nd sacral nerve
11. 第 1 骶神经 1st sacral nerve
12. 腰骶干 lumbosacral trunk
13. 左臀下动、静脉 left inferior gluteal artery and vein
14. 左输卵管 left uterine tube
15. 左卵巢 left ovary
16. 髂腰肌 iliopsoas
17. 髂骨翼 ala of ilium
18. 臀小肌 gluteus minimuss
19. 臀中肌 gluteus medius
20. 臀大肌 gluteus maximus
21. 第 4 骶神经 4th sacral nerve
22. 第 4 骶椎 4th sacral vertebra
23. S3-4 椎间盘 S3-4 intervertebral disc
24. 梨状肌 piriformis
25. 第 3 骶神经 3rd sacral nerve
26. 右臀上动、静脉 right superior gluteal artery and vein
27. 右臀下动脉 right inferior gluteal artery
28. 右臀下静脉 right inferior gluteal vein
29. 右髂外静脉 right external iliac vein
30. 右髂外动脉 right external iliac artery
31. 右输卵管 right uterine tube
32. 右卵巢 right ovary
33. 子宫底 fundus of uterus
34. 子宫体 body of uterus
35. 膀胱 urinary bladder
36. 子宫腔 cavity of uterus
37. 子宫内膜 endometrium

关键结构：梨状肌，子宫底，卵巢。

此断面经过 S3-4 椎间盘（临床上常写作 S3/4 椎间盘）。

第 4 骶椎椎体前方见梨状肌，梨状肌起于第 2~4 骶椎骶前孔外侧，经坐骨大切迹上缘，穿坐骨大孔出骨盆，止于股骨大转子梨状肌窝。其功能为大腿外伸时使髋关节外旋，屈曲时使髋关节外展。髂骨缩小，其与骶骨之间形成坐骨大孔。坐骨大孔被其分为梨状肌上孔和下孔，梨状肌上孔有臀上神经、臀上血管通过；梨状肌下孔有坐骨神经、股后皮神经、臀下神经、阴部神经和臀下血管、阴部内血管通过。由于梨状肌穿越坐骨大孔的中心并是孔内最大的结构，因此是骶丛和坐骨神经定位的标志。在 CT 图像上，梨状肌呈软组织密度；在 MR 图像上，T1WI 及 T2WI 呈中等信号。此断面梨状肌前方见臀上动、静脉经梨状肌下孔出入盆腔与臀区之间。两侧髂腰肌位于髂骨体内侧面，股神经沿髂腰肌向下延伸，髂外动、静脉位于髂腰肌内侧。右侧输卵管及右侧卵巢位于臀下动、静脉内侧。在此断面子宫底及左侧卵巢、输卵管出现，子宫底位于右侧卵巢后内侧，左侧卵巢及输卵管位于左侧髂外静脉与臀下动脉之间。

女性盆部与会阴连续横断层 29（FH.8810）

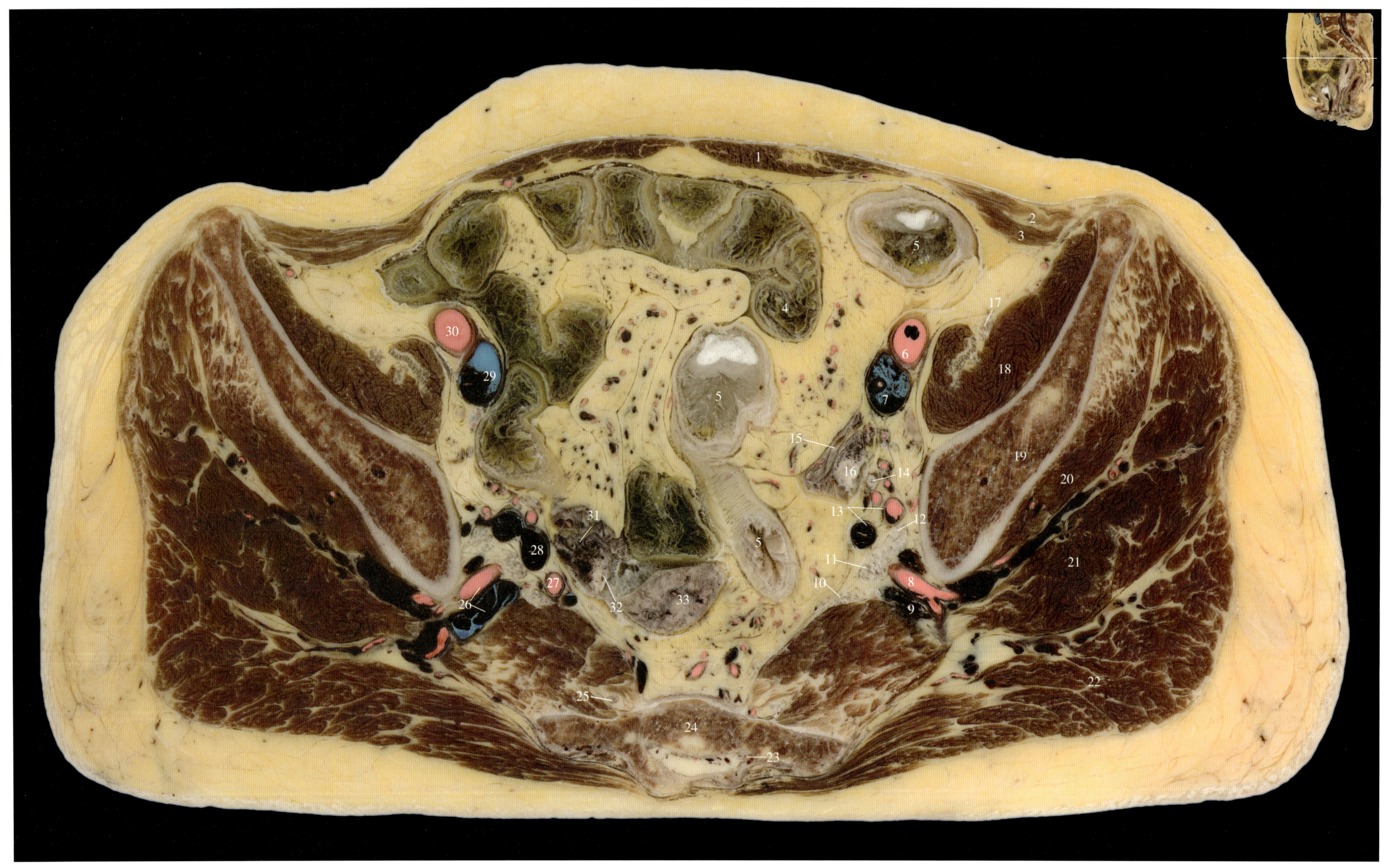

A. 断层标本图像

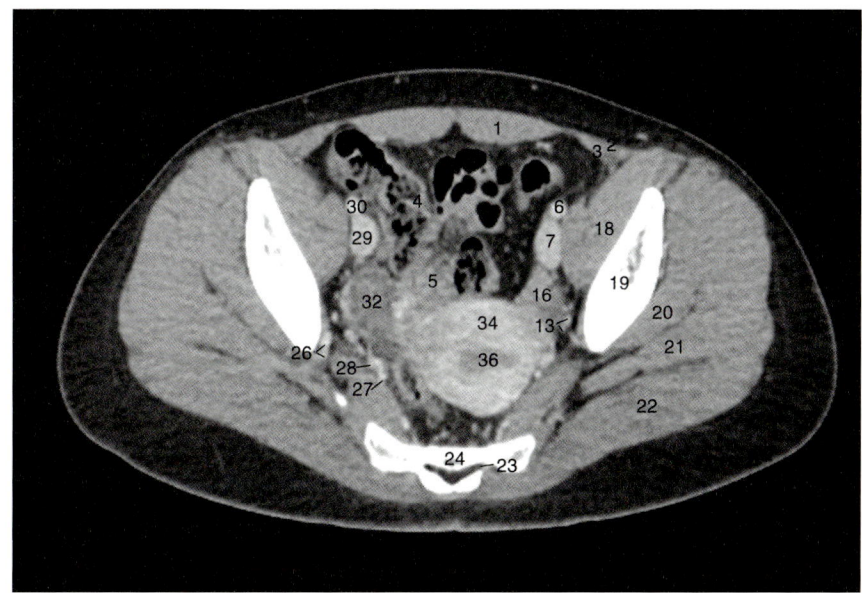

B. CT 增强图像

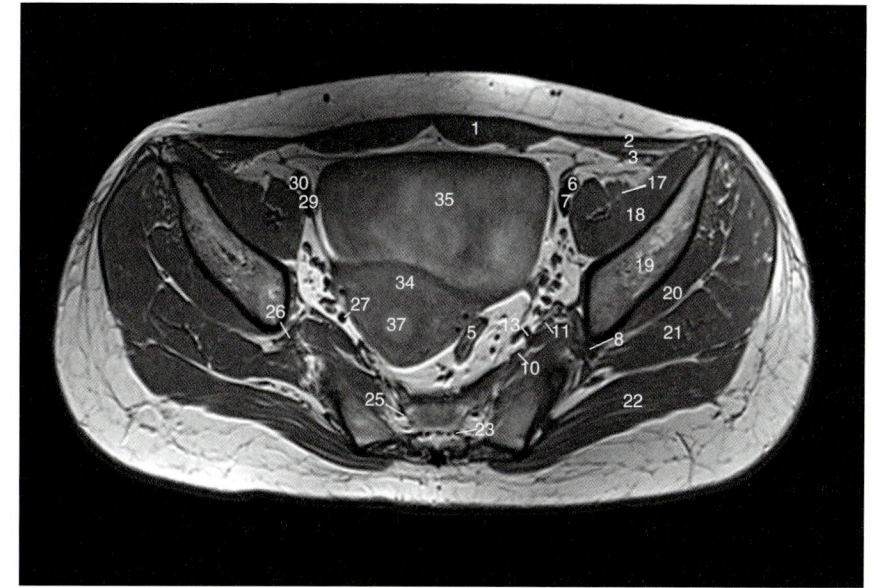

C. MR T1WI

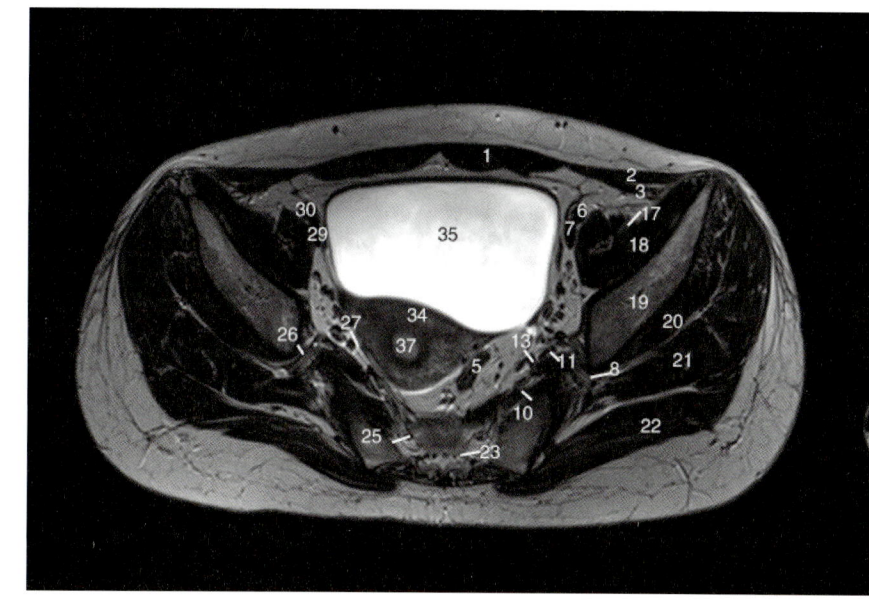

D. MR T2WI

1. 腹直肌 rectus abdominis
2. 腹内斜肌 obliquus internus abdominis
3. 腹横肌 transversus abdominis
4. 回肠 ileum
5. 乙状结肠 sigmoid colon
6. 左髂外动脉 left external iliac artery
7. 左髂外静脉 left external iliac vein
8. 左臀上动脉 left superior gluteal artery
9. 左臀上静脉 left superior gluteal vein
10. 第 2 骶神经 2nd sacral nerve
11. 第 1 骶神经 1st sacral nerve
12. 腰骶干 lumbosacral trunk
13. 左臀下动、静脉 left inferior gluteal artery and vein
14. 左输尿管 left ureter
15. 左输卵管 left uterine tube
16. 左卵巢 left ovary
17. 股神经 femoral nerve
18. 髂腰肌 iliopsoas
19. 髂骨翼 ala of ilium
20. 臀小肌 gluteus minimuss
21. 臀中肌 gluteus medius
22. 臀大肌 gluteus maximus
23. 第 4 骶神经 4th sacral nerve
24. 第 4 骶椎 4th sacral vertebra
25. 第 3 骶神经 3rd sacral nerve
26. 右臀上动、静脉 right superior gluteal artery and vein
27. 右臀下动脉 right inferior gluteal artery
28. 右臀下静脉 right inferior gluteal vein
29. 右髂外静脉 right external iliac vein
30. 右髂外动脉 right external iliac artery
31. 右输卵管 right uterine tube
32. 右卵巢 right ovary
33. 子宫底 fundus of uterus
34. 子宫体 body of uterus
35. 膀胱 urinary bladder
36. 子宫腔 cavity of uterus
37. 子宫内膜 endometrium

关键结构：髂外动脉，梨状肌，卵巢。

此断面经过第 4 骶椎椎体上份。

第 4 骶椎椎体前方见梨状肌，腰骶干、第 1 骶神经、第 2 骶神经由前外侧向后内侧依次位于梨状肌前方并相互靠近。第 3 骶神经位于骶椎与梨状肌之间。髂骨体继续缩小，两侧髂腰肌位于髂骨体内侧面，股神经沿髂腰肌向下延伸，两侧臀下动、静脉继续通过坐骨大孔向外移行，两侧臀上动、静脉向盆腔后方移行。髂外动、静脉位于髂腰肌内侧，呈前后方向排列。髂外动脉是髂总动脉的自然延续，沿腰大肌内缘外侧下降，达到髂前上棘与耻骨连线的中点处，在腹股沟韧带后方进入股部改称为股动脉。右髂外动脉前为回肠末端，左髂外动脉前为乙状结肠，髂筋膜薄层包裹髂动、静脉，髂血管前方和内侧有许多淋巴结。除一些小分支外，髂外动脉在腹股沟韧带上方发出 2 支较大的动脉：腹壁下动脉和旋髂深动脉。腹壁下动脉与腹壁上动脉和下几对肋间后动脉吻合。旋髂深动脉与旋股外侧动脉、髂腰动脉和臀上动脉吻合[5]。右侧输卵管及右侧卵巢位于臀下动、静脉内侧，此断面右侧卵巢已近消失，子宫底及左侧卵巢在断面中继续增大。

女性盆部与会阴连续横断层 30（FH.8790）

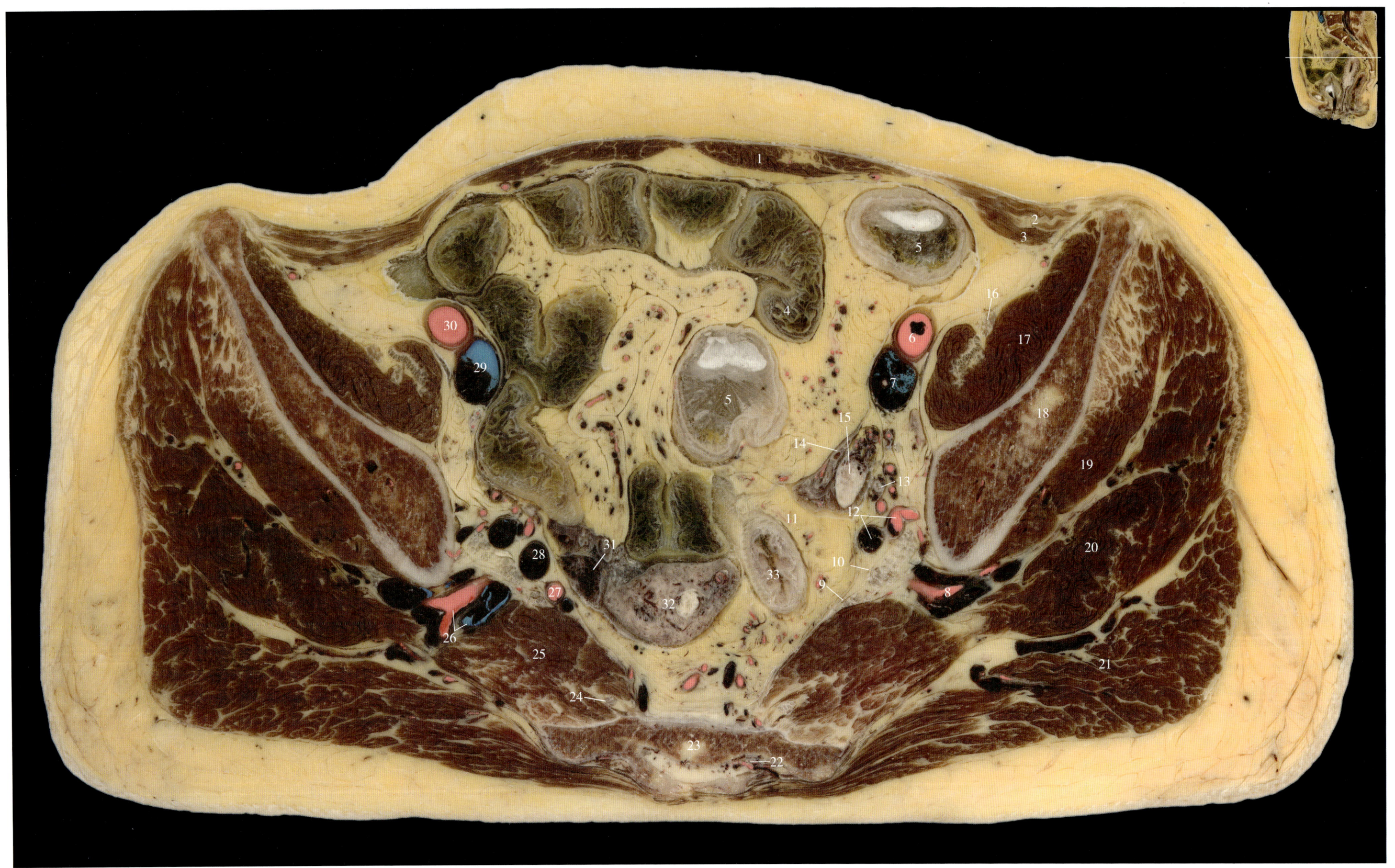

A. 断层标本图像

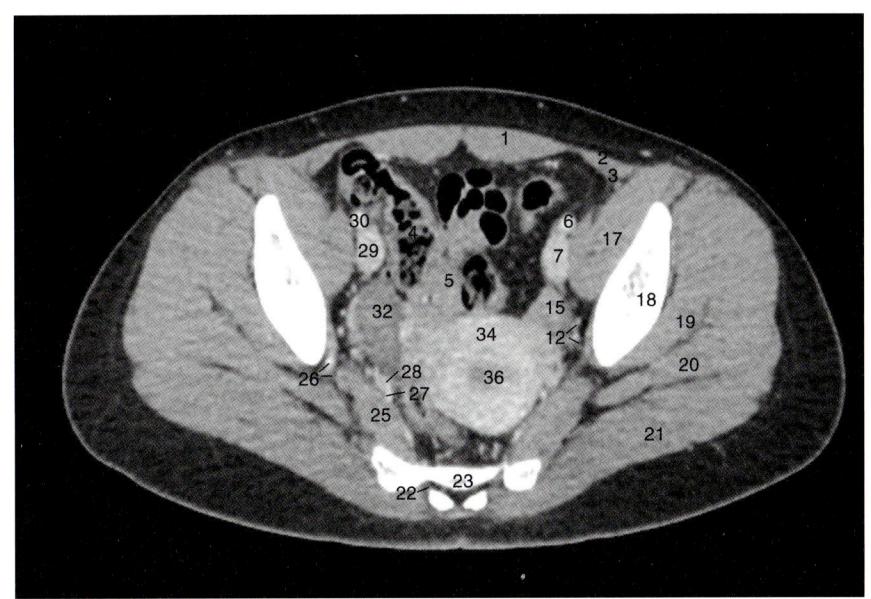
B. CT 增强图像

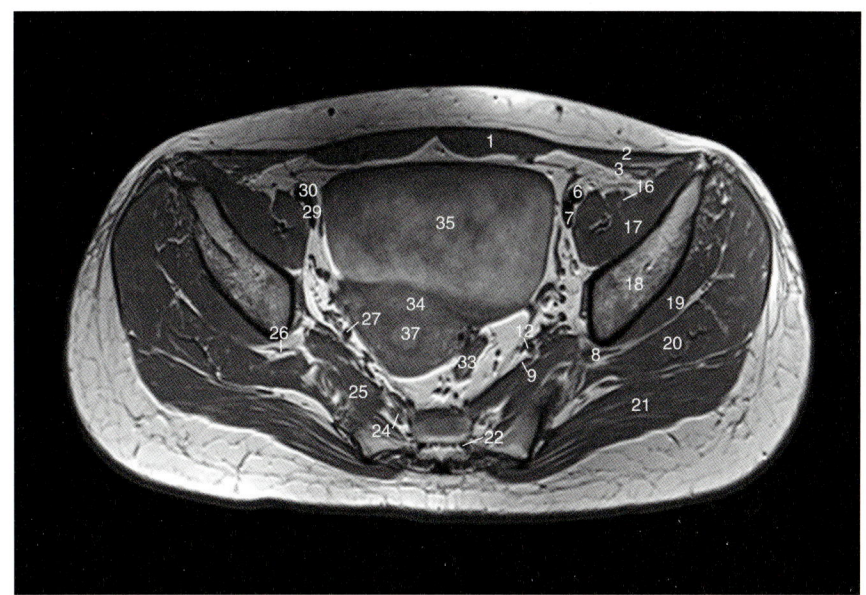
C. MR T1WI

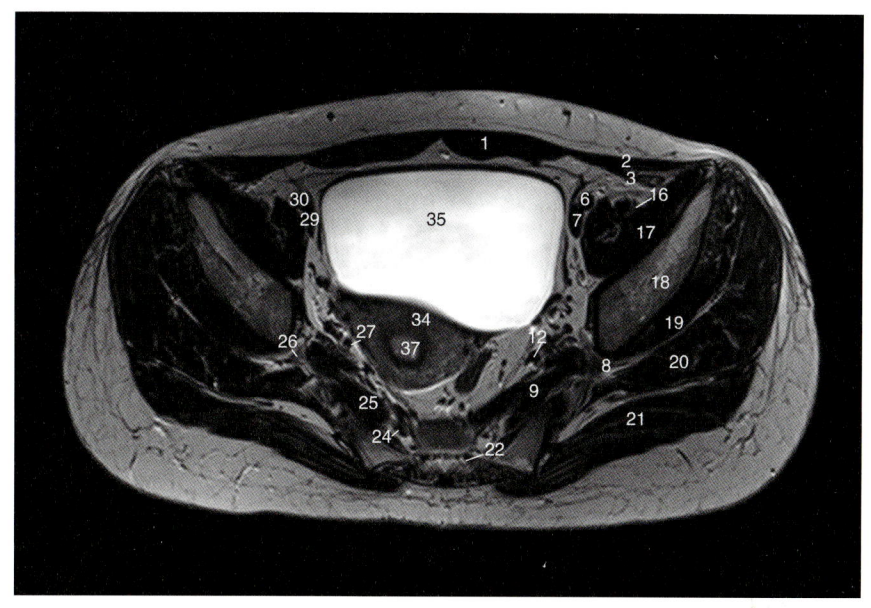
D. MR T2WI

关键结构：坐骨神经，髂外静脉，梨状肌。

此断面经过第 4 骶椎椎体上份。

第 4 骶椎椎体前方见梨状肌，此断面中腰骶干、第 1 骶神经已经完全融合形成坐骨神经，其与第 2 骶神经由前外侧向后内侧位于梨状肌前方，坐骨神经从骶丛发出后，经梨状肌下孔出盆腔至臀大肌深面，在坐骨结节与大转子连线的中点深面下行到达股后区，继而行于股二头肌长头的深面，一般在腘窝上方分为胫神经和腓总神经两大终支。髂外动、静脉位于髂腰肌内侧，呈前后方向排列，髂外静脉是股静脉近端的延续，长约为 9.44（4.50~15.50）cm，左侧长为 8.25 cm ± 1.23 cm，右侧长为 7.93 cm ± 2.01 cm。左侧外径为 13.15 cm ± 0.23 mm，右侧外径为 13.72 cm ± 0.17 mm[16]。髂外静脉自腹股沟韧带的后方，沿着盆腔上行并在骶髂关节的前方汇入髂内静脉从而形成髂总静脉。髂外动脉的疾病经常使其在与静脉接触的位置黏附在一起，特别是在右侧，血管壁可以融合，使分离它们变得危险[5]。通常髂外静脉没有静脉瓣膜，但可有单一的瓣膜存在；属支有腹壁下静脉、旋髂深静脉和耻静脉。盆腔内，左髂窝及骶骨前方见乙状结肠，其余部分为回肠襻。

1. 腹直肌 rectus abdominis
2. 腹内斜肌 obliquus internus abdominis
3. 腹横肌 transversus abdominis
4. 回肠 ileum
5. 乙状结肠 sigmoid colon
6. 左髂外动脉 left external iliac artery
7. 左髂外静脉 left external iliac vein
8. 左臀上动、静脉 left superior gluteal artery and vein
9. 第 2 骶神经 2nd sacral nerve
10. 坐骨神经 sciatic nerve
11. 乙状结肠系膜 sigmoid mesocolon
12. 左臀下动、静脉 left inferior gluteal artery and vein
13. 左输尿管 left ureter
14. 左输卵管 left uterine tube
15. 左卵巢 left ovary
16. 股神经 femoral nerve
17. 髂腰肌 iliopsoas
18. 髂骨翼 ala of ilium
19. 臀小肌 gluteus minimuss
20. 臀中肌 gluteus medius
21. 臀大肌 gluteus maximus
22. 第 4 骶神经 4th sacral nerve
23. 第 4 骶椎 4th sacral vertebra
24. 第 3 骶神经 3rd sacral nerve
25. 梨状肌 piriformis
26. 右臀上动、静脉 right superior gluteal artery and vein
27. 右臀下动脉 right inferior gluteal artery
28. 右臀下静脉 right inferior gluteal vein
29. 右髂外静脉 right external iliac vein
30. 右髂外动脉 right external iliac artery
31. 右输卵管 right uterine tube
32. 子宫底 fundus of uterus
33. 直肠 rectum
34. 子宫体 body of uterus
35. 膀胱 urinary bladder
36. 子宫腔 cavity of uterus
37. 子宫内膜 endometrium

女性盆部与会阴连续横断层 31（FH.8770）

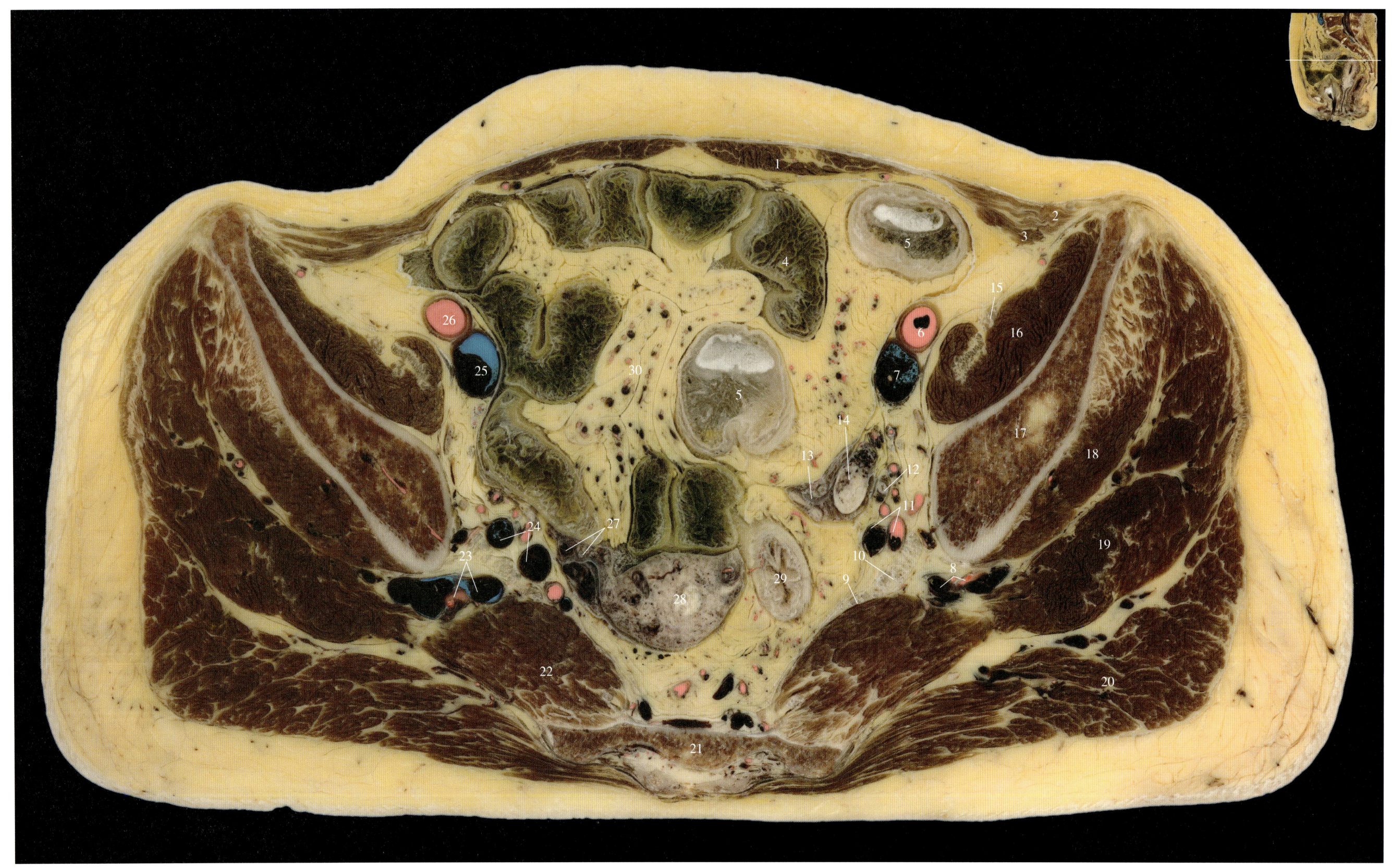

A. 断层标本图像

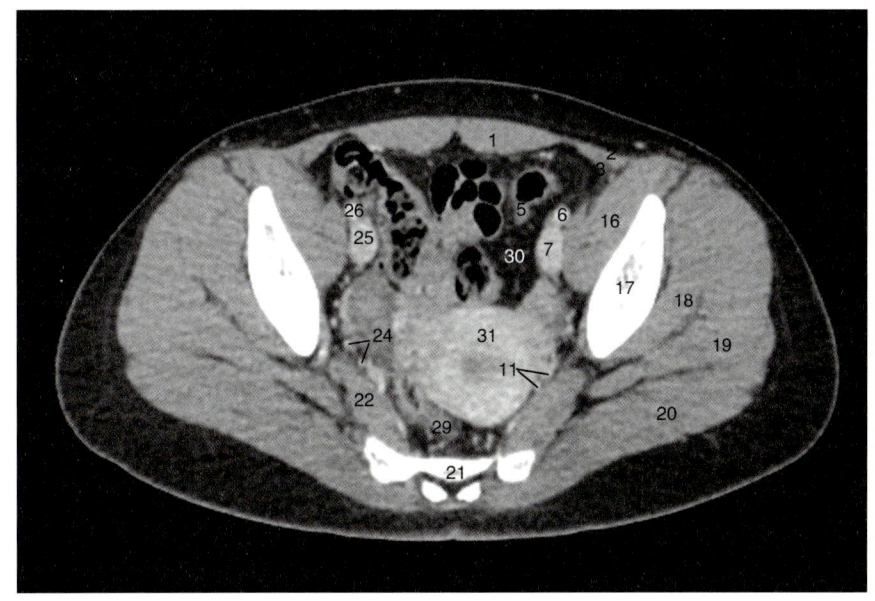
B. CT 增强图像

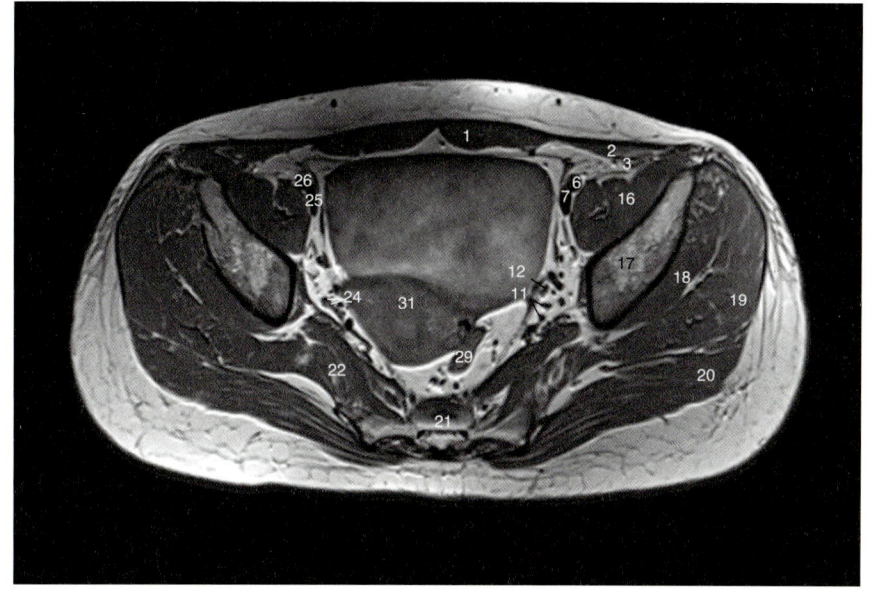
C. MR T1WI

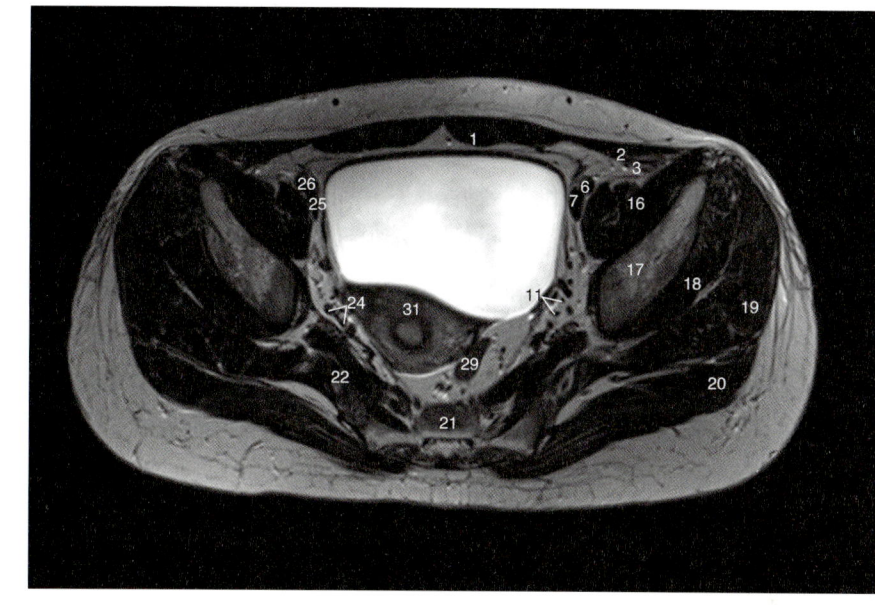
D. MR T2WI

1. 腹直肌 rectus abdominis
2. 腹内斜肌 obliquus internus abdominis
3. 腹横肌 transversus abdominis
4. 回肠 ileum
5. 乙状结肠 sigmoid colon
6. 左髂外动脉 left external iliac artery
7. 左髂外静脉 left external iliac vein
8. 左臀上动、静脉 left superior gluteal artery and vein
9. 第3骶神经 3rd sacral nerve
10. 坐骨神经 sciatic nerve
11. 左臀下动、静脉 left inferior gluteal artery and vein
12. 左输尿管 left ureter
13. 左输卵管 left uterine tube
14. 左卵巢 left ovary
15. 股神经 femoral nerve
16. 髂腰肌 iliopsoas
17. 髂骨翼 ala of ilium
18. 臀小肌 gluteus minimus
19. 臀中肌 gluteus medius
20. 臀大肌 gluteus maximus
21. 第4骶椎 4th sacral vertebra
22. 梨状肌 piriformis
23. 右臀上动、静脉 right superior gluteal artery and vein
24. 右髂内静脉属支 tributary of right internal iliac vein
25. 右髂外静脉 right external iliac vein
26. 右髂外动脉 right external iliac artery
27. 右卵巢动、静脉 right ovarian artery and vein
28. 子宫底 fundus of uterus
29. 直肠 rectum
30. 肠系膜及肠系膜动、静脉 mesentery and mesenteric artery and vein
31. 子宫体 body of uterus

关键结构：子宫，卵巢，输卵管。

此断面经过第4骶椎椎体中份。

断面中部为骨盆骨性结构，由后正中的第4骶椎和其前方两侧的髂骨翼围成。骨盆前方自中线向两侧由腹直肌、腹内斜肌、腹横肌保护。盆腔内主要被回肠、乙状结肠、直肠、子宫、左卵巢及脂肪组织占据。此断面仍可见子宫底，其断面呈类椭圆形。子宫是女性盆腔中最重要的器官之一，具有孕育胚胎及参与女性内分泌等功能。成人未孕子宫呈前后稍扁、倒置的梨形，大小与年龄及生育有关，未产者长7~9 cm、宽4~5 cm、厚2~3 cm，重50g。子宫自上而下分为底、体与颈3个部分[1]。宫体上部与左、右输卵管相接处为子宫角。两侧髂骨翼前方紧贴髂腰肌，盆腔内还见两侧髂外动、静脉，右侧髂内动、静脉，两侧臀上动、静脉、臀下动、静脉，右卵巢动、静脉，左输卵管，左输尿管，股神经，第3骶神经，坐骨神经断面。骨盆后外侧肌肉组织从内侧向外侧依次为臀小肌、臀中肌、梨状肌、臀大肌。

女性盆部与会阴连续横断层 32（FH.8750）

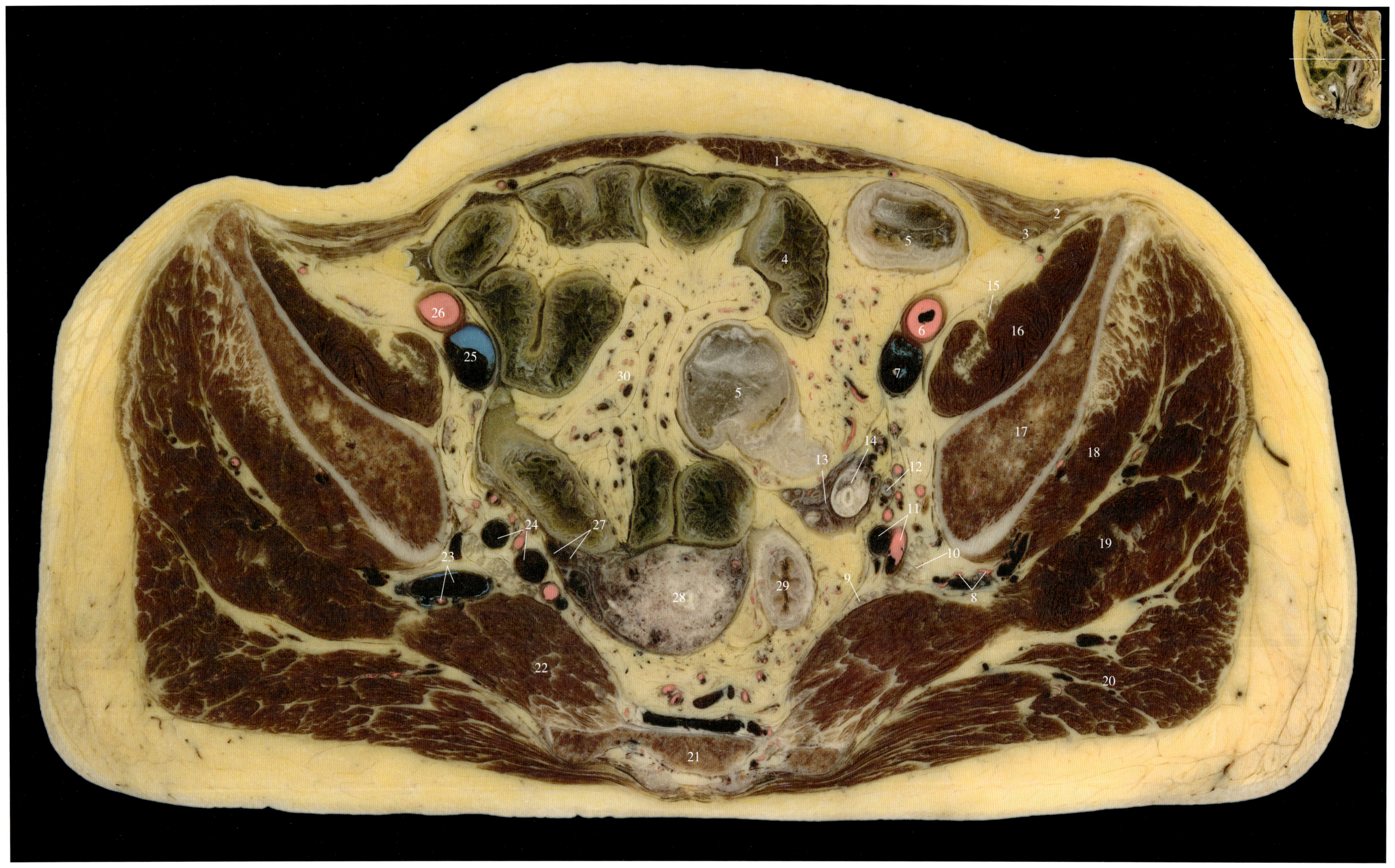

A. 断层标本图像

1. 腹直肌 rectus abdominis
2. 腹内斜肌 obliquus internus abdominis
3. 腹横肌 transversus abdominis
4. 回肠 ileum
5. 乙状结肠 sigmoid colon
6. 左髂外动脉 left external iliac artery
7. 左髂外静脉 left external iliac vein
8. 左臀下动、静脉 left inferior gluteal artery and vein
9. 第3骶神经 3rd sacral nerve
10. 坐骨神经 sciatic nerve
11. 左臀下动、静脉 left inferior gluteal artery and vein
12. 左输尿管 left ureter
13. 左输卵管 left uterine tube
14. 左卵巢 left ovary
15. 股神经 femoral nerve
16. 髂腰肌 iliopsoas
17. 髂骨翼 ala of ilium
18. 臀小肌 gluteus minimus
19. 臀中肌 gluteus medius
20. 臀大肌 gluteus maximus
21. 第4骶椎 4th sacral vertebra
22. 梨状肌 piriformis
23. 右臀上动、静脉 right superior gluteal artery and vein
24. 右髂内静脉属支 tributary of right internal iliac vein
25. 右髂外静脉 right external iliac vein
26. 右髂外动脉 right external iliac artery
27. 右卵巢动、静脉 right ovarian artery and vein
28. 子宫底 fundus of uterus
29. 直肠 rectum
30. 肠系膜及肠系膜动、静脉 mesentery and mesenteric artery and vein
31. 子宫内膜 endometrium
32. 阴道 vaginaa
33. 右卵巢 right ovary
34. 坐骨 ischium
35. 闭孔内肌 obturator internus
36. 坐骨肛门窝 ischioanal fossa
37. 股骨头 femoral head
38. 子宫体 body of uterus
39. 子宫结合带 uterine junction zone
40. 子宫肌层 myometrium of uterus

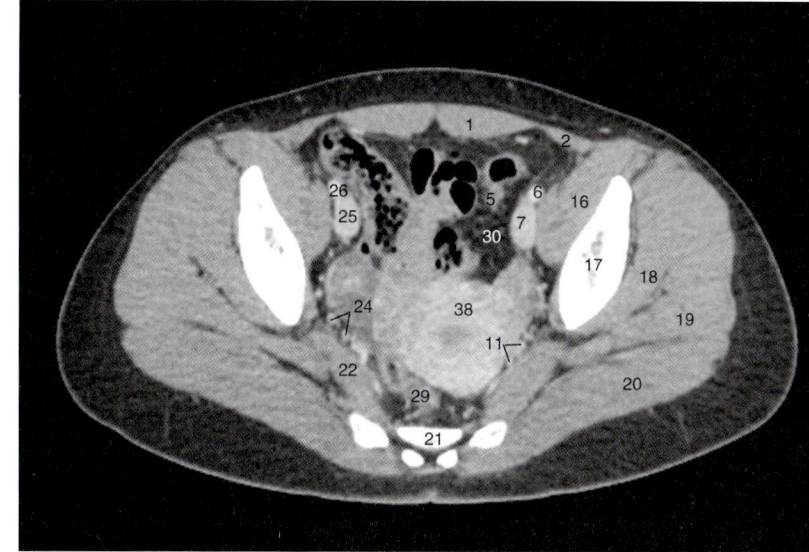

B. CT 增强图像

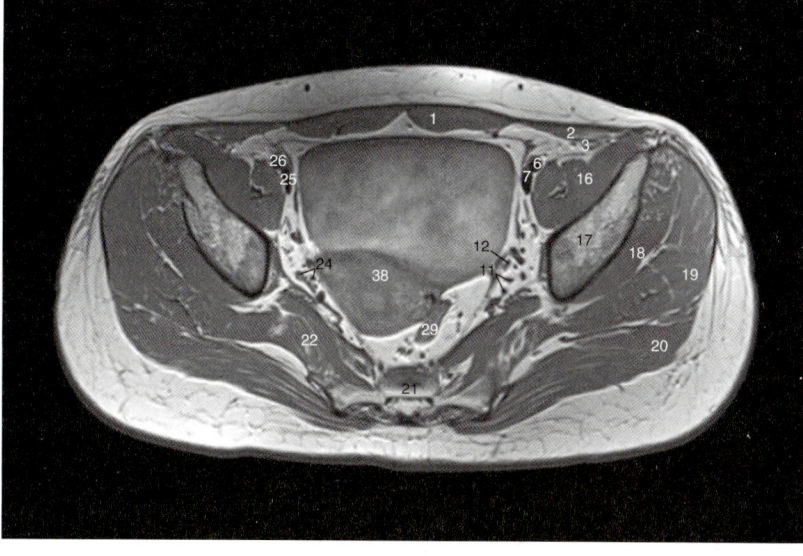

C. MR T1WI

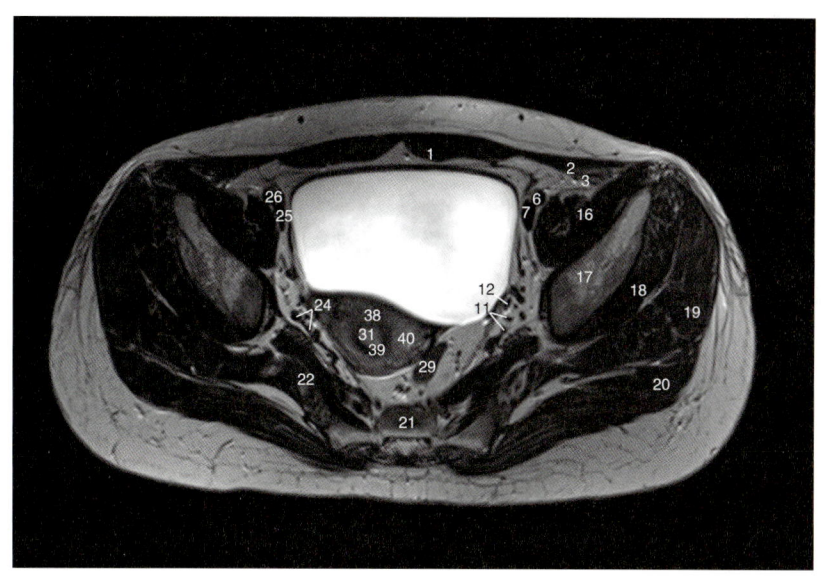

D. MR T2WI

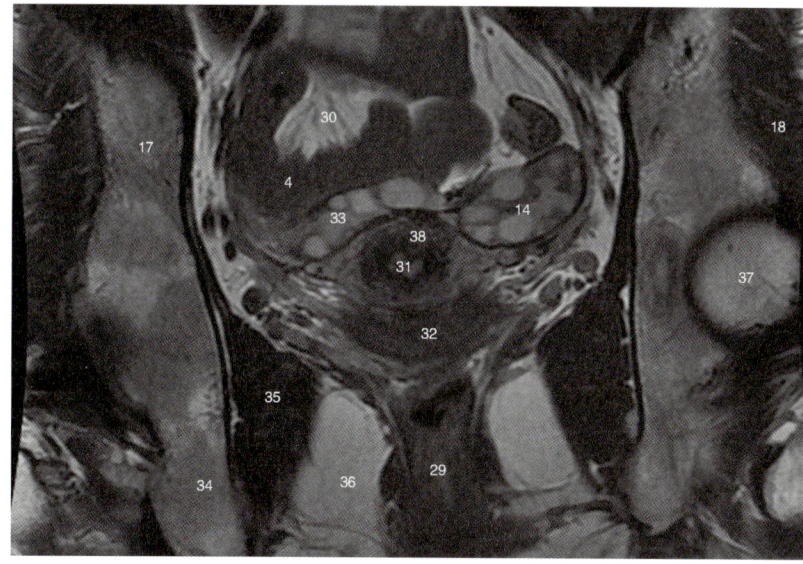

E. 子宫宫底部冠状位 T2WI

关键结构：卵巢，子宫底，输卵管。

此断面经过第4骶椎椎体中份。

较前一断面变化不大。髂骨翼断面缩短，子宫体及左侧卵巢断面增大。卵巢为女性生殖腺，是产生女性生殖细胞卵子和分泌女性激素的器官，呈扁卵圆形，位于子宫两侧，左右各一，被子宫阔韧带后叶所覆盖包绕，即卵巢系膜。内侧通过卵巢固有韧带与子宫相连，外侧通过骨盆漏斗韧带与骨盆壁相连，该韧带内有卵巢血管、淋巴管和神经通行。卵巢为实性器官，由皮质、髓质和卵巢门组成。皮质由生殖上皮、处于不同发育阶段的卵泡和间质组成，是卵巢的主要功能结构；髓质位于卵巢中间，含有血管、淋巴管、神经纤维和结缔组织。卵巢门位于卵巢的前缘中部，是卵巢血管、淋巴管和神经出入的部位。卵巢大小和形状因年龄不同而异。幼年的卵巢小而表面光滑。性成熟期卵巢最大，表面因多次排卵出现瘢痕而凹凸不平。成人卵巢长度左侧为 2.93 cm，右侧为 2.88 cm；宽度左侧为 1.48 cm，右侧为 1.38 cm；厚度左侧为 0.82 cm，右侧为 0.83 cm。卵巢从 35~40 岁开始逐渐缩小，直至老年期。绝经后妇女的卵巢为生育期妇女的 1/2。卵巢大小也与卵泡发育周期变化相关。CT 可显示部分育龄期卵巢，表现为子宫角两侧椭圆形的略低密度，增强扫描轻度强化。MR T2WI 可清晰显示 87%~95% 的育龄期卵巢，卵泡位于周边呈圆形高信号，卵巢内部中央基质呈低信号[1]。

女性盆部与会阴连续横断层 33（FH.8730）

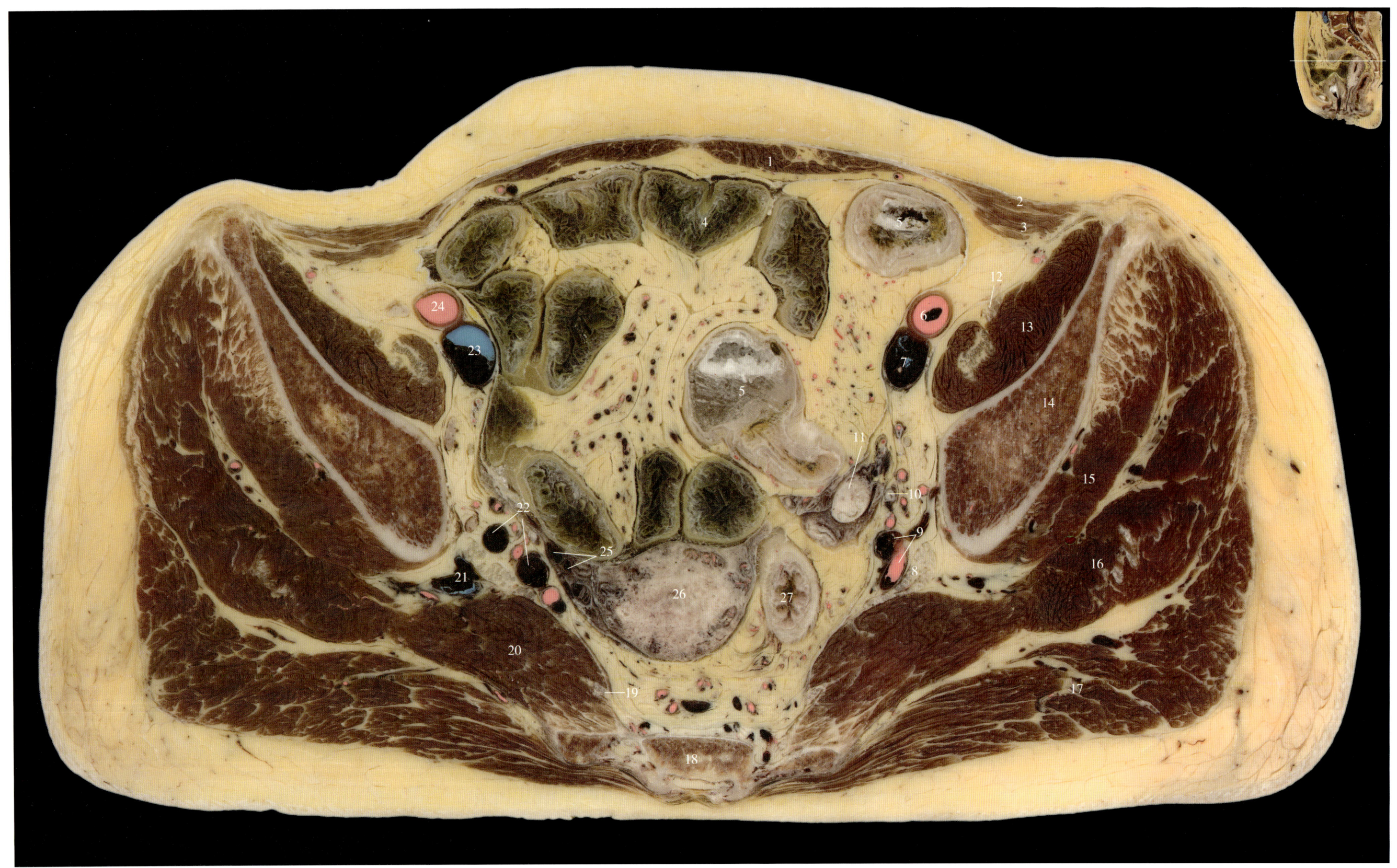

A. 断层标本图像

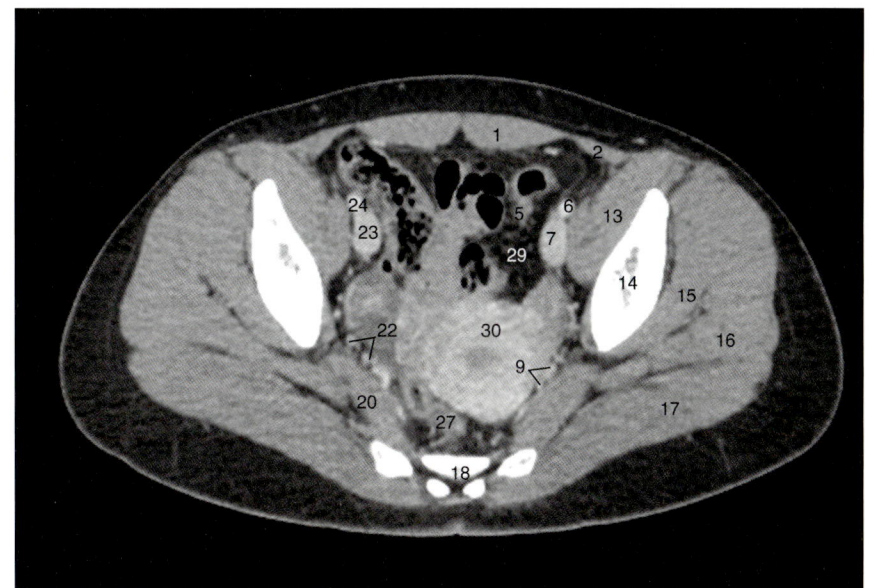

B. CT 增强图像

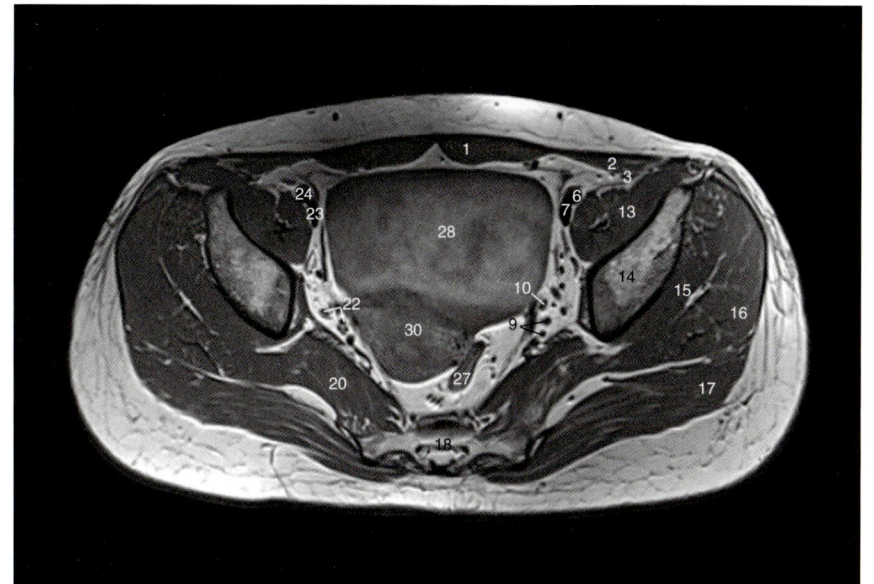

C. MR T1WI

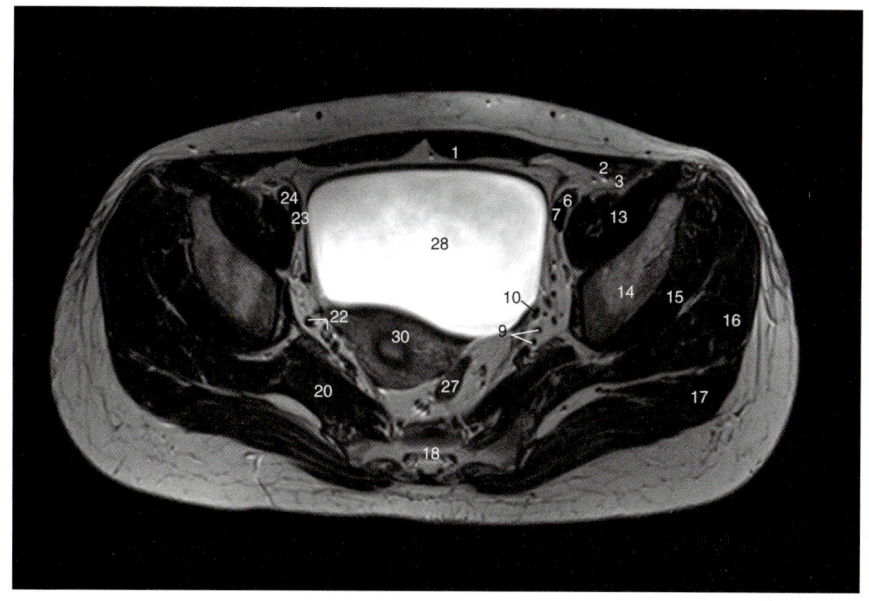

D. MR T2WI

关键结构：直肠，子宫，卵巢。

此断面经过第 4 骶椎椎体下份。

盆腔内肠管仍占据主要空间，乙状结肠被切为前、后两个呈类椭圆形的断面。直肠断面呈卵圆形，居于乙状结肠后断面的后方、子宫体的左侧。直肠上端平第 3 骶椎处接续乙状结肠，沿骶骨和尾骨的前面下行，穿过盆膈，下端以肛门而终，全长约 11 cm。其行程在矢状面上有两个弯曲，骶曲与骶骨盆面曲度一致，凸弯向后，会阴曲在尾骨尖处，凸弯向前。盆膈以上的部分称为直肠盆部，下段肠腔膨大，称为直肠壶腹。盆膈以下的部分缩窄称为肛管或直肠肛门部。直肠壶腹内面的黏膜，形成上、中、下 3 条半月状的直肠横襞，中直肠横襞位于前右侧壁，大而恒定，相当于腹膜返折的水平。在通过乙状肠镜检查确定直肠肿瘤与腹膜腔的位置关系时，常以此横襞作为标志。3 条横襞有支持粪便的作用。CT 图像上，直肠壁在周围低密度脂肪组织、肠腔内更低密度气体及不规则形肠内容物衬托下显示清晰。MR T1WI 及 T2WI 图像上，直肠壁在周围高信号脂肪组织及直肠内低信号气体映衬下显示清晰。T2WI 高分辨序列显示直肠壁呈 3 层结构，最内层略低信号为黏膜层，中间高信号为黏膜下层，外层低信号代表肌层。MRI 对直肠癌的局部分期评估具有重要价值[1, 20]。

1. 腹直肌 rectus abdominis
2. 腹内斜肌 obliquus internus abdominis
3. 腹横肌 transversus abdominis
4. 回肠 ileum
5. 乙状结肠 sigmoid colon
6. 左髂外动脉 left external iliac artery
7. 左髂外静脉 left external iliac vein
8. 坐骨神经 sciatic nerve
9. 左臀下动、静脉 left inferior gluteal artery and vein
10. 左输尿管 left ureter
11. 左卵巢 left ovary
12. 股神经 femoral nerve
13. 髂腰肌 iliopsoas
14. 髂骨翼 ala of ilium
15. 臀小肌 gluteus minimus
16. 臀中肌 gluteus medius
17. 臀大肌 gluteus maximus
18. 第 4 骶椎 4th sacral vertebra
19. 第 4 骶神经 4th sacral nerve
20. 梨状肌 piriformis
21. 右臀上静脉 right superior gluteal vein
22. 右髂内静脉属支 tributaries of right internal iliac vein
23. 右髂外静脉 right external iliac vein
24. 右髂外动脉 right external iliac artery
25. 右卵巢动、静脉 right ovarian artery and vein
26. 子宫底 fundus of uterus
27. 直肠 rectum
28. 膀胱 urinary bladder
29. 肠系膜及肠系膜动、静脉 mesentery and mesenteric artery and vein
30. 子宫体 body of uterus

女性盆部与会阴连续横断层 34（FH.8710）

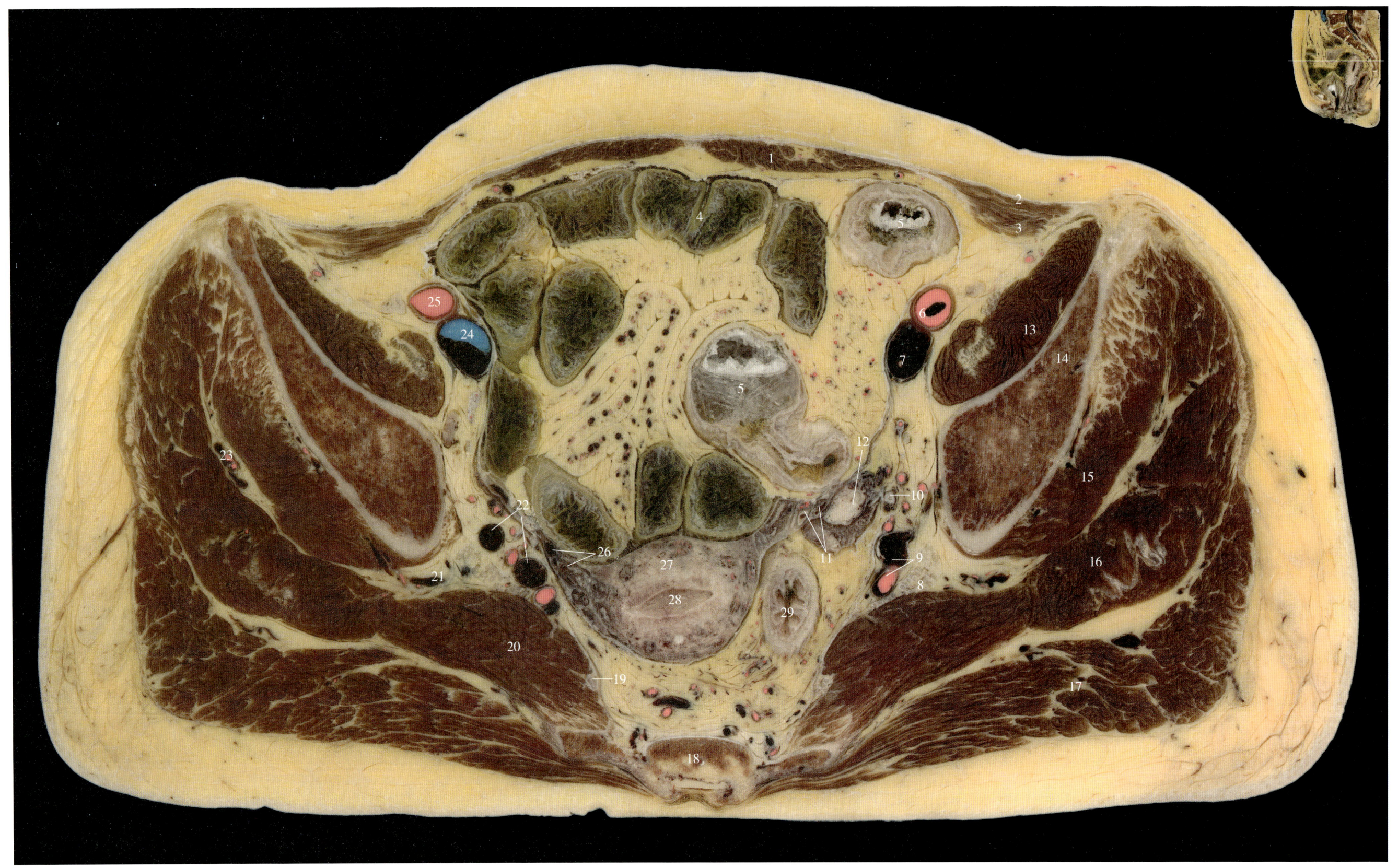

A. 断层标本图像

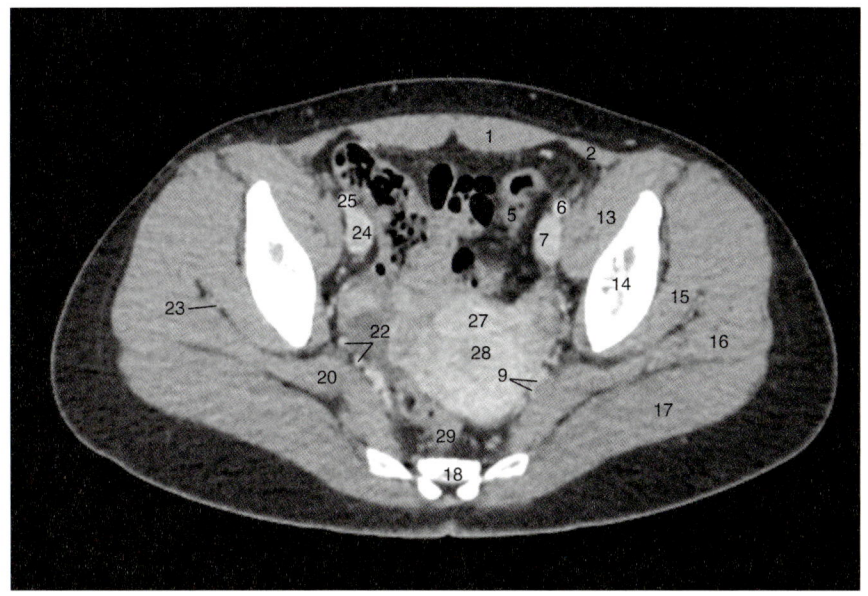

B. CT 增强图像

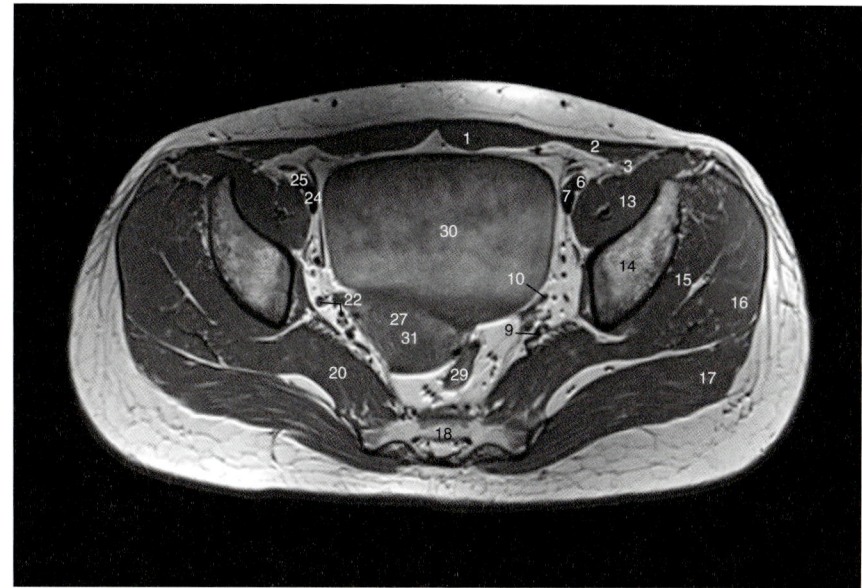

C. MR T1WI

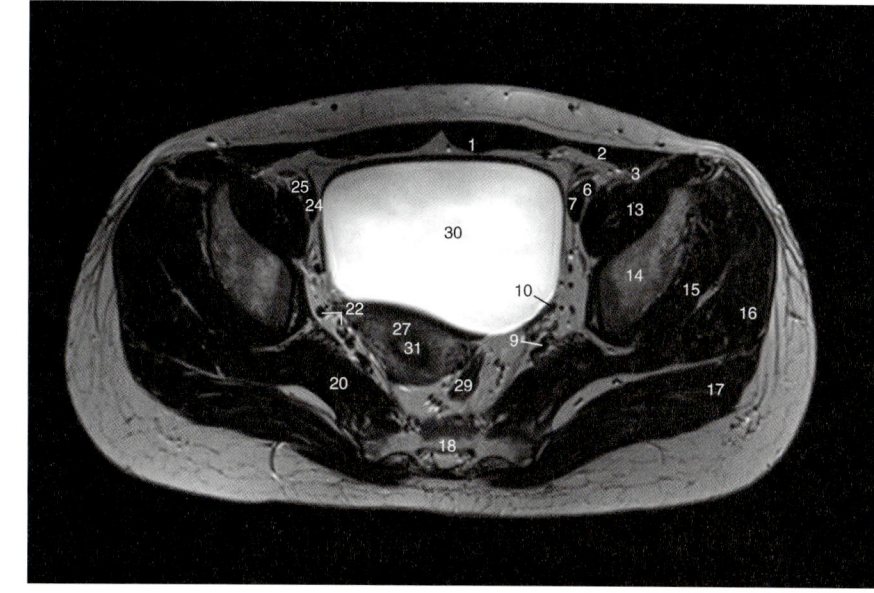

D. MR T2WI

1. 腹直肌 rectus abdominis
2. 腹内斜肌 obliquus internus abdominis
3. 腹横肌 transversus abdominis
4. 回肠 ileum
5. 乙状结肠 sigmoid colon
6. 左髂外动脉 left external iliac artery
7. 左髂外静脉 left external iliac vein
8. 坐骨神经 sciatic nerve
9. 左臀下动、静脉 left inferior gluteal artery and vein
10. 左输尿管 left ureter
11. 左卵巢动、静脉 left ovarian artery and vein
12. 左卵巢 left ovary
13. 髂腰肌 iliopsoas
14. 髂骨翼 ala of ilium
15. 臀小肌 gluteus minimus
16. 臀中肌 gluteus medius
17. 臀大肌 gluteus maximus
18. 第4骶椎 4th sacral vertebra
19. 第4骶神经 4th sacral nerve
20. 梨状肌 piriformis
21. 右臀上动、静脉 right superior gluteal artery and vein
22. 右髂内静脉属支 tributary of right internal iliac vein
23. 右臀上动、静脉分支 branches of right superior gluteal artery and vein
24. 右髂外静脉 right external iliac vein
25. 右髂外动脉 right external iliac artery
26. 右卵巢动、静脉 right ovarian artery and vein
27. 子宫体 body of uterus
28. 子宫腔 cavity of uterus
29. 直肠 rectum
30. 膀胱 urinary bladder
31. 子宫内膜 endometrium

关键结构：卵巢，卵巢动、静脉，子宫腔。

此断面经过第4骶椎体下份。

与上一断面相延续，变化不大。梨状肌位于第4骶椎前方两侧，其内侧缘出现第4骶神经断面，梨状肌前缘见坐骨神经断面。右侧臀小肌与臀中肌之间见右臀上动、静脉断面。此断面出现子宫腔，子宫腔断面呈扁平裂隙状。左侧卵巢断面继续缩小，包绕在其周围的结构为卵巢系膜，是子宫阔韧带后叶的一部分，连于卵巢前缘，较短，内有出入卵巢的血管、淋巴管和神经通过[21]。左卵巢内侧见左卵巢动、静脉断面。国内一项卵巢动脉造影研究显示，95.8%卵巢动脉开口发自腹主动脉前外侧壁，异位开口（副肾动脉、肠系膜下动脉、肾上腺下动脉）占4.2%。左侧卵巢动脉平均直径为0.9 mm ± 0.3 mm，≤ 1.1 mm 者占 98.3%；右侧平均直径为 0.8 mm ± 0.3 mm，≤ 1.1 mm 者占 95.2%。有盆腔疾病患者左侧卵巢动脉直径为 1.7 mm ± 1.1 mm，≥ 1.2 mm 者占 56.2%；右侧为 1.8 mm ± 1.2 mm，≥ 1.2 mm 者占 47.5%。在有盆腔疾病（肿瘤、孕产相关出血性疾病）的患者中，至少有一侧卵巢动脉参与供血者占 35.8%。对参与病变供血的卵巢动脉行栓塞术有助于提高疗效[7, 8]。

女性盆部与会阴连续横断层 35（FH.8690）

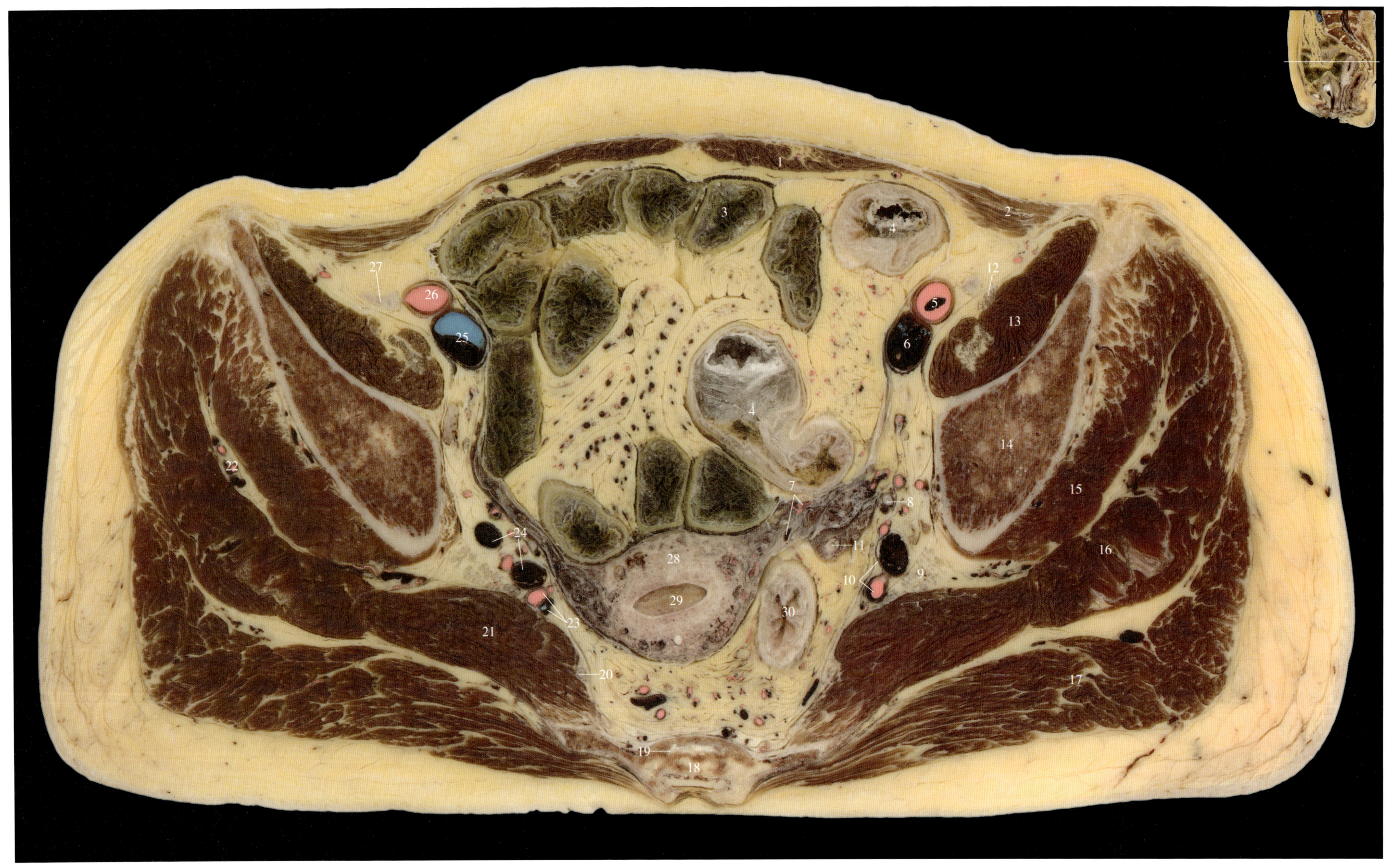

A. 断层标本图像

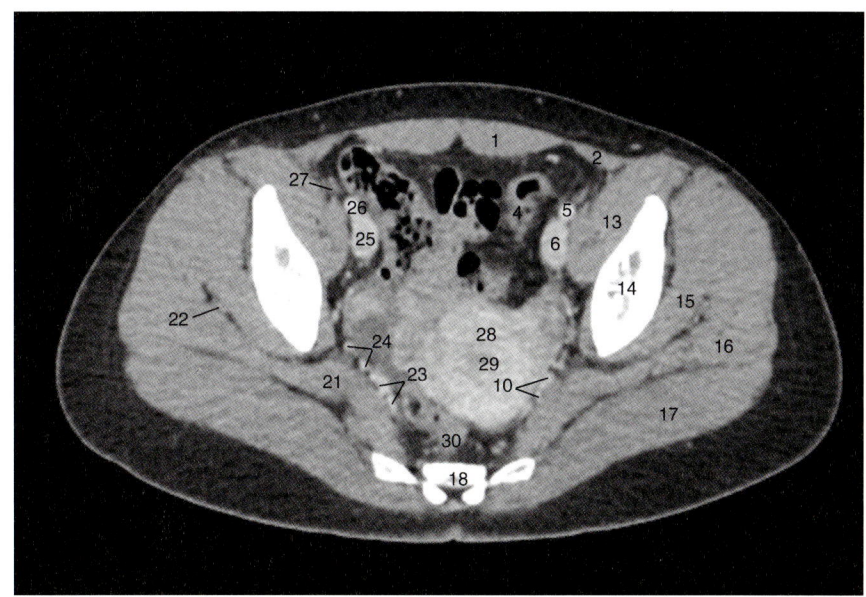
B. CT 增强图像

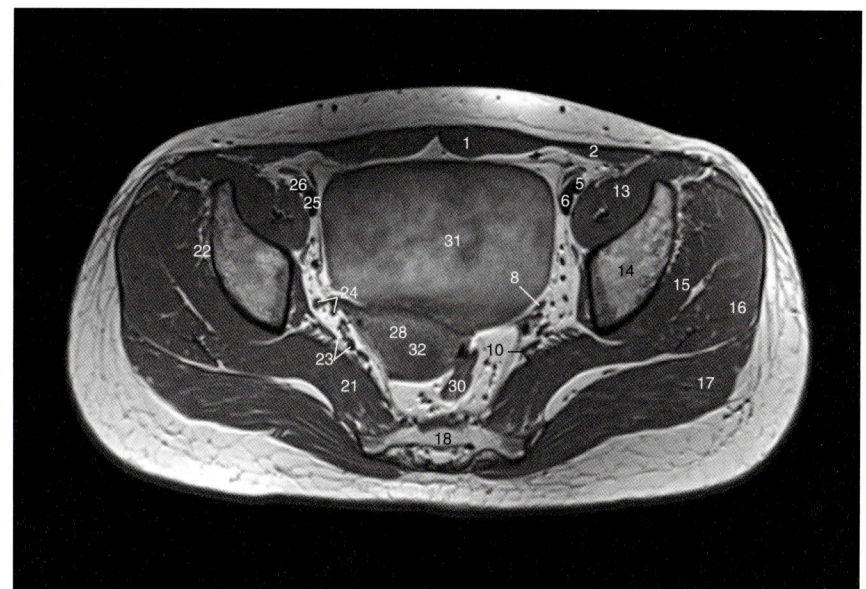
C. MR T1WI

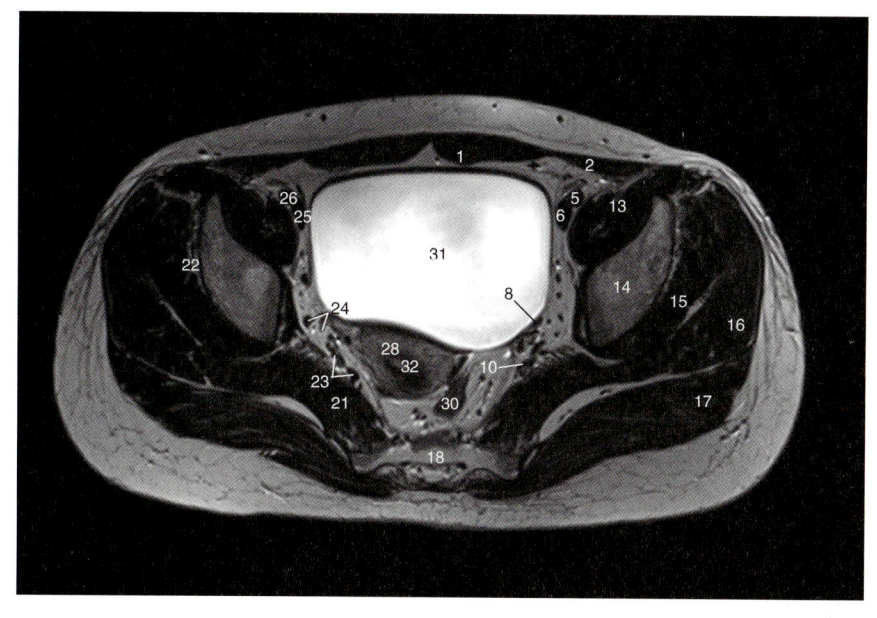
D. MR T2WI

关键结构：髂骨体，髂外淋巴结，髂外动、静脉。

此断面经过第 5 骶椎椎体上份。

第 5 骶椎前方见少许 S4-5 椎间盘断面。髂骨翼逐渐消失，向下延续为髂骨体，近似扇形。两侧髂腰肌位于髂骨体前内侧。髂腰肌断面的前内方自内侧向外侧分别为髂外静脉、髂外动脉及股神经的断面。髂外动脉沿腰大肌内侧缘下行，穿血管腔隙至股部。女性髂外动脉起始部前方有卵巢血管越过，末段前上方有子宫圆韧带斜向越过[22]。两侧髂外动脉外侧见髂外淋巴结断面，其主要功能为收纳腹股沟深浅淋巴结的输出管及下肢和腹前壁下部、膀胱、前列腺、子宫等部分盆内脏器的淋巴液。髂外淋巴结由 3 个亚组组成：外侧、中间和内侧亚组。外侧亚组包括沿髂外动脉侧面分布的淋巴结；中间亚组包括位于髂外动脉和髂外静脉之间的淋巴结，也称为闭孔淋巴结；内侧亚组包含位于髂外静脉内侧和后方的淋巴结[23]。

1. 腹直肌 rectus abdominis
2. 腹内斜肌 obliquus internus abdominis
3. 回肠 ileum
4. 乙状结肠 sigmoid colon
5. 左髂外动脉 left external iliac artery
6. 左髂外静脉 left external iliac vein
7. 左卵巢动、静脉 left ovarian artery and vein
8. 左输尿管 left ureter
9. 坐骨神经 sciatic nerve
10. 左臀下动、静脉 left inferior gluteal artery and vein
11. 左卵巢 left ovary
12. 股神经 femoral nerve
13. 髂腰肌 iliopsoas
14. 髂骨体 body of ilium
15. 臀小肌 gluteus minimus
16. 臀中肌 gluteus medius
17. 臀大肌 gluteus maximus
18. 第 5 骶椎 5th sacral vertebra
19. S4-5 椎间盘 S4-5 intervertebral disc
20. 第 4 骶神经 4th sacral nerve
21. 梨状肌 piriformis
22. 右臀上动、静脉分支 branches of right superior gluteal artery and vein
23. 右臀下动、静脉 right inferior gluteal artery and vein
24. 右髂内静脉属支 tributary of right internal iliac vein
25. 右髂外静脉 right external iliac vein
26. 右髂外动脉 right external iliac artery
27. 右髂外淋巴结 right external iliac lymph nodes
28. 子宫体 body of uterus
29. 子宫腔 cavity of uterus
30. 直肠 rectum
31. 膀胱 urinary bladder
32. 子宫内膜 endometrium

女性盆部与会阴连续横断层 36（FH.8670）

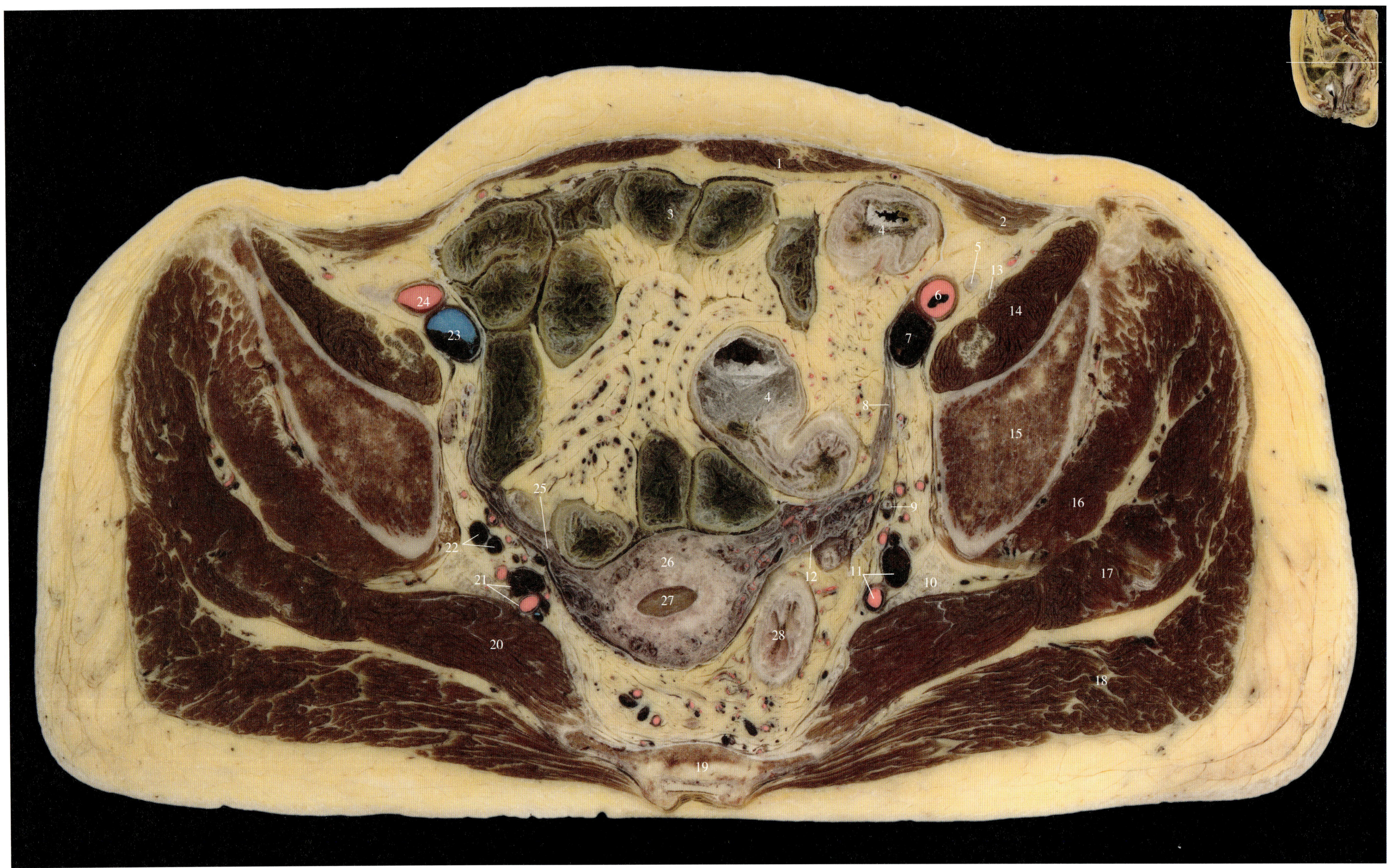

A. 断层标本图像

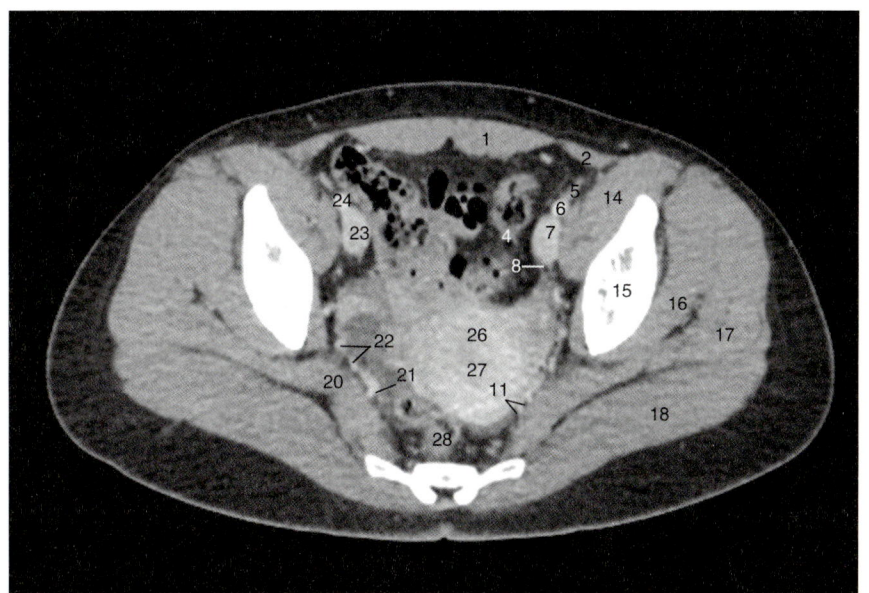
B. CT 增强图像

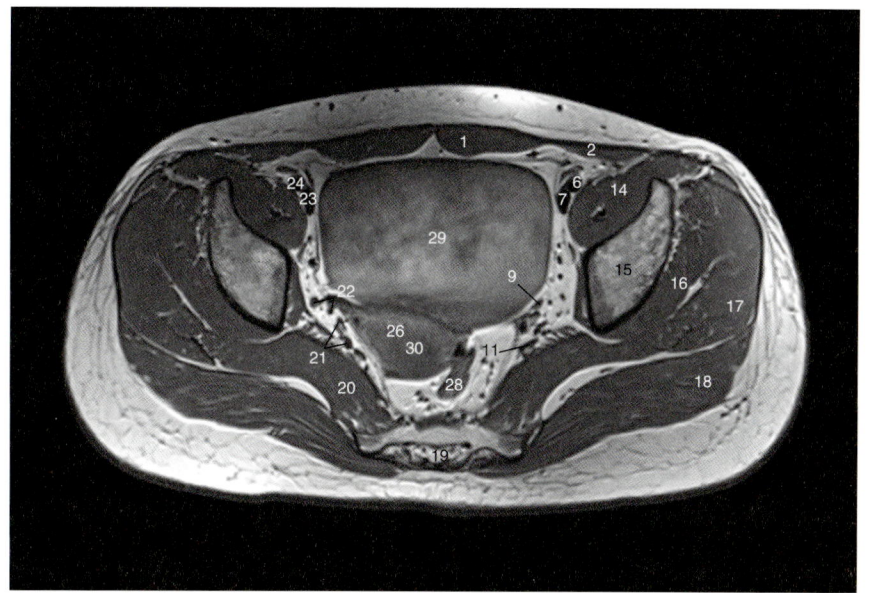
C. MR T1WI

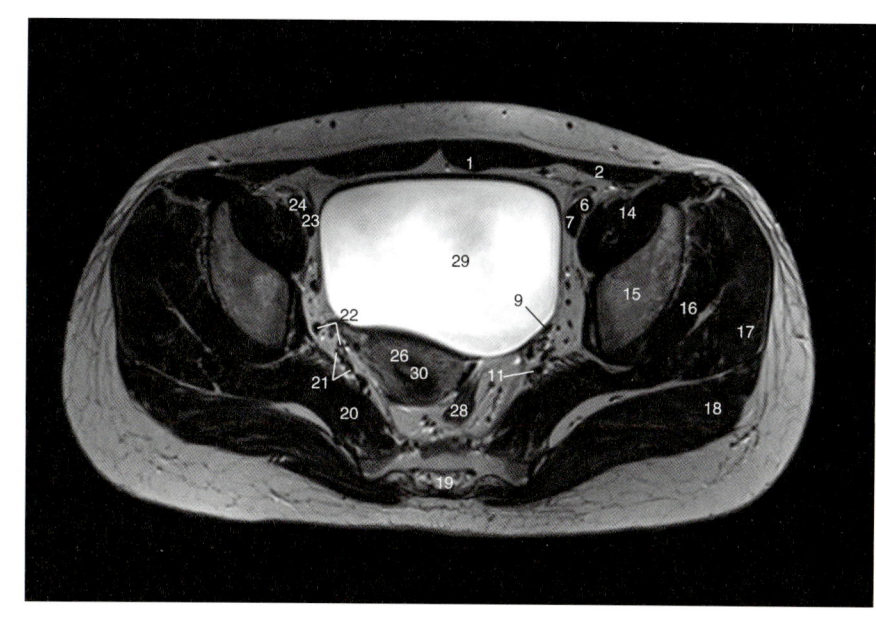
D. MR T2WI

1. 腹直肌 rectus abdominis
2. 腹内斜肌 obliquus internus abdominis
3. 回肠 ileum
4. 乙状结肠 sigmoid colon
5. 左髂外淋巴结 left external iliac lymph nodes
6. 左髂外动脉 left external iliac artery
7. 左髂外静脉 left external iliac vein
8. 子宫圆韧带 round ligament of uterus
9. 左输尿管 left ureter
10. 坐骨神经 sciatic nerve
11. 左臀下动、静脉 left inferior gluteal artery and vein
12. 左输卵管 left uterine tube
13. 股神经 femoral nerve
14. 髂腰肌 iliopsoas
15. 髂骨体 body of ilium

16. 臀小肌 gluteus minimus
17. 臀中肌 gluteus medius
18. 臀大肌 gluteus maximus
19. 第5骶椎 5th sacral vertebra
20. 梨状肌 piriformis
21. 右臀下动、静脉 right inferior gluteal artery and vein
22. 右髂内静脉属支 tributary of right internal iliac vein
23. 右髂外静脉 right external iliac vein
24. 右髂外动脉 right external iliac artery
25. 右输卵管 right uterine tube
26. 子宫体 body of uterus
27. 子宫腔 cavity of uterus
28. 直肠 rectum
29. 膀胱 urinary bladder
30. 子宫内膜 endometrium

关键结构：输卵管，子宫圆韧带，子宫体。

此断面经过第5骶椎上份。

子宫断面呈椭圆形居盆腔中后方，子宫腔断面呈橄榄形。左卵巢在此断面几乎消失不见。左输卵管在此断面显示较为清晰。输卵管是一对细长而弯曲的肌性管道，全长6~15 cm，直径约0.5 mm，位于子宫阔韧带的上缘，被输卵管系膜包绕，内侧端开口于子宫角，外侧端游离开口于腹膜腔，与卵巢相邻。输卵管走行弯曲，由内向外侧分四部分：间质部、峡部、壶腹部、漏斗部，末端边缘形成多个细长的指状突起，称为输卵管伞。卵子通常在壶腹部与精子结合成受精卵，经输卵管子宫口入子宫腔，植入子宫内膜发育成胎儿[1]。盆腔炎症可导致输卵管粘连而引起部分阻塞，受精卵可能无法到达子宫，种植在输卵管黏膜上形成异位妊娠，壶腹部最常发生。输卵管妊娠破裂引起的出血可导致胚胎死亡并会危及母亲生命[24]。因输卵管纤细，CT及MRI均不易识别。子宫输卵管碘油造影及低浓度过氧化氢子宫输卵管声学造影可确定输卵管是否畅通及阻塞部位[1]。子宫圆韧带在本断面显示清晰。子宫借韧带、阴道、尿生殖膈和盆底肌等保持其正常位置，韧带是其重要固定装置，包括子宫阔韧带、子宫圆韧带、子宫主韧带和子宫骶韧带，将分别在后续断面对其展开介绍[25]。

女性盆部与会阴连续横断层 37（FH.8650）

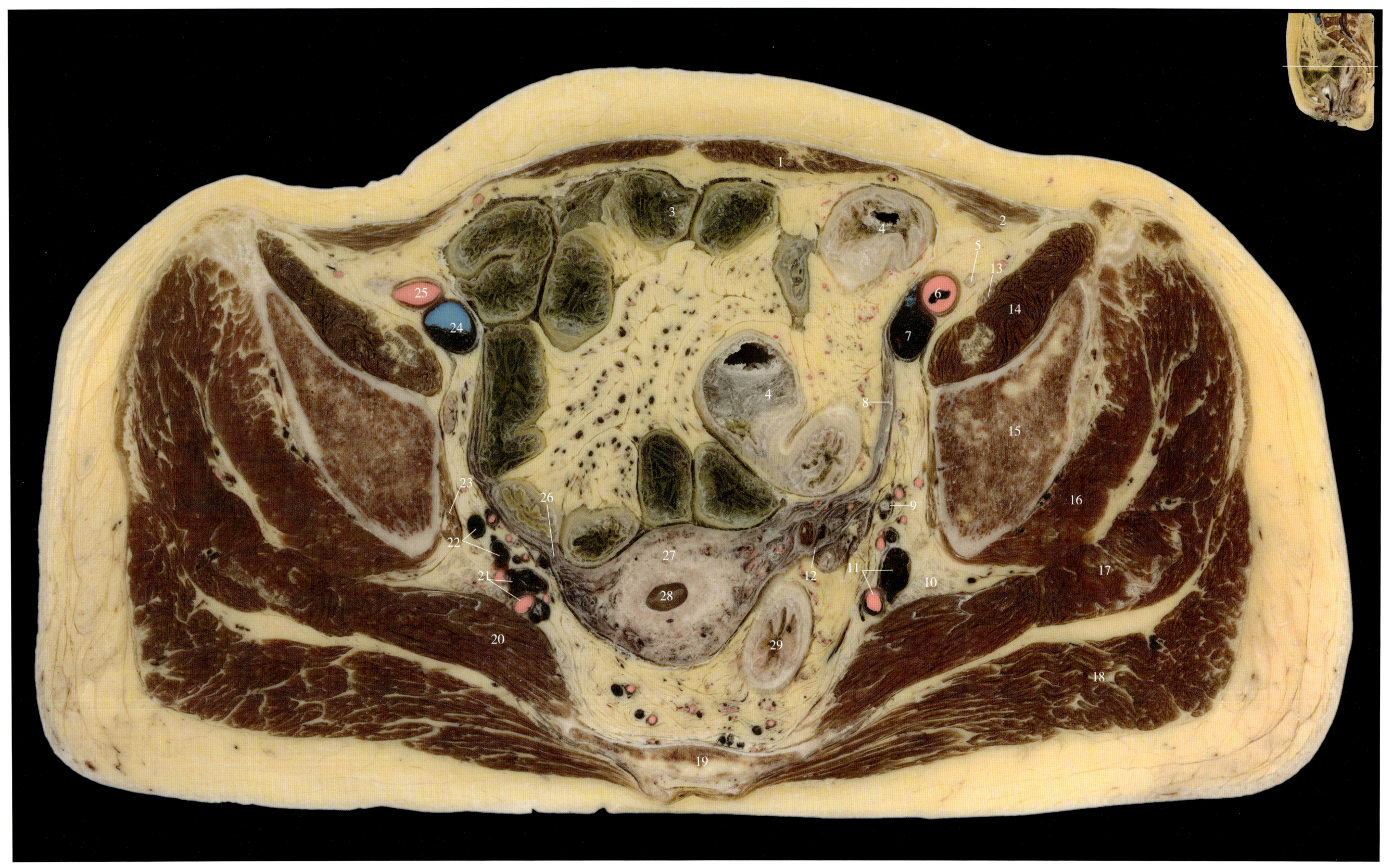

A. 断层标本图像

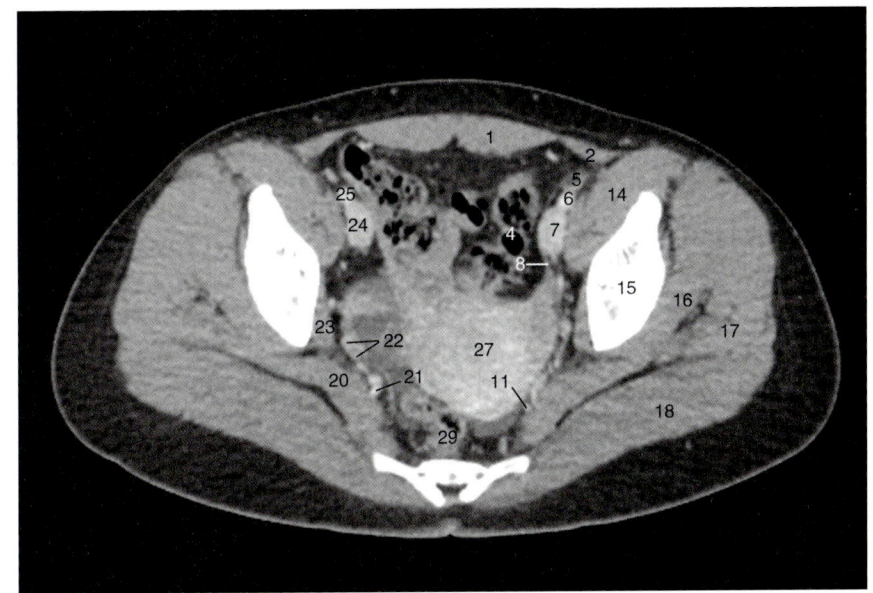
B. CT 增强图像

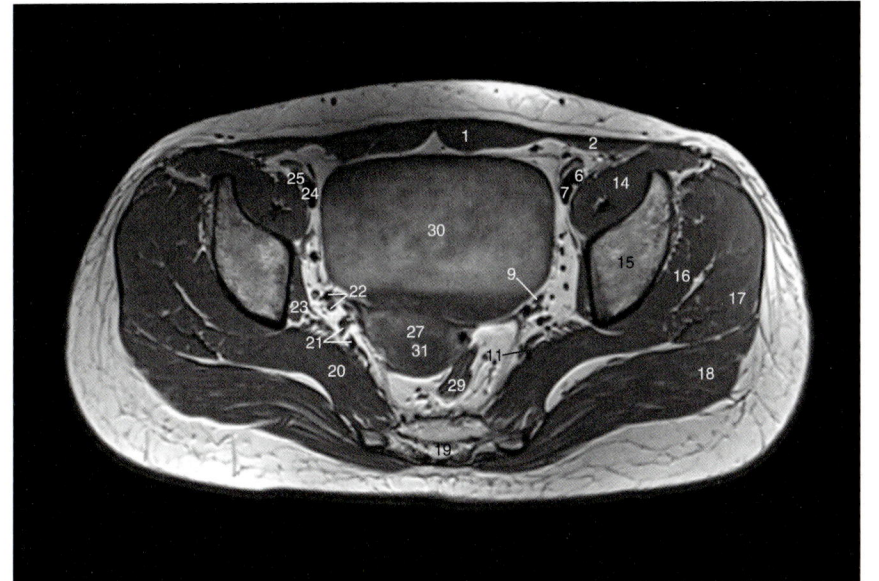
C. MR T1WI

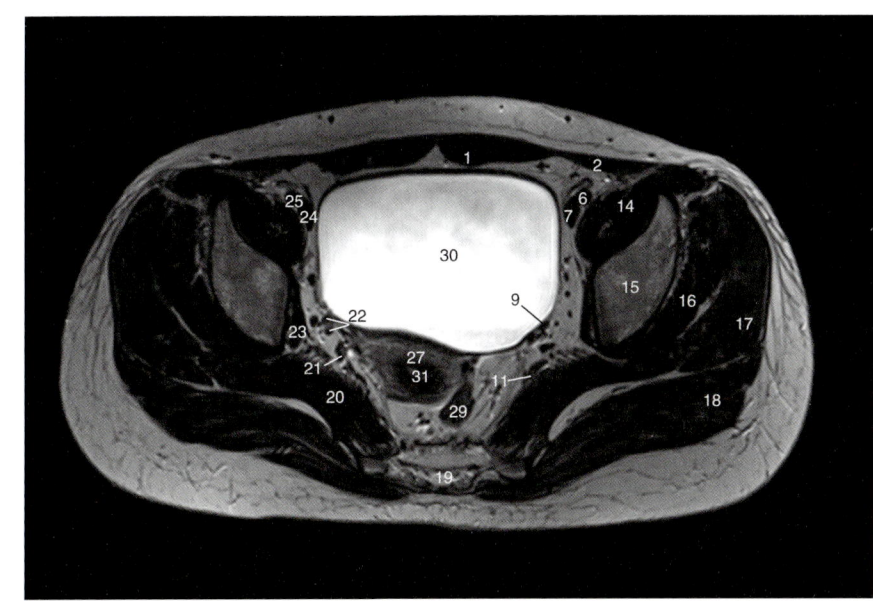
D. MR T2WI

1. 腹直肌 rectus abdominis
2. 腹内斜肌 obliquus internus abdominis
3. 回肠 ileum
4. 乙状结肠 sigmoid colon
5. 左髂外淋巴结 left external iliac lymph nodes
6. 左髂外动脉 left external iliac artery
7. 左髂外静脉 left external iliac vein
8. 子宫圆韧带 round ligament of uterus
9. 左输尿管 left ureter
10. 坐骨神经 sciatic nerve
11. 左臀下动、静脉 left inferior gluteal artery and vein
12. 左输卵管 left uterine tube
13. 股神经 femoral nerve
14. 髂腰肌 iliopsoas
15. 髂骨体 body of ilium
16. 臀小肌 gluteus minimus
17. 臀中肌 gluteus medius
18. 臀大肌 gluteus maximus
19. 第 5 骶椎 5th sacral vertebra
20. 梨状肌 piriformis
21. 右臀下动、静脉 right inferior gluteal artery and vein
22. 右髂内静脉属支 right tributary of internal iliac vein
23. 闭孔内肌 obturator internus
24. 右髂外静脉 right external iliac vein
25. 右髂外动脉 right external iliac artery
26. 右输卵管 right uterine tube
27. 子宫体 body of uterus
28. 子宫腔 cavity of uterus
29. 直肠 rectum
30. 膀胱 urinary bladder
31. 子宫内膜 endometrium

关键结构：闭孔内肌，子宫体，子宫内膜。

此断面经过第 5 骶椎椎体中份。

较前一断面的重要变化为闭孔内肌开始出现。闭孔内肌为盆壁肌组成肌肉之一，位于骨盆侧壁前份，起自闭孔膜内面及周围骨面，止于股骨大转子内侧、股骨转子窝前方，由腰骶干和第 1、2 骶神经支配[26]。在横断面上，闭孔内肌位于两侧髂骨体内侧。子宫断面呈椭圆形居盆腔中后方，子宫腔断面呈椭圆形。宫腔表面覆盖的黏膜为子宫内膜，出生时，子宫内膜较薄，厚度仅为 0.2~0.4 cm，表面有一层立方上皮，间质稀疏。在婴幼儿至青春期前，子宫内膜腺体呈单层矮立方状，处于静止状态。当女性 17~18 岁时，子宫形状与生育年龄的形状接近，子宫内膜开始增生、变厚，可达 0.7~0.8 cm，其间可见血管生成，并开始伴随卵巢周期激素发生变化。在初潮 1~2 年内，由于卵巢无排卵，子宫内膜为增生期反应。至卵巢排卵，子宫内膜开始有分泌期变化，出现周期性脱落[21]。生育期子宫内膜分为 3 层，自宫腔面向外依次为致密层、海绵层和基底层，前二者为功能层，厚度约占 2/3，受卵巢分泌激素的影响，发生周期性脱落。基底层约占 1/3，不发生脱落，月经后向宫腔再生黏膜。MR T2WI 图像能显示育龄期子宫内膜依月经周期发生的厚度变化，矢状位 T2WI 显示最清晰。子宫内膜在增生早期最薄，厚度约为 2 mm；分泌中、晚期增厚，可达 10 mm。绝经期后子宫内膜变薄。育龄期妇女子宫内膜厚度 >10 mm、绝经后妇女 >4 mm，认为存在子宫内膜异常可能[1]。

女性盆部与会阴连续横断层 38（FH.8630）

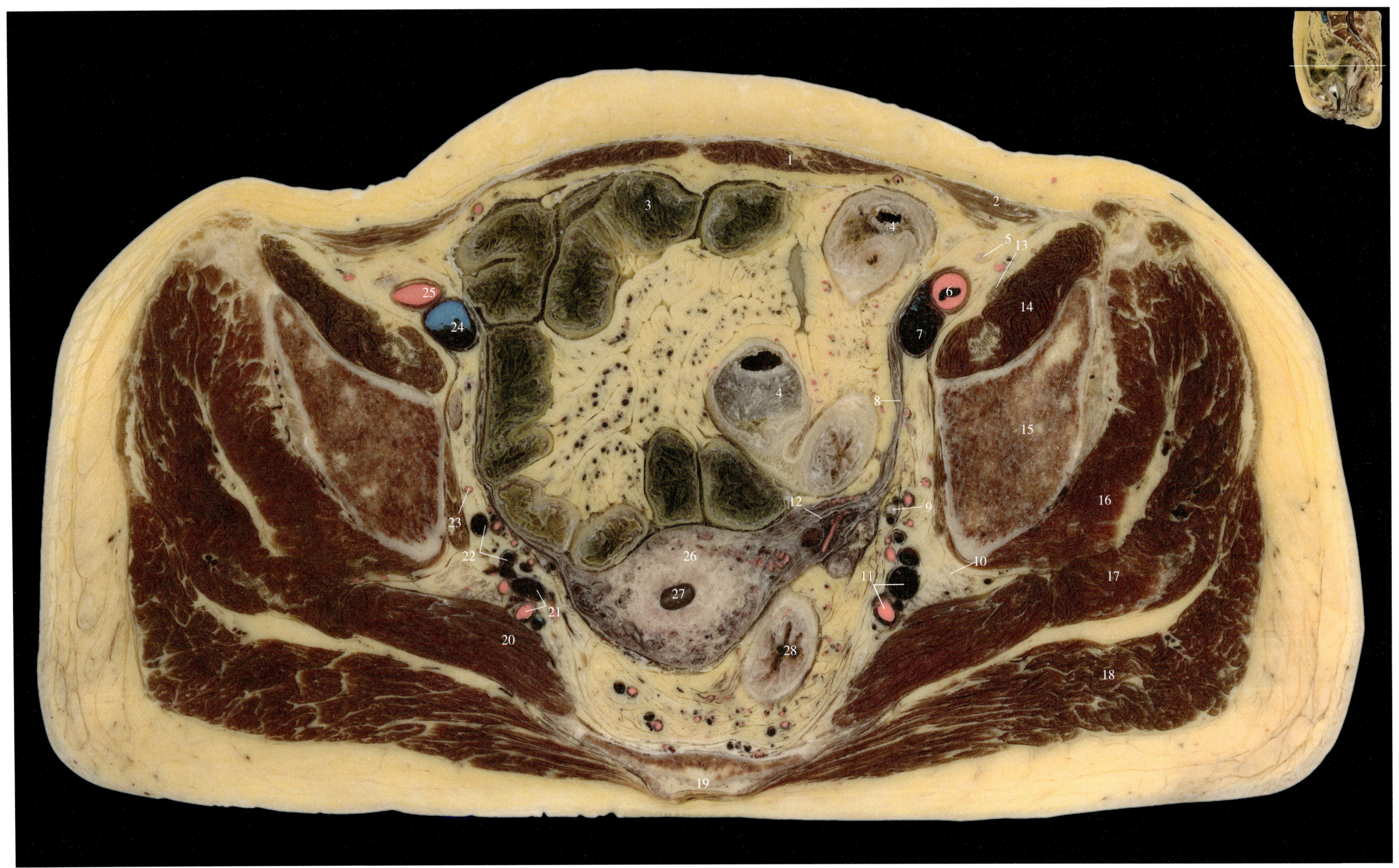

A. 断层标本图像

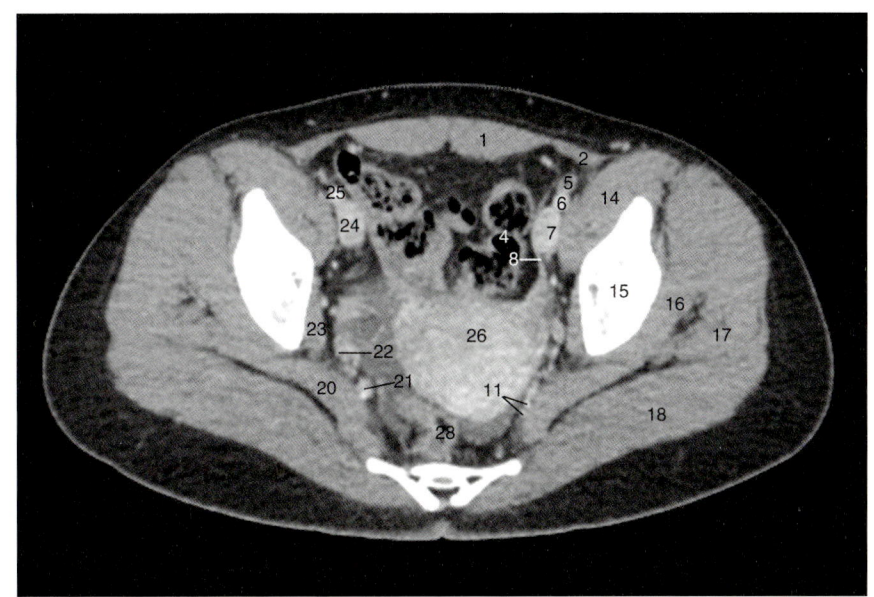

B. CT 增强图像

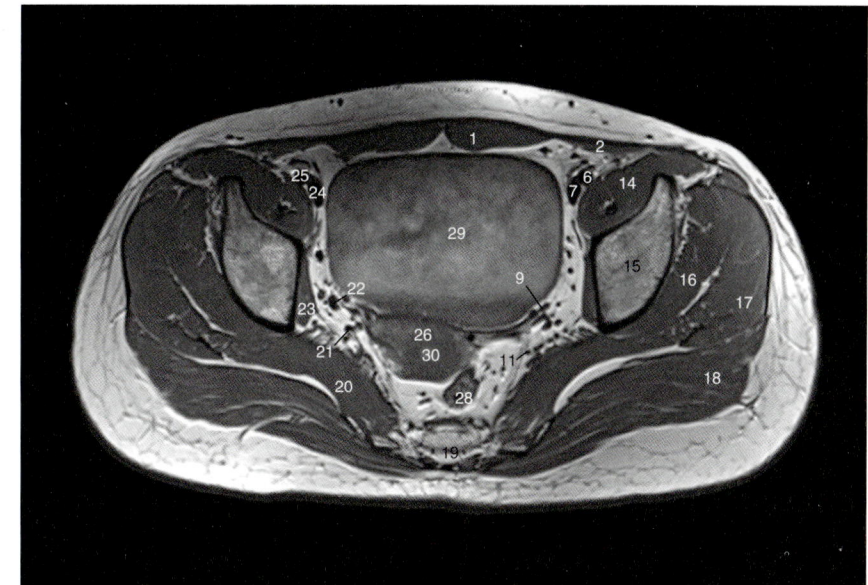

C. MR T1WI

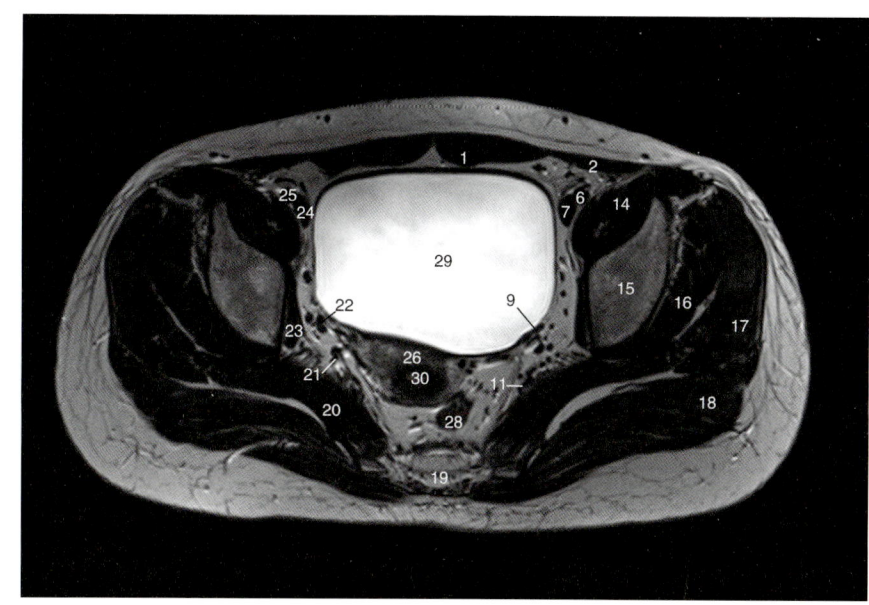

D. MR T2WI

1. 腹直肌 rectus abdominis
2. 腹内斜肌 obliquus internus abdominis
3. 回肠 ileum
4. 乙状结肠 sigmoid colon
5. 左髂外淋巴结 left external iliac lymph nodes
6. 左髂外动脉 left external iliac artery
7. 左髂外静脉 left external iliac vein
8. 子宫圆韧带 round ligament of uterus
9. 左输尿管 left ureter
10. 坐骨神经 sciatic nerve
11. 左臀下动、静脉 left inferior gluteal artery and vein
12. 左输卵管 left uterine tube
13. 股神经 femoral nerve
14. 髂腰肌 iliopsoas
15. 髂骨体 body of ilium
16. 臀小肌 gluteus minimus
17. 臀中肌 gluteus medius
18. 臀大肌 gluteus maximus
19. 第 5 骶椎 5th sacral vertebra
20. 梨状肌 piriformis
21. 右臀下动、静脉 right inferior gluteal artery and vein
22. 右髂内静脉属支 right tributary of internal iliac vein
23. 闭孔内肌 obturator internus
24. 右髂外静脉 right external iliac vein
25. 右髂外动脉 right external iliac artery
26. 子宫体 body of uterus
27. 子宫腔 cavity of uterus
28. 直肠 rectum
29. 膀胱 urinary bladder
30. 子宫内膜 endometrium

关键结构：髂骨体，子宫体，子宫圆韧带。

此断面经过第 5 骶椎椎体下份。

断面中部为骨盆腔，在该断面由位于后正中的第 5 骶椎和两侧近似扇形的髂骨体围成。髂骨体内侧见闭孔内肌断面，较上一断面略增大。盆腔前方自中线向两侧依次见腹直肌、腹内斜肌断面。盆腔内中后部重要结构为子宫，子宫体及子宫腔断面均呈椭圆形。子宫体前方主要由肠管、肠系膜、脂肪组织占据，偏左侧颜色浅者为乙状结肠断面，偏右侧呈暗绿色为回肠断面。子宫体右侧见右侧髂内动、静脉断面。子宫体左后方见卵圆形直肠断面。盆腔内另见位于髂骨体前方的髂腰肌、髂外静脉、髂外动脉、髂外淋巴结及股神经的断面，位于子宫左侧的左输卵管、子宫圆韧带、左输尿管及左臀下动、静脉断面。

女性盆部与会阴连续横断层 39（FH.8610）

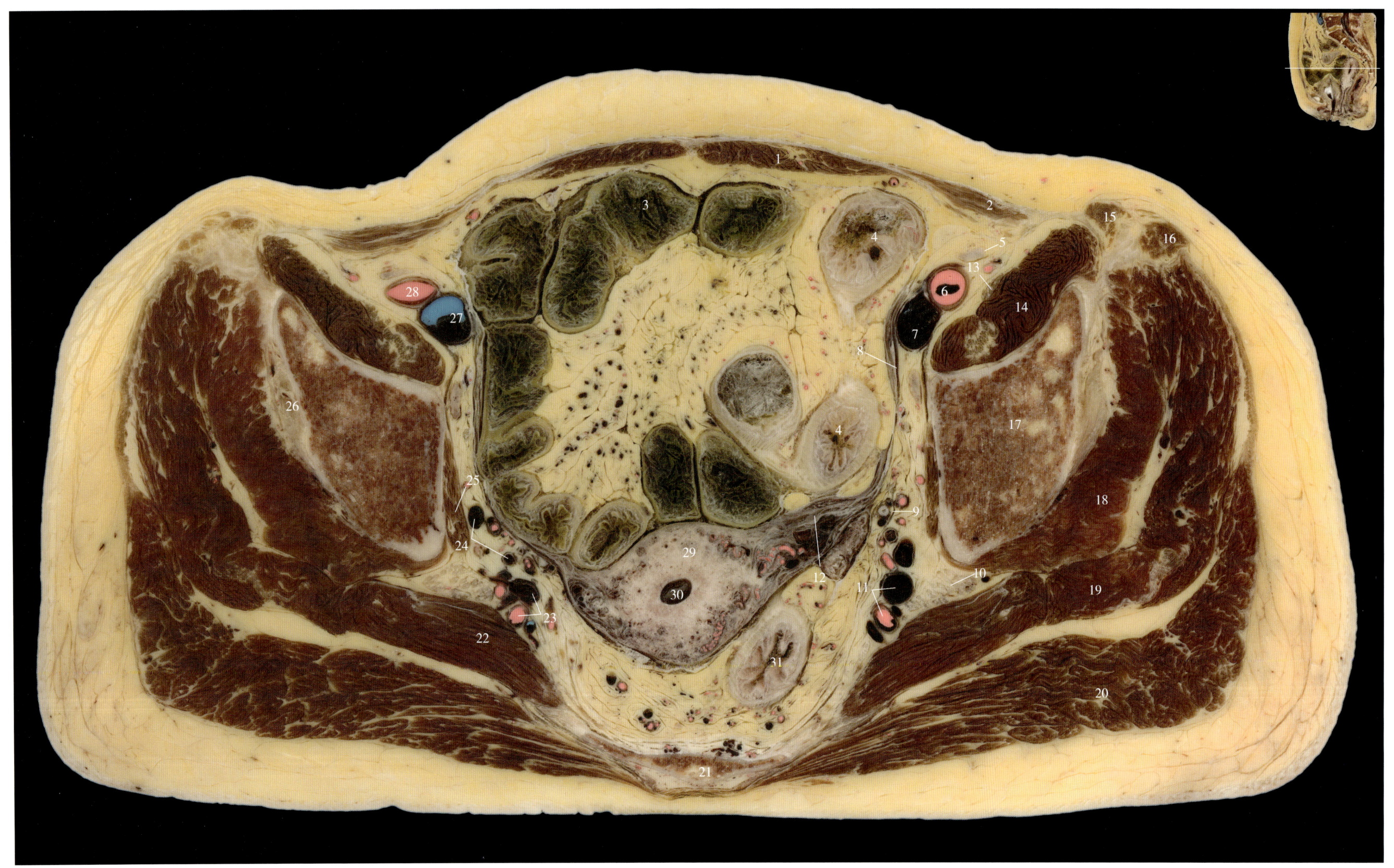

A. 断层标本图像

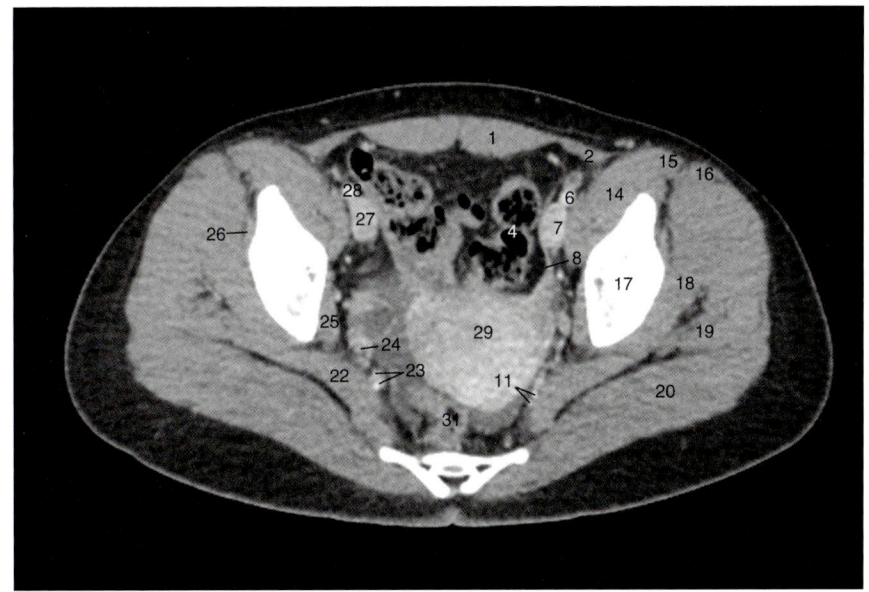

B. CT 增强图像

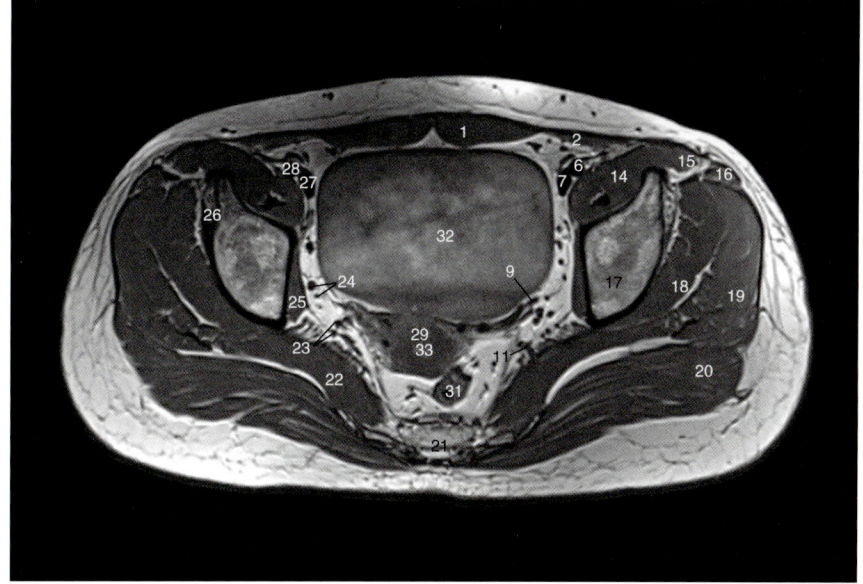

C. MR T1WI

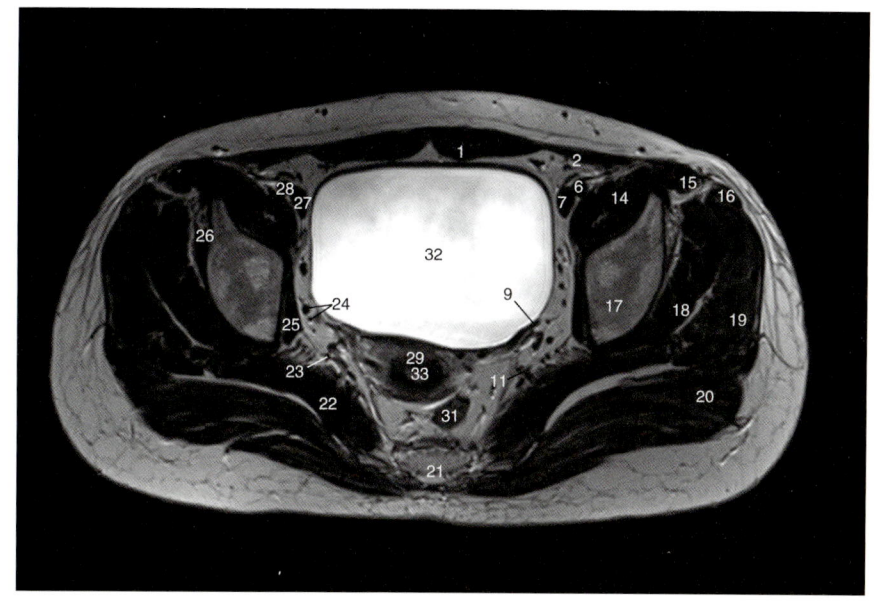

D. MR T2WI

关键结构：子宫圆韧带，缝匠肌，阔筋膜张肌，髂股韧带。

1. 腹直肌 rectus abdominis
2. 腹内斜肌 obliquus internus abdominis
3. 回肠 ileum
4. 乙状结肠 sigmoid colon
5. 左髂外淋巴结 left external iliac lymph nodes
6. 左髂外动脉 left external iliac artery
7. 左髂外静脉 left external iliac vein
8. 子宫圆韧带 round ligament of uterus
9. 左输尿管 left ureter
10. 坐骨神经 sciatic nerve
11. 左臀下动、静脉 left inferior gluteal artery and vein
12. 左输卵管 left uterine tube
13. 股神经 femoral nerve
14. 髂腰肌 iliopsoas
15. 缝匠肌 sartorius
16. 阔筋膜张肌 tensor fasciae latae
17. 髂骨体 body of ilium
18. 臀小肌 gluteus minimus
19. 臀中肌 gluteus medius
20. 臀大肌 gluteus maximus
21. 第 5 骶椎 5th sacral vertebra
22. 梨状肌 piriformis
23. 右臀下动、静脉 right inferior gluteal artery and vein
24. 右髂内静脉属支 right tributary of internal iliac vein
25. 闭孔内肌 obturator internus
26. 髂股韧带 iliofemoral ligament
27. 右髂外静脉 right external iliac vein
28. 右髂外动脉 right external iliac artery
29. 子宫体 body of uterus
30. 子宫腔 cavity of uterus
31. 直肠 rectum
32. 膀胱 urinary bladder
33. 子宫内膜 endometrium

此断面经过第 5 骶椎椎体下份。

髂骨体断面继续缩短呈近似扇形，子宫体断面继续增大。子宫和两侧盆壁之间见圆索状的子宫圆韧带，由结缔组织和平滑肌纤维构成，长度为 12~14 cm，起自子宫角的下方（或输卵管子宫口的下方），在阔韧带前叶的覆盖下向前外侧弯行，由腹环进入腹股沟管，出皮下环后分散为纤维束，止于阴阜和大阴唇皮下，分为盆段、腹段和腹股沟段。对维持子宫前倾起重要作用。子宫圆韧带有淋巴管分布，子宫的恶性肿瘤可经此韧带转移至腹股沟浅淋巴结近侧群[21]。在本断层，于左髂腰肌外侧、左臀小肌和臀中肌前方自内侧向外侧依次见缝匠肌和阔筋膜张肌断面出现。缝匠肌是人体最长的肌肉，起自髂前上棘，向前内下方走行，止于胫骨体上端内侧，起屈曲、内收、外旋髋关节及屈曲并内收膝关节的作用[25]。阔筋膜张肌同样起自髂前上棘，而向下走行止于胫骨外侧髁，起紧张阔筋膜并屈髋关节作用。本断层髂股韧带已出现，位于髂骨体与臀小肌之间，髋关节即将出现，髋关节囊周围有许多韧带，髂股韧带位于关节囊前部，起自髂前下棘，止于股骨转子间线，呈"Y"形，维持直立及防止关节向前脱位[12]。

女性盆部与会阴连续横断层 40（FH.8590）

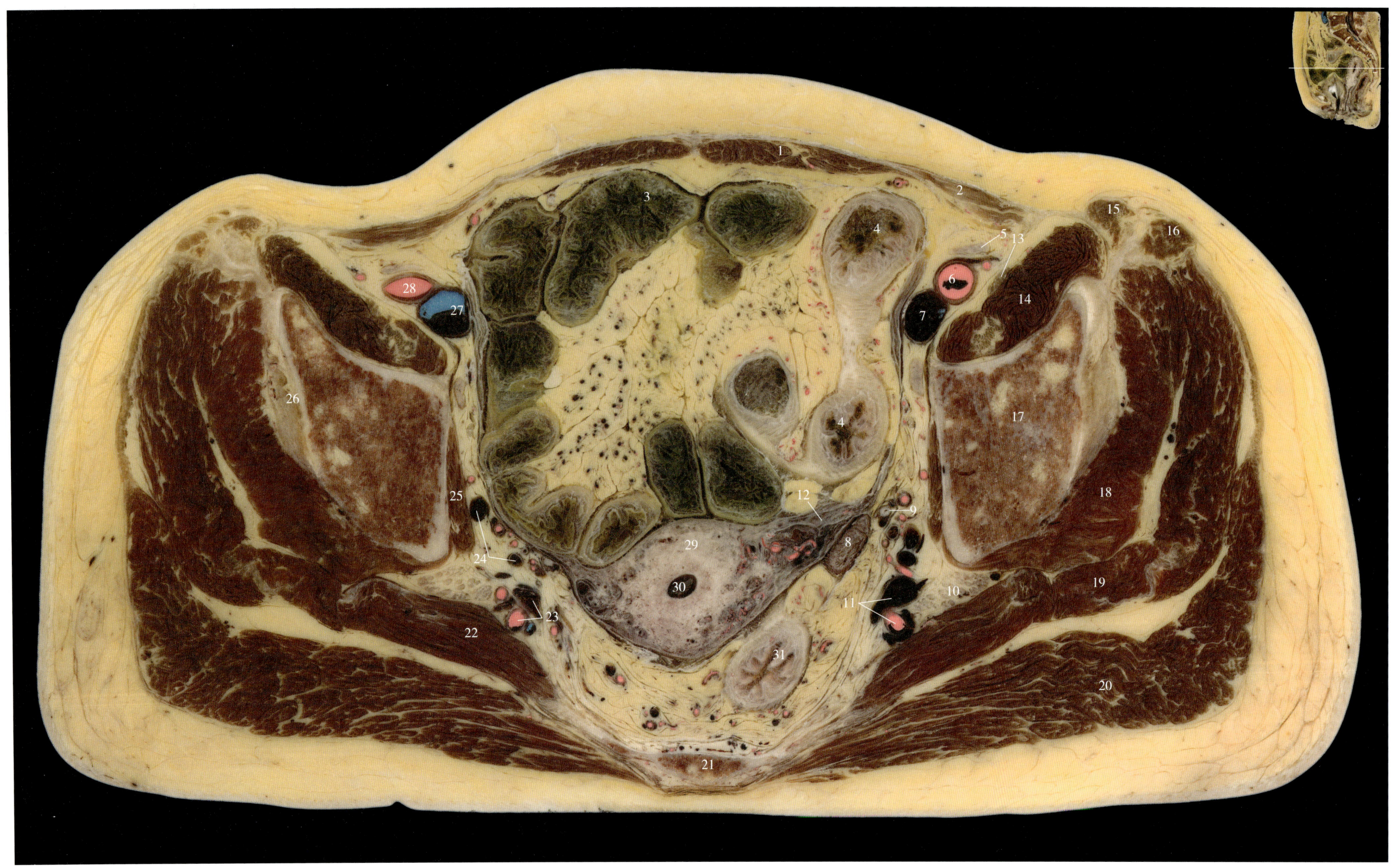

A. 断层标本图像

1. 腹直肌 rectus abdominis
2. 腹内斜肌 obliquus internus abdominis
3. 回肠 ileum
4. 乙状结肠 sigmoid colon
5. 左髂外淋巴结 left external iliac lymph nodes
6. 左髂外动脉 left external iliac artery
7. 左髂外静脉 left external iliac vein
8. 左卵巢 left ovary
9. 左输尿管 left ureter
10. 坐骨神经 sciatic nerve
11. 左臀下动、静脉 left inferior gluteal artery and vein
12. 左输卵管 left uterine tube
13. 股神经 femoral nerve
14. 髂腰肌 iliopsoas
15. 缝匠肌 sartorius
16. 阔筋膜张肌 tensor fasciae latae
17. 髂骨体 body of ilium
18. 臀小肌 gluteus minimus
19. 臀中肌 gluteus medius
20. 臀大肌 gluteus maximus
21. 尾骨 coccyx
22. 梨状肌 piriformis
23. 右臀下动、静脉 right inferior gluteal artery and vein
24. 右髂内静脉属支 right tributary of internal iliac vein
25. 闭孔内肌 obturator internus
26. 髂股韧带 iliofemoral ligament
27. 右髂外静脉 right external iliac vein
28. 右髂外动脉 right external iliac artery
29. 子宫体 body of uterus
30. 子宫腔 cavity of uterus
31. 直肠 rectum
32. 膀胱 urinary bladder
33. 子宫底 fundus of uterus
34. 子宫颈 neck of uterus
35. 宫颈黏膜 cervical mucosa
36. 阴道 vagina
37. 子宫内膜 endometrium
38. 子宫结合带 uterine junction zone
39. 子宫肌层 myometrium of uterus

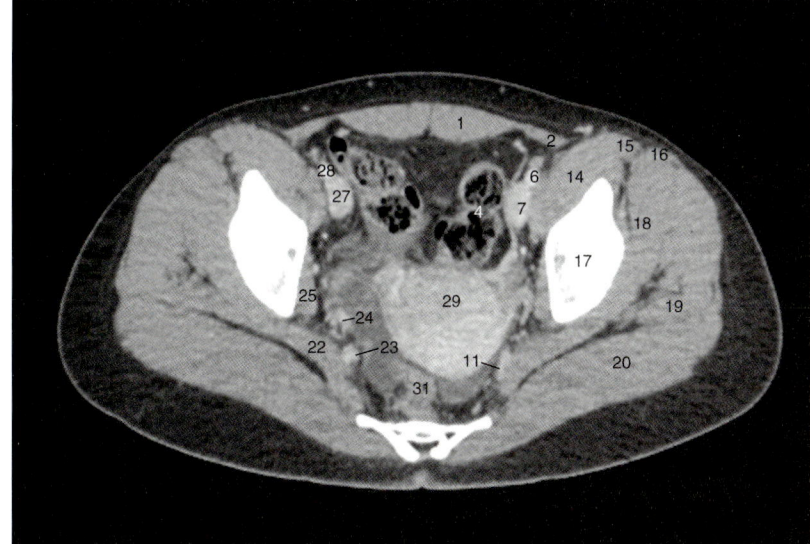

B. CT 增强图像

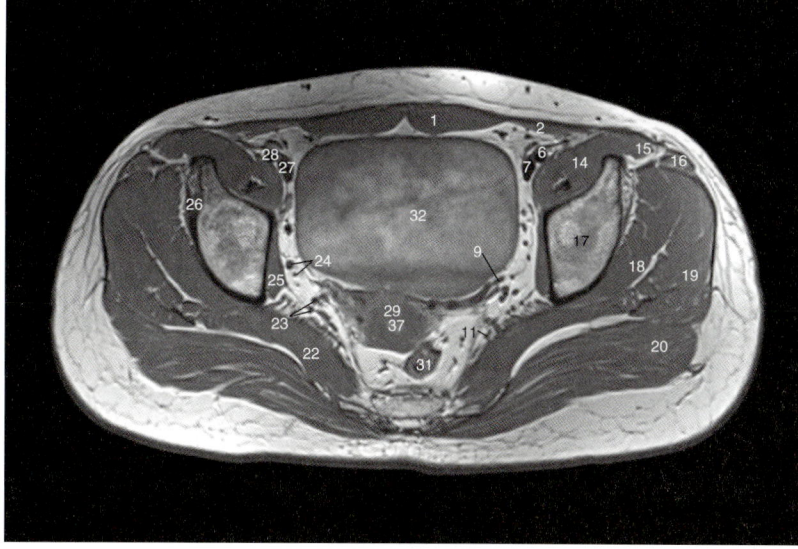

C. MR T1WI

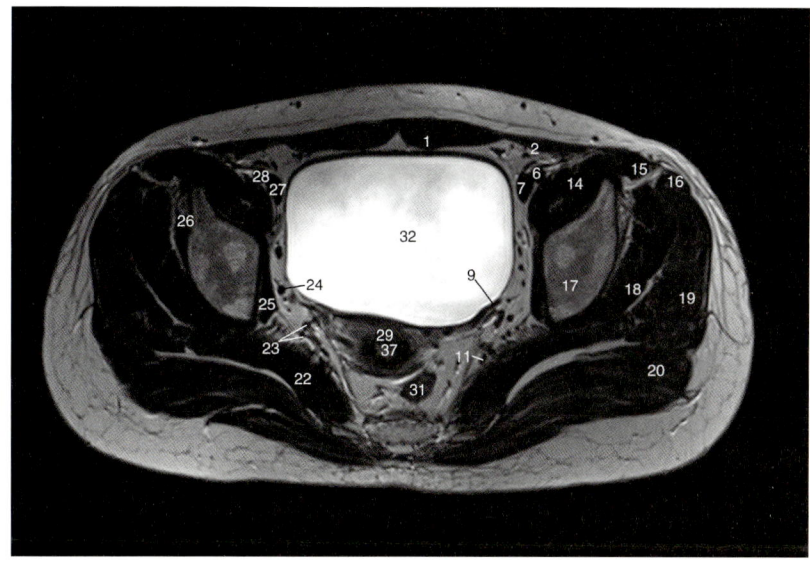

D. MR T2WI

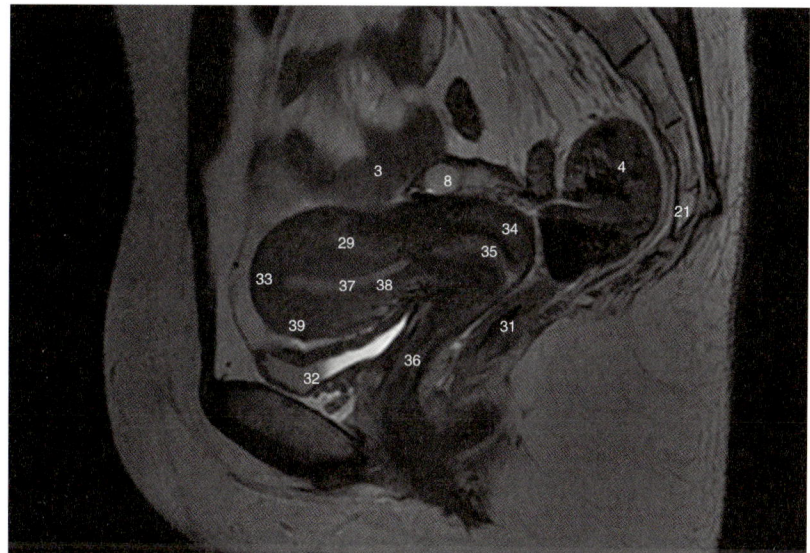

E. 子宫正中矢状位 T2WI

关键结构：尾骨，子宫体，乙状结肠。

此断面经过尾骨上份。尾骨位于骶骨下方，略呈三角形，由 3~5 节尾椎融合而成，一般在 30~40 岁才融合完成，在人类为退化之骨。坐位时，尾骨并不着力，而系坐骨结节负重。尾骨下端尖，上端为底，尾骨的形状可有很多变异，两侧可不对称，其曲度可前弯或向一侧倾斜。骶尾关节可发生骨性融合，这在老年女性更为多见。尾骨可以改变骨盆出口形状，如尾骨不能活动，分娩时可发生骨折[27]。盆腔内，子宫断面在本层达到最大横径，国人解剖学数值显示，经产妇子宫的位置前位约占 25.5%，中位约 33.7%，后位约 40.8%[16]。矢状位 MRI 可以直观地显示子宫的位置及结构。子宫体呈椭圆形或锥形，向前下逐渐变细过渡至子宫颈。子宫在 T1WI 呈较均匀一致信号，有时宫腔呈略低信号。T2WI 能显示子宫内不同结构，呈不同信号强度分层表现。宫体自宫腔向外呈 4 层 T2WI 不同信号强度，依次为高信号的子宫内膜、低信号的子宫肌层（MR 图像上称结合带）、中等信号的子宫肌层、线样低信号的浆膜层。子宫结合带在标本上并没有精确的解剖部位，T2WI 低信号由子宫内肌层结构致密、含水量低所致。结合带厚度一般 <8 mm，子宫腺肌病时往往增厚[1]。此断面子宫体左前方两个乙状结肠断面已汇合，呈哑铃形。

81

女性盆部与会阴连续横断层 41（FH.8570）

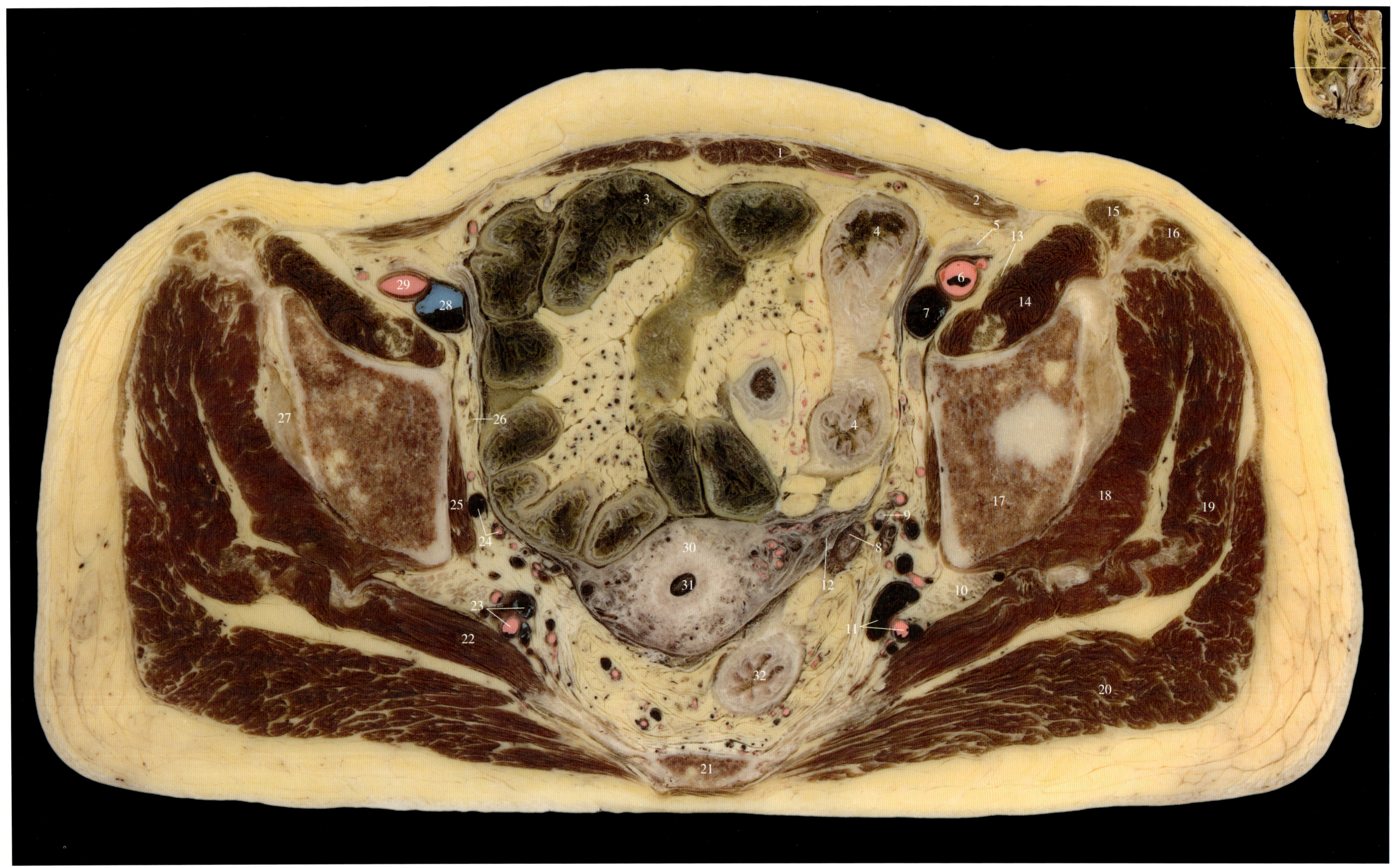

A. 断层标本图像

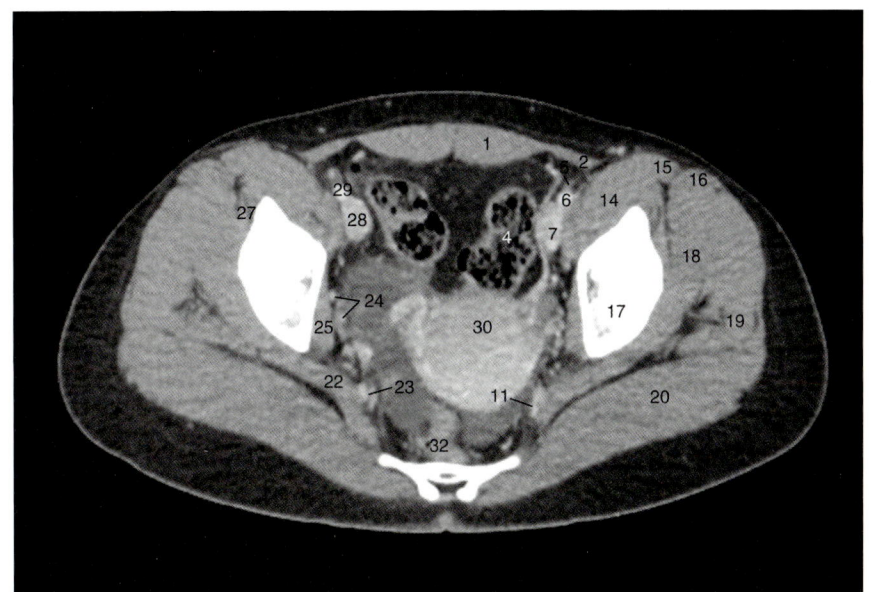
B. CT 增强图像

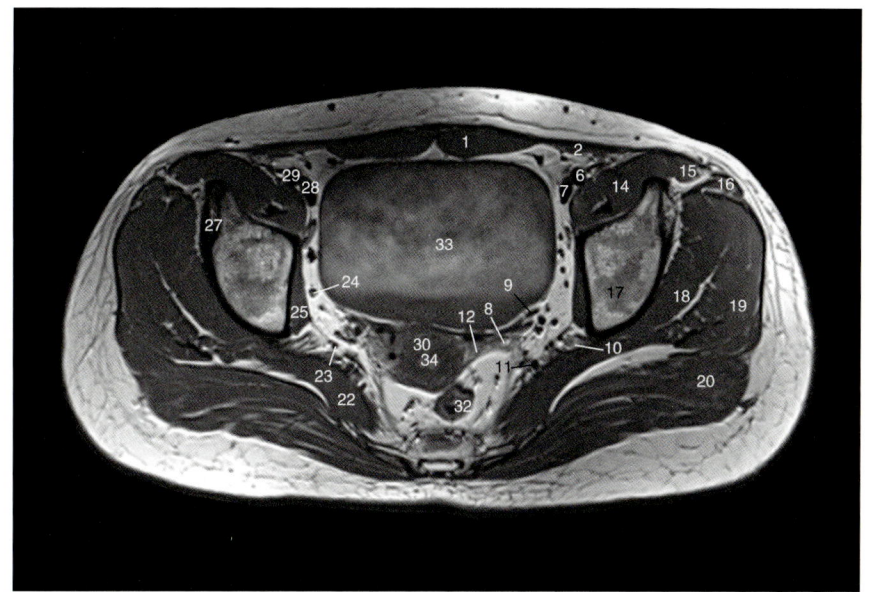
C. MR T1WI

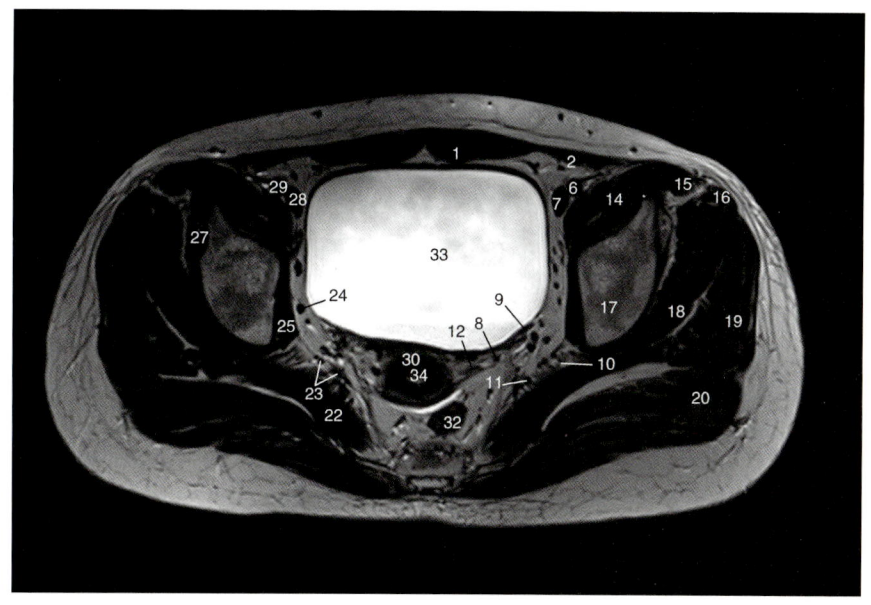
D. MR T2WI

1. 腹直肌 rectus abdominis
2. 腹内斜肌 obliquus internus abdominis
3. 回肠 ileum
4. 乙状结肠 sigmoid colon
5. 左髂外淋巴结 left external iliac lymph nodes
6. 左髂外动脉 left external iliac artery
7. 左髂外静脉 left external iliac vein
8. 左卵巢 left ovary
9. 左输尿管 left ureter
10. 坐骨神经 sciatic nerve
11. 左臀下动、静脉 left inferior gluteal artery and vein
12. 左输卵管 left uterine tube
13. 股神经 femoral nerve
14. 髂腰肌 iliopsoas
15. 缝匠肌 sartorius
16. 阔筋膜张肌 tensor fasciae latae
17. 髂骨体 body of ilium
18. 臀小肌 gluteus minimus
19. 臀中肌 gluteus medius
20. 臀大肌 gluteus maximus
21. 尾骨 coccyx
22. 梨状肌 piriformis
23. 右臀下动、静脉 right inferior gluteal artery and vein
24. 闭孔动、静脉 obturator artery and vein
25. 闭孔内肌 obturator internus
26. 闭孔神经 obturator nerve
27. 髂股韧带 iliofemoral ligament
28. 右髂外静脉 right external iliac vein
29. 右髂外动脉 right external iliac artery
30. 子宫体 body of uterus
31. 子宫腔 cavity of uterus
32. 直肠 rectum
33. 膀胱 urinary bladder
34. 子宫内膜 endometrium

关键结构：闭孔动、静脉，闭孔神经，乙状结肠。

此断面经过尾骨上份。较前一断面变化不大。其中髂骨体内侧的闭孔内肌断面逐渐明显，闭孔内肌内侧见闭孔动、静脉及闭孔神经断面。闭孔动脉多数为1支（98.6%），少数为2支，起始部位比较分散，一般是髂内动脉前干的分支（33.7%），起始于脐动脉稍下方，沿盆侧壁前行，经盆内筋膜与壁腹膜之间，上有同名神经下有同名静脉伴行，达盆壁前、中1/3交界处，穿闭膜管出骨盆，分为前支和后支，前支至股内侧的内收肌群，后支至髋关节、股方肌。有时闭孔动脉阙如，可见副闭孔动脉。凡直接或间接起自髂外动脉或股动脉者，均为副闭孔动脉，其出现率按例数统计约为17.95%。副闭孔动脉多数经股环外侧至闭膜管出盆者，占62.12%；经股环内侧者，占28.03%；经股环中间者，占9.85%。行闭孔淋巴结清扫时，应注意识别副闭孔动脉，以免损伤后造成闭孔窝内出血[21]。闭孔静脉与闭孔动脉伴行，回流至髂内静脉。闭孔神经起自腰丛，与闭孔血管伴行出闭膜管后分前、后两支分别支配内收肌群及闭孔外肌、大收肌[22]。在盆腔手术如清扫盆腔侧壁淋巴结时容易损伤闭孔神经，引起大腿内收肌疼痛性痉挛和大腿内侧区感觉丧失[24]。

女性盆部与会阴连续横断层 42（FH.8550）

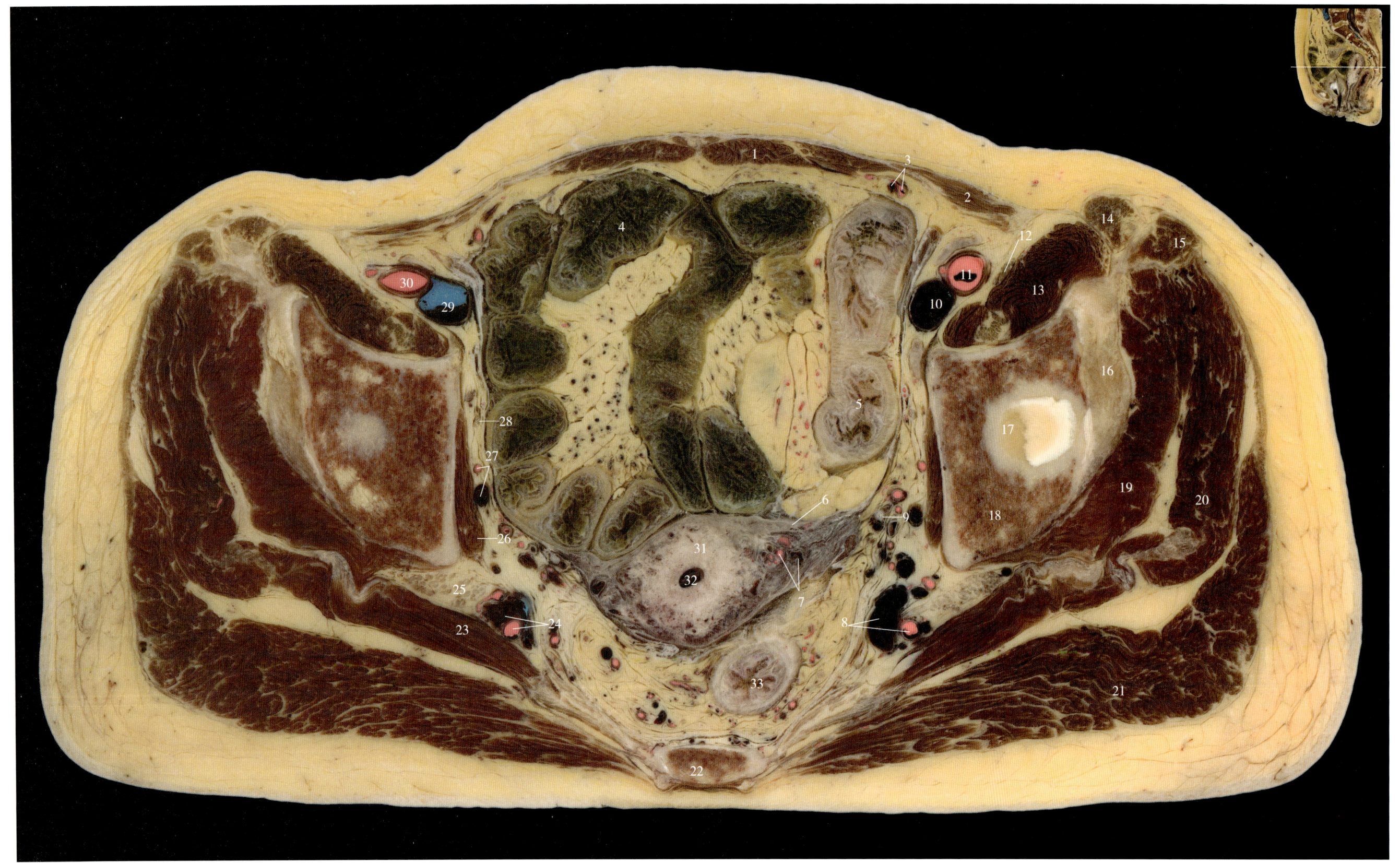

A. 断层标本图像

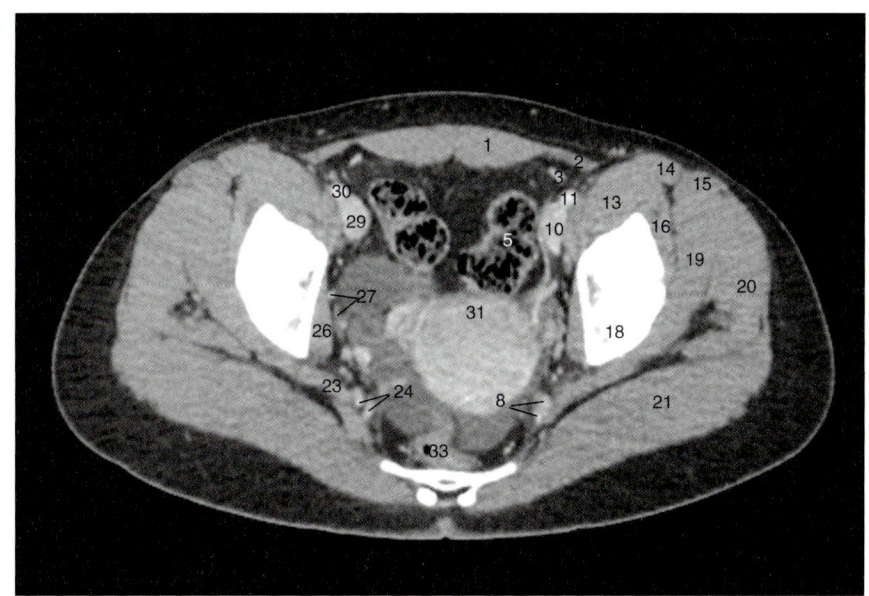

B. CT 增强图像

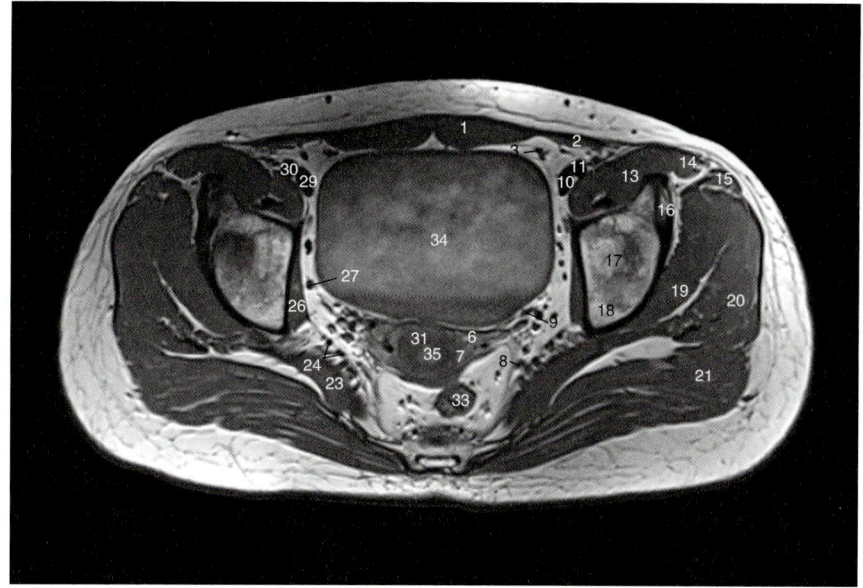

C. MR T1WI

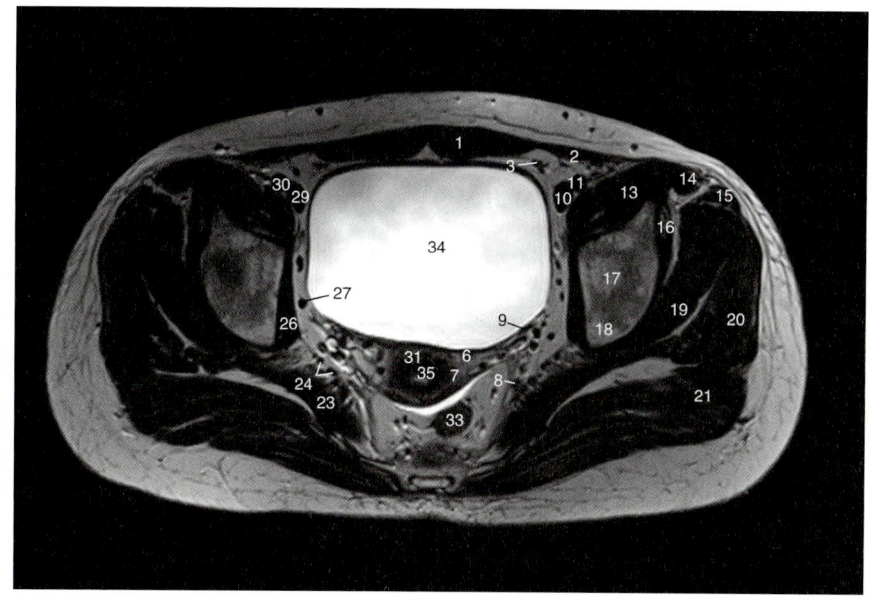

D. MR T2WI

1. 腹直肌 rectus abdominis	19. 臀小肌 gluteus minimus
2. 腹内斜肌 obliquus internus abdominis	20. 臀中肌 gluteus medius
3. 腹壁下动、静脉 inferior epigastric artery and vein	21. 臀大肌 gluteus maximus
4. 回肠 ileum	22. 尾骨 coccyx
5. 乙状结肠 sigmoid colon	23. 梨状肌 piriformis
6. 子宫阔韧带前叶 anterior layer of cardinal ligament of uterus	24. 右臀下动、静脉 right inferior gluteal artery and vein
7. 子宫动、静脉 uterine artery and vein	25. 坐骨神经 sciatic nerve
8. 左臀下动、静脉 left inferior gluteal artery and vein	26. 闭孔内肌 obturator internus
9. 左输尿管 left ureter	27. 闭孔动、静脉 obturator artery and vein
10. 左股静脉 left femoral vein	28. 闭孔神经 obturator nerve
11. 左股动脉 left femoral artery	29. 右股静脉 right femoral vein
12. 股神经 femoral nerve	30. 右股动脉 right femoral artery
13. 髂腰肌 iliopsoas	31. 子宫体 body of uterus
14. 缝匠肌 sartorius	32. 子宫腔 cavity of uterus
15. 阔筋膜张肌 tensor fasciae latae	33. 直肠 rectum
16. 髂股韧带 iliofemoral ligament	34. 膀胱 urinary bladder
17. 髋臼 acetabulum	35. 子宫内膜 endometrium
18. 坐骨体 body of ischium	

关键结构：髋臼，子宫阔韧带。

此断面经过尾骨上份。

在本断层，由髂骨、耻骨、坐骨体部汇合而成的髋臼开始出现。髋臼呈半球深凹状包围股骨头，直径为 30~50 mm，边缘覆盖厚约为 2 mm 的半月形透明关节软骨，中央髋臼窝无关节软骨覆盖，为股骨头韧带出入处[12, 22]。双侧髂外动脉在此断面延续为股动脉，其旁见小血管断面，追踪发现该分支血管行向上内方，入腹直肌鞘后层与腹直肌之间，升至脐部，证实为腹壁下动脉，是髂外动脉重要分支之一。与股动脉伴行的为股静脉，汇入髂外静脉。盆腔内结构较前一断面变化不大，主要见肠管、子宫、脂肪组织及血管、神经。断面上子宫前后壁外周的条索状结构为子宫阔韧带，由覆盖于子宫前后的双层腹膜在其两侧汇合而成，分为前叶和后叶，冠状位呈翼状，其内包裹卵巢、输卵管、子宫圆韧带、血管、淋巴管、神经等。上缘游离，包裹输卵管，其外侧 1/3 移行于卵巢悬韧带。下缘和外侧缘与盆底和盆侧壁的腹膜相续，内侧缘与子宫前、后面的腹膜相续。以其附着部位，分为子宫系膜、输卵管系膜、卵巢系膜 3 个部分。前、后叶之间有子宫动静脉、淋巴管、神经等。其作用是限制子宫向两侧倾倒[1]。

女性盆部与会阴连续横断层 43（FH.8530）

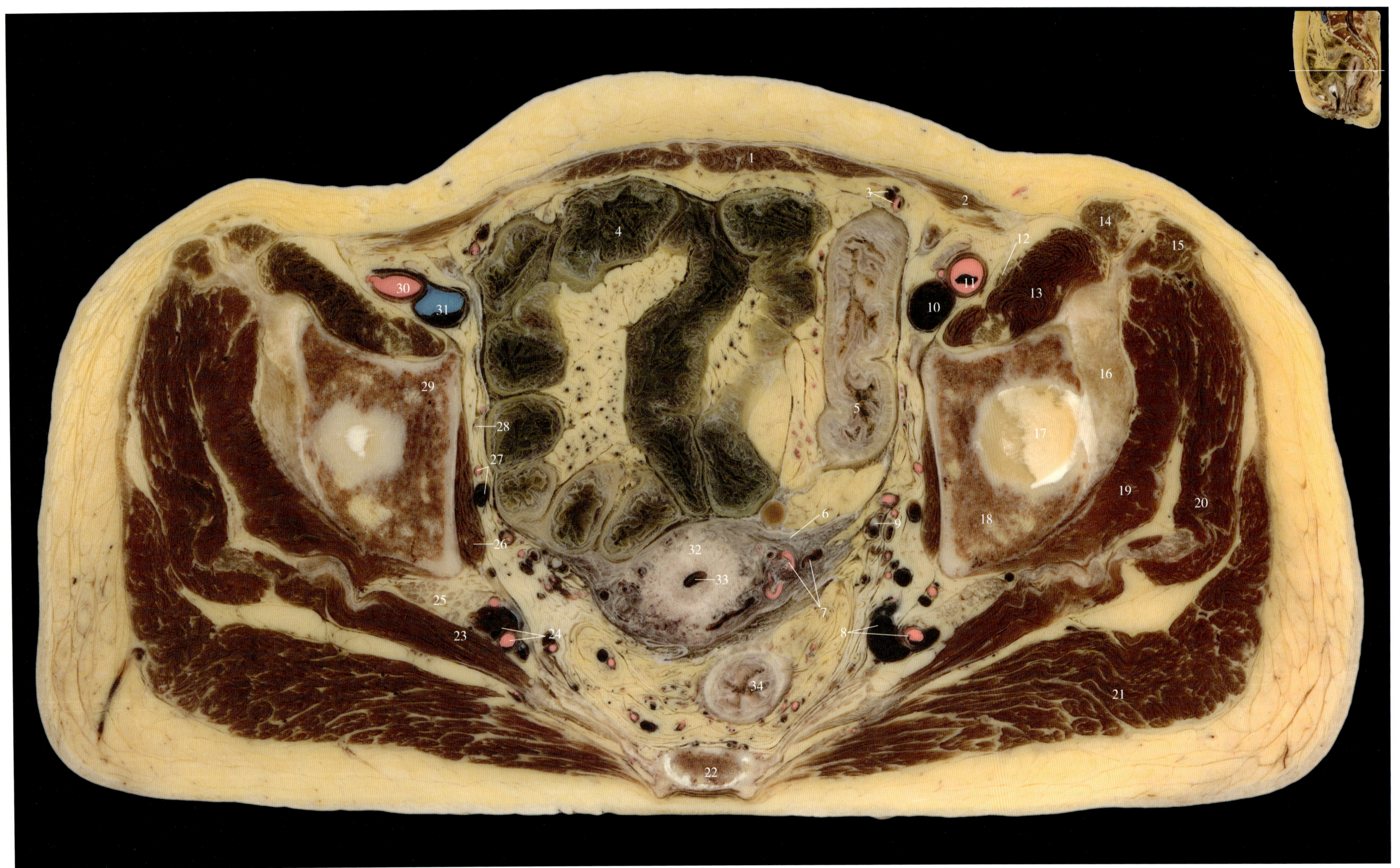

A. 断层标本图像

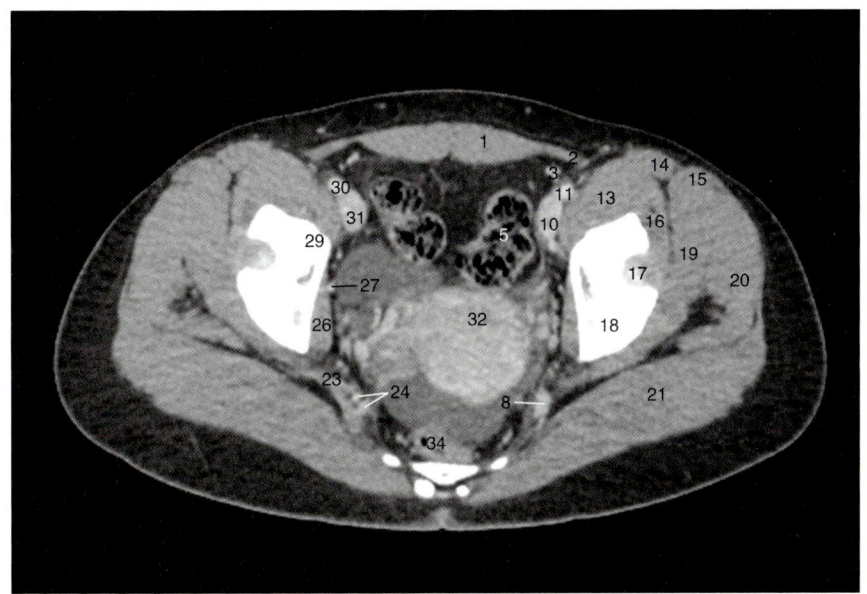
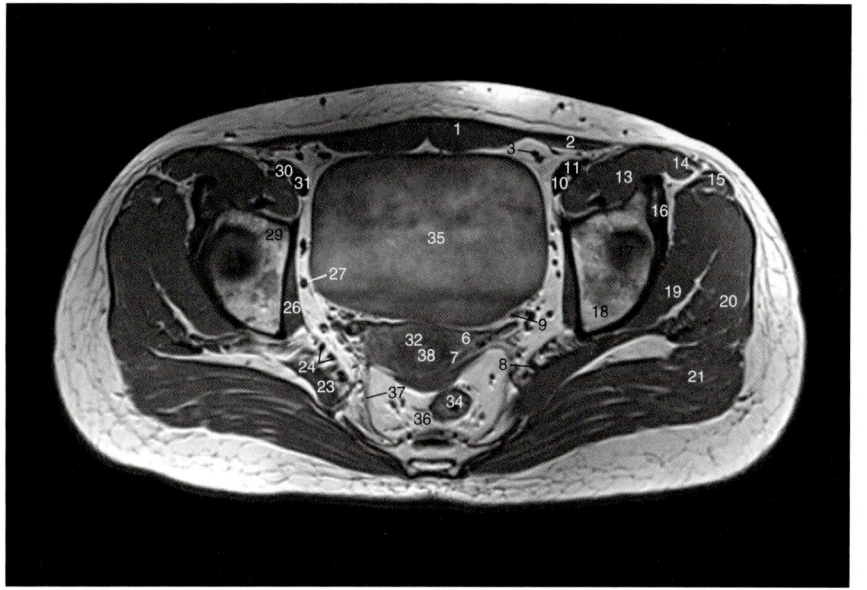
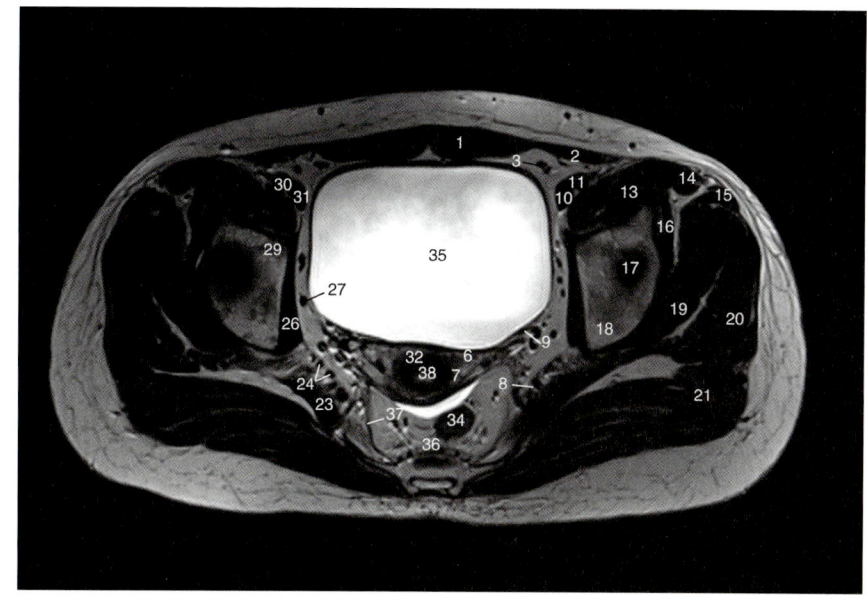

B. CT 增强图像　　　　　　　　　　　　C. MR T1WI　　　　　　　　　　　　D. MR T2WI

1. 腹直肌 rectus abdominis
2. 腹内斜肌 obliquus internus abdominis
3. 腹壁下动、静脉 inferior epigastric artery and vein
4. 回肠 ileum
5. 乙状结肠 sigmoid colon
6. 子宫阔韧带前叶 anterior layer of cardinal ligament of uterus
7. 子宫动、静脉 uterine artery and vein
8. 左臀下动、静脉 left inferior gluteal artery and vein
9. 左输尿管 left ureter
10. 左股静脉 left femoral vein
11. 左股动脉 left femoral artery
12. 股神经 femoral nerve
13. 髂腰肌 iliopsoas
14. 缝匠肌 sartorius
15. 阔筋膜张肌 tensor fasciae latae
16. 髂股韧带 iliofemoral ligament
17. 股骨头 femoral head
18. 坐骨体 body of ischium
19. 臀小肌 gluteus minimus
20. 臀中肌 gluteus medius
21. 臀大肌 gluteus maximus
22. 尾骨 coccyx
23. 梨状肌 piriformis
24. 右臀下动、静脉 right inferior gluteal artery and vein
25. 坐骨神经 sciatic nerve
26. 闭孔内肌 obturator internus
27. 闭孔动、静脉 obturator artery and vein
28. 闭孔神经 obturator nerve
29. 耻骨 pubis
30. 右股动脉 right femoral artery
31. 右股静脉 right femoral vein
32. 子宫体 body of uterus
33. 子宫腔 cavity of uterus
34. 直肠 rectum
35. 膀胱 urinary bladder
36. 直肠系膜 mesorectum
37. 直肠系膜筋膜 mesorectal fascia
38. 子宫内膜 endometrium

关键结构：股骨头，耻骨，乙状结肠。

此断面经过尾骨上份，与髋臼相关节的股骨头开始出现。股骨头呈 2/3 球形，表面被关节软骨覆盖，非常光滑，其顶部偏后有一小凹陷，为股骨头凹，是股骨头韧带附着处。当出现股骨颈骨折、长期使用激素等情形时，可造成股骨头缺血坏死，人工髋关节置换术目前已成为一项成熟的治疗手段。子宫体左前方的乙状结肠断面完全汇合，呈长条形。乙状结肠在左髂嵴处起自降结肠，沿左髂窝转入盆腔内，呈"乙"形或"S"形弯曲，至第 3 骶椎平面移行为直肠。乙状结肠长度变化很大，平均 40~45 cm。临床常用乙状结肠代阴道术治疗先天性无阴道症。乙状结肠是先天性巨结肠症、结肠肿瘤、结肠憩室等疾病的好发部位。CT 可清晰地显示乙状结肠的形态及肠壁变化，当结肠内有足够的气体或对比剂时，CT 显示肠壁厚度一般不超过 5 mm，如果 ＞ 6 mm，提示结肠病变[1]。此外，乙状结肠通过乙状结肠系膜连于腹后壁。乙状结肠系膜是双层腹膜结构，根部附于左髂窝和骨盆左后壁，系膜内含有乙状结肠血管、直肠上血管、淋巴管和神经丛等[21]。乙状结肠系膜在肠中部活动范围较大，向两端逐渐变短消失，故乙状结肠与降结肠和直肠相连处较固定，中部活动范围大，所以易发生乙状结肠扭转[1]。

女性盆部与会阴连续横断层 44（FH.8510）

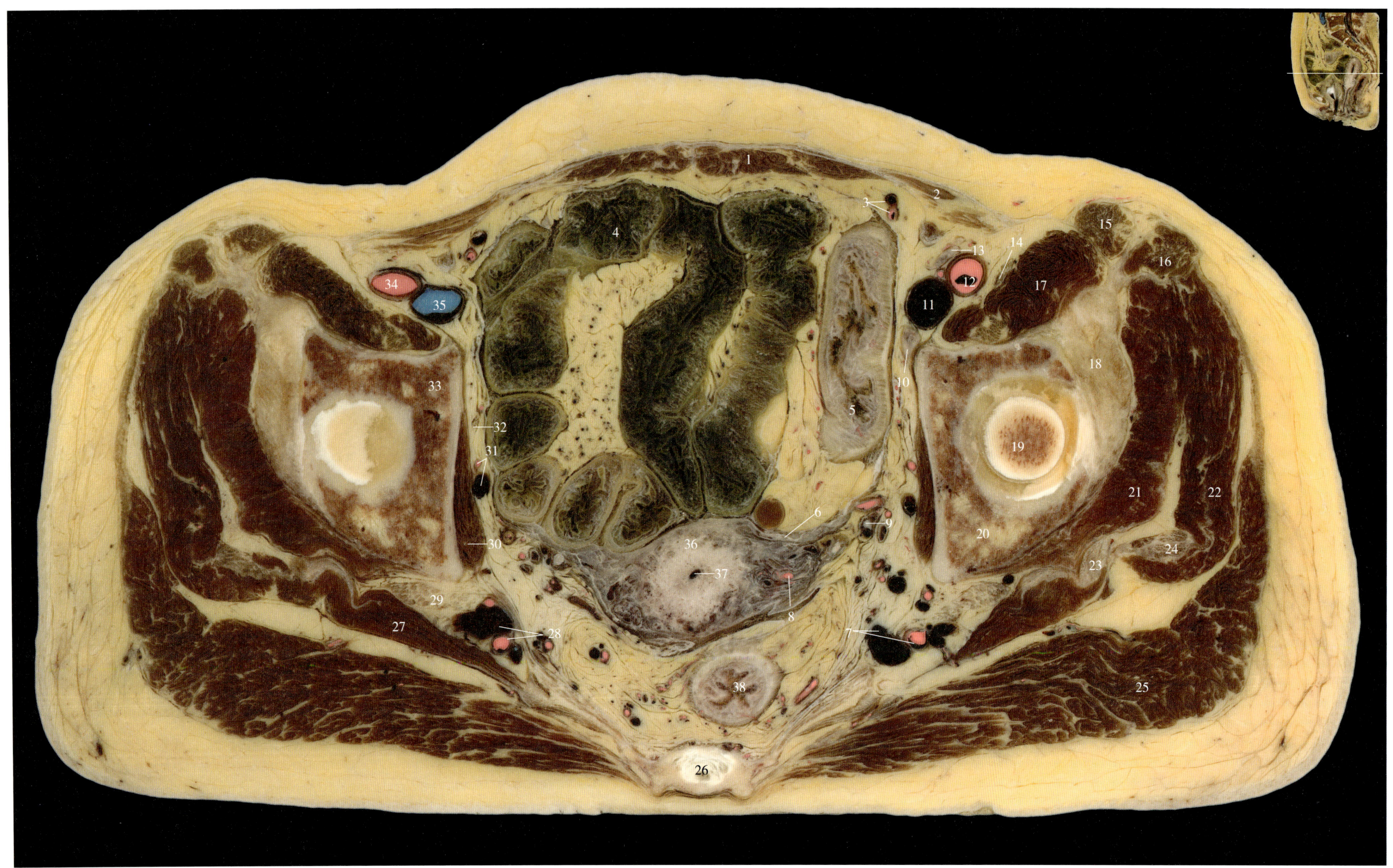

A. 断层标本图像

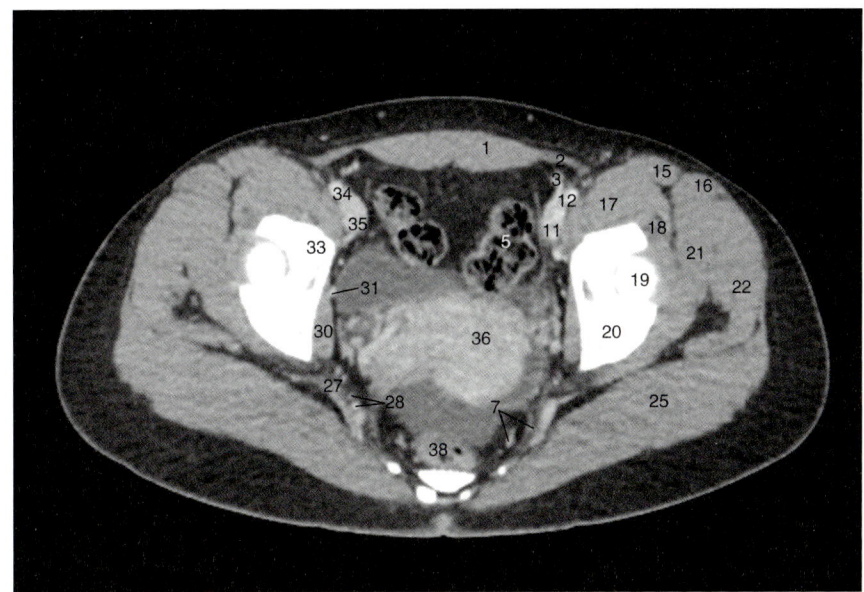
B. CT 增强图像

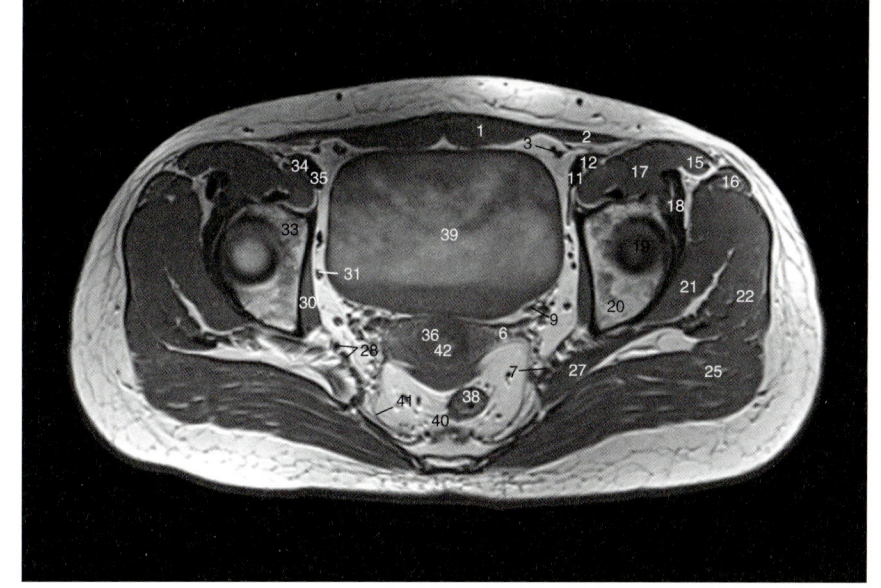
C. MR T1WI

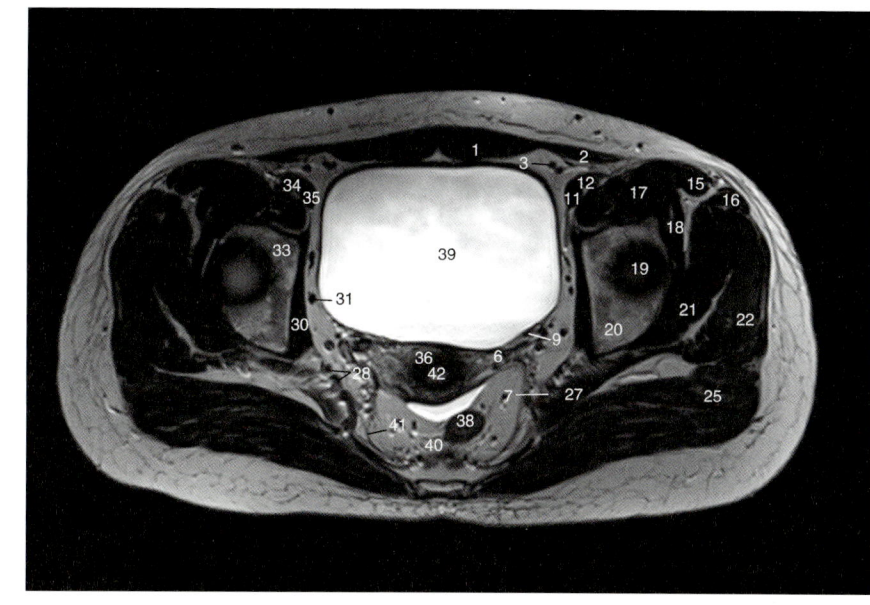
D. MR T2WI

1. 腹直肌 rectus abdominis
2. 腹内斜肌 obliquus internus abdominis
3. 腹壁下动、静脉 inferior epigastric artery and vein
4. 回肠 ileum
5. 乙状结肠 sigmoid colon
6. 子宫阔韧带前叶 anterior layer of cardinal ligament of uterus
7. 左臀下动、静脉 left inferior gluteal artery and vein
8. 子宫动脉 uterine artery
9. 左输尿管 left ureter
10. 腹股沟深淋巴结 deep inguinal lymph node
11. 左股静脉 left femoral vein
12. 左股动脉 left femoral artery
13. 腹股沟浅淋巴结 superficial inguinal lymph nodes
14. 股神经 femoral nerve
15. 缝匠肌 sartorius
16. 阔筋膜张肌 tensor fasciae latae
17. 髂腰肌 iliopsoas
18. 髂股韧带 iliofemoral ligament
19. 股骨头 femoral head
20. 坐骨体 body of ischium
21. 臀小肌 gluteus minimus
22. 臀中肌 gluteus medius
23. 梨状肌肌腱 tendon of piriformis
24. 臀中肌肌腱 tendon of gluteus medius
25. 臀大肌 gluteus maximus
26. 尾骨 coccyx
27. 梨状肌 piriformis
28. 右臀下动、静脉 right inferior gluteal artery and vein
29. 坐骨神经 sciatic nerve
30. 闭孔内肌 obturator internus
31. 闭孔动、静脉 obturator artery and vein
32. 闭孔神经 obturator nerve
33. 耻骨体 body of pubis
34. 右股动脉 right femoral artery
35. 右股静脉 right femoral vein
36. 子宫颈 neck of uterus
37. 子宫颈管 canal of cervix of uterus
38. 直肠 rectum
39. 膀胱 urinary bladder
40. 直肠系膜 mesorectum
41. 直肠系膜筋膜 mesorectal fascia
42. 子宫内膜 endometrium

关键结构：子宫颈。

　　此断面经过尾骨上份。子宫断面较前明显缩小，呈类椭圆形居盆腔中后方，由子宫体逐渐延续为较窄呈圆柱状的子宫颈，子宫腔断面缩小，逐渐呈梭形，为子宫颈管。子宫体与子宫颈的比例随着年龄增长而变化。出生时，子宫体与子宫颈比例为1:2，呈哑铃形。至10岁左右，子宫体与子宫颈比例约为1:1。在10～16岁青春期，受卵巢分泌的雌激素影响，子宫发育明显，子宫体长度增加，子宫体各层肌肉如环形肌、纵形及斜形肌形成，子宫体与子宫颈比例逐渐变为2:1，子宫形状逐渐由三角形发育成梨形[21]。子宫颈在CT平扫呈软组织密度，增强扫描因间质成分多而强化程度低于宫体。超声是判断子宫发育状况的首选检查方法。子宫颈MRI检查可以清晰显示解剖结构。T1WI图像上整个子宫及子宫颈表现为均匀一致的中等信号。MR T2WI 显示宫颈结构清晰，自宫颈管向外呈4层不同信号，依次为明显高信号的宫颈管内黏液、稍高信号的宫颈黏膜皱襞、低信号的宫颈内基质环（与子宫结合带相连续）、中等信号的宫颈肌层[1]。子宫骶韧带是维持子宫颈位置的重要支持结构，由结缔组织和平滑肌纤维构成，从子宫颈后面向后呈弓形绕过直肠两侧，附于第2、3骶椎前面的筋膜，其表面有腹膜覆盖，形成直肠子宫襞，其功能是向后上方牵引子宫颈，防止子宫前移，维持子宫前屈位[1]。在臀小肌、臀中肌和梨状肌围成的间隙内，股骨大转子开始出现，为臀小肌、臀中肌、闭孔内肌等的止点，并且是髋部手术重要的解剖标志。

女性盆部与会阴连续横断层 45（FH.8490）

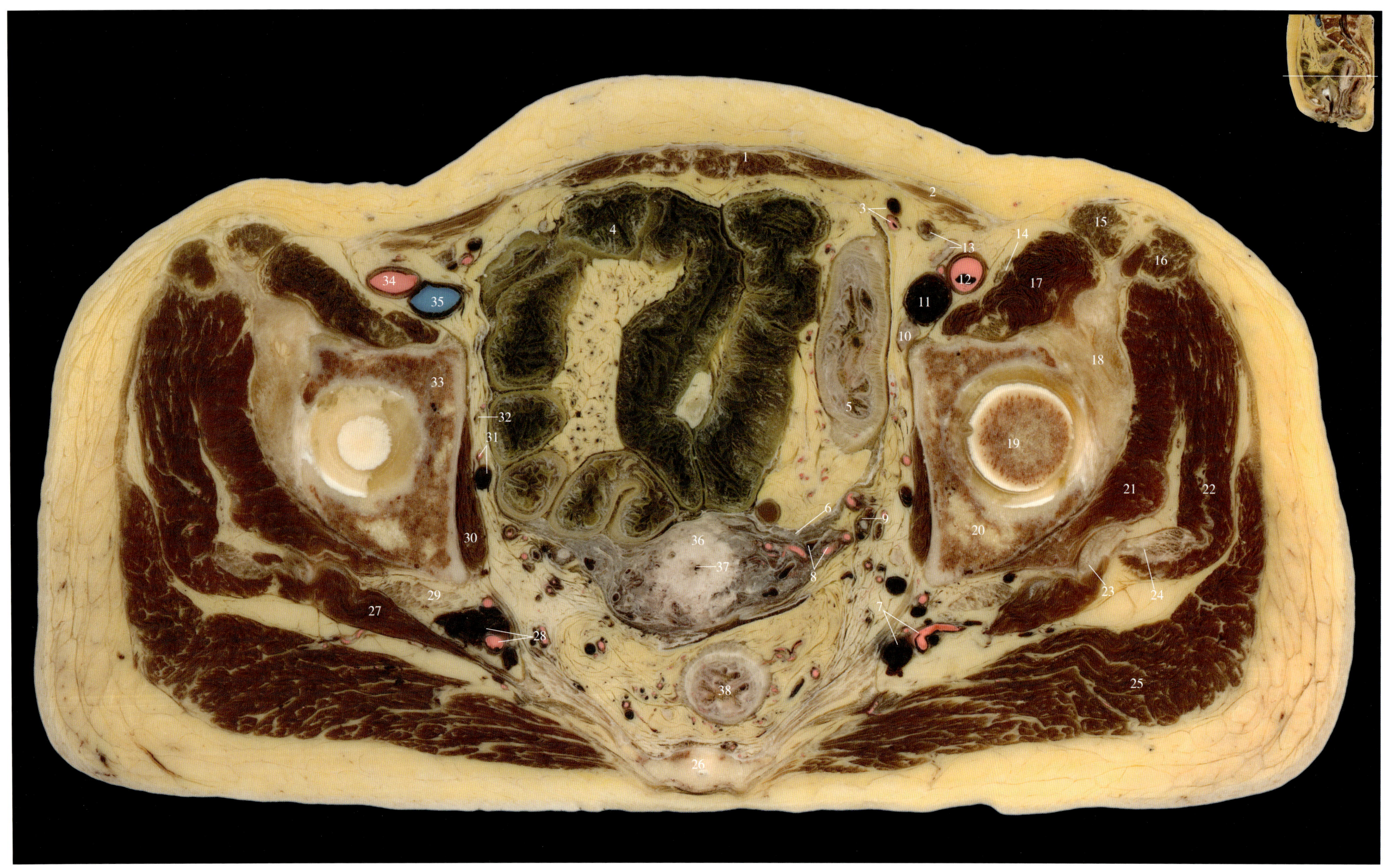

A. 断层标本图像

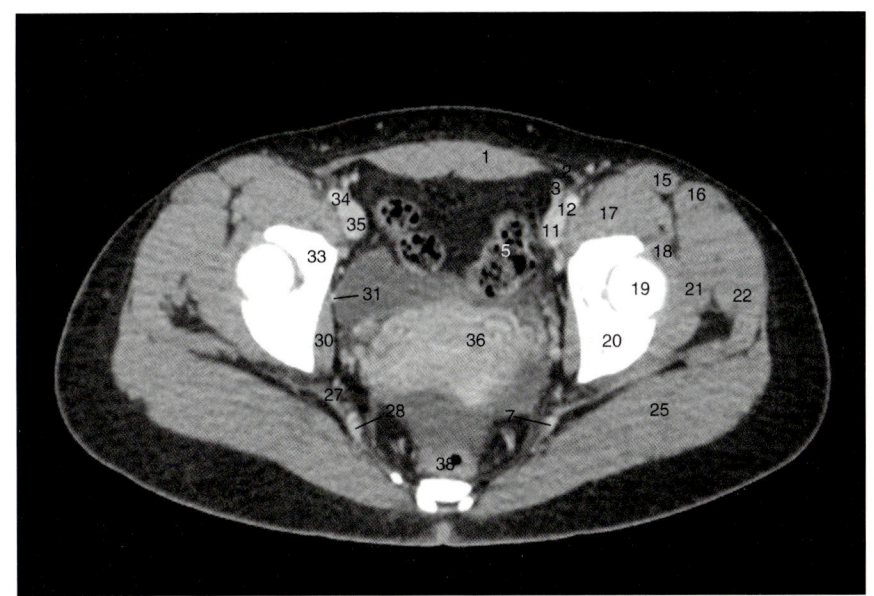
B. CT 增强图像

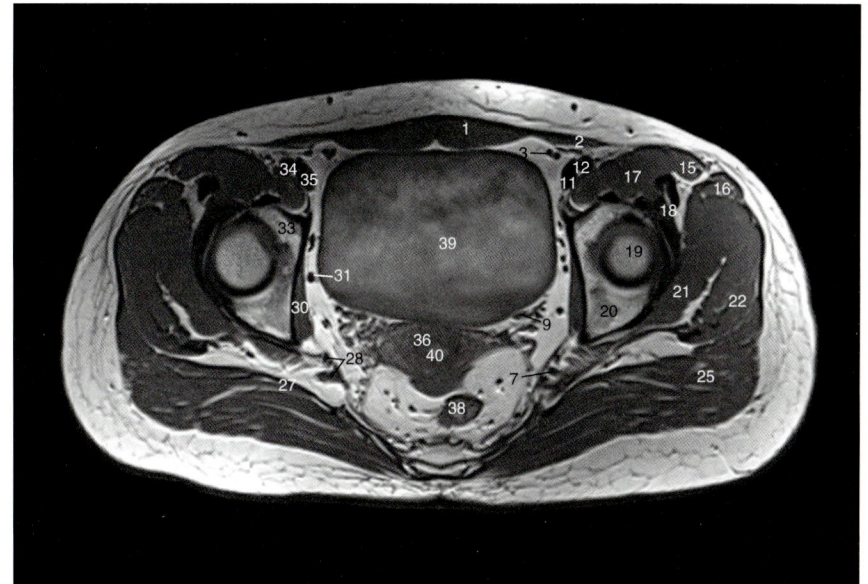
C. MR T1WI

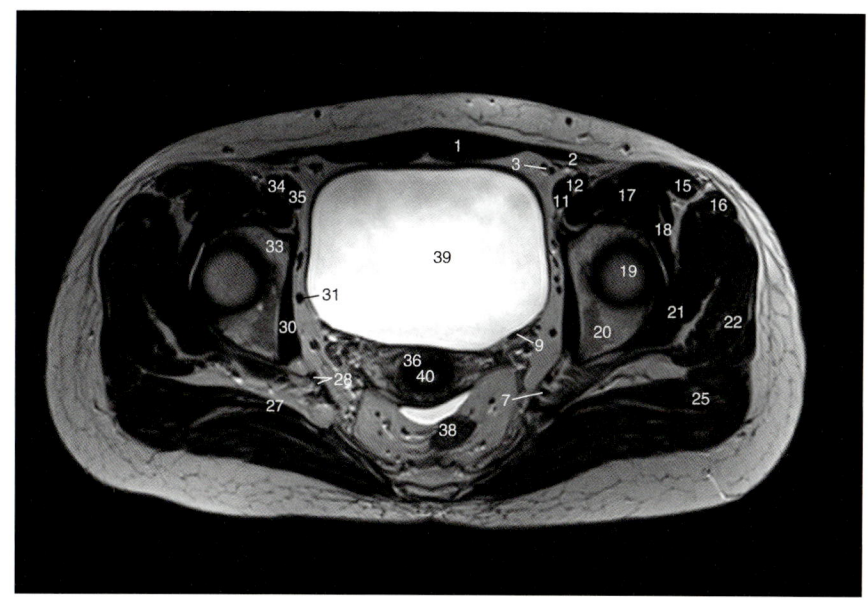
D. MR T2WI

1. 腹直肌 rectus abdominis
2. 腹内斜肌 obliquus internus abdominis
3. 腹壁下动、静脉 inferior epigastric artery and vein
4. 回肠 ileum
5. 乙状结肠 sigmoid colon
6. 子宫阔韧带 broad ligament of uterus
7. 左臀下动、静脉 left inferior gluteal artery and vein
8. 子宫动、静脉 uterine artery and vein
9. 左输尿管 left ureter
10. 腹股沟深淋巴结 deep inguinal lymph node
11. 左股静脉 left femoral vein
12. 左股动脉 left femoral artery
13. 腹股沟浅淋巴结 superficial inguinal lymph nodes
14. 股神经 femoral nerve
15. 缝匠肌 sartorius
16. 阔筋膜张肌 tensor fasciae latae
17. 髂腰肌 iliopsoas
18. 髂股韧带 iliofemoral ligament
19. 股骨头 femoral head
20. 坐骨体 body of ischium

21. 臀小肌 gluteus minimus
22. 臀中肌 gluteus medius
23. 梨状肌肌腱 tendon of piriformis
24. 臀中肌肌腱 tendon of gluteus medius
25. 臀大肌 gluteus maximus
26. 尾骨 coccyx
27. 梨状肌 piriformis
28. 右臀下动、静脉 right inferior gluteal artery and vein
29. 坐骨神经 sciatic nerve
30. 闭孔内肌 obturator internus
31. 闭孔动、静脉 obturator artery and vein
32. 闭孔神经 obturator nerve
33. 耻骨体 body of pubis
34. 右股动脉 right femoral artery
35. 右股静脉 right femoral vein
36. 子宫颈 neck of uterus
37. 子宫颈管 canal of cervix of uterus
38. 直肠 rectum
39. 膀胱 urinary bladder
40. 子宫内膜 endometrium

关键结构：腹股沟深、浅淋巴结。

此断面经过尾骨上份。其前方两侧见断面逐渐缩小的梨状肌。梨状肌前方为近似扇形的髋骨，近中心部位见断面逐渐增大的圆形股骨头。自前一断面起，髂腰肌断面的前内方自内侧向外侧见腹股沟深、浅淋巴结断面。腹股沟浅淋巴结位于腹股沟韧带前的皮下组织内，伴股浅静脉和大隐静脉，呈"T"形排列[2]。其中的前哨淋巴结位于隐股点处，大隐静脉在这里流入股总静脉。腹股沟深淋巴结位于股血管周围，位置最高的位于股环处，并且较大；低位的淋巴结数量不等，沿股静脉近侧段和大隐静脉注入股静脉处排列。此群淋巴结收纳下肢的深淋巴管、股部和外阴部的深淋巴管，及腹股沟下浅淋巴结的输出管，经子宫圆韧带及腹股沟淋巴结，其输出管注入髂外淋巴结及闭孔淋巴结。区分腹股沟深淋巴结和髂外淋巴结内链的解剖学标志是腹股沟韧带和腹壁下血管和旋髂血管的起源[23, 28]。盆腔内子宫颈断面呈类椭圆形居盆腔中后方，逐渐缩小。

女性盆部与会阴连续横断层 46（FH.8470）

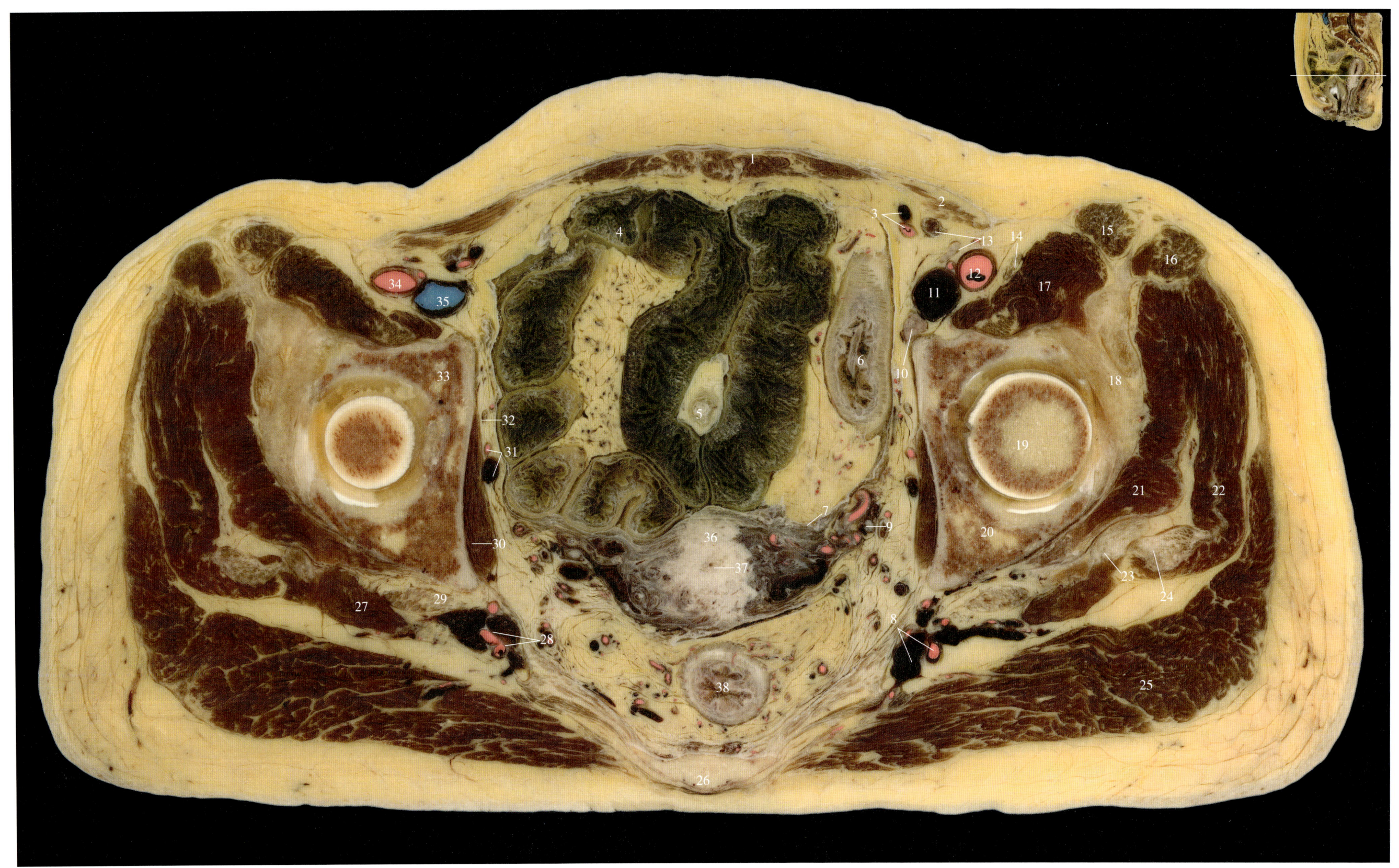

A. 断层标本图像

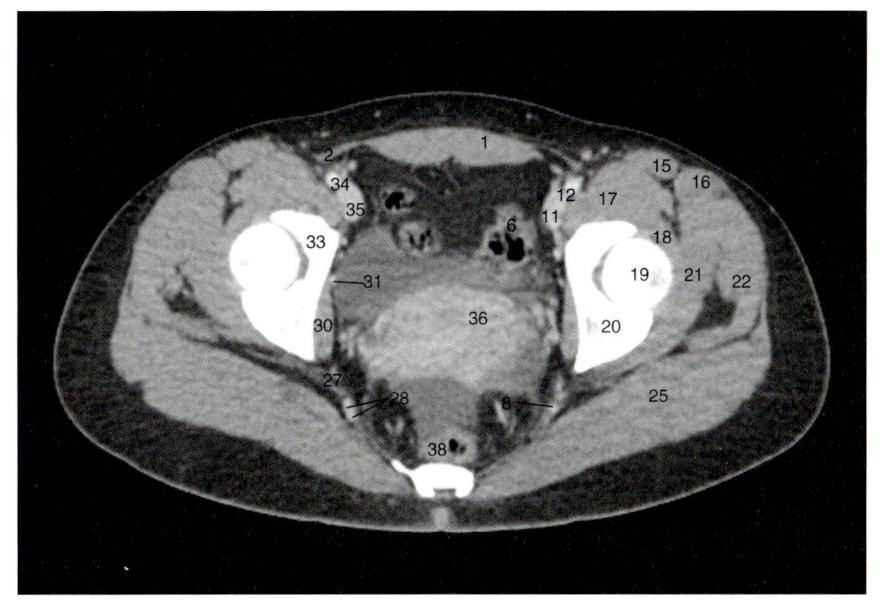

B. CT 增强图像

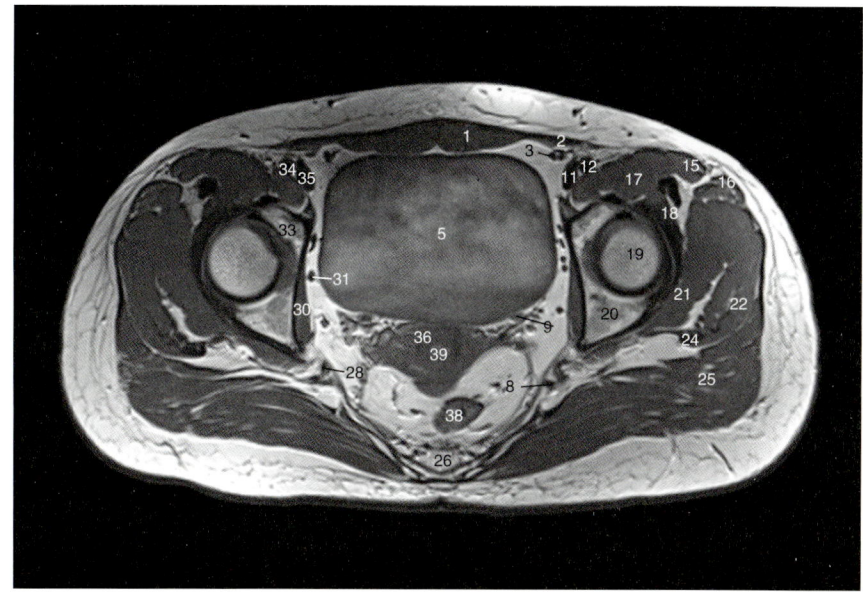

C. MR T1WI

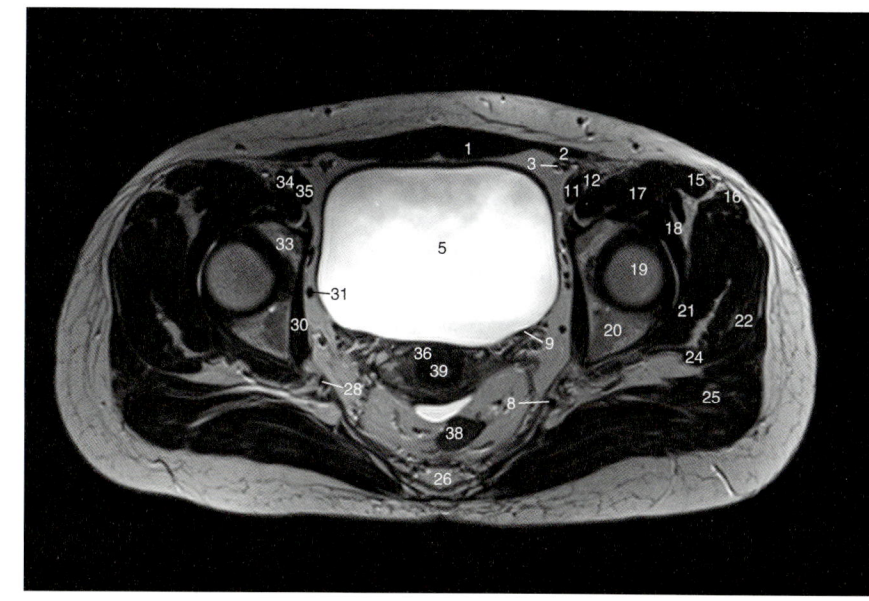

D. MR T2WI

关键结构：膀胱，子宫主韧带，子宫颈。

此断面经过尾骨中份，较前一断面变化不大，重点区别在于盆腔中部未充盈状态的膀胱开始出现。而在 CT 和 MR 图像上，由于志愿者的膀胱处于充盈状态，已于更高位断面出现。梨状肌断面逐渐缩短、缩小，股骨头断面逐渐增大。子宫颈居盆腔中后方，断面逐渐缩小，中心见裂隙状的子宫颈管。子宫颈两侧有子宫主韧带，又称子宫颈横韧带、子宫旁组织，位于子宫阔韧带的下部深面，由结缔组织和平滑肌纤维构成，连于子宫颈与盆侧壁之间，呈扇形，功能是固定子宫颈位置，防止子宫向下脱垂。此韧带内有盆内血管、淋巴管和神经走行[21]。

1. 腹直肌 rectus abdominis
2. 腹内斜肌 obliquus internus abdominis
3. 腹壁下动、静脉 inferior epigastric artery and vein
4. 回肠 ileum
5. 膀胱 urinary bladder
6. 乙状结肠 sigmoid colon
7. 子宫阔韧带 broad ligament of uterus
8. 左臀下动、静脉 left inferior gluteal artery and vein
9. 左输尿管 left ureter
10. 腹股沟深淋巴结 deep inguinal lymph node
11. 左股静脉 left femoral vein
12. 左股动脉 left femoral artery
13. 腹股沟浅淋巴结 superficial inguinal lymph nodes
14. 股神经 femoral nerve
15. 缝匠肌 sartorius
16. 阔筋膜张肌 tensor fasciae latae
17. 髂腰肌 iliopsoas
18. 髂股韧带 iliofemoral ligament
19. 股骨头 femoral head
20. 坐骨体 body of ischium
21. 臀小肌 gluteus minimus
22. 臀中肌 gluteus medius
23. 梨状肌肌腱 tendon of piriformis
24. 臀中肌肌腱 tendon of gluteus medius
25. 臀大肌 gluteus maximus
26. 尾骨 coccyx
27. 梨状肌 piriformis
28. 右臀下动、静脉 right inferior gluteal artery and vein
29. 坐骨神经 sciatic nerve
30. 闭孔内肌 obturator internus
31. 闭孔动、静脉 obturator artery and vein
32. 闭孔神经 obturator nerve
33. 耻骨体 body of pubis
34. 右股动脉 right femoral artery
35. 右股静脉 right femoral vein
36. 子宫颈 neck of uterus
37. 子宫颈管 canal of cervix of uterus
38. 直肠 rectum
39. 子宫内膜 endometrium

93

女性盆部与会阴连续横断层 47（FH.8450）

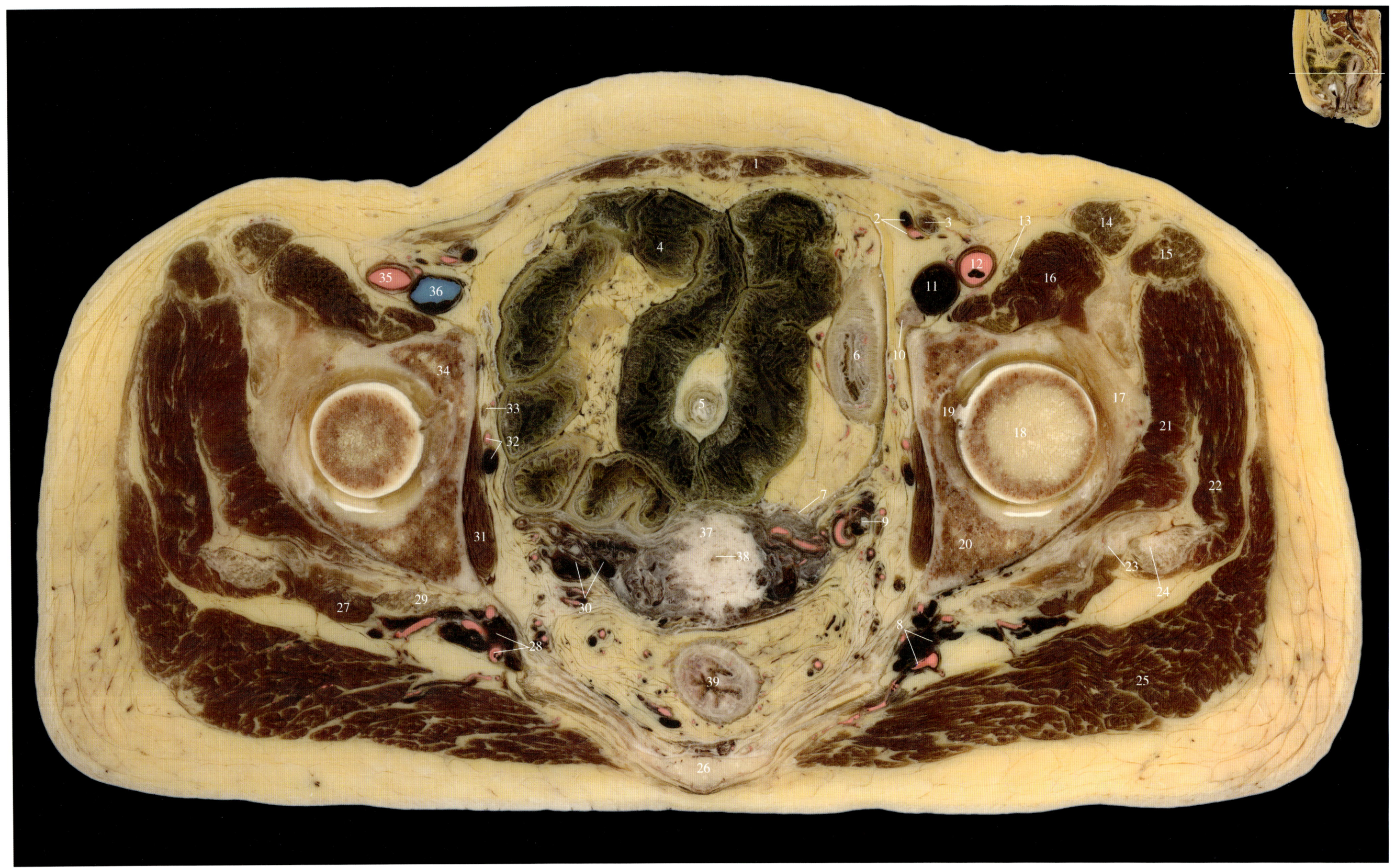

A. 断层标本图像

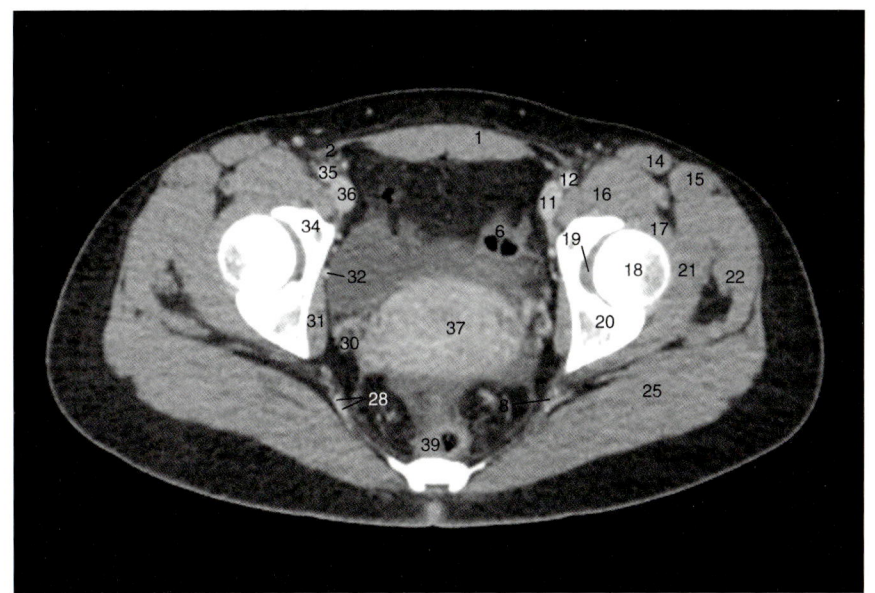
B. CT 增强图像

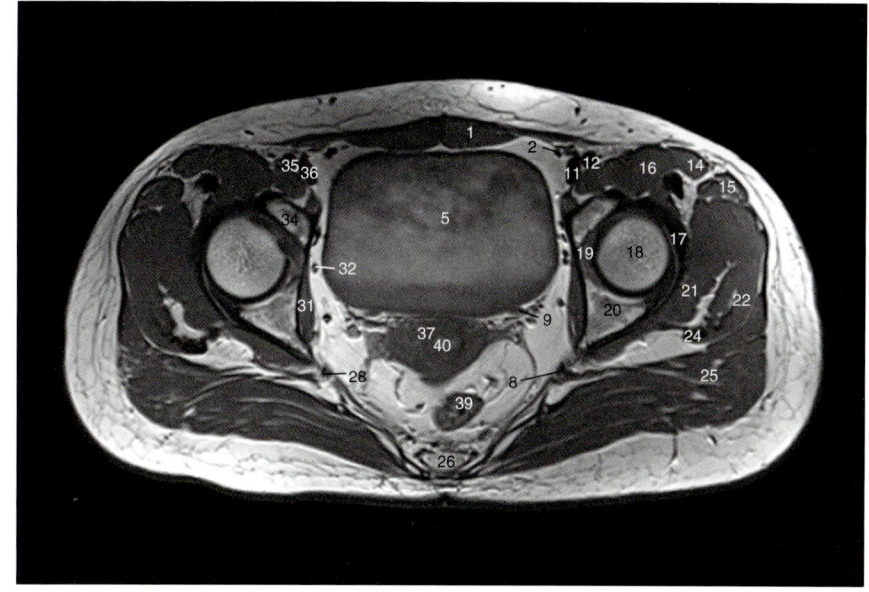
C. MR T1WI

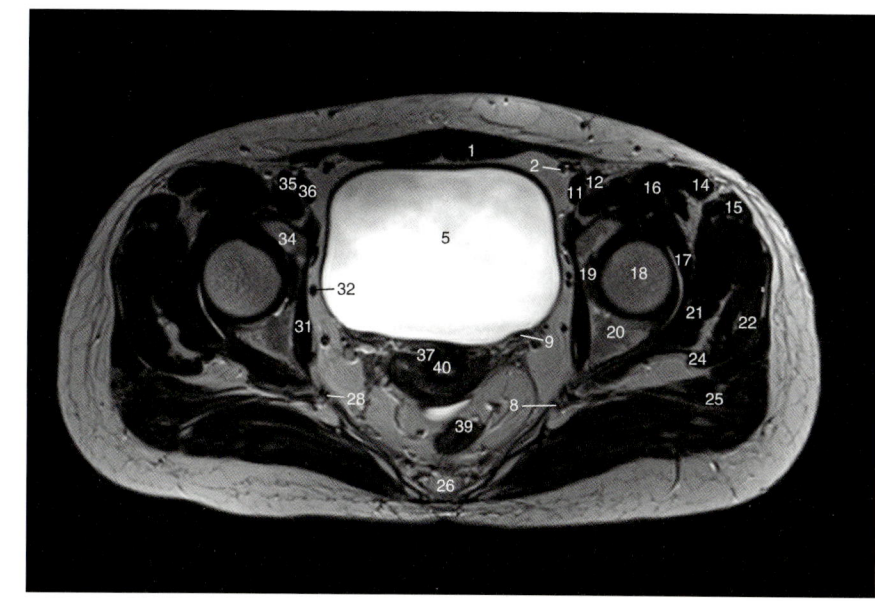
D. MR T2WI

1. 腹直肌 rectus abdominis
2. 腹壁下动、静脉 inferior epigastric artery and vein
3. 腹股沟浅淋巴结 superficial inguinal lymph nodes
4. 回肠 ileum
5. 膀胱 urinary bladder
6. 乙状结肠 sigmoid colon
7. 子宫阔韧带 broad ligament of uterus
8. 左臀下动、静脉 left inferior gluteal artery and vein
9. 左输尿管 left ureter
10. 腹股沟深淋巴结 deep inguinal lymph node
11. 左股静脉 left femoral vein
12. 左股动脉 left femoral artery
13. 股神经 femoral nerve
14. 缝匠肌 sartorius
15. 阔筋膜张肌 tensor fasciae latae
16. 髂腰肌 iliopsoas
17. 髂股韧带 iliofemoral ligament
18. 股骨头 femoral head
19. 髋臼窝 acetabular fossa
20. 坐骨体 body of ischium

21. 臀小肌 gluteus minimus
22. 臀中肌 gluteus medius
23. 梨状肌肌腱 tendon of piriformis
24. 臀中肌肌腱 tendon of gluteus medius
25. 臀大肌 gluteus maximus
26. 尾骨 coccyx
27. 梨状肌 piriformis
28. 右臀下动、静脉 right inferior gluteal artery and vein
29. 坐骨神经 sciatic nerve
30. 子宫阴道静脉丛 uterovaginaal venous plexus
31. 闭孔内肌 obturator internus
32. 闭孔动、静脉 obturator artery and vein
33. 闭孔神经 obturator nerve
34. 耻骨体 body of pubis
35. 右股动脉 right femoral artery
36. 右股静脉 right femoral vein
37. 子宫颈 neck of uterus
38. 子宫颈管 canal of cervix of uterus
39. 直肠 rectum
40. 宫颈黏膜 cervical mucosa

关键结构：子宫阴道静脉丛，子宫颈。

此断面经过尾骨中份。子宫颈居盆腔中后方，断面逐渐缩小，中心见裂隙状的子宫颈管。子宫颈两侧见许多细小的血管断面，为子宫静脉丛，向上、向前、向后分别与蔓状静脉丛、膀胱静脉丛和直肠静脉丛相连，向下与阴道静脉丛相接，形成复杂的血管网结构，合称子宫阴道静脉丛，汇合成子宫静脉注入髂内静脉。这些静脉丛大多位于盈虚变化很大的脏器周围的疏松结缔组织中，静脉丛的壁很薄，其面积为动脉的10~15倍。彼此吻合的静脉丛，如同网篮一样围绕各脏器。在静脉之间，有动脉穿过，呈海绵状间隙。由于以上特点，手术过程中静脉丛容易损伤出血，做压迫、缝扎止血时，应慎重处理[21]。子宫颈左前方仍可见少许乙状结肠断面，右前方为回肠断面，包绕膀胱。子宫颈后方见类圆形直肠断面。子宫颈侧后方见臀下动、静脉断面。两侧盆壁内面见闭孔内肌断面。闭孔内肌内侧见闭孔动、静脉及闭孔神经断面。两侧髂腰肌位于耻骨体前方。髂腰肌断面的前内方自内侧向外侧分别见腹股沟深淋巴结、髂外静脉、髂外动脉及股神经的断面。本断面中梨状肌断面继续缩小，即将消失。

女性盆部与会阴连续横断层 48（FH.8430）

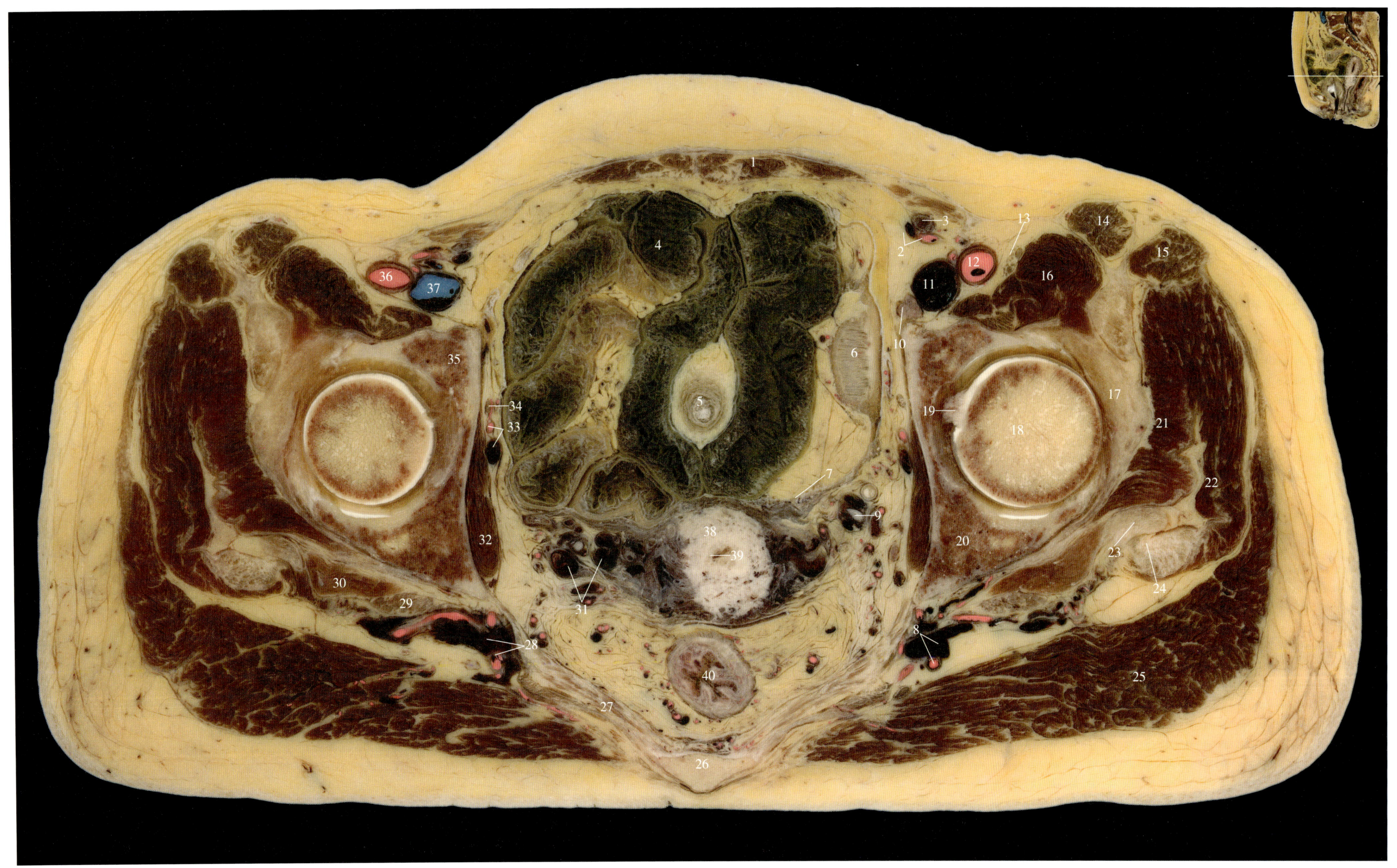

A. 断层标本图像

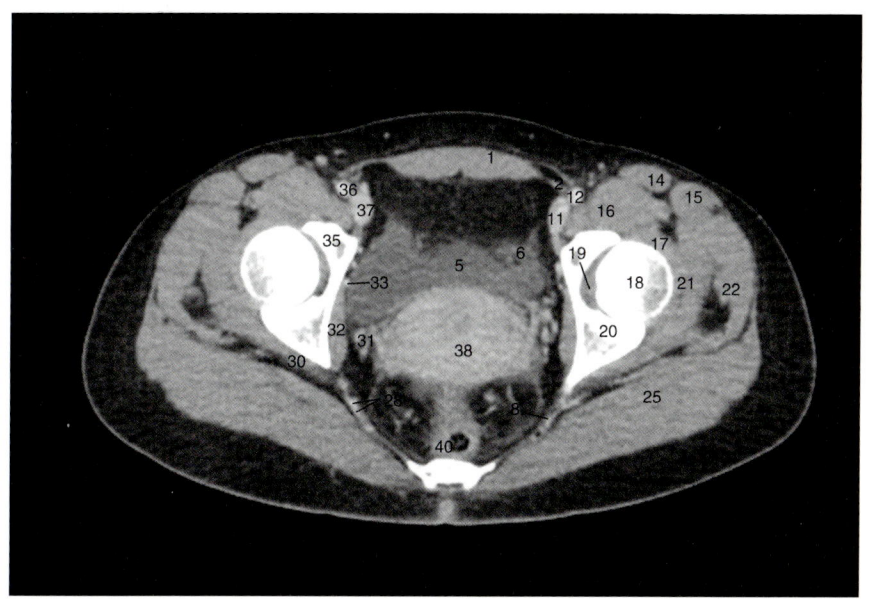
B. CT 增强图像

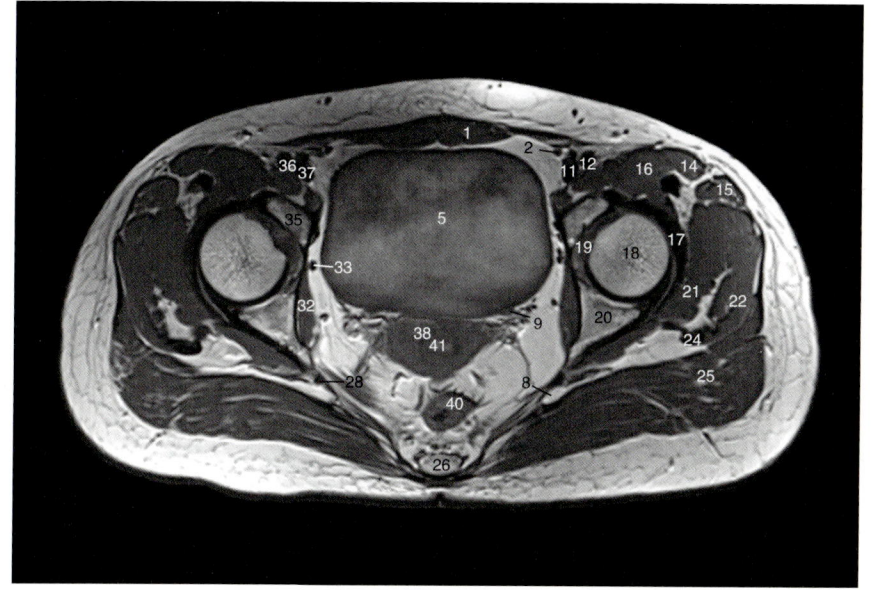
C. MR T1WI

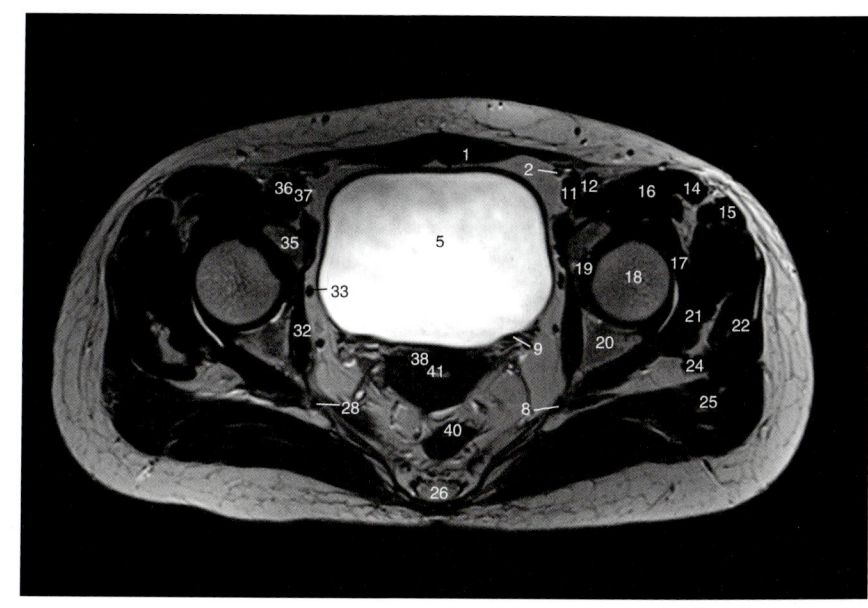
D. MR T2WI

1. 腹直肌 rectus abdominis
2. 腹壁下动、静脉 inferior epigastric artery and vein
3. 腹股沟浅淋巴结 superficial inguinal lymph nodes
4. 回肠 ileum
5. 膀胱 urinary bladder
6. 乙状结肠 sigmoid colon
7. 子宫阔韧带 broad ligament of uterus
8. 左臀下动、静脉 left inferior gluteal artery and vein
9. 左输尿管 left ureter
10. 腹股沟深淋巴结 deep inguinal lymph node
11. 左股静脉 left femoral vein
12. 左股动脉 left femoral artery
13. 股神经 femoral nerve
14. 缝匠肌 sartorius
15. 阔筋膜张肌 tensor fasciae latae
16. 髂腰肌 iliopsoas
17. 髂股韧带 iliofemoral ligament
18. 股骨头 femoral head
19. 股骨头韧带 ligament of head of femur
20. 坐骨体 body of ischium
21. 臀小肌 gluteus minimus

22. 臀中肌 gluteus medius
23. 上孖肌肌腱 tendon of gemellus superior
24. 臀中肌肌腱 tendon of gluteus medius
25. 臀大肌 gluteus maximus
26. 尾骨 coccyx
27. 肛提肌 levator ani
28. 右臀下动、静脉 right inferior gluteal artery and vein
29. 坐骨神经 sciatic nerve
30. 上孖肌 gemellus superior
31. 子宫阴道静脉丛 uterovaginaal venous plexus
32. 闭孔内肌 obturator internus
33. 闭孔动、静脉 obturator artery and vein
34. 闭孔神经 obturator nerve
35. 耻骨体 body of pubis
36. 右股动脉 right femoral artery
37. 右股静脉 right femoral vein
38. 子宫颈 neck of uterus
39. 子宫颈管 canal of cervix of uterus
40. 直肠 rectum
41. 宫颈黏膜 cervical mucosa

关键结构：上孖肌，肛提肌，股骨头韧带。

此断面经过尾骨中份。

其前方两侧呈倒"八"形的肛提肌条带状断面开始出现。梨状肌几乎全部消失，股骨大转子内侧见新出现的上孖肌断面。上孖肌位于闭孔内肌上方，起自坐骨棘，止于股骨大转子内侧表面，受骶丛分支（L4~S2）支配。坐骨神经在其上方穿过，本断层在上孖肌断面旁见粗大的坐骨神经断面。在后面的断面还将看到下孖肌。这两对肌肉就像双生子分别位于闭孔内肌的上下方。下孖肌起自坐骨结节和闭孔内肌肌腱，止于股骨转子窝，受骶丛分支（L4~S2）支配。上孖肌、下孖肌与闭孔内肌、梨状肌、股方肌共同组成髋关节短外旋肌群，使髋关节外旋，单独讨论上孖肌和下孖肌临床意义不大[26]。上孖肌前方为耻骨体和坐骨体组合成的髋骨，髋臼窝内见断面逐渐增大的圆形股骨头，股骨头内侧偏前见股骨头韧带出现，止于股骨头凹。股骨头外侧及后方从内侧向外侧依次为髂股韧带、臀小肌、臀中肌、臀大肌，臀小肌和臀中肌之间见臀中肌肌腱、股骨大转子和上孖肌。盆腔前方自中线向两侧依次见腹直肌、腹内斜肌、缝匠肌和阔筋膜张肌断面。

女性盆部与会阴连续横断层 49（FH.8410）

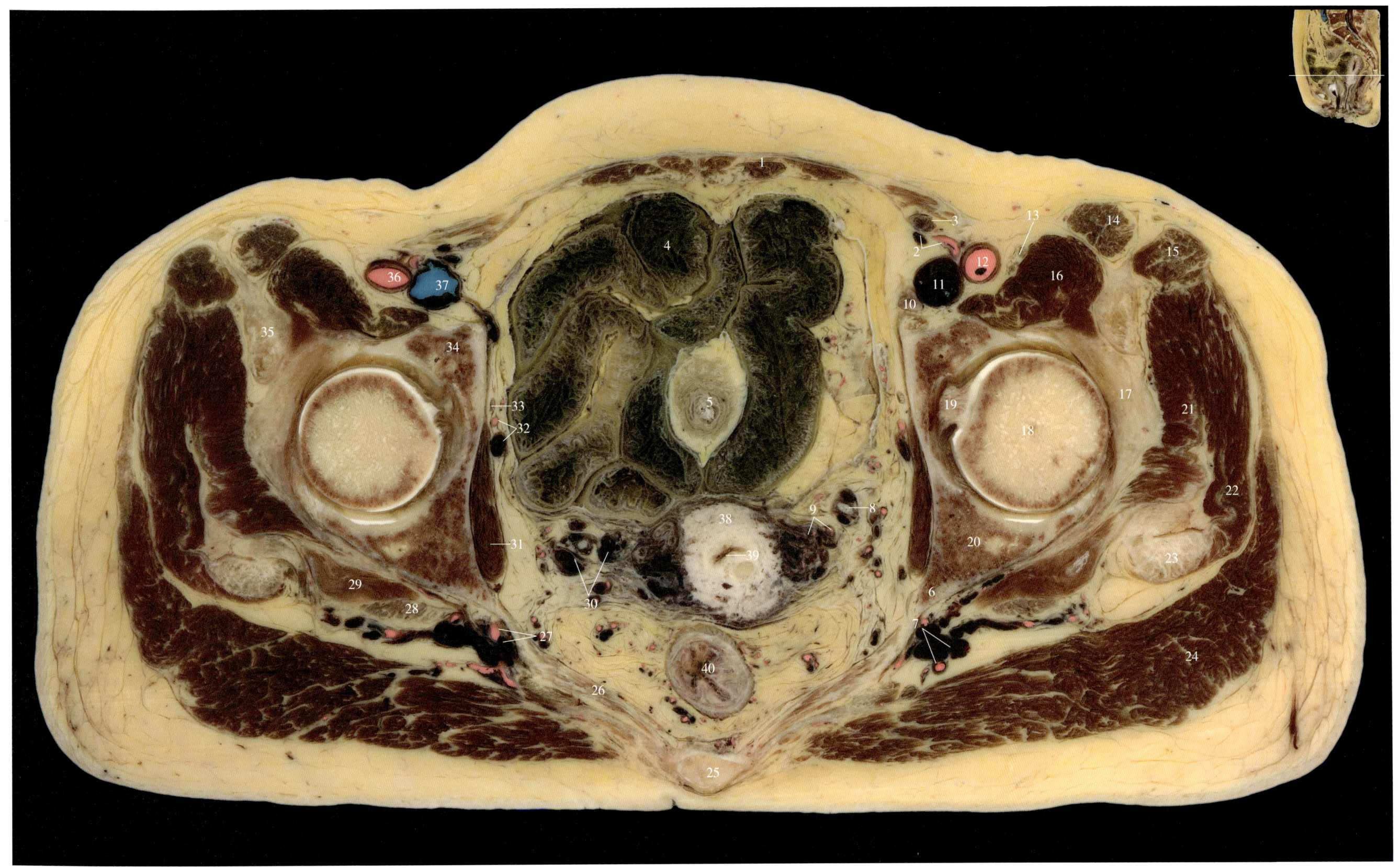

A. 断层标本图像

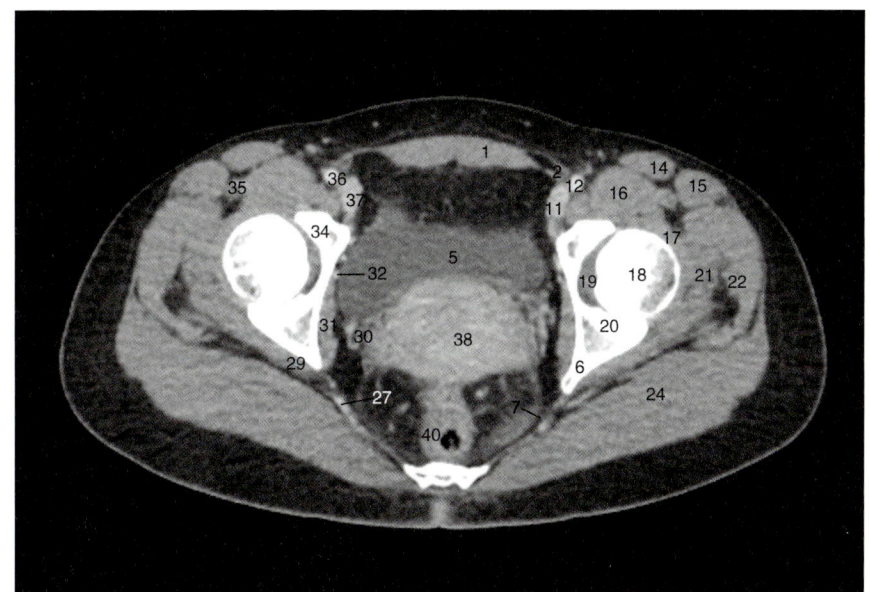
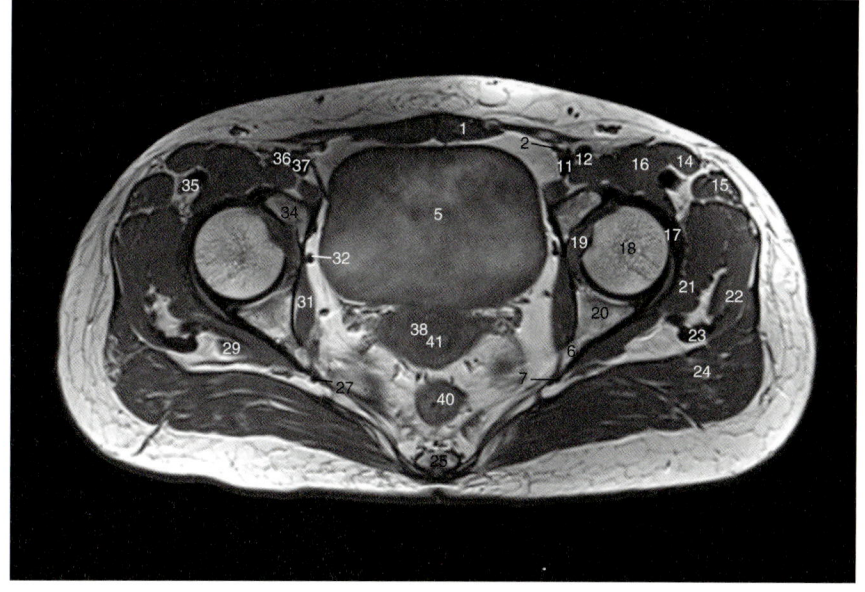
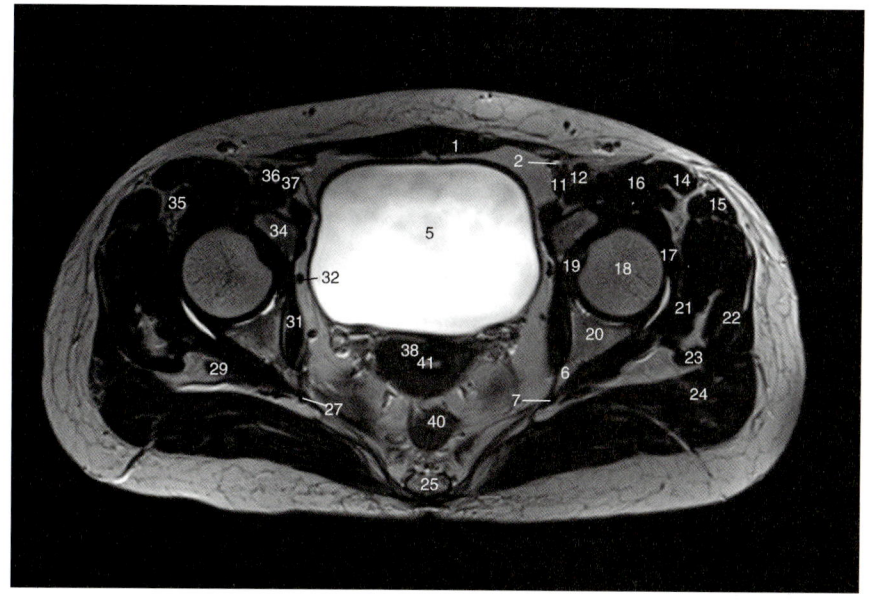

B. CT 增强图像　　　　　　　　　　　C. MR T1WI　　　　　　　　　　　D. MR T2WI

1. 腹直肌 rectus abdominis
2. 腹壁下动、静脉 inferior epigastric artery and vein
3. 腹股沟浅淋巴结 superficial inguinal lymph nodes
4. 回肠 ileum
5. 膀胱 urinary bladder
6. 坐骨棘 ischial spine
7. 左臀下动、静脉 left inferior gluteal artery and vein
8. 左输尿管 left ureter
9. 子宫动、静脉 uterine artery and vein
10. 腹股沟深淋巴结 deep inguinal lymph node
11. 左股静脉 left femoral vein
12. 左股动脉 left femoral artery
13. 股神经 femoral nerve
14. 缝匠肌 sartorius
15. 阔筋膜张肌 tensor fasciae latae
16. 髂腰肌 iliopsoas
17. 髂股韧带 iliofemoral ligament
18. 股骨头 femoral head
19. 股骨头韧带 ligament of head of femur
20. 坐骨体 body of ischium
21. 臀小肌 gluteus minimus
22. 臀中肌 gluteus medius
23. 臀中肌肌腱 tendon of gluteus medius
24. 臀大肌 gluteus maximus
25. 尾骨 coccyx
26. 肛提肌 levator ani
27. 右臀下动、静脉 right inferior gluteal artery and vein
28. 坐骨神经 sciatic nerve
29. 上孖肌 gemellus superior
30. 子宫阴道静脉丛 uterovaginaal venous plexus
31. 闭孔内肌 obturator internus
32. 闭孔动、静脉 obturator artery and vein
33. 闭孔神经 obturator nerve
34. 耻骨体 body of pubis
35. 股直肌 rectus femoris
36. 右股动脉 right femoral artery
37. 右股静脉 right femoral vein
38. 子宫颈 neck of uterus
39. 子宫颈管 canal of cervix of uterus
40. 直肠 rectum
41. 宫颈黏膜 cervical mucosa

关键结构：坐骨棘，子宫动、静脉。

此断面经过尾骨中份。盆腔两侧的坐骨体向下延伸，坐骨棘开始出现，为坐骨大切迹和坐骨小切迹之间的骨性突起，不仅是上孖肌的附着点，两侧坐骨棘间距在产科工作中也有着指导意义。肛提肌出现，股骨头断面继续增大。在髂腰肌、缝匠肌、阔筋膜张肌、臀小肌和髂股韧带之间的腔隙内，股直肌断面开始出现。盆腔内子宫颈断面继续缩小，膀胱逐渐增大，乙状结肠断面消失。子宫旁见子宫动、静脉断面。子宫动脉是女性特有动脉，为髂内动脉前干分支，在腹膜后沿盆侧壁向下向前走行，经阔韧带基底部、子宫旁组织达到子宫外侧，于距子宫颈内口水平约 2 cm 处横跨输尿管达到子宫侧缘，沿子宫侧缘迂曲上行，称为子宫体支。主干至子宫角部分为宫底支（分布于子宫底部）、卵巢支（与卵巢动脉末梢吻合）和输卵管支（分布于输卵管）。在宫颈内口水平，子宫动脉分出一些侧支，供应膀胱、阴道上部、宫颈[21]。国内一项用三维 DSA 研究显示，69% 的子宫动脉起源于髂内动脉前干，19.1% 起源于髂内动脉主干，9.5% 发自阴部内动脉，2.4% 起源于臀下动脉。子宫动脉开口和走行在对侧斜位于 25°~35° 投照时的显示效果佳，有助于介入治疗选择性插管[29]。

女性盆部与会阴连续横断层 50（FH.8390）

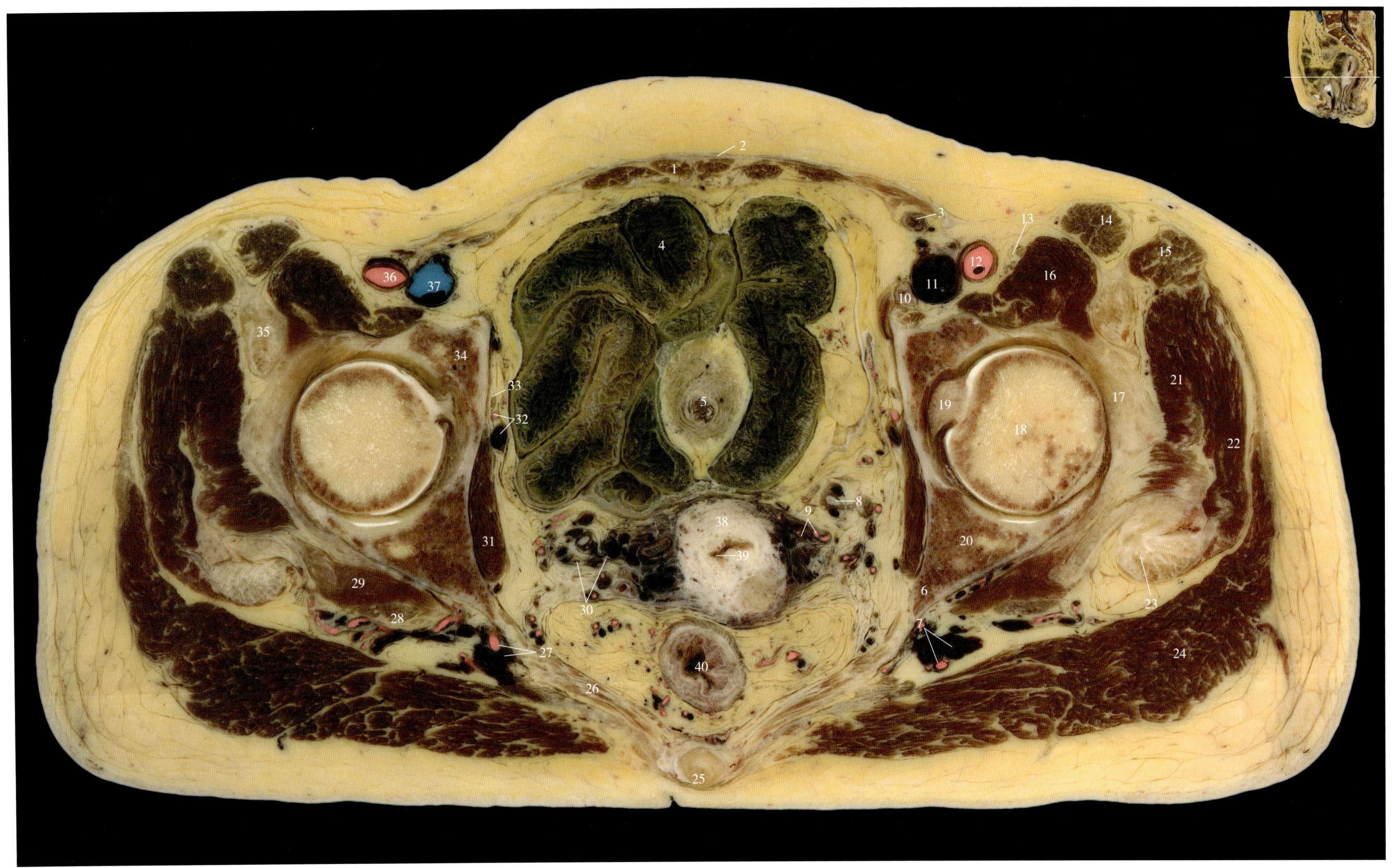

A. 断层标本图像

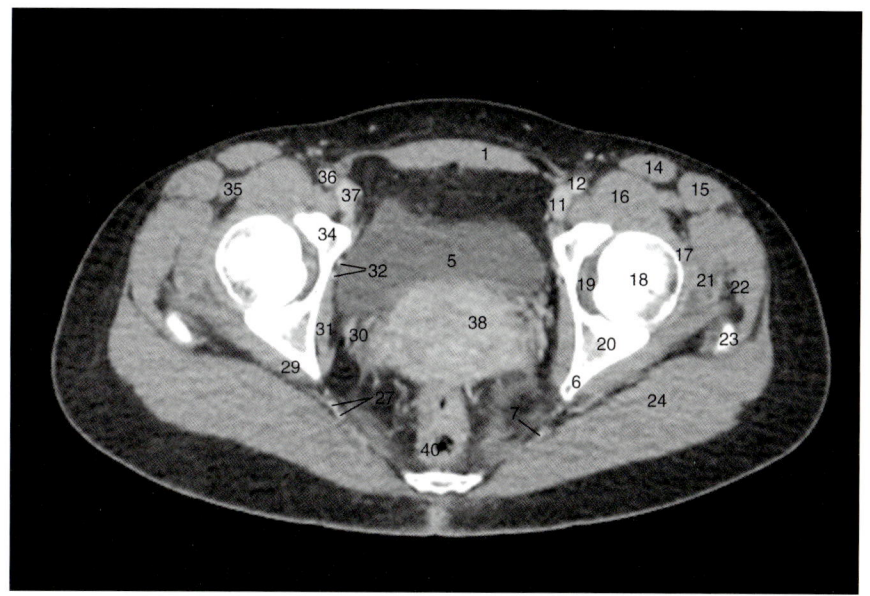
B. CT 增强图像

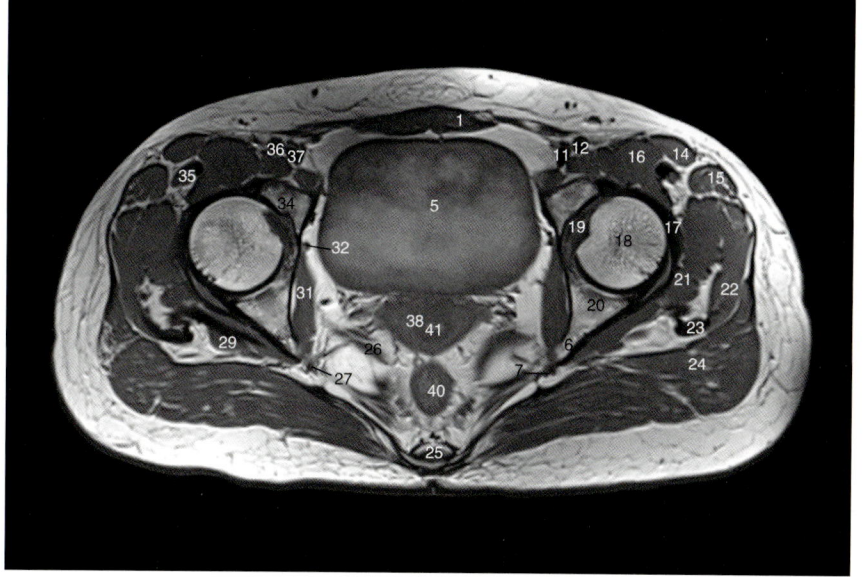
C. MR T1WI

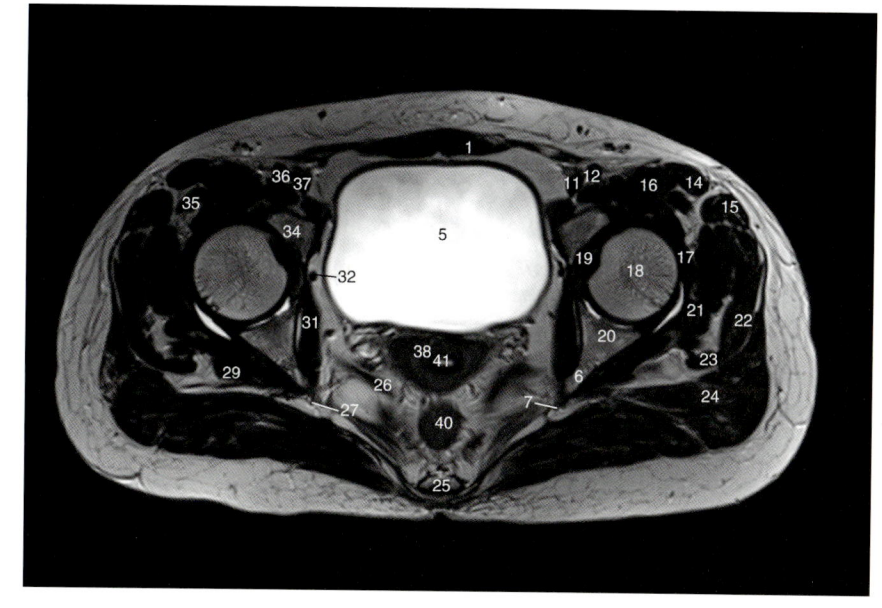
D. MR T2WI

1. 腹直肌 rectus abdominis
2. 腹直肌鞘 sheath of rectus abdominis
3. 腹股沟浅淋巴结 superficial inguinal lymph nodes
4. 回肠 ileum
5. 膀胱 urinary bladder
6. 坐骨棘 ischial spine
7. 左臀下动、静脉 left inferior gluteal artery and vein
8. 左输尿管 left ureter
9. 子宫动、静脉 uterine artery and vein
10. 腹股沟深淋巴结 deep inguinal lymph node
11. 左股静脉 left femoral vein
12. 左股动脉 left femoral artery
13. 股神经 femoral nerve
14. 缝匠肌 sartorius
15. 阔筋膜张肌 tensor fasciae latae
16. 髂腰肌 iliopsoas
17. 髂股韧带 iliofemoral ligament
18. 股骨头 femoral head
19. 股骨头韧带 ligament of head of femur
20. 坐骨体 body of ischium
21. 臀小肌 gluteus minimus

22. 臀中肌 gluteus medius
23. 臀中肌肌腱 tendon of gluteus medius
24. 臀大肌 gluteus maximus
25. 尾骨 coccyx
26. 肛提肌 levator ani
27. 右臀下动、静脉 right inferior gluteal artery and vein
28. 坐骨神经 sciatic nerve
29. 上孖肌 gemellus superior
30. 子宫阴道静脉丛 uterovaginaal venous plexus
31. 闭孔内肌 obturator internus
32. 闭孔动、静脉 obturator artery and vein
33. 闭孔神经 obturator nerve
34. 耻骨体 body of pubis
35. 股直肌 rectus femoris
36. 右股动脉 right femoral artery
37. 右股静脉 right femoral vein
38. 子宫颈 neck of uterus
39. 子宫颈管 canal of cervix of uterus
40. 直肠 rectum
41. 宫颈黏膜 cervical mucosa

关键结构：腹直肌鞘，子宫颈。

此断面经过尾骨中份。

膀胱继续增大，子宫颈断面逐渐缩小，坐骨棘和股骨头断面继续增大。盆腔前壁的腹直肌鞘在该断面显示较清楚。腹直肌鞘由腹壁的 3 层扁肌肌腱膜包绕腹直肌构成，呈封套状。鞘分前、后 2 层，前层由腹外斜肌肌腱膜与腹内斜肌肌腱膜的前层相互融合构成；后层由腹内斜肌肌腱膜的后层与腹横肌肌腱膜相互融合构成。在脐下 4~5 cm 以下，鞘后层的腱膜全部移至前层，参与前层的构成，因此鞘后层下部阙如，中断之处形成一弓状游离下缘，称弓状线。弓状线以下，腹直肌后面直接与腹横筋膜相贴，腹直肌的后面由浅入深仅有腹横筋膜、腹膜外筋膜和壁腹膜。孕妇在妊娠的后几个月，由于腹盆腔压力不断增加，可使弓状线以下的腹直肌从中线向两侧分离，严重者子宫前壁仅覆以腹膜、筋膜和皮肤。腹直肌鞘内含有腹直肌，锥状肌，下 5 对肋间神经、肋下神经，肋间后动、静脉、肋下动、静脉，以及腹壁上、下动、静脉等[21]。锥状肌为腹直肌下端前面的三角形小扁肌，位于腹直肌鞘内、白线的两侧，以腱性纤维起于耻骨结节与耻骨联合之间，肌纤维斜向内上方止于白线，达脐与耻骨联合连线的中点以下。此肌由肋下神经支配，有紧张白线的功能。该肌在有袋类动物比较发达，在人类此肌已经退化甚至阙如，其功能不甚重要[30]。

女性盆部与会阴连续横断层 51（FH.8370）

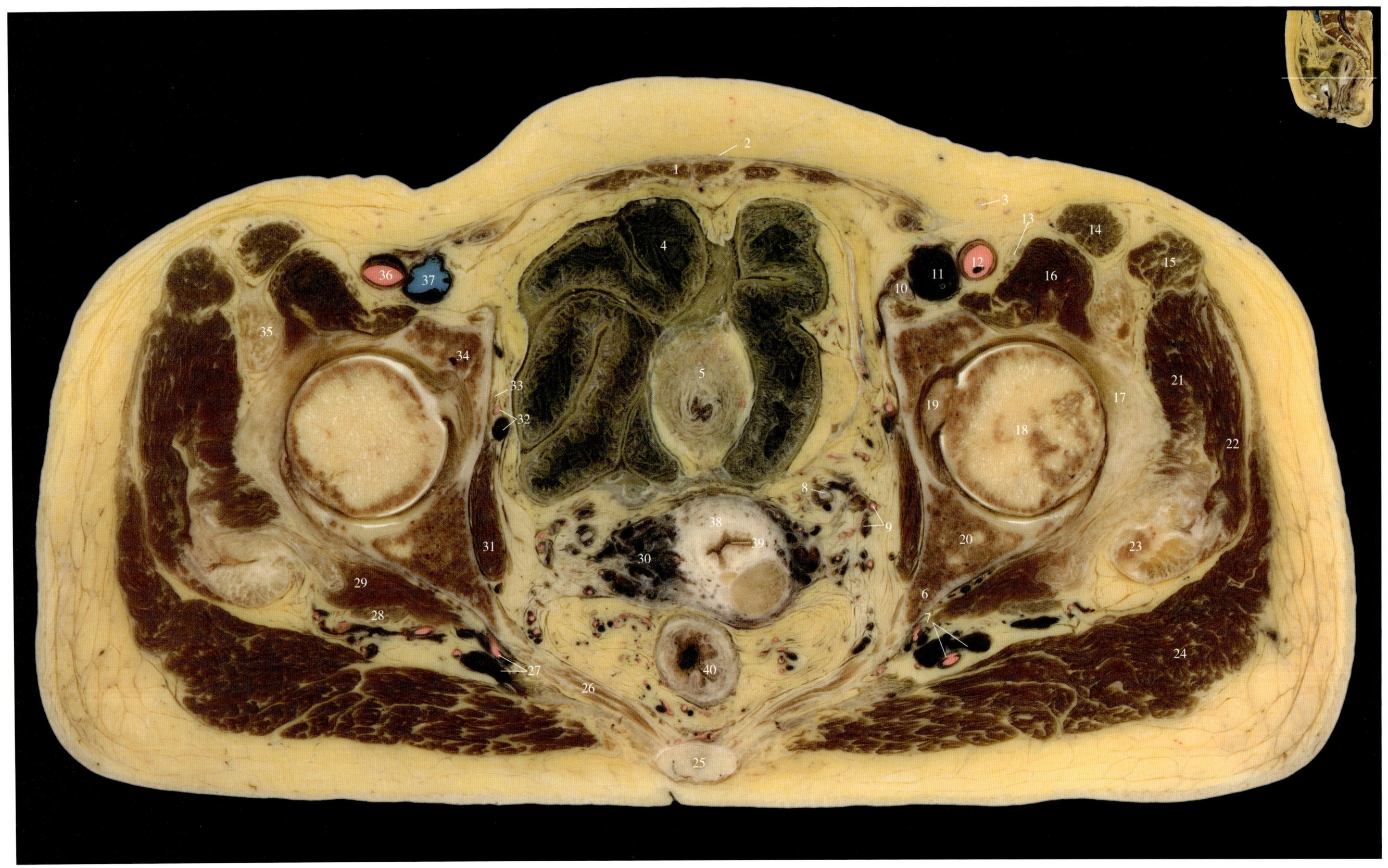

A. 断层标本图像

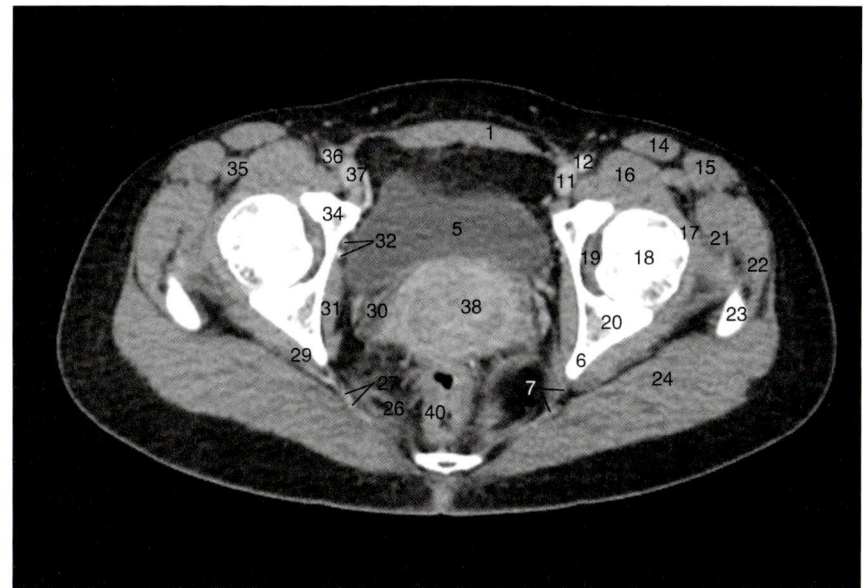
B. CT 增强图像

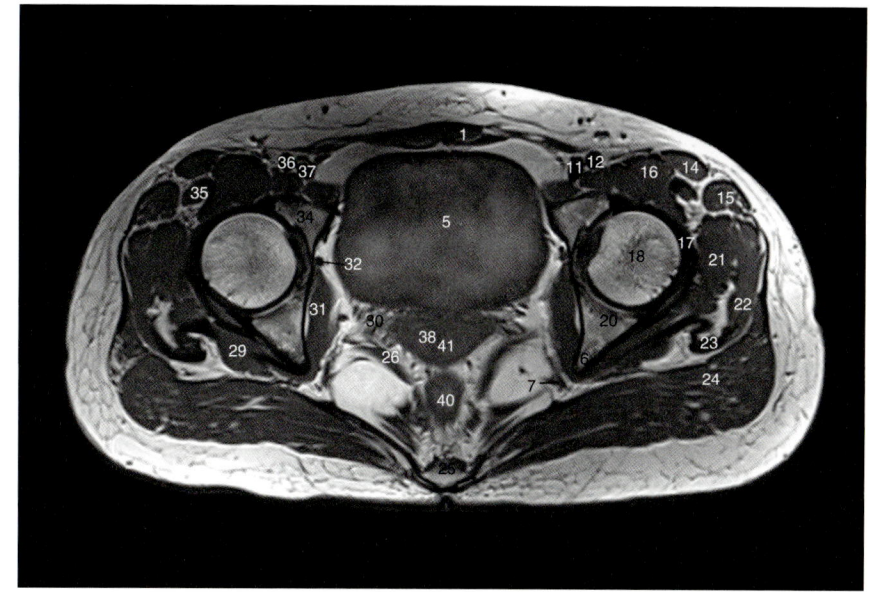
C. MR T1WI

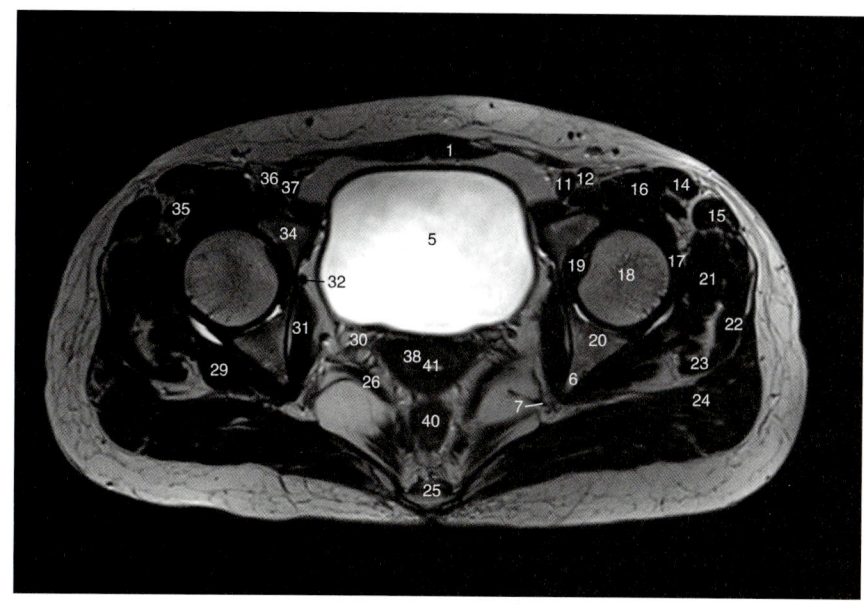
D. MR T2WI

1. 腹直肌 rectus abdominis
2. 腹直肌鞘 sheath of rectus abdominis
3. 腹股沟浅淋巴结 superficial inguinal lymph nodes
4. 回肠 ileum
5. 膀胱 urinary bladder
6. 坐骨棘 ischial spine
7. 左臀下动、静脉 left inferior gluteal artery and vein
8. 左输尿管 left ureter
9. 子宫动、静脉 uterine artery and vein
10. 腹股沟深淋巴结 deep inguinal lymph node
11. 左股静脉 left femoral vein
12. 左股动脉 left femoral artery
13. 股神经 femoral nerve
14. 缝匠肌 sartorius
15. 阔筋膜张肌 tensor fasciae latae
16. 髂腰肌 iliopsoas
17. 髂股韧带 iliofemoral ligament
18. 股骨头 femoral head
19. 股骨头韧带 ligament of head of femur
20. 坐骨体 body of ischium
21. 臀小肌 gluteus minimus
22. 臀中肌 gluteus medius
23. 股骨大转子 greater trochanter
24. 臀大肌 gluteus maximus
25. 尾骨 coccyx
26. 肛提肌 levator ani
27. 右臀下动、静脉 right inferior gluteal artery and vein
28. 坐骨神经 sciatic nerve
29. 上孖肌 gemellus superior
30. 子宫阴道静脉丛 uterovaginaal venous plexus
31. 闭孔内肌 obturator internus
32. 闭孔动、静脉 obturator artery and vein
33. 闭孔神经 obturator nerve
34. 耻骨体 body of pubis
35. 股直肌 rectus femoris
36. 右股动脉 right femoral artery
37. 右股静脉 right femoral vein
38. 子宫颈 neck of uterus
39. 子宫颈管 canal of cervix of uterus
40. 直肠 rectum
41. 宫颈黏膜 cervical mucosa

关键结构：子宫颈，膀胱。

此断面经过尾骨中份。较前一断面变化不大。子宫颈居盆腔中后方，断面逐渐缩小，中心见裂隙状的子宫颈管。在本标本子宫颈左后壁见一大一小两个棕黄色卵圆形肿物断面，边界光滑、清楚，可能为宫颈肌瘤或宫颈管囊肿。宫颈肌瘤的发生率约占子宫肌瘤的10%，B超是首选检查方法。肌壁间肌瘤在超声上多表现为低回声结节，较大的肌瘤伴后方回声衰减，肌瘤内部回声特征取决于肌瘤结缔组织纤维含量及有无变性。MRI 能准确判断肌瘤的大小、数目和位置。典型表现为肌层内边界清楚 T2WI 低信号结节或肿块，单发或多发，增强扫描不均匀持续强化，延迟强化较均匀。宫颈囊肿为宫颈管腺开口堵塞导致分泌物潴留而成，多数无临床症状[21]。宫颈囊肿在 MRI 上的典型表现为边界清楚的长 T1、长 T2 信号，增强扫描不强化。尾骨居于盆部后壁中央，其前方两侧的肛提肌断面逐渐增大。坐骨棘和耻骨体包绕的股骨头断面继续增大，股骨头内侧偏前见股骨头韧带断面。盆腔前方中线两侧见腹直肌，其两侧的腹内斜肌几乎消失不见。

女性盆部与会阴连续横断层 52（FH.8350）

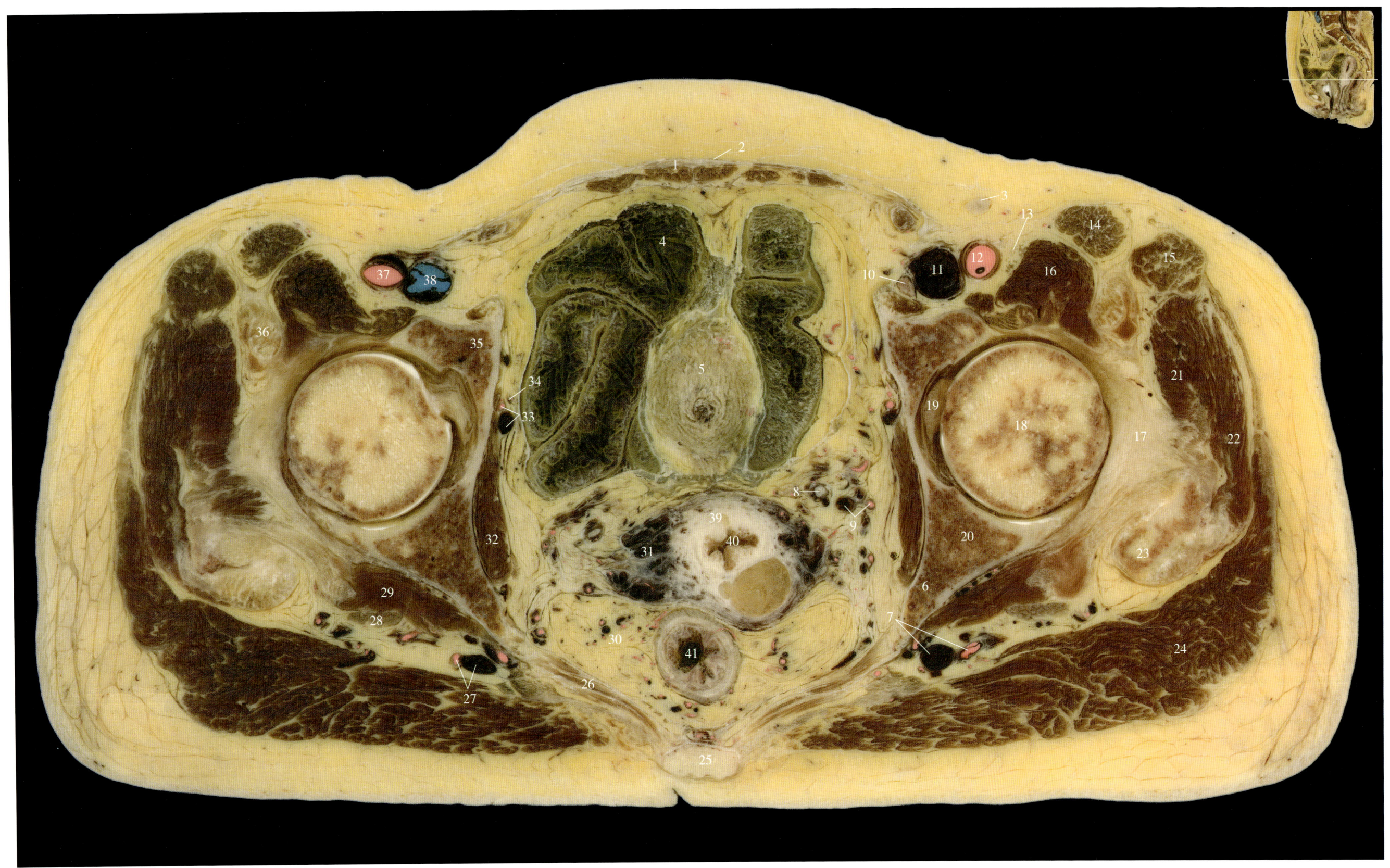

A. 断层标本图像

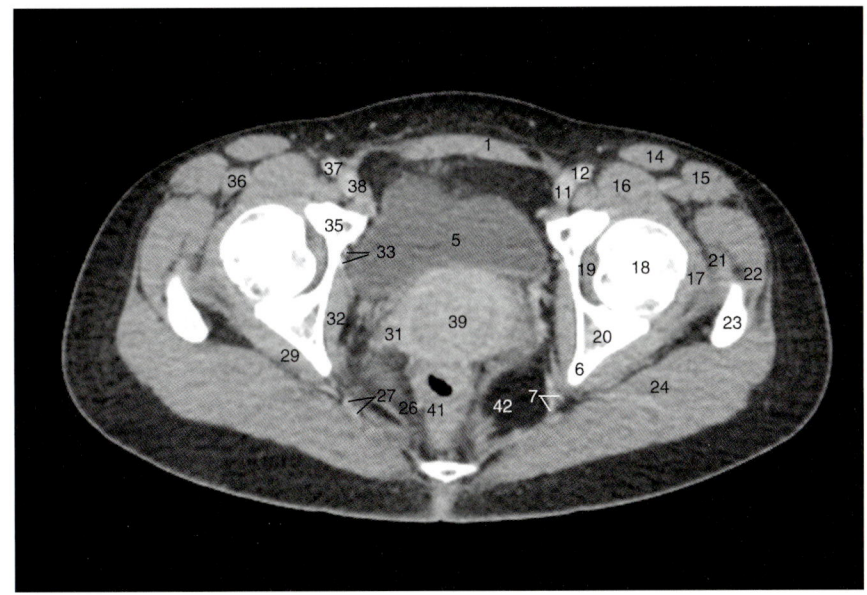
B. CT 增强图像

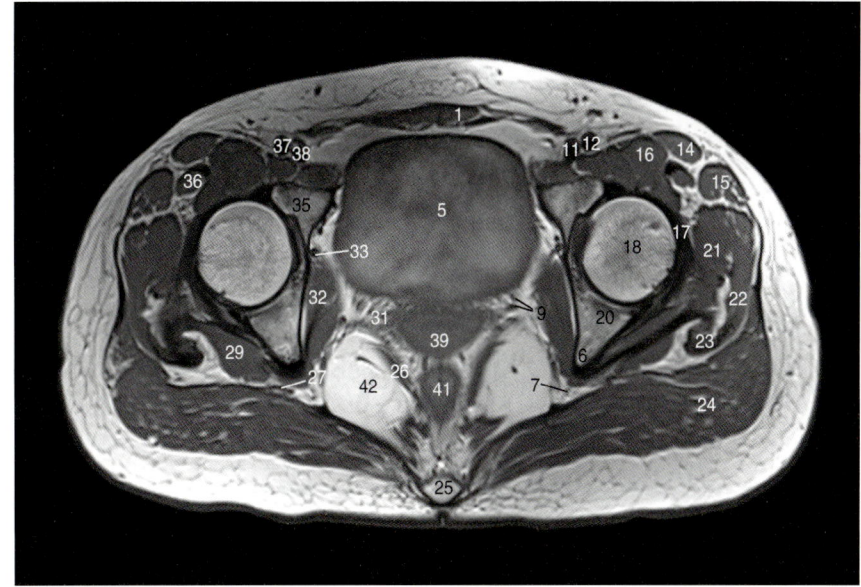
C. MR T1WI

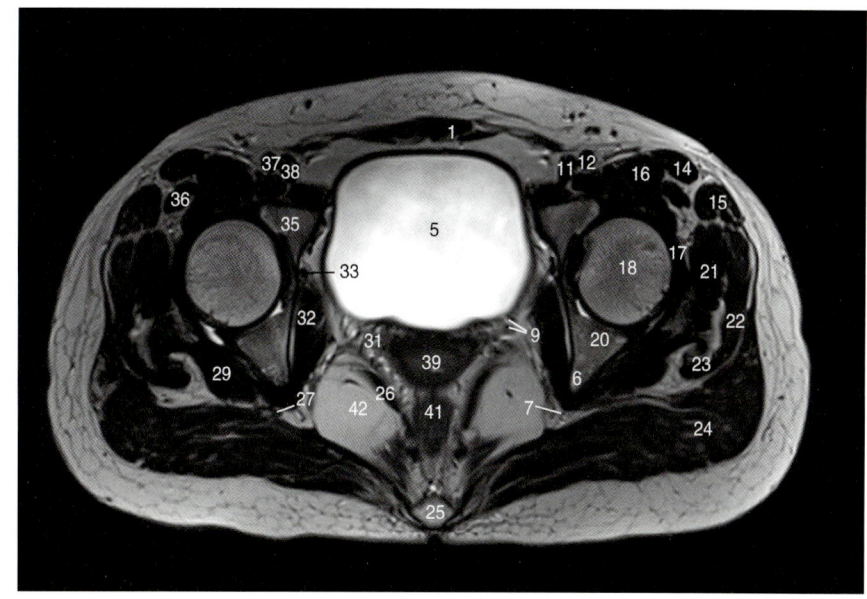
D. MR T2WI

1. 腹直肌 rectus abdominis
2. 腹直肌鞘 sheath of rectus abdominis
3. 腹股沟浅淋巴结 superficial inguinal lymph nodes
4. 回肠 ileum
5. 膀胱 urinary bladder
6. 坐骨棘 ischial spine
7. 左臀下动、静脉 left inferior gluteal artery and vein
8. 左输尿管 left ureter
9. 子宫动、静脉 uterine artery and vein
10. 腹股沟深淋巴结 deep inguinal lymph node
11. 左股静脉 left femoral vein
12. 左股动脉 left femoral artery
13. 股神经 femoral nerve
14. 缝匠肌 sartorius
15. 阔筋膜张肌 tensor fasciae latae
16. 髂腰肌 iliopsoas
17. 髂股韧带 iliofemoral ligament
18. 股骨头 femoral head
19. 股骨头韧带 ligament of head of femur
20. 坐骨体 body of ischium
21. 臀小肌 gluteus minimus
22. 臀中肌 gluteus medius
23. 股骨大转子 greater trochanter
24. 臀大肌 gluteus maximus
25. 尾骨 coccyx
26. 肛提肌 levator ani
27. 右臀下动、静脉 right inferior gluteal artery and vein
28. 坐骨神经 sciatic nerve
29. 上孖肌 gemellus superior
30. 直肠系膜 mesorectum
31. 子宫阴道静脉丛 uterovaginaal venous plexus
32. 闭孔内肌 obturator internus
33. 闭孔动、静脉 obturator artery and vein
34. 闭孔神经 obturator nerve
35. 耻骨体 body of pubis
36. 股直肌 rectus femoris
37. 右股动脉 right femoral artery
38. 右股静脉 right femoral vein
39. 子宫颈 neck of uterus
40. 子宫颈管 canal of cervix of uterus
41. 直肠 rectum
42. 坐骨肛门窝 ischioanal fossa

关键结构：坐骨肛门窝，膀胱，直肠。

　　此断面经过尾骨下份。较前一断面变化不大。肛提肌和股骨头断面逐渐增大。盆腔内膀胱断面逐渐增大，子宫颈断面逐渐缩小。子宫颈后方可见类圆形直肠断面。CT 及 MR 图像显示直肠两侧富含脂肪组织的区域为坐骨肛门窝。坐骨肛门窝是盆膈下方肛管和坐骨之间的楔形腔隙，在横断面上大致呈倒立的三角形，由筋膜包围形成，其下方为会阴皮肤，上方为盆膈；在肛尾韧带上方，两侧坐骨肛门窝相互交通。在上方，它的顶端位于肛提肌在闭孔筋膜的起点处；内侧为肛提肌和肛门外括约肌及其筋膜，外侧为闭孔内肌及其筋膜，后方为骶结节韧带和臀大肌下缘，前方为尿生殖膈后缘。坐骨肛门窝内充填大量脂肪组织，脂肪内含有许多纤维隔，像海绵一样具有缓冲功能，保护肛管。坐骨肛门窝是脓肿的好发部位，且容易向周围蔓延。当脓液穿入直肠穿通皮肤时，即形成肛瘘[21]。在 CT 图像上，坐骨肛门窝为坐骨结节、肛管和臀大肌所围成的三角形低密度区域。MR T1 和 T2 加权图像上，直肠内气体呈黑色，坐骨肛门窝内脂肪呈白色，直肠壁呈灰色，易于辨识[1]。

女性盆部与会阴连续横断层 53（FH.8330）

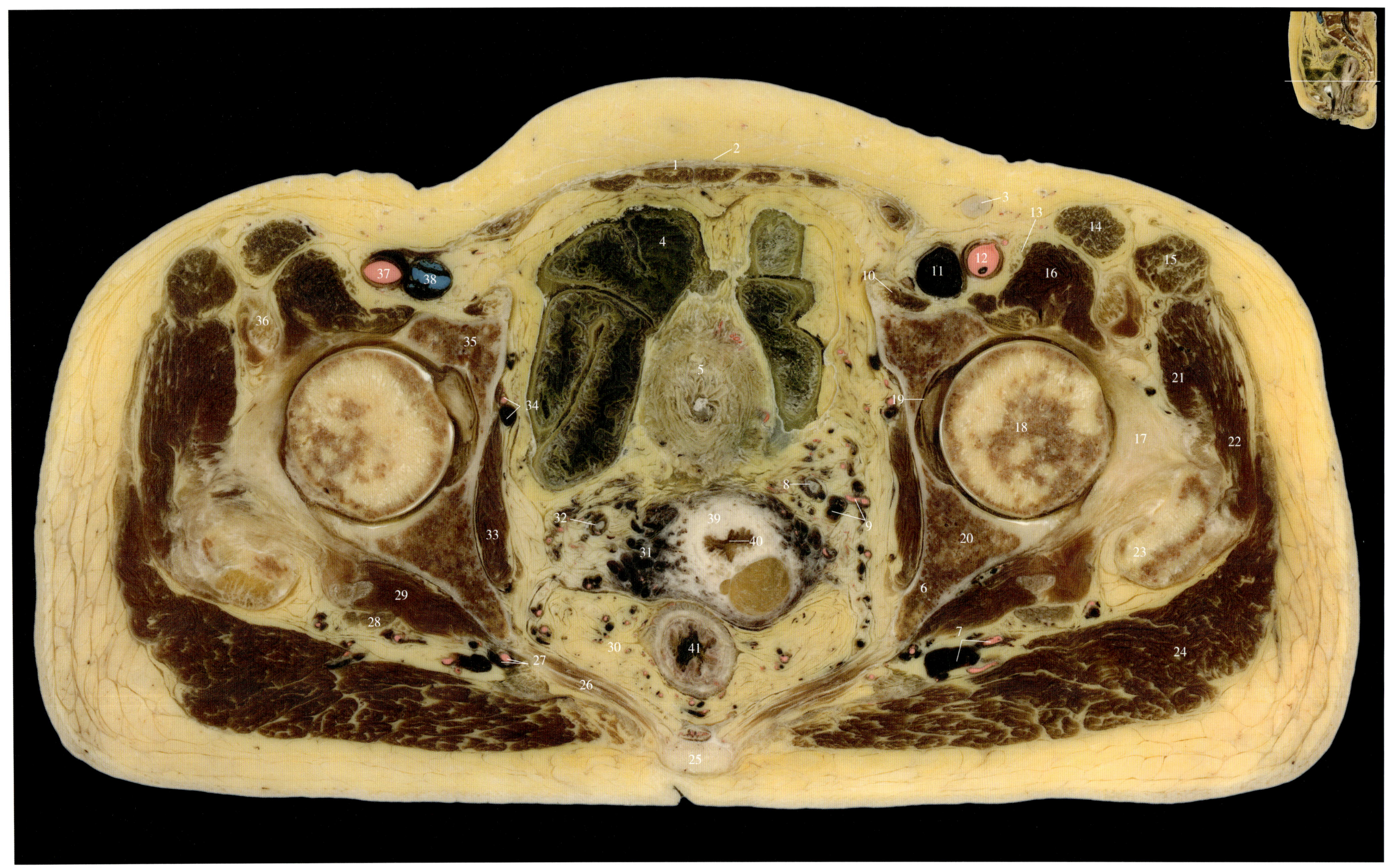

A. 断层标本图像

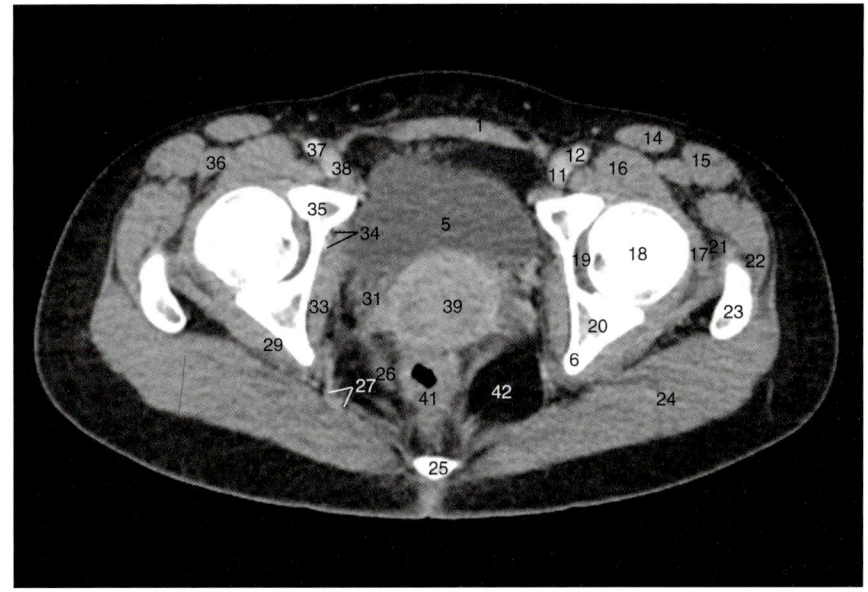
B. CT 增强图像

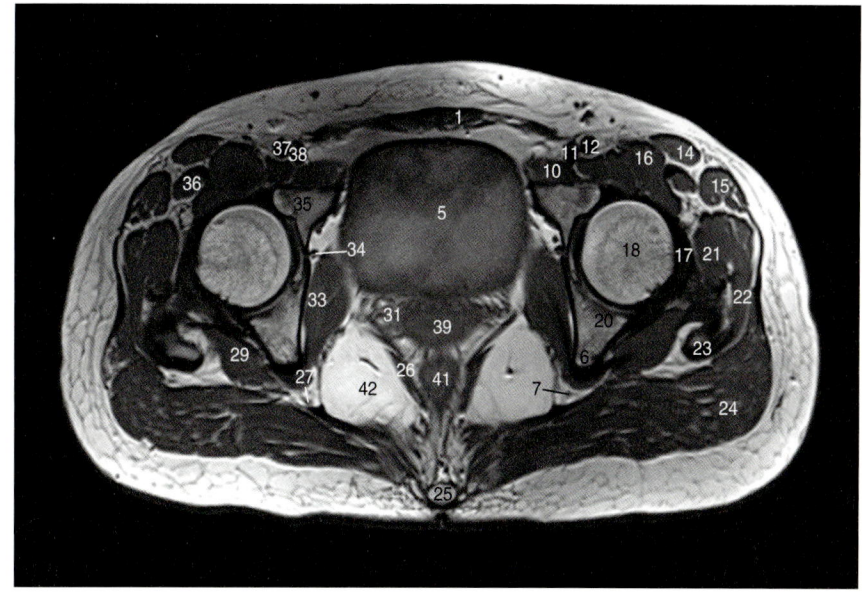
C. MR T1WI

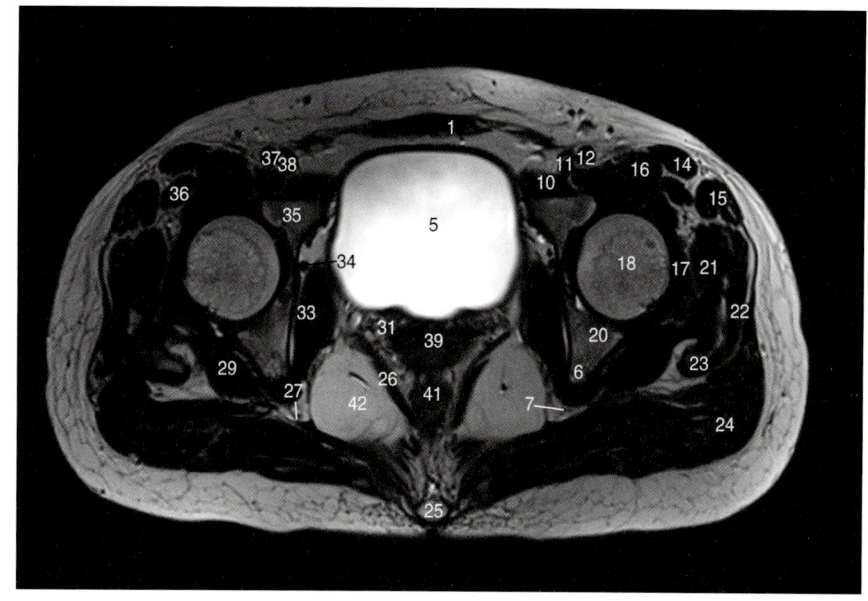
D. MR T2WI

1. 腹直肌 rectus abdominis
2. 腹直肌鞘 sheath of rectus abdominis
3. 腹股沟浅淋巴结 superficial inguinal lymph nodes
4. 回肠 ileum
5. 膀胱 urinary bladder
6. 坐骨棘 ischial spine
7. 左臀下动、静脉 left inferior gluteal artery and vein
8. 左输尿管 left ureter
9. 子宫动、静脉 uterine artery and vein
10. 耻骨体 body of pubis
11. 左股静脉 left femoral vein
12. 左股动脉 left femoral artery
13. 股神经 femoral nerve
14. 缝匠肌 sartorius
15. 阔筋膜张肌 tensor fasciae latae
16. 髂腰肌 iliopsoas
17. 髂股韧带 iliofemoral ligament
18. 股骨头 femoral head
19. 股骨头韧带 ligament of head of femur
20. 坐骨体 body of ischium
21. 臀小肌 gluteus minimus
22. 臀中肌 gluteus medius
23. 股骨大转子 greater trochanter
24. 臀大肌 gluteus maximus
25. 尾骨 coccyx
26. 肛提肌 levator ani
27. 右阴部内动、静脉 right internal pudendal artery and vein
28. 坐骨神经 sciatic nerve
29. 上孖肌 gemellus superior
30. 直肠系膜 mesorectum
31. 子宫阴道静脉丛 uterovaginaal venous plexus
32. 右输尿管 right ureter
33. 闭孔内肌 obturator internus
34. 闭孔动、静脉 obturator artery and vein
35. 耻骨体 body of pubis
36. 股直肌 rectus femoris
37. 右股动脉 right femoral artery
38. 右股静脉 right femoral vein
39. 子宫颈 neck of uterus
40. 子宫颈管 canal of cervix of uterus
41. 直肠 rectum
42. 坐骨肛门窝 ischioanal fossa

关键结构：耻骨肌，坐骨肛门窝，直肠。

此断面经过尾骨下份。

断面中部为盆腔，子宫颈居于中后方，断面继续缩小，中心见不规则裂隙状的子宫颈管。子宫颈两侧见子宫阴道静脉丛的无数小断面及输尿管和子宫动、静脉断面。子宫颈前方见回肠断面，包绕逐渐增大的膀胱。子宫颈后方见类圆形直肠断面。坐骨棘与直肠之间为坐骨肛门窝，被脂肪组织充填。盆腔两侧为耻骨体和坐骨体形成的骨性盆壁。紧贴耻骨体前方、股静脉内侧见耻骨肌断面出现。耻骨肌为长方形的短肌，位于大腿上部前面的皮下，髂腰肌的内侧，长收肌的外侧，其深面紧贴短收肌和闭孔外肌。此肌为股三角的后壁，并与髂腰肌共同形成髂耻窝。起自耻骨梳和耻骨上支，肌束斜向后下外方，绕过股骨颈向后，借扁腱止于股骨小转子以下的耻骨肌线。耻骨肌收缩使大腿屈曲、内收和旋外。耻骨肌受股神经的分支（L2、L3）支配，偶尔也由闭孔神经的分支（L3）支配[30]。耻骨肌外侧依次见腹股沟深淋巴结、股静脉、股动脉、股神经、髂腰肌、缝匠肌和阔筋膜张肌的断面。盆腔前方中线处见腹直肌及包裹它的腹直肌鞘。

女性盆部与会阴连续横断层 54（FH.8310）

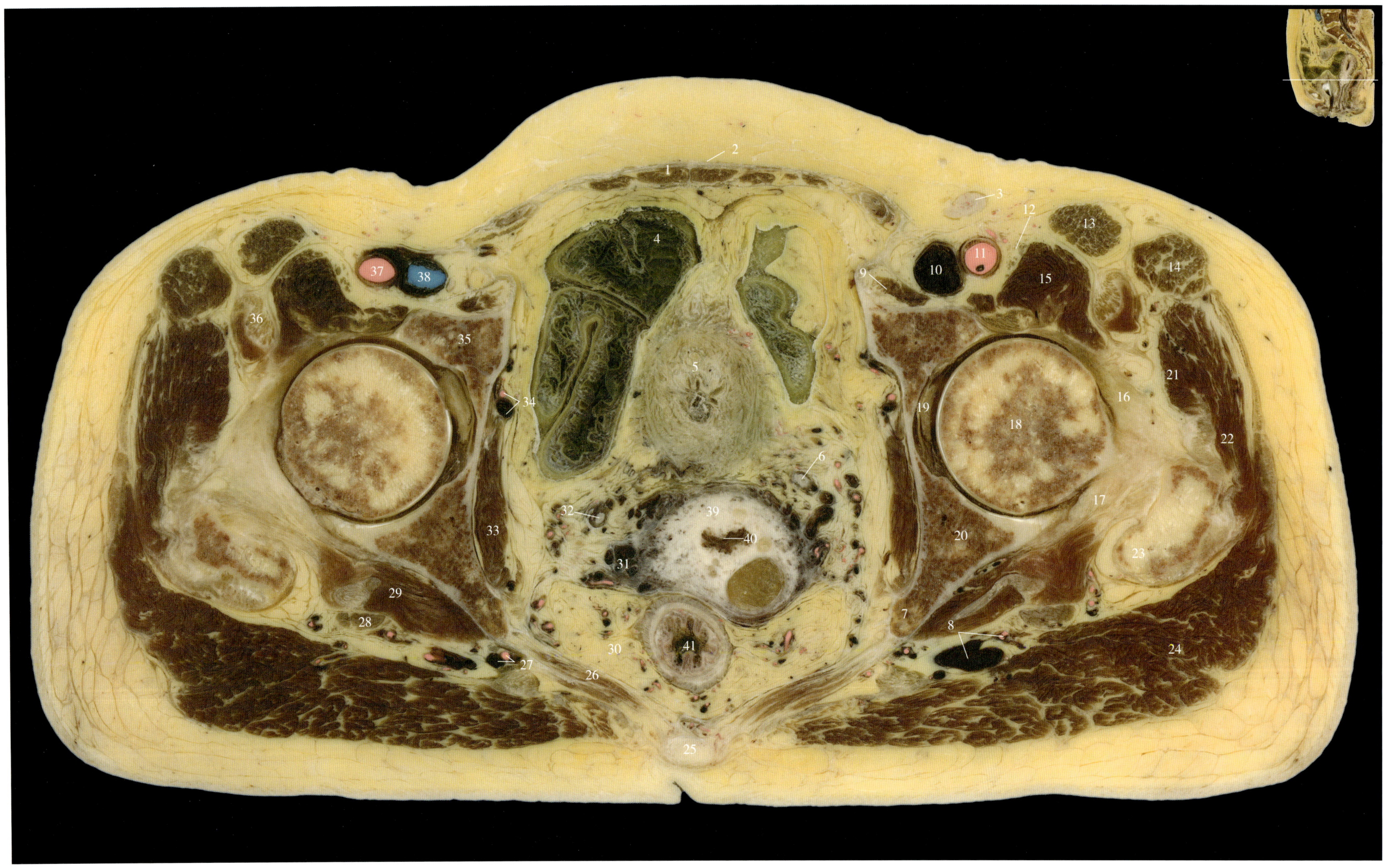

A. 断层标本图像

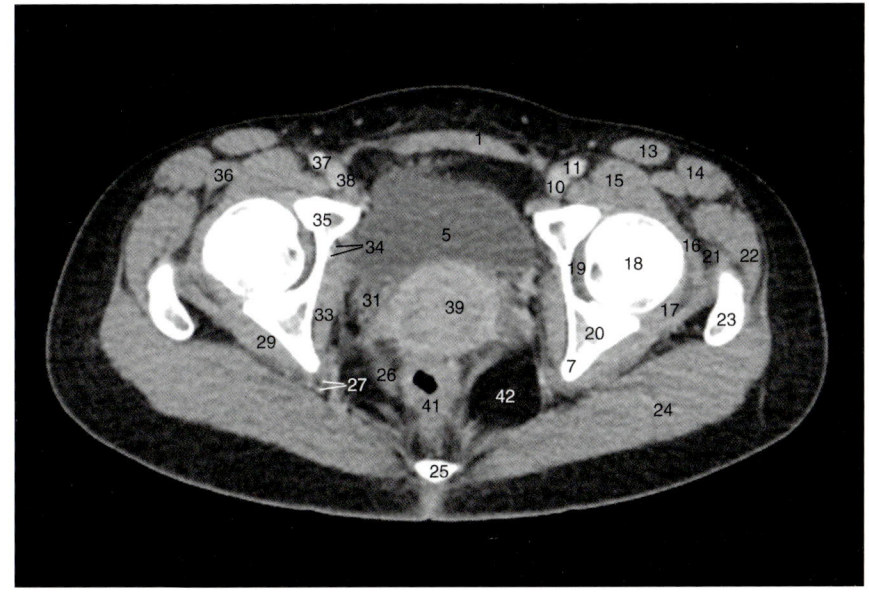
B. CT 增强图像

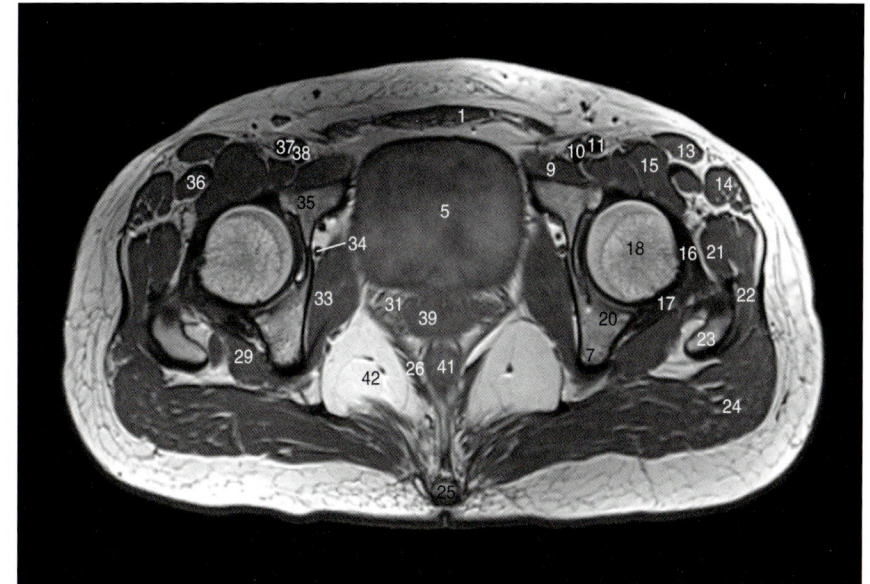
C. MR T1WI

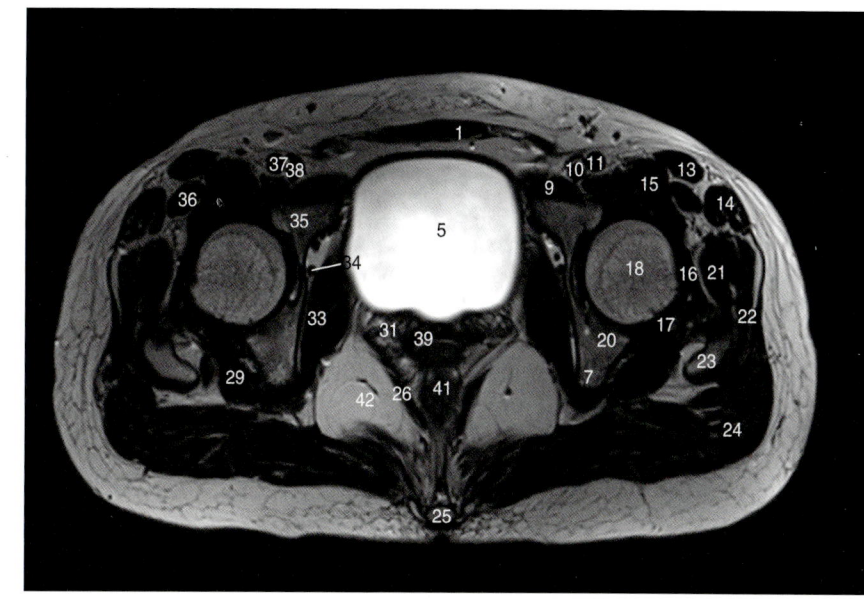
D. MR T2WI

1. 腹直肌 rectus abdominis
2. 腹直肌鞘 sheath of rectus abdominis
3. 腹股沟浅淋巴结 superficial inguinal lymph nodes
4. 回肠 ileum
5. 膀胱 urinary bladder
6. 左输尿管 left ureter
7. 坐骨棘 ischial spine
8. 左臀下动、静脉 left inferior gluteal artery and vein
9. 耻骨体 body of pubis
10. 左股静脉 left femoral vein
11. 左股动脉 left femoral artery
12. 股神经 femoral nerve
13. 缝匠肌 sartorius
14. 阔筋膜张肌 tensor fasciae latae
15. 髂腰肌 iliopsoas
16. 髂股韧带 iliofemoral ligament
17. 坐股韧带 ischiofemoral ligament
18. 股骨头 femoral head
19. 股骨头韧带 ligament of head of femur
20. 坐骨体 body of ischium
21. 臀小肌 gluteus minimus
22. 臀中肌 gluteus medius
23. 股骨大转子 greater trochanter
24. 臀大肌 gluteus maximus
25. 尾骨 coccyx
26. 肛提肌 levator ani
27. 右阴部内动、静脉 right internal pudendal artery and vein
28. 坐骨神经 sciatic nerve
29. 上孖肌 gemellus superior
30. 直肠系膜 mesorectum
31. 子宫阴道静脉丛 uterovaginaal venous plexus
32. 右输尿管 right ureter
33. 闭孔内肌 obturator internus
34. 闭孔动、静脉 obturator artery and vein
35. 耻骨体 body of pubis
36. 股直肌 rectus femoris
37. 右股动脉 right femoral artery
38. 右股静脉 right femoral vein
39. 子宫颈 neck of uterus
40. 子宫颈管 canal of cervix of uterus
41. 直肠 rectum
42. 坐骨肛门窝 ischioanal fossa

关键结构：坐股韧带，子宫颈，膀胱。

此断面经过尾骨下份、股骨头中份。尾骨居于盆部后壁中央，其前方两侧的肛提肌断面逐渐增大。坐骨棘和耻骨体包绕的股骨头断面达到最高水平，股骨头内侧偏前见股骨头韧带断面。股骨头外侧及后方从内侧向外侧依次为髂股韧带、股直肌、臀小肌、臀中肌、臀大肌，坐骨棘后方、臀大肌前方见上孖肌和臀下动、静脉，臀中肌和上孖肌之间见坐股韧带及股骨大转子。坐股韧带较薄，位于髋关节后面，与关节囊紧密愈合，起自髋臼的后部与下部，向外上方经股骨颈的后面，一部分纤维移行于轮匝带，另一部分则附于股骨大转子的根部。此韧带限制大腿的内收及旋内运动。盆腔内的结构较前一断面变化不大，从前至后依次见回肠、膀胱、子宫颈、直肠。膀胱与子宫颈夹角处见两侧输尿管断面。

109

女性盆部与会阴连续横断层 55（FH.8290）

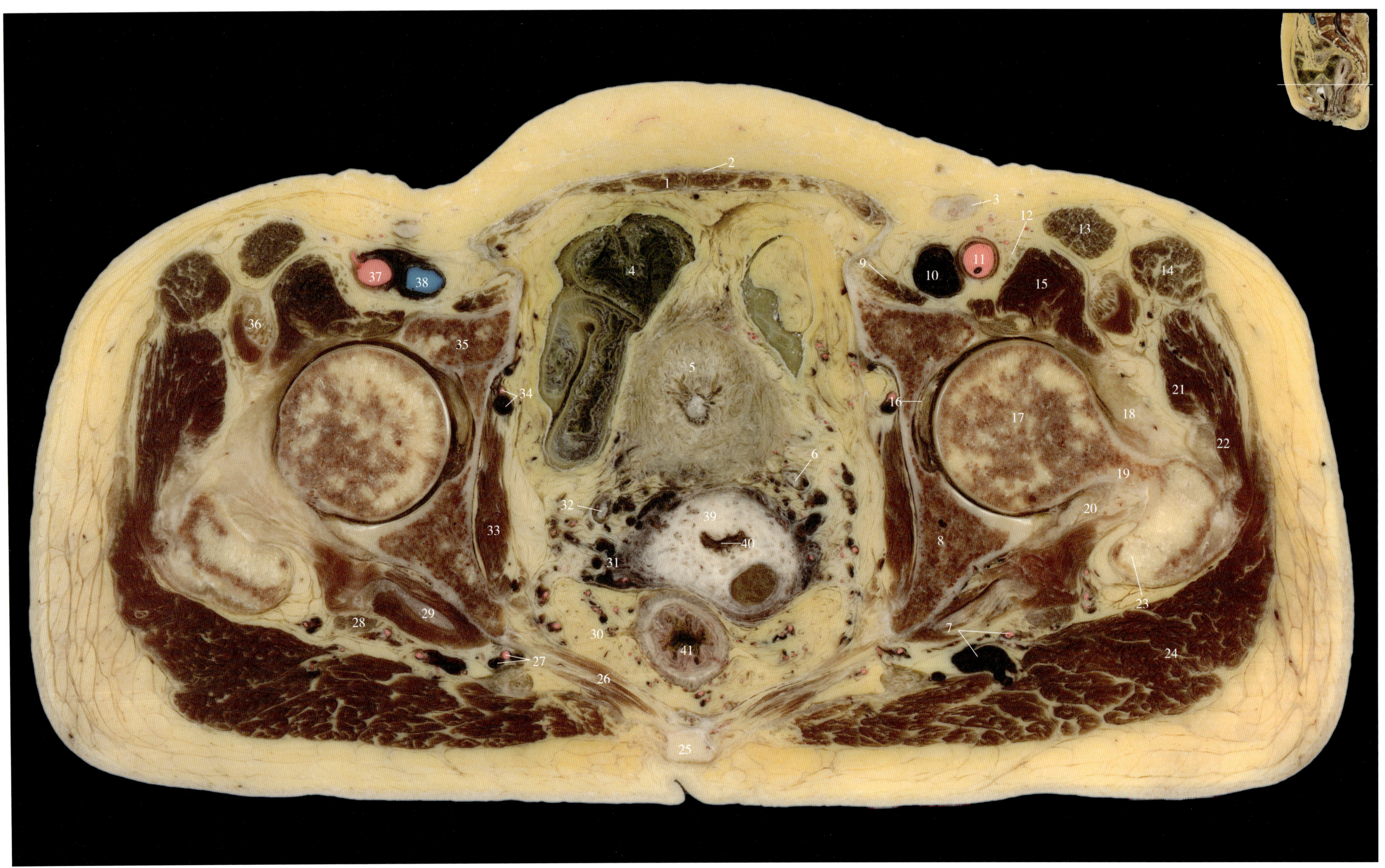

A. 断层标本图像

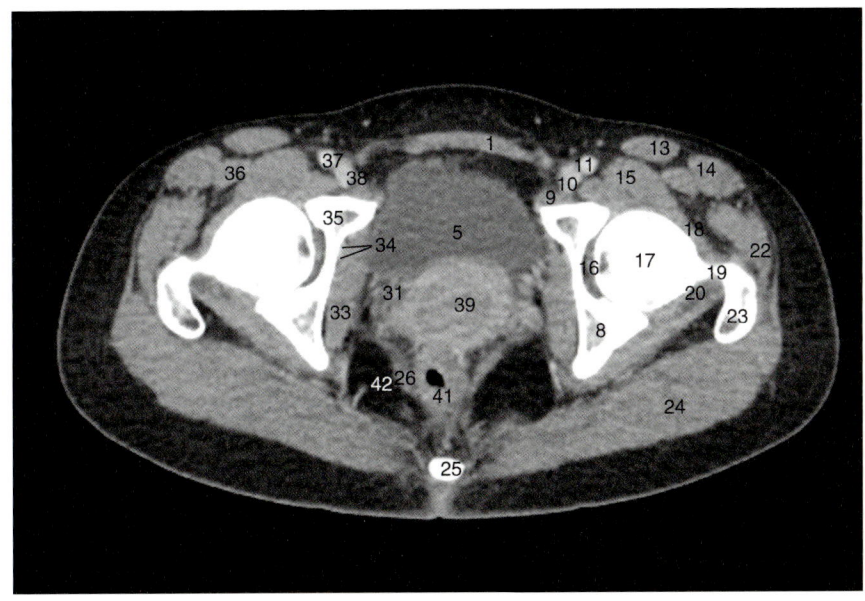

B. CT 增强图像

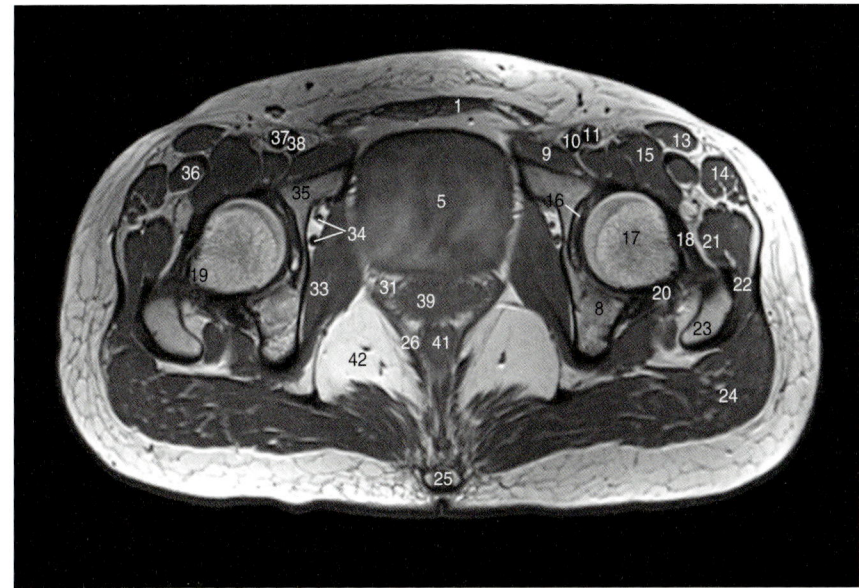

C. MR T1WI

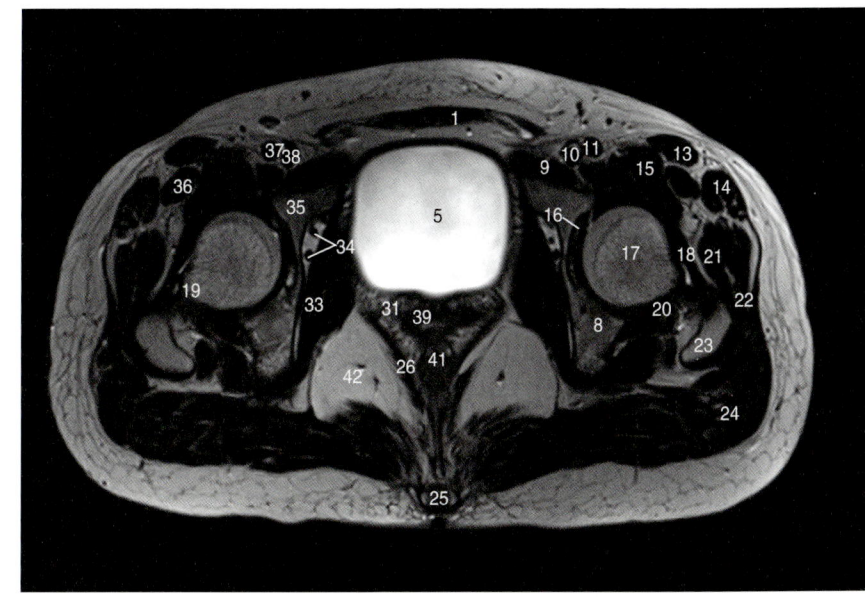

D. MR T2WI

1. 腹直肌 rectus abdominis
2. 腹直肌鞘 sheath of rectus abdominis
3. 腹股沟浅淋巴结 superficial inguinal lymph nodes
4. 回肠 ileum
5. 膀胱 urinary bladder
6. 左输尿管 left ureter
7. 左臀下动、静脉 left inferior gluteal artery and vein
8. 坐骨体 body of ischium
9. 耻骨体 body of pubis
10. 左股静脉 left femoral vein
11. 左股动脉 left femoral artery
12. 股神经 femoral nerve
13. 缝匠肌 sartorius
14. 阔筋膜张肌 tensor fasciae latae
15. 髂腰肌 iliopsoas
16. 股骨头韧带 ligament of head of femur
17. 股骨头 femoral head
18. 髂股韧带 iliofemoral ligament
19. 股骨颈 neck of femur
20. 坐股韧带 ischiofemoral ligament
21. 臀小肌 gluteus minimus

22. 臀中肌 gluteus medius
23. 股骨大转子 greater trochanter
24. 臀大肌 gluteus maximus
25. 尾骨 coccyx
26. 肛提肌 levator ani
27. 右阴部内动、静脉 right internal pudendal artery and vein
28. 坐骨神经 sciatic nerve
29. 闭孔内肌肌腱 tendon of obturator internus
30. 直肠系膜 mesorectum
31. 子宫阴道静脉丛 uterovaginaal venous plexus
32. 右输尿管 right ureter
33. 闭孔内肌 obturator internus
34. 闭孔动、静脉 obturator artery and vein
35. 耻骨体 body of pubis
36. 股直肌 rectus femoris
37. 右股动脉 right femoral artery
38. 右股静脉 right femoral vein
39. 子宫颈 neck of uterus
40. 子宫颈管 canal of cervix of uteri
41. 直肠 rectum
42. 坐骨肛门窝 ischioanal fossa

关键结构：股骨颈，股骨头韧带，股骨大转子。

此断面经过尾骨下份。

股骨颈开始出现，股骨颈为连接股骨头与股骨干之间狭细的部分，被髋关节囊的韧带包裹，前方为髂股韧带，后方为坐股韧带。60 岁以上的老年人由于骨质疏松等原因，摔倒时由于股骨颈力量薄弱，容易发生骨折。女性比男性更易发生。由于覆盖在股骨颈的骨膜菲薄，骨生成的能力极其有限，因此股骨颈骨折的治疗较棘手。股骨头的营养动脉来自旋股内侧动脉，与股骨颈平行进入股骨头。当股骨颈发生骨折时，这些营养动脉极易受到损伤，血管破裂会导致股骨头变性坏死及关节出血[24,25]。本断层中央为髂骨体和尾骨围成的骨盆腔，盆腔内从前向后依次见回肠、膀胱、子宫颈、直肠。回肠受胆汁影响呈暗绿色。膀胱子宫夹角内见输尿管断面。子宫颈旁见数个小血管断面，为子宫阴道静脉丛。盆腔两侧紧贴耻骨体见闭孔动、静脉和闭孔内肌。盆腔前界由腹直肌和腹直肌鞘包围保护，后界为肛提肌连接尾骨和坐骨棘。髋关节前方为股动脉、股静脉、股神经、耻骨肌、髂腰肌、缝匠肌、阔筋膜张肌、髂腰肌断面，外后方依次见臀小肌、臀中肌、股骨大转子、上孖肌、坐骨神经、臀大肌断面，及位于臀大肌前方的臀下动、静脉。

女性盆部与会阴连续横断层 56（FH.8270）

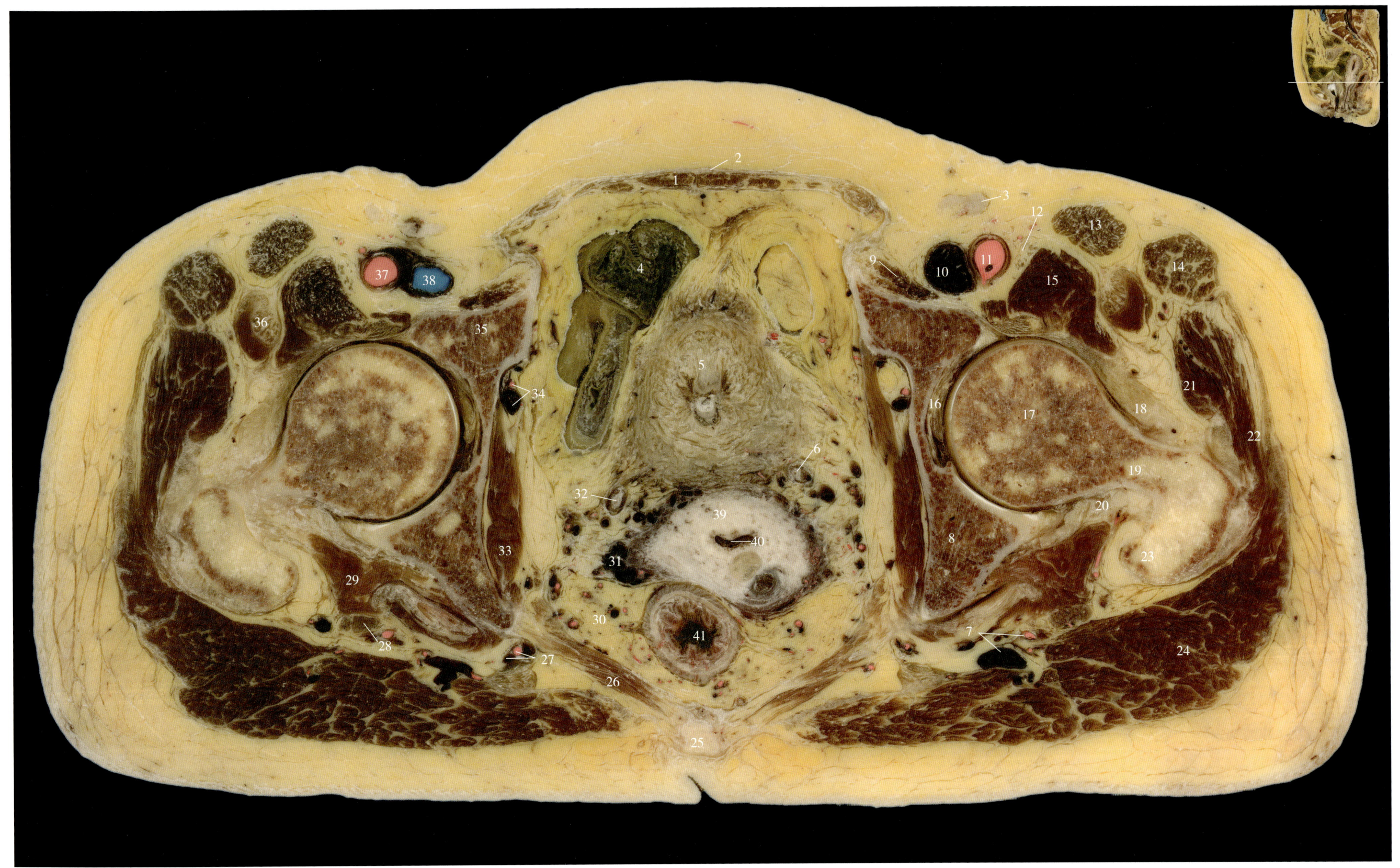

A. 断层标本图像

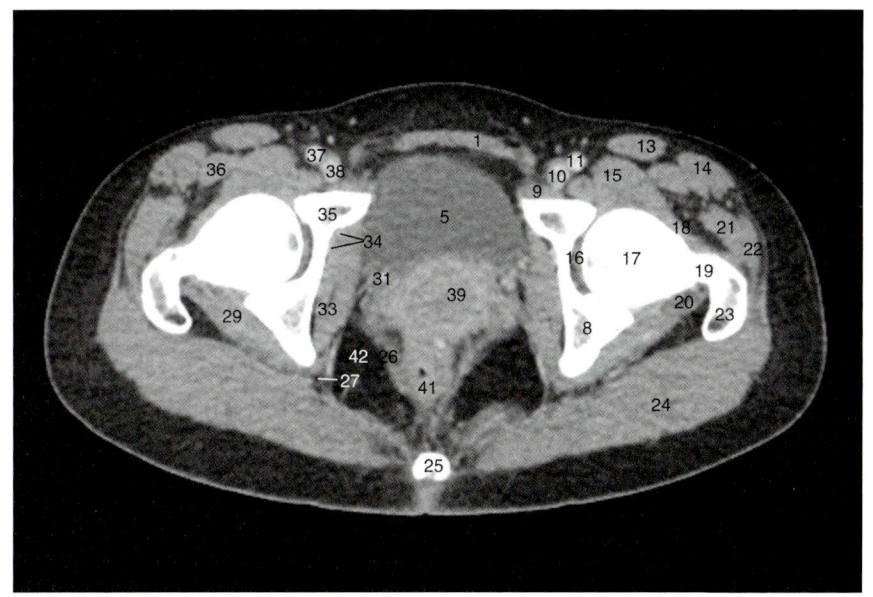

B. CT 增强图像

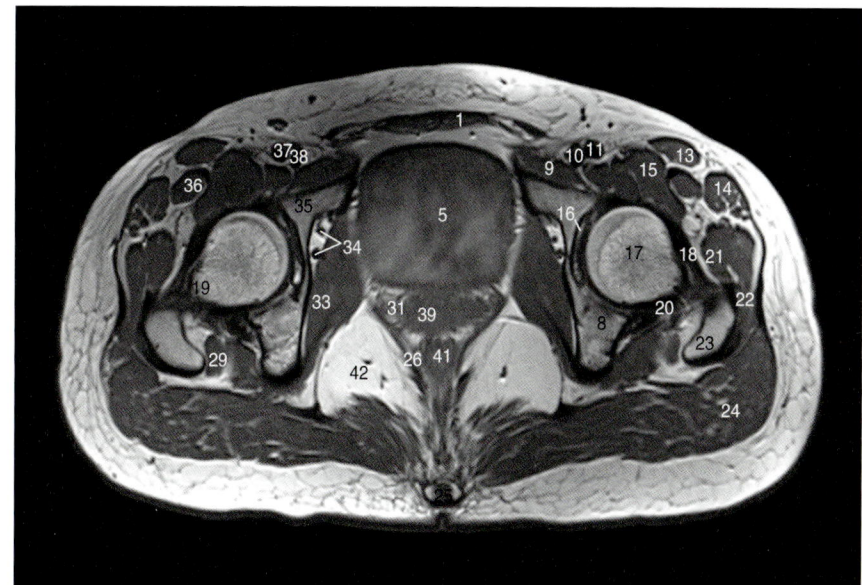

C. MR T1WI

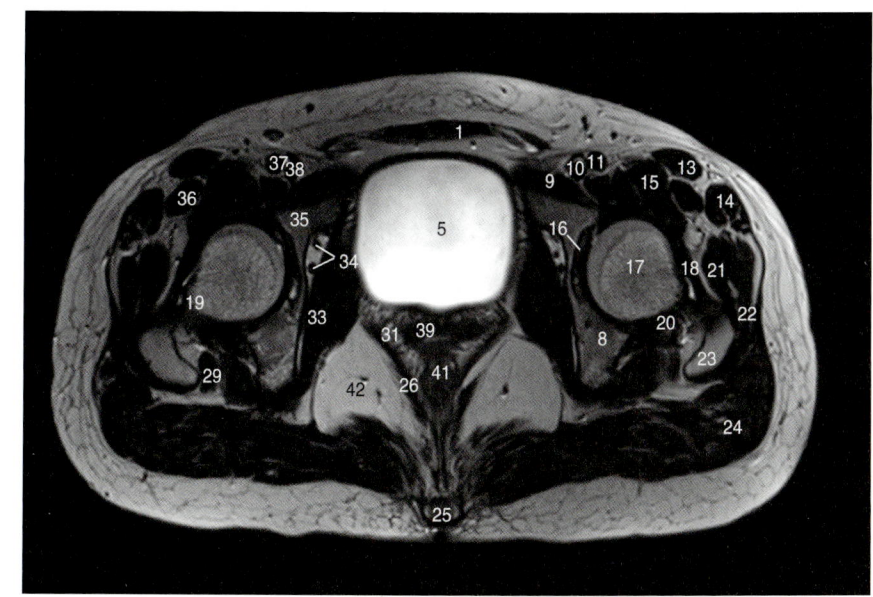

D. MR T2WI

1. 腹直肌 rectus abdominis
2. 腹直肌鞘 sheath of rectus abdominis
3. 腹股沟浅淋巴结 superficial inguinal lymph nodes
4. 回肠 ileum
5. 膀胱 urinary bladder
6. 左输尿管 left ureter
7. 左臀下动、静脉 left inferior gluteal artery and vein
8. 坐骨体 body of ischium
9. 耻骨肌 pectineus
10. 左股静脉 left femoral vein
11. 左股动脉 left femoral artery
12. 股神经 femoral nerve
13. 缝匠肌 sartorius
14. 阔筋膜张肌 tensor fasciae latae
15. 髂腰肌 iliopsoas
16. 股骨头韧带 ligament of head of femur
17. 股骨头 femoral head
18. 髂股韧带 iliofemoral ligament
19. 股骨颈 neck of femur
20. 坐股韧带 ischiofemoral ligament
21. 臀小肌 gluteus minimus
22. 臀中肌 gluteus medius
23. 股骨大转子 greater trochanter
24. 臀大肌 gluteus maximus
25. 尾骨 coccyx
26. 肛提肌 levator ani
27. 右阴部内动、静脉 right internal pudendal artery and vein
28. 坐骨神经 sciatic nerve
29. 下孖肌 gemellus inferior
30. 直肠系膜 mesorectum
31. 子宫阴道静脉丛 uterovaginaal venous plexus
32. 右输尿管 right ureter
33. 闭孔内肌 obturator internus
34. 闭孔动、静脉 obturator artery and vein
35. 耻骨体 body of pubis
36. 股直肌 rectus femoris
37. 右股动脉 right femoral artery
38. 右股静脉 right femoral vein
39. 子宫颈 neck of uterus
40. 子宫颈管 canal of cervix of uterus
41. 直肠 rectum
42. 坐骨肛门窝 ischioanal fossa

关键结构：下孖肌，肛提肌，膀胱。

此断面经过尾骨下份。上孖肌消失，下孖肌开始出现。这对双生子已经一同介绍过，此处不再赘述。本断层的肛提肌显示较清楚。肛提肌为一对阔肌复合体，包含耻尾肌、耻骨直肠肌和髂尾肌，起自耻骨盆面、坐骨棘及二者之间的肛提肌肌腱弓，在中线处汇合终止于会阴中心腱、肛尾韧带和尾骨尖，两侧联合形成漏斗状，封闭大部分小骨盆下口。在本断层可见肛提肌呈条状，一端连于尾骨，另一端分两束分别进入耻骨盆面和坐骨方向。肛提肌是构成盆底肌最重要的肌肉，各部共同收缩可以向上提拉盆底，此外，其在有意识控制排尿、节制排便及承托子宫中发挥重要作用[24]。在分娩过程中，盆底承托胎儿头部，会阴、肛提肌、盆筋膜都可能受到损伤，特别是构成肛提肌主要部分的耻尾肌常常会撕裂。由于分娩时的过度牵拉和撕裂，可使肛提肌和盆筋膜的作用减弱，从而引起膀胱颈和尿道位置的改变。这些变化可导致压力性尿失禁，即腹内压升高（如咳嗽）时出现尿滴流[21, 24]。可行手术治疗，近年来提倡的尿道中段吊带术式对膀胱功能及容量正常、未合并明显膀胱膨出的解剖性压力性尿失禁患者，取得满意疗效[31]。通过塑化切片技术进行女性盆底肌计算机重建模型、女盆3D重建模型，MRI弥散张量成像等技术可以对女性骨盆底解剖结构进行3D可视化和量化，以帮助理解盆底结构[32-34]。

女性盆部与会阴连续横断层 57（FH.8250）

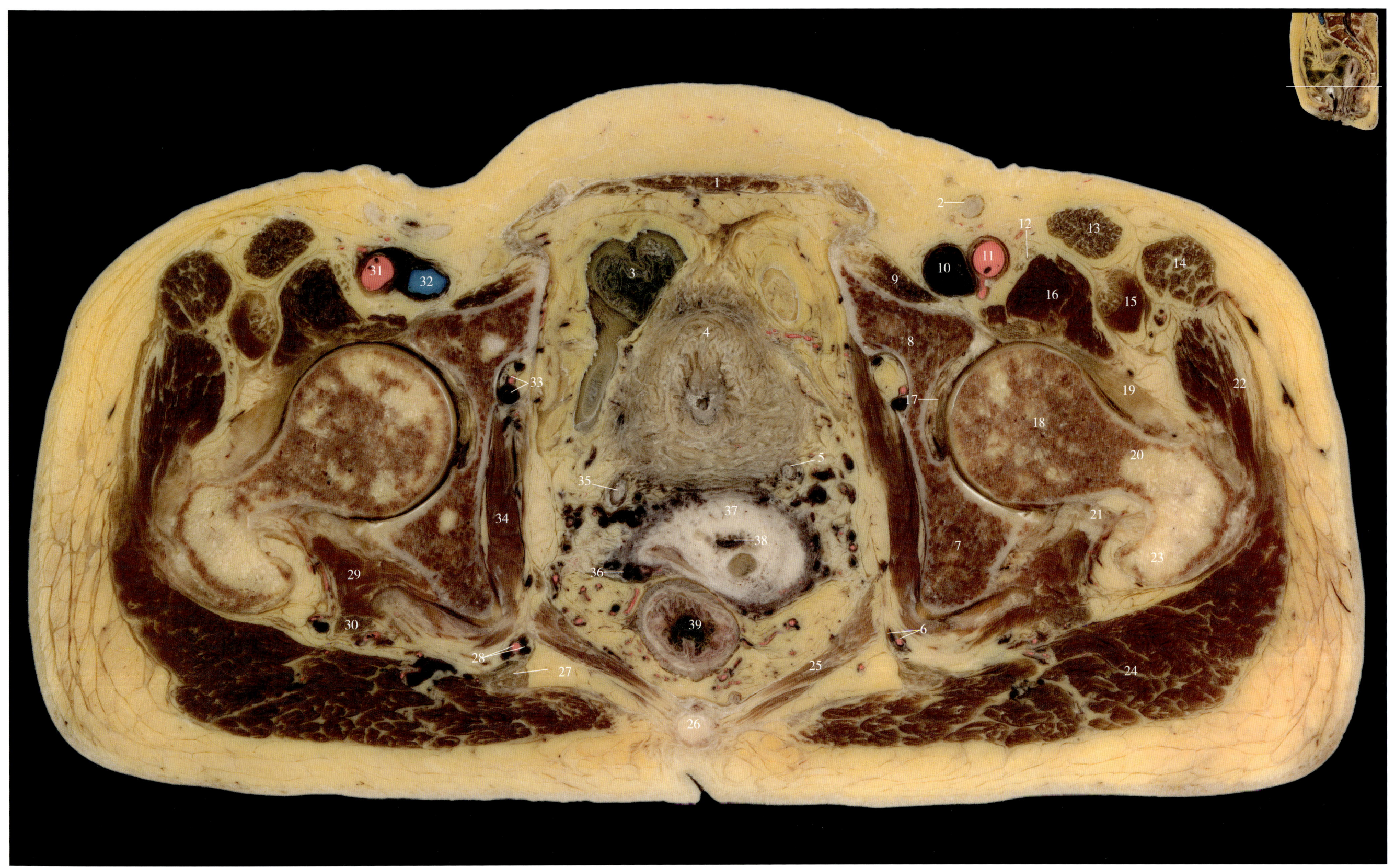

A. 断层标本图像

114

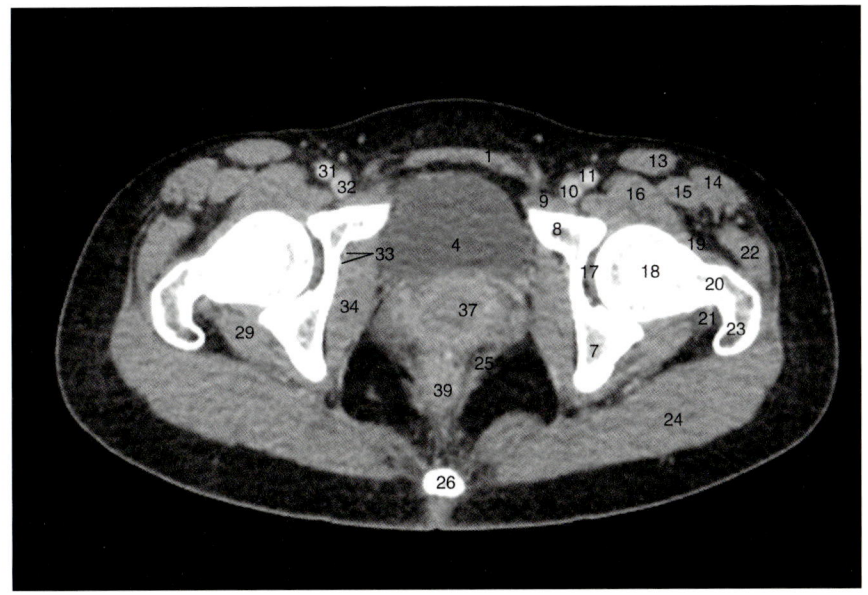
B. CT 增强图像

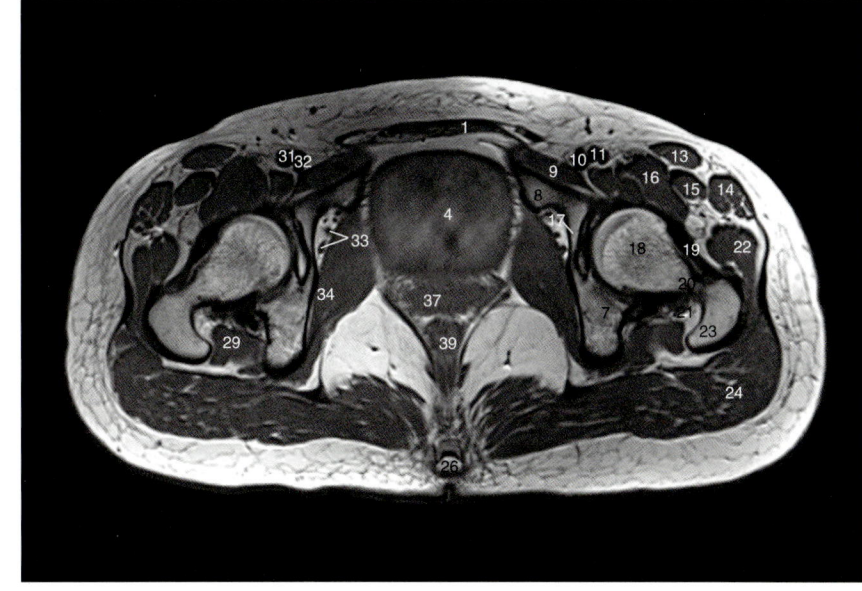
C. MR T1WI

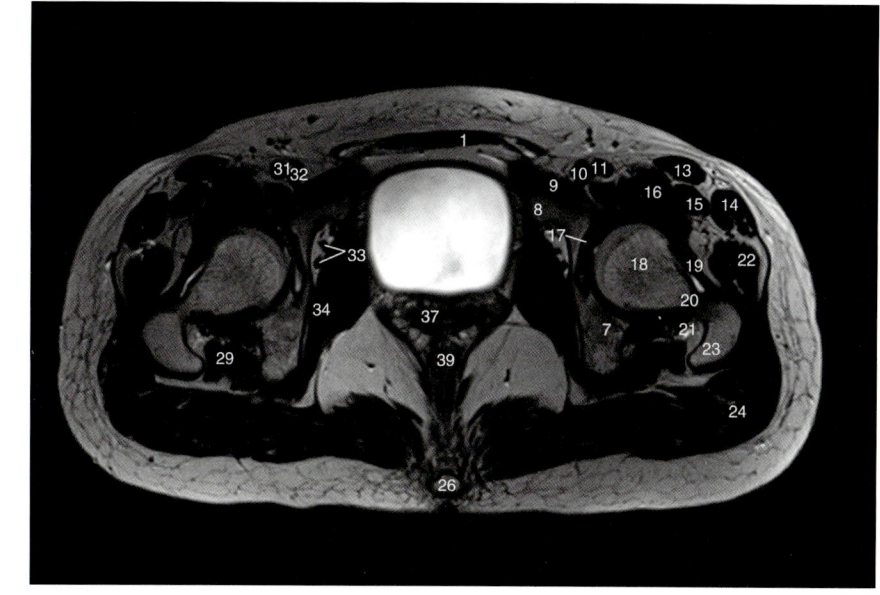
D. MR T2WI

1. 腹直肌 rectus abdominis
2. 腹股沟浅淋巴结 superficial inguinal lymph nodes
3. 回肠 ileum
4. 膀胱 urinary bladder
5. 左输尿管 left ureter
6. 左阴部内动、静脉 left internal pudendal artery and vein
7. 坐骨体 body of ischium
8. 耻骨体 body of pubis
9. 耻骨肌 pectineus
10. 左股静脉 left femoral vein
11. 左股动脉 left femoral artery
12. 股神经 femoral nerve
13. 缝匠肌 sartorius
14. 阔筋膜张肌 tensor fasciae latae
15. 股直肌 rectus femoris
16. 髂腰肌 iliopsoas
17. 股骨头韧带 ligament of head of femur
18. 股骨头 femoral head
19. 髂股韧带 iliofemoral ligament
20. 股骨颈 neck of femur
21. 坐股韧带 ischiofemoral ligament
22. 臀中肌 gluteus medius
23. 股骨大转子 greater trochanter
24. 臀大肌 gluteus maximus
25. 肛提肌 levator ani
26. 尾骨 coccyx
27. 骶结节韧带 sacrotuberous ligament
28. 右阴部内动、静脉 right internal pudendal artery and vein
29. 下孖肌 gemellus inferior
30. 坐骨神经 sciatic nerve
31. 右股动脉 right femoral artery
32. 右股静脉 right femoral vein
33. 闭孔动、静脉 obturator artery and vein
34. 闭孔内肌 obturator internus
35. 右输尿管 right ureter
36. 子宫阴道静脉丛 uterovaginaal venous plexus
37. 子宫颈 neck of uterus
38. 子宫颈管 canal of cervix of uterus
39. 直肠 rectum

关键结构：膀胱，输尿管。

此断面经过尾骨下份。膀胱断面继续增大，膀胱位于小骨盆腔的前部，膀胱空虚时呈三棱锥体形，分尖、体、底和颈四部分。尖部朝向前上方，底部朝向后下方，尖部与底部之间为体部。膀胱的最下部为膀胱颈部。各部之间无明确界限。其形状、大小、位置和壁的厚度随尿液充盈程度而异。成人膀胱容量300~500 mL尿液。膀胱前方为耻骨联合。女性膀胱后方与子宫、阴道相邻。膀胱空虚时完全位于盆腔内，充满时上缘可升至耻骨联合上缘以上，相应的膀胱腹膜翻折线亦随之上移，膀胱前外侧壁则直接邻贴腹前壁。临床上常利用这种解剖关系，在耻骨联合上缘之上进行膀胱穿刺或做手术切口，可不伤及腹膜。儿童的膀胱位置较高，位于腹腔内，到6岁左右逐渐降至盆腔。在CT及MR图像上，适度充盈状态下的膀胱壁光滑均匀，厚度2~3 mm。膀胱子宫角内见输尿管断面，其中左侧输尿管已走行至膀胱壁外，即将进入。输尿管CT平扫为2个低密度的圆点，直径约4 mm，增强后排泄期呈明显的高密度（充满含对比剂的尿液）[1]。在盆腔手术时易损伤输尿管，由于子宫动脉在靠近阴道侧弯处从前上方跨过输尿管，卵巢血管和输尿管在经过骨盆入口时非常接近，因此结扎子宫动脉、卵巢动脉或直肠上动脉时，可误夹输尿管，此外在分离直肠外侧韧带、切除盆腔较大肿瘤时，均可能伤及盆部输尿管，应引起注意[1]。

女性盆部与会阴连续横断层 58（FH.8230）

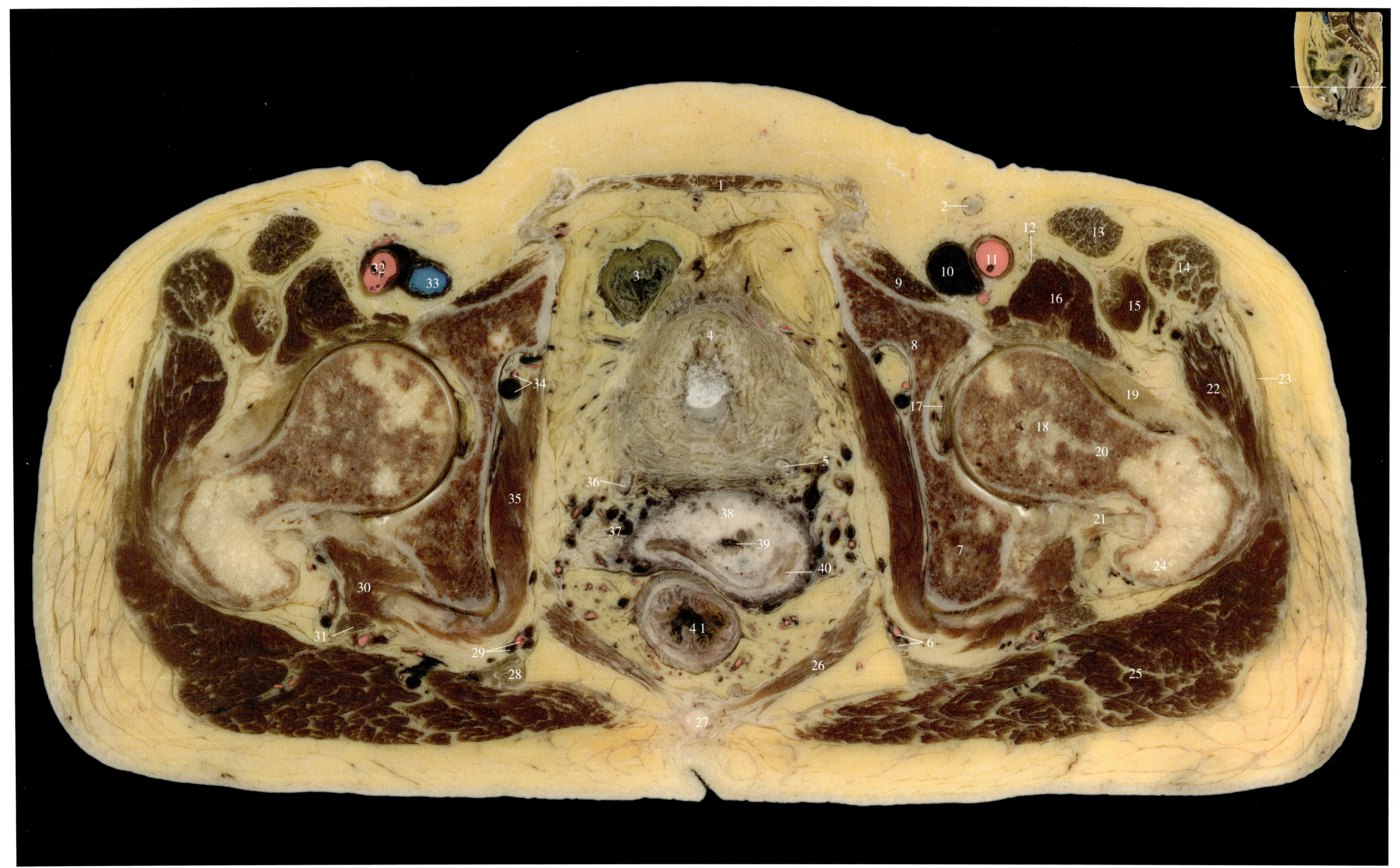

A. 断层标本图像

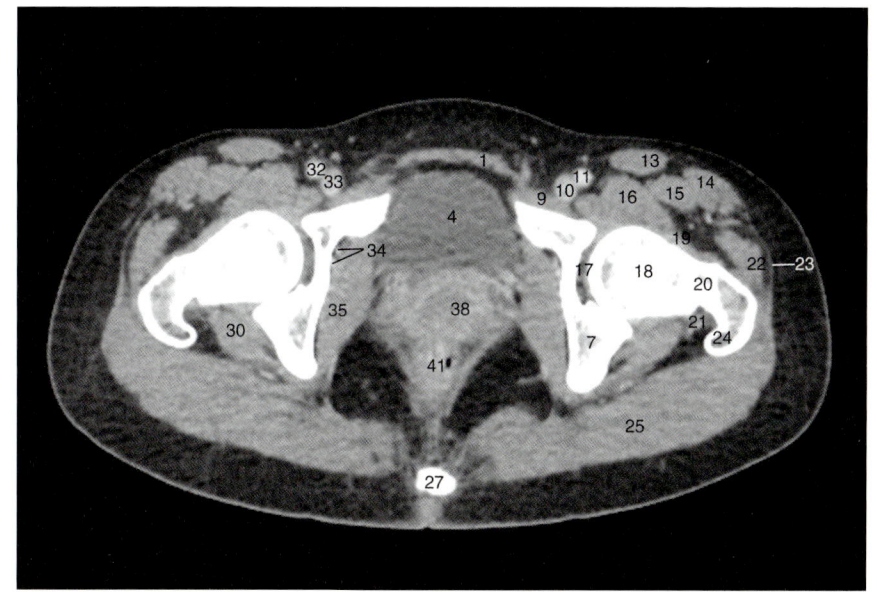
B. CT 增强图像

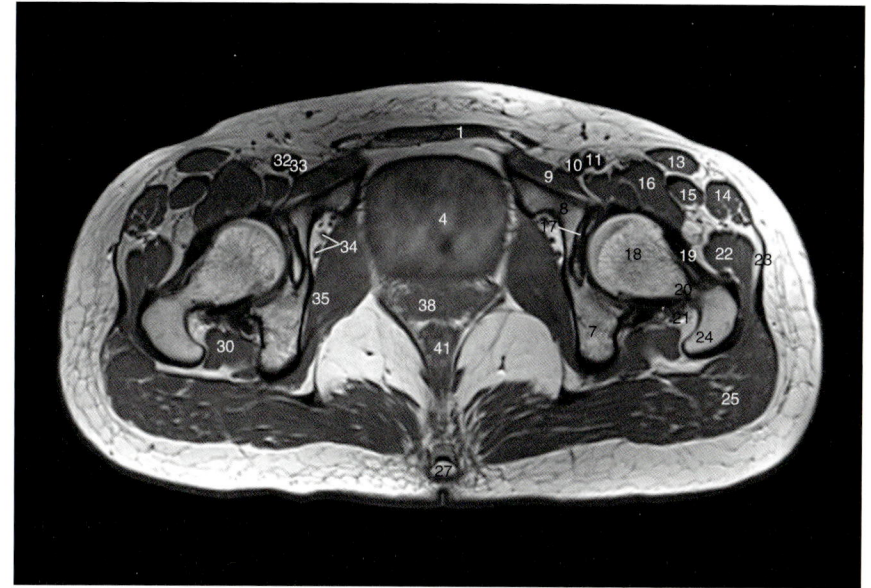
C. MR T1WI

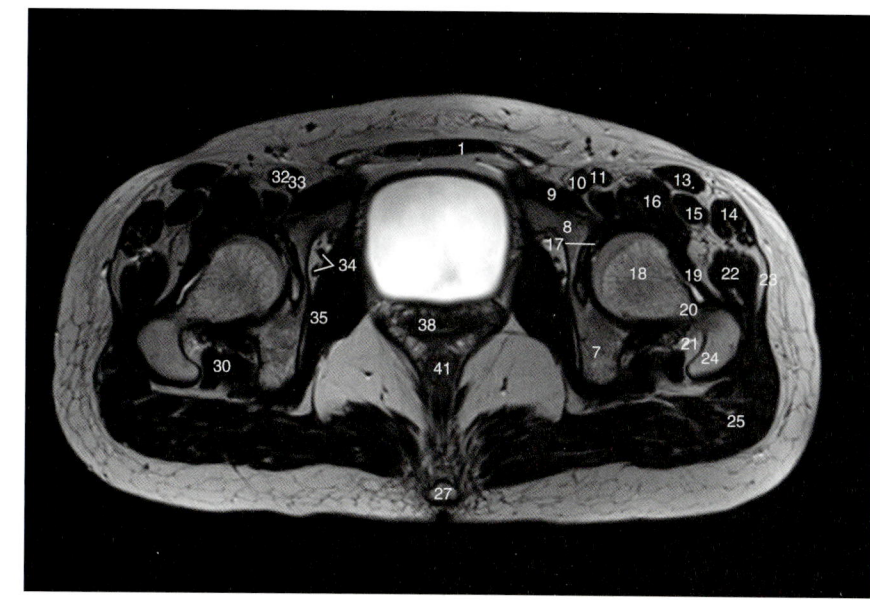
D. MR T2WI

1. 腹直肌 rectus abdominis
2. 腹股沟浅淋巴结 superficial inguinal lymph nodes
3. 回肠 ileum
4. 膀胱 urinary bladder
5. 左输尿管 left ureter
6. 左阴部内动、静脉 left internal pudendal artery and vein
7. 坐骨体 body of ischium
8. 耻骨体 body of pubis
9. 耻骨肌 pectineus
10. 左股静脉 left femoral vein
11. 左股动脉 left femoral artery
12. 股神经 femoral nerve
13. 缝匠肌 sartorius
14. 阔筋膜张肌 tensor fasciae latae
15. 股直肌 rectus femoris
16. 髂腰肌 iliopsoas
17. 股骨头韧带 ligament of head of femur
18. 股骨头 femoral head
19. 髂股韧带 iliofemoral ligament
20. 股骨颈 neck of femur
21. 坐股韧带 ischiofemoral ligament
22. 臀中肌 gluteus medius
23. 阔筋膜 fasciae lata
24. 股骨大转子 greater trochanter
25. 臀大肌 gluteus maximus
26. 肛提肌 levator ani
27. 尾骨 coccyx
28. 骶结节韧带 sacrotuberous ligament
29. 右阴部内动、静脉 right internal pudendal artery and vein
30. 下孖肌 gemellus inferior
31. 坐骨神经 sciatic nerve
32. 右股动脉 right femoral artery
33. 右股静脉 right femoral vein
34. 闭孔动、静脉 obturator artery and vein
35. 闭孔内肌 obturator internus
36. 右输尿管 right ureter
37. 子宫阴道静脉丛 uterovaginaal venous plexus
38. 子宫颈 neck of uterus
39. 子宫颈管 canal of cervix of uterus
40. 阴道穹后部 posterior part of fornix of vaginaa
41. 直肠 rectum

关键结构：阴道穹后部，子宫颈。

此断面经过尾骨尖。断面中部为骨盆腔，从前至后依次见回肠、膀胱、子宫颈和直肠。两侧输尿管刚进入膀胱后壁。子宫颈中心见不规则裂隙状的子宫颈管，其后方见弧形裂隙状阴道穹后部的断面。子宫颈与阴道壁之间形成的环形腔隙称阴道穹，其中阴道穹后部较深，与子宫直肠陷凹紧邻。MRI T2 加权图像上子宫颈中心的高信号区相当于子宫颈黏液及子宫颈上皮。在 MRI 矢状面中，76% 的受检者其阴道穹后部可与子宫颈阴道部相区分；在横断面图像，仅当阴道穹内有液体或气体时才能与子宫颈阴道部区分。在 MR 影像上阴道穹前部可与宫颈前唇区分，但显示率低，在矢状成像中仅 26%，而且仅能用矢状断面来显示[1]。阴道穹后部与直肠子宫陷凹之间仅相隔阴道壁和一层菲薄的腹膜，当直肠子宫陷凹积血、积液时，可经阴道后穹穿刺或切开引流进行诊断或治疗[21]。

女性盆部与会阴连续横断层 59（FH.8210）

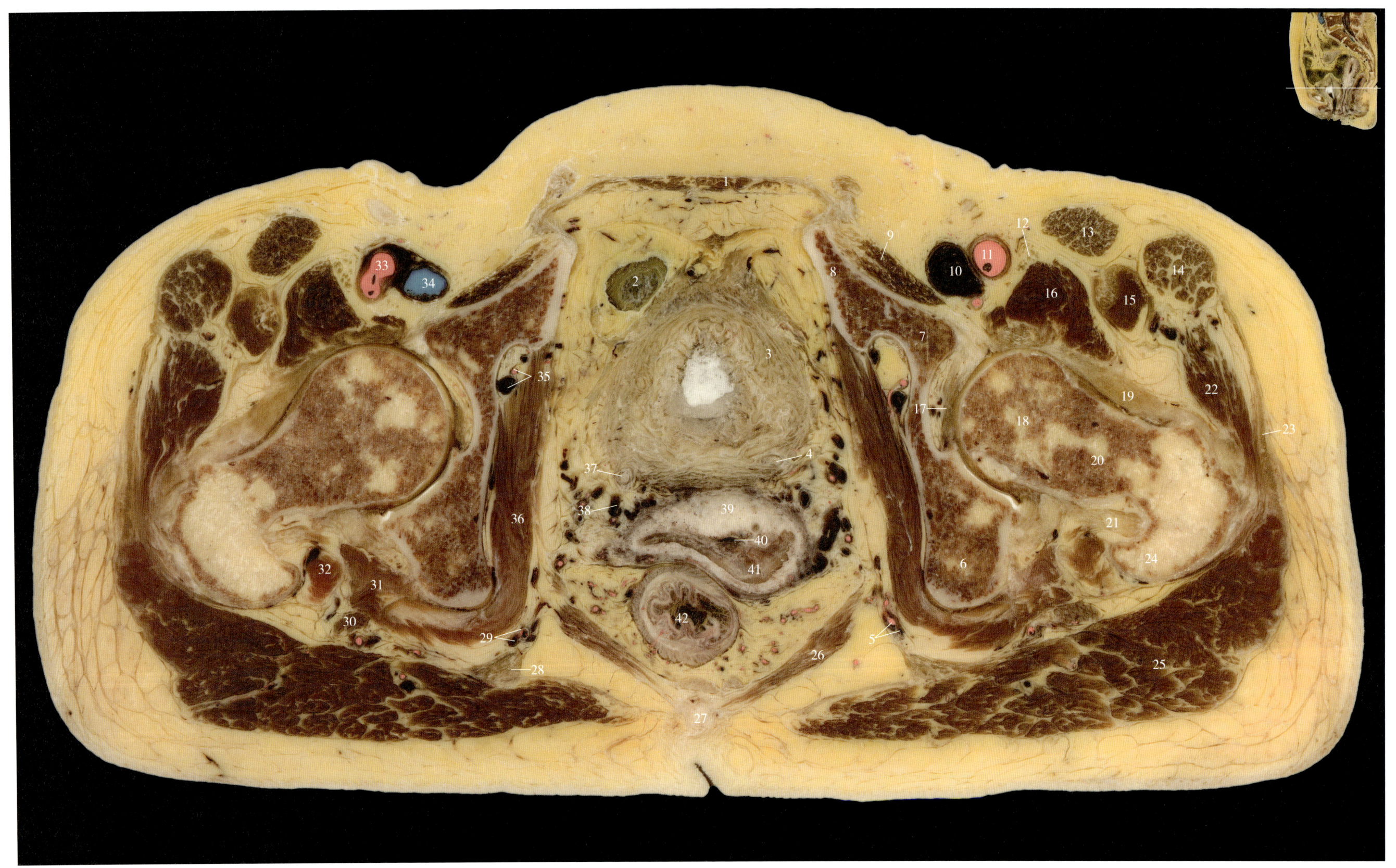

A. 断层标本图像

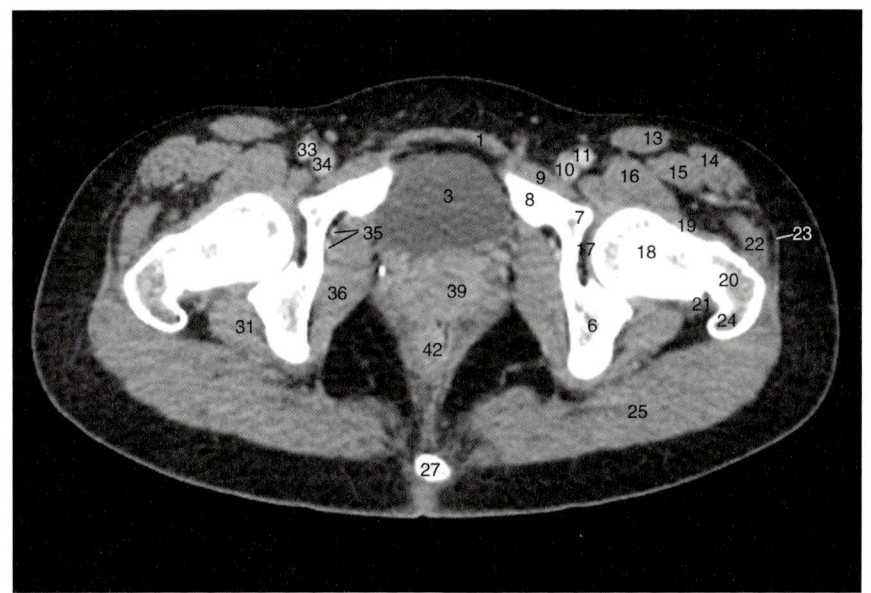

B. CT 增强图像

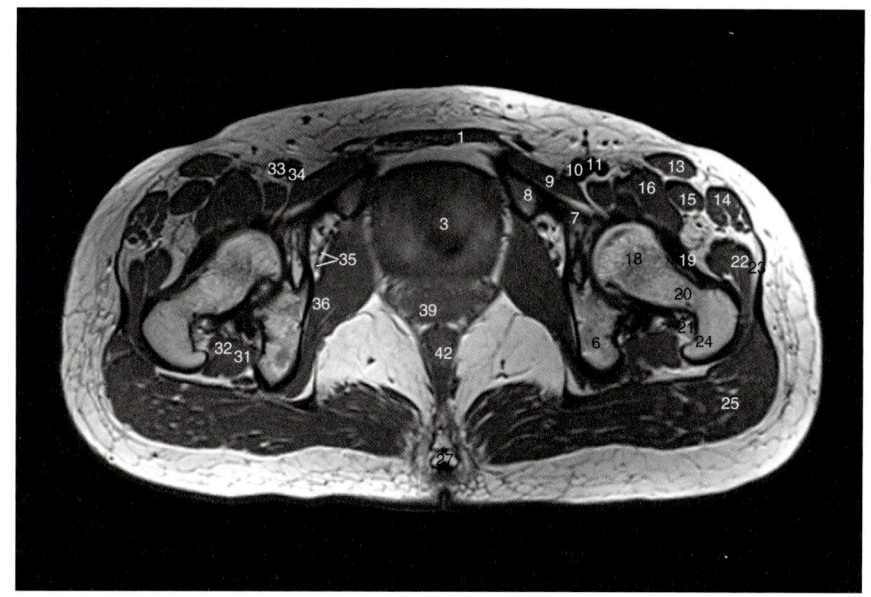

C. MR T1WI

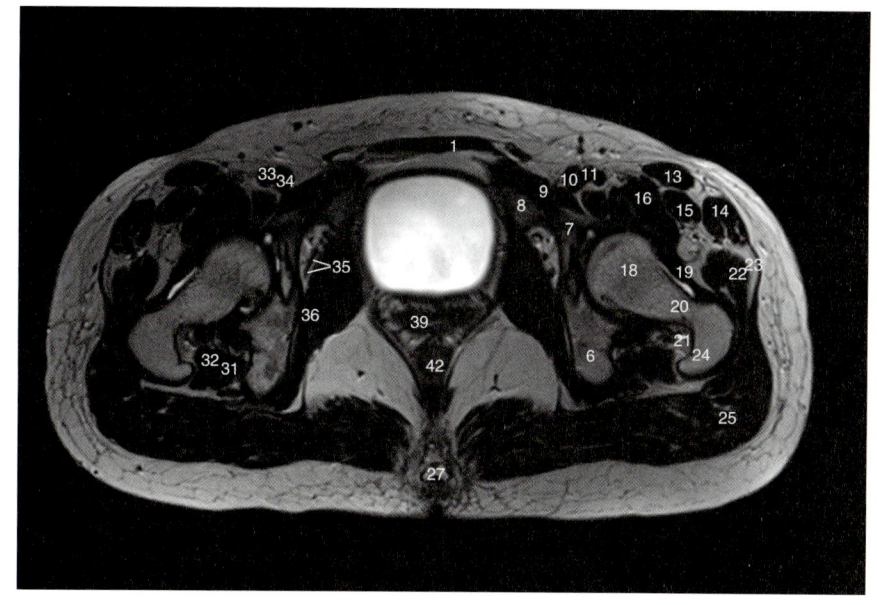

D. MR T2WI

1. 腹直肌 rectus abdominis
2. 回肠 ileum
3. 膀胱 urinary bladder
4. 左输尿管 left ureter
5. 左阴部内动、静脉 left internal pudendal artery and vein
6. 坐骨体 body of ischium
7. 耻骨体 body of pubis
8. 耻骨上支 superior ramus of pubis
9. 耻骨肌 pectineus
10. 左股静脉 left femoral vein
11. 左股动脉 left femoral artery
12. 股神经 femoral nerve
13. 缝匠肌 sartorius
14. 阔筋膜张肌 tensor fasciae latae
15. 股直肌 rectus femoris
16. 髂腰肌 iliopsoas
17. 股骨头韧带 ligament of head of femur
18. 股骨头 femoral head
19. 髂股韧带 iliofemoral ligament
20. 股骨颈 neck of femur
21. 坐股韧带 ischiofemoral ligament

22. 臀中肌 gluteus medius
23. 阔筋膜 fasciae lata
24. 股骨大转子 greater trochanter
25. 臀大肌 gluteus maximus
26. 肛提肌 levator ani
27. 尾骨 coccyx
28. 骶结节韧带 sacrotuberous ligament
29. 右阴部内动、静脉 right internal pudendal artery and vein
30. 坐骨神经 sciatic nerve
31. 下孖肌 gemellus inferior
32. 股方肌 quadratus femoris
33. 右股动脉 right femoral artery
34. 右股静脉 right femoral vein
35. 闭孔血管、神经 obturator vessels and nerve
36. 闭孔内肌 obturator internus
37. 右输尿管 right ureter
38. 子宫阴道静脉丛 uterovaginaal venous plexus
39. 子宫颈 neck of uterus
40. 子宫颈管 canal of cervix of uterus
41. 阴道穹后部 posterior part of fornix of vaginaa
42. 直肠 rectum

关键结构：尾骨尖，耻骨上支，阴道穹后部。

此断面经过尾骨尖。耻骨体向前延伸出耻骨上支，耻骨上、下支及坐骨支围成闭孔结构。当发生交通事故，骨盆受到撞击、碾压时，容易发生骨盆骨折。骨盆骨折根据形态改变分为压缩型、分离型和中间型，根据骨盆环稳定性分为稳定性骨折和不稳定性骨折。耻骨支、坐骨支属于骨盆的薄弱部分，当骨盆受到侧方外力或前后方向同时撞击时容易发生耻骨支、坐骨支骨折，但其属于前环骨折，不破坏骨盆稳定性，但错位的断端可能引起膀胱及周围其他血管、神经等损伤[27, 30]。盆腔内，膀胱断面达到最大直径。阴道穹后部显示清晰。其余结构较前一断面变化不大。

女性盆部与会阴连续横断层 60（FH.8190）

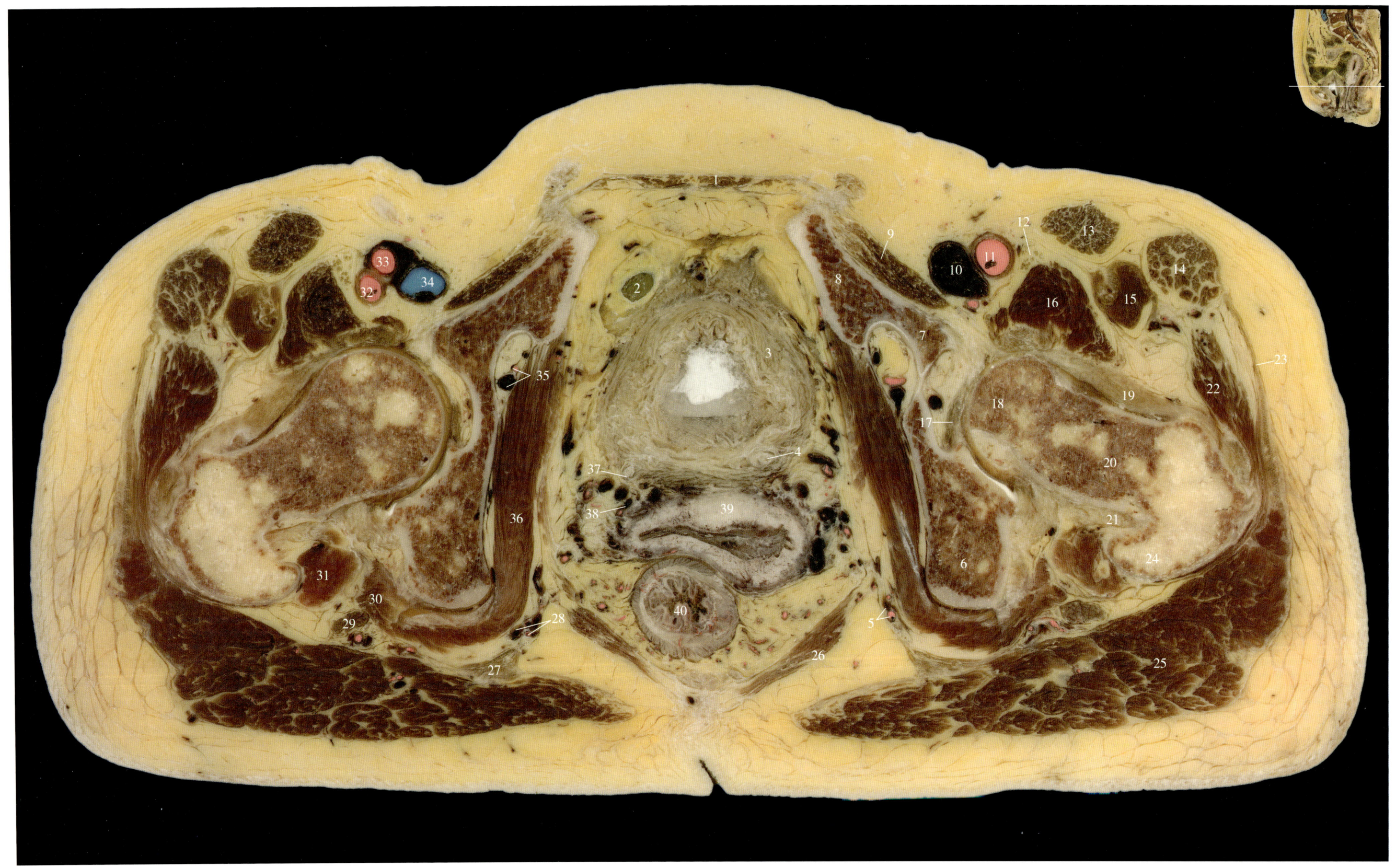

A. 断层标本图像

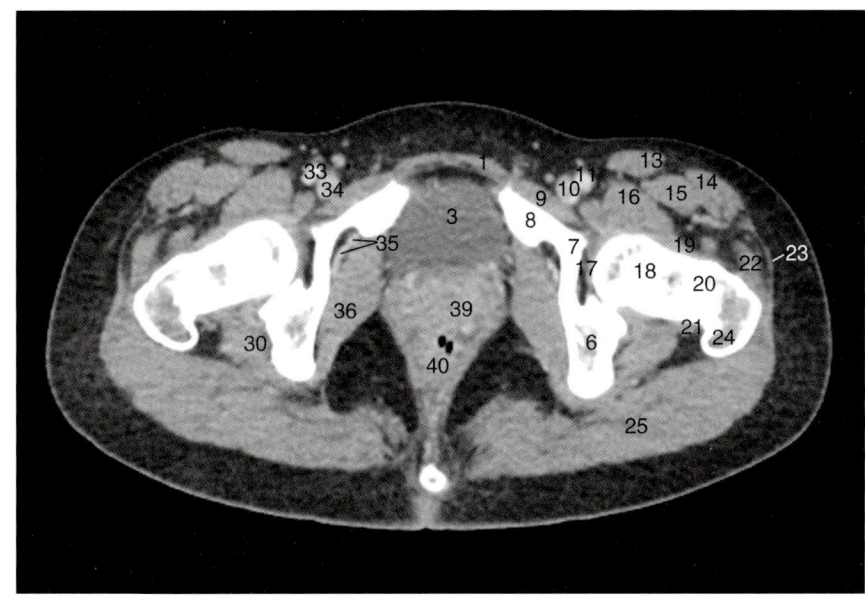
B. CT 增强图像

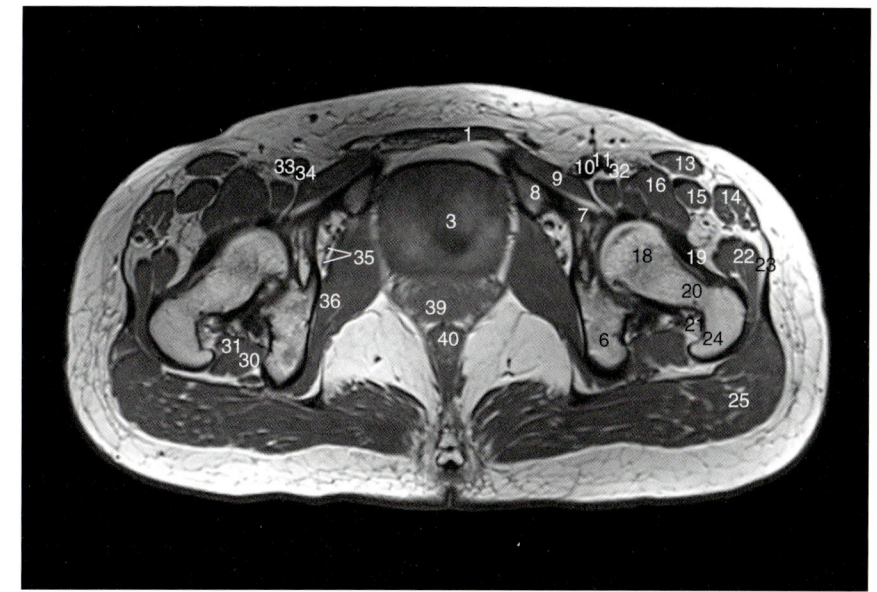
C. MR T1WI

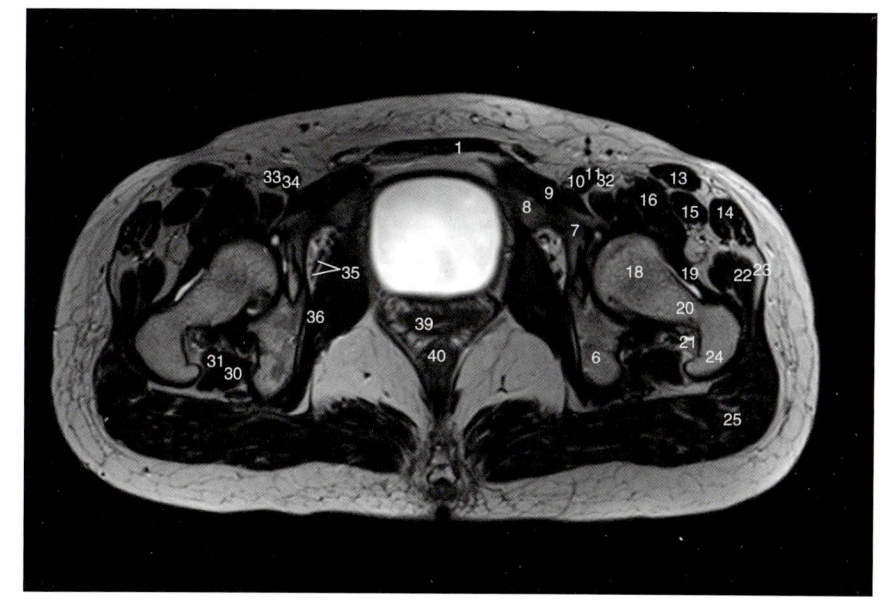
D. MR T2WI

1. 腹直肌 rectus abdominis
2. 回肠 ileum
3. 膀胱 urinary bladder
4. 左输尿管 left ureter
5. 左阴部内动、静脉 left internal pudendal artery and vein
6. 坐骨体 body of ischium
7. 耻骨体 body of pubis
8. 耻骨上支 superior ramus of pubis
9. 耻骨肌 pectineus
10. 左股静脉 left femoral vein
11. 左股动脉 left femoral artery
12. 股神经 femoral nerve
13. 缝匠肌 sartorius
14. 阔筋膜张肌 tensor fasciae latae
15. 股直肌 rectus femoris
16. 髂腰肌 iliopsoas
17. 股骨头韧带 ligament of head of femur
18. 股骨头 femoral head
19. 髂股韧带 iliofemoral ligament
20. 股骨颈 neck of femur
21. 坐股韧带 ischiofemoral ligament

22. 臀中肌 gluteus medius
23. 阔筋膜 fasciae lata
24. 股骨大转子 greater trochanter
25. 臀大肌 gluteus maximus
26. 肛提肌 levator ani
27. 骶结节韧带 sacrotuberous ligament
28. 右阴部内动、静脉 right internal pudendal artery and vein
29. 坐骨神经 sciatic nerve
30. 下孖肌 gemellus inferior
31. 股方肌 quadratus femoris
32. 股深动脉 deep femoral artery
33. 右股动脉 right femoral artery
34. 右股静脉 right femoral vein
35. 闭孔动、静脉 obturator artery and vein
36. 闭孔内肌 obturator internus
37. 右输尿管 right ureter
38. 子宫阴道静脉丛 uterovaginaal venous plexus
39. 阴道 vaginaa
40. 直肠 rectum

关键结构：输尿管，闭膜管，股深动脉，阴道。

此断面尾骨已消失不见。子宫颈向下延续为阴道。膀胱壁内可见左、右输尿管壁内段的断面。输尿管壁内段斜贯膀胱壁，长约为 1.5 cm，为输尿管的第三处生理狭窄，当肾结石随尿液下行时，容易嵌顿在此狭窄处，并产生绞痛和排尿障碍[1]。膀胱充盈时该段管腔闭合，阻止尿液回流[12]。耻骨体与闭孔内肌之间围成的类椭圆形腔隙为闭膜管。闭膜管位于耻骨上支的下方，由耻骨闭孔沟与闭孔内肌围成，孔的方向是自外上向前下方，长为 2~2.5 cm，有内、外两口，内口由闭孔沟的起端与闭孔内肌及其筋膜围成，外口位于耻骨肌的深面，由闭孔沟的末端与闭孔外肌及其筋膜围成。管内通过闭孔神经及血管[21]。盆腔外，右侧股动脉已发出股深动脉，为股动脉向深部发出的最大分支。

女性盆部与会阴连续横断层 61（FH.8170）

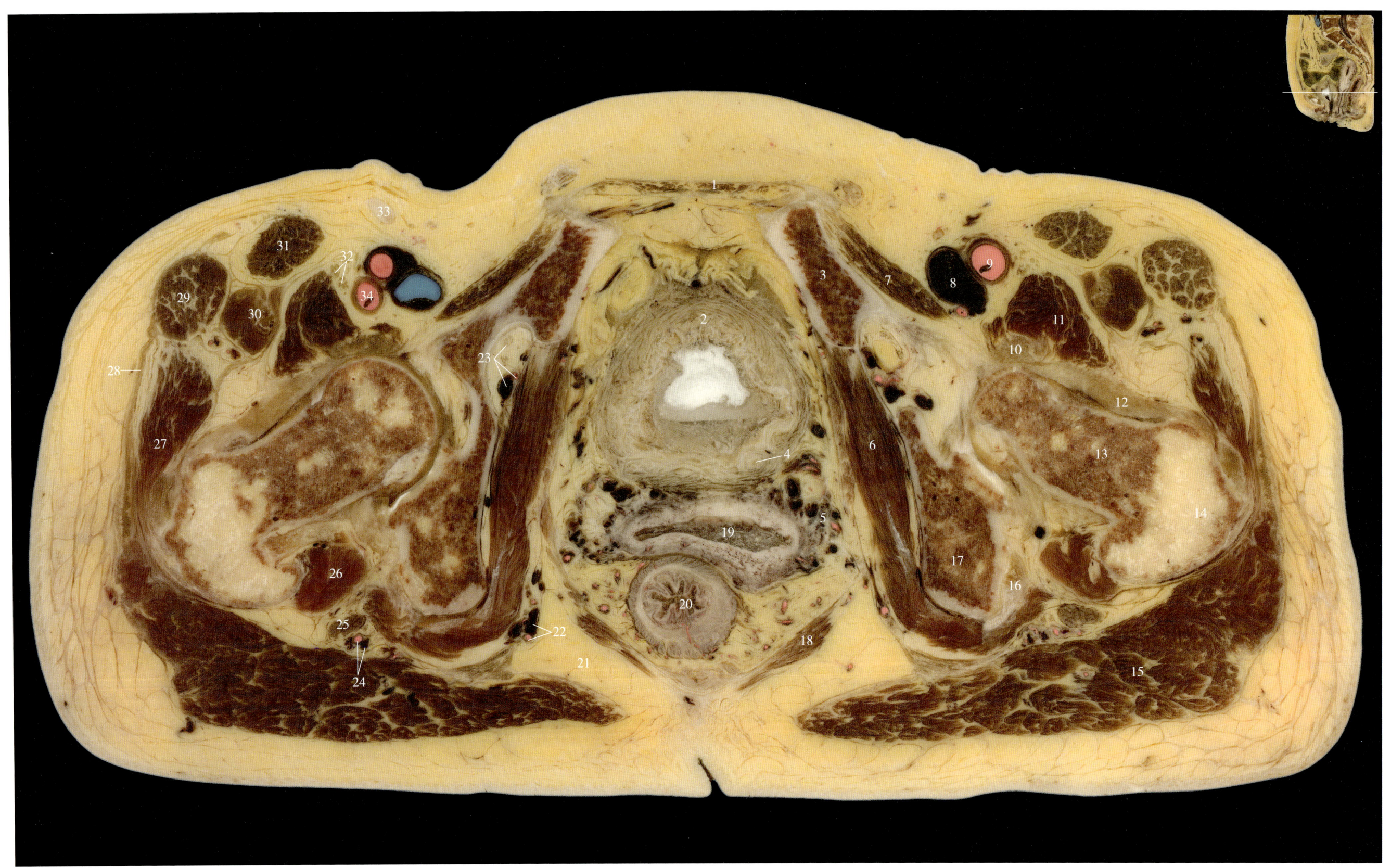

A. 断层标本图像

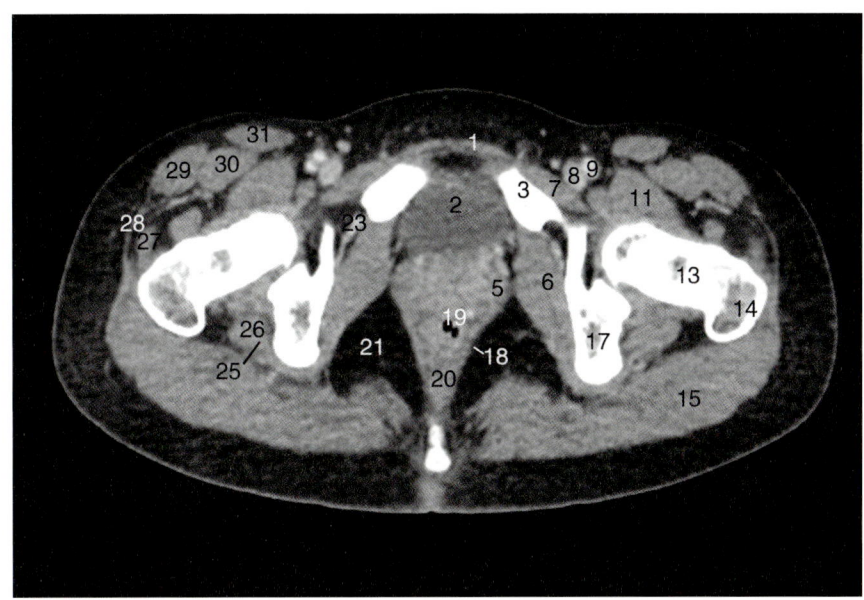
B. CT 增强图像

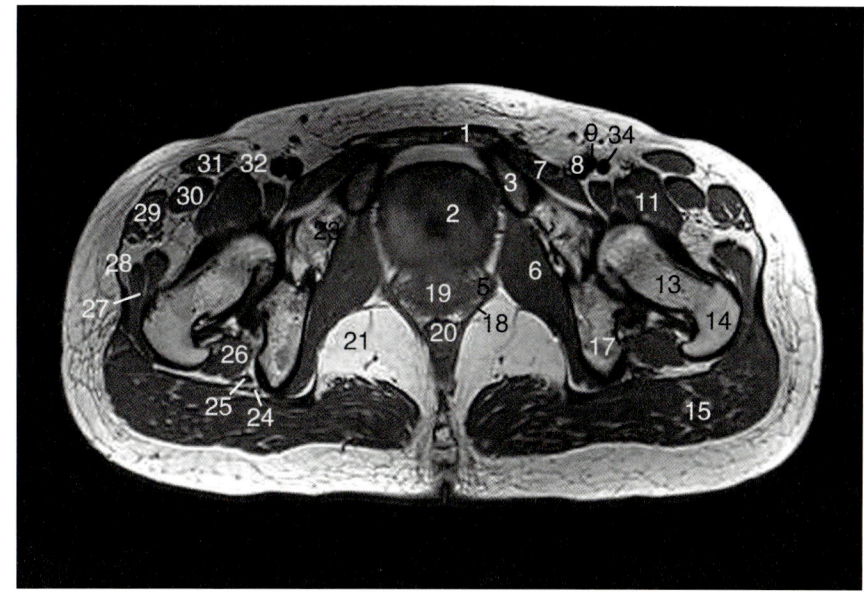
C. MR T1WI

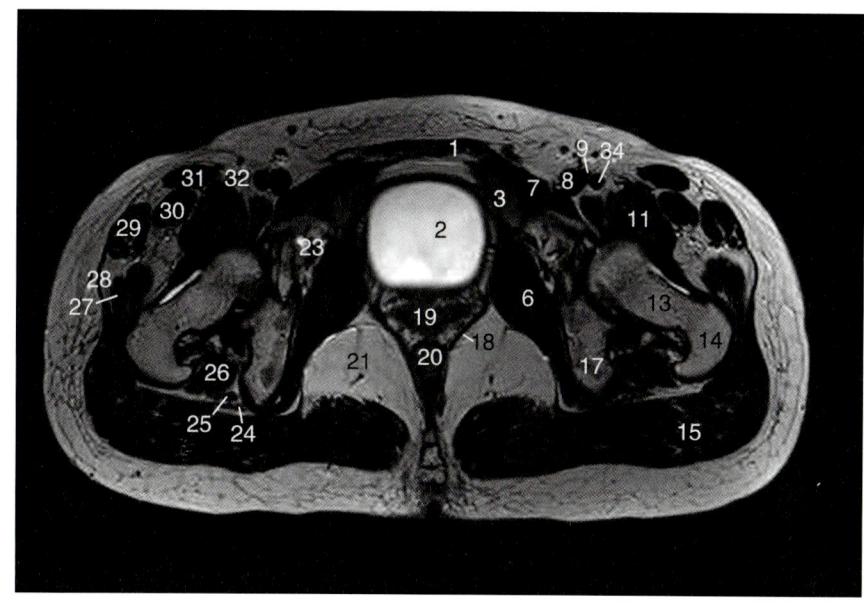
D. MR T2WI

关键结构：输尿管壁内部，膀胱三角，阴道。

1. 腹直肌 rectus abdominis
2. 膀胱 urinary bladder
3. 耻骨上支 superior ramus of pubis
4. 输尿管壁内部 intramural part of ureter
5. 阴道静脉丛 vaginaal venous plexus
6. 闭孔内肌 obturator internus
7. 耻骨肌 pectineus
8. 股静脉 femoral vein
9. 股动脉 femoral artery
10. 髂腰肌肌腱 iliopsoas tendon
11. 髂腰肌 iliopsoas
12. 髂股韧带 iliofemoral ligament
13. 股骨颈 neck of femur
14. 股骨大转子 greater trochanter
15. 臀大肌 gluteus maximus
16. 股二头肌、半腱肌和半膜肌总腱 tendons of biceps femoris, semitendinous and semimembranousus
17. 坐骨体 body of ischium
18. 肛提肌 levator ani
19. 阴道 vaginaa
20. 直肠 rectum
21. 坐骨肛门窝 ischioanal fossa
22. 阴部内动、静脉 internal pudental artery and vein
23. 闭孔动、静脉和神经 obturator artery, vein and nerve
24. 臀下动、静脉 inferior gluteal artery and vein
25. 坐骨神经 sciatic nerve
26. 股方肌 quadratus femoris
27. 臀中肌 gluteus medius
28. 阔筋膜 fasciae lata
29. 阔筋膜张肌 tensor fasciae latae
30. 股直肌 rectus femoris
31. 缝匠肌 sartorius
32. 股神经 femoral nerve
33. 腹股沟浅淋巴结 superficial inguinal lymph nodes
34. 股深动脉 deep femoral artery

　　此断面经股骨头下份。断面中央部狭窄的盆腔内，由前向后依次可见膀胱、阴道和直肠的断面。阴道为中段断面，其周围见大小不等的阴道静脉丛断面。直肠断面后方见肛提肌，呈细长条状自尾骨前外侧始、向前外方延伸直达闭孔内肌内侧缘。两侧肛提肌在断面上呈"V"形。膀胱的左后壁可见斜穿膀胱壁的输尿管壁内部。输尿管壁内部长约为 1.5 cm，当膀胱充盈时，壁内部的管腔闭合，加之输尿管的蠕动，因此有阻止尿液逆流入输尿管的作用。若壁内部过短或肌组织发育不良，则可发生尿液回流。在壁内部炎症及水肿，或因脊髓损伤而影响其神经支配时，也可发生尿液回流。儿童时期的壁内部较短，也有尿液回流现象，但随着生长发育，壁内部不断延长，肌层不断增厚，因此大部分的回流现象即自然消失[12]。此处是输尿管最狭窄处，也是常见的结石滞留部位。输尿管壁内部的开口为输尿管口，左、右输尿管口和尿道内口之间的三角形区域为膀胱三角，此处缺少黏膜下层组织，无论膀胱充盈还是空虚，始终保持平滑。膀胱三角是肿瘤、结核和炎症的好发部位[12]。

女性盆部与会阴连续横断层 62（FH.8150）

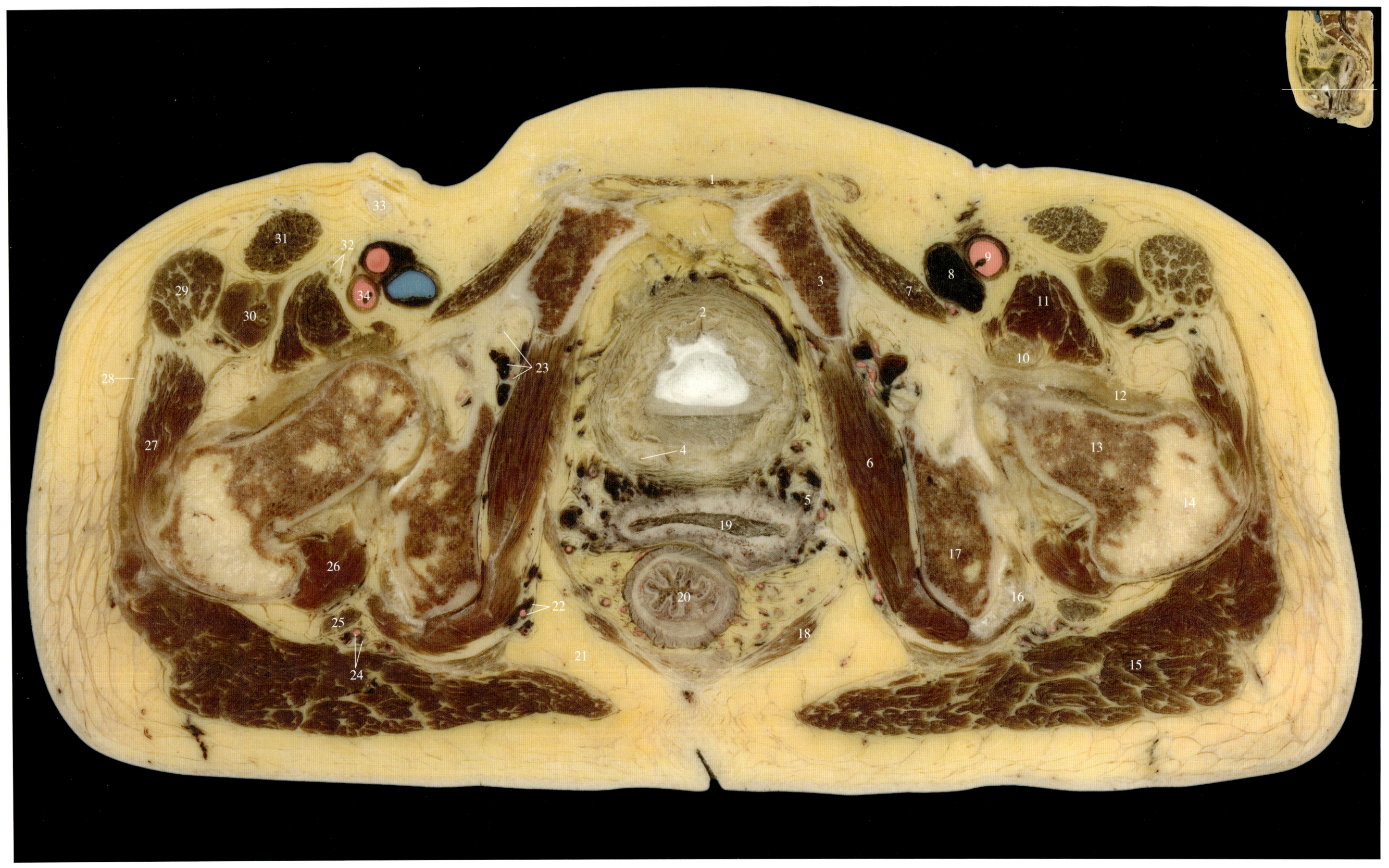

A. 断层标本图像

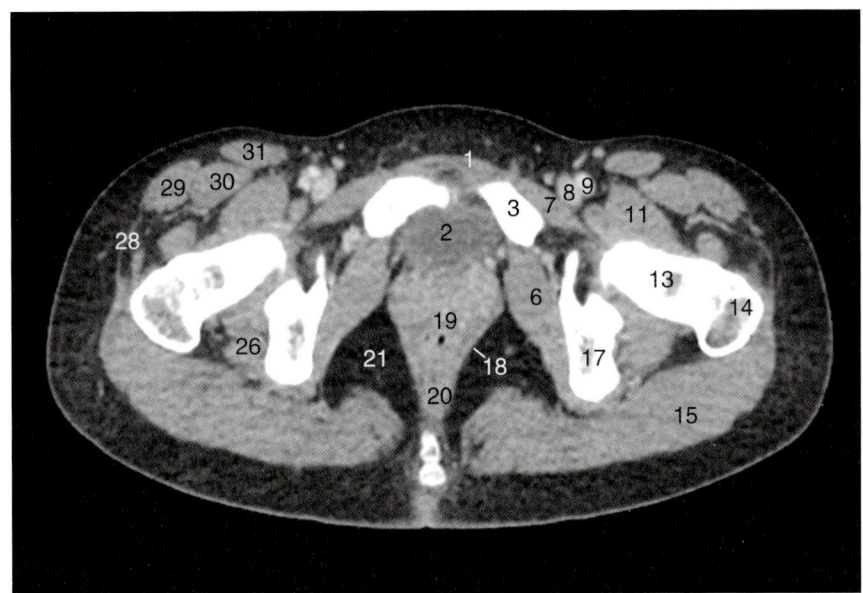
B. CT 增强图像

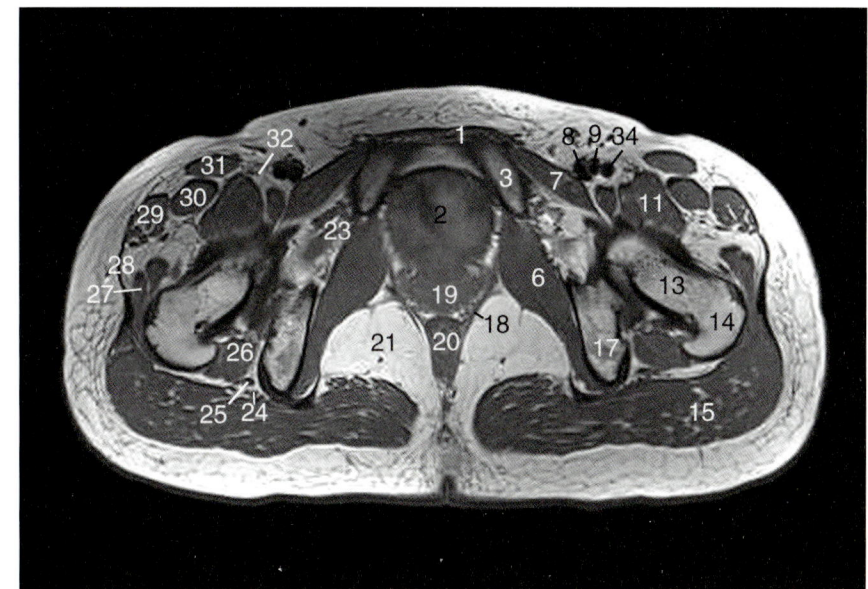
C. MR T1WI

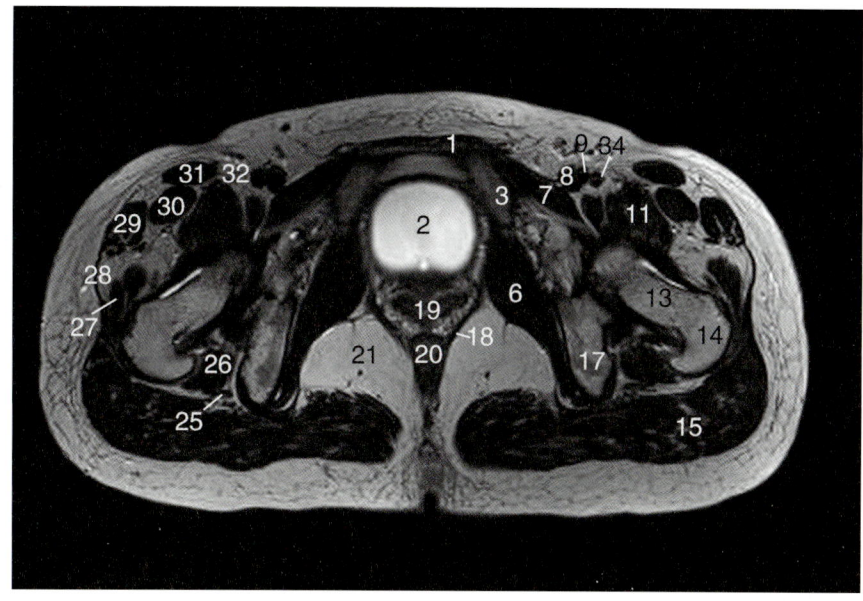
D. MR T2WI

关键结构：阴道，膀胱，直肠。

此断面股骨头几近消失。盆腔前壁由腹直肌下端构成，盆腔后方有肛提肌。侧壁由两侧耻骨上支、坐骨及闭孔内肌构成。两侧耻骨上支呈"八"形排列，逐渐向中线靠拢。盆腔内从前向后依次可见膀胱、阴道和直肠。尾骨尖前方的直肠为末端断面，再向下的断面，直肠向后下绕过尾骨尖，在矢状面上形成直肠骶曲，穿过盆膈移行为肛管。阴道分为上、中、下三段，分别以阴道穹侧部、膀胱底和尿道为标志[1]。CT横断图像上阴道表现为类圆形软组织密度，偶见中心低密度区，代表阴道腔隙及分泌液。MRI矢状面T2WI显示阴道效果较好，能清晰地分辨阴道与膀胱、直肠的关系。T2WI显示阴道中心部位呈细条样高信号，为阴道内黏液，周围环以低信号壁。低信号的阴道壁易于同高信号阴道黏液及周围脂肪相区别。T1WI不易区分阴道壁与阴道腔隙及黏液，但阴道壁与外周脂肪有优良的对比。

1. 腹直肌 rectus abdominis
2. 膀胱 urinary bladder
3. 耻骨上支 superior ramus of pubis
4. 输尿管壁内部 intramural part of ureter
5. 阴道静脉丛 vaginaal venous plexus
6. 闭孔内肌 obturator internus
7. 耻骨肌 pectineus
8. 股静脉 femoral vein
9. 股动脉 femoral artery
10. 髂腰肌肌腱 iliopsoas tendon
11. 髂腰肌 iliopsoas
12. 髂股韧带 iliofemoral ligament
13. 股骨颈 neck of femur
14. 股骨大转子 greater trochanter
15. 臀大肌 gluteus maximus
16. 股二头肌、半腱肌和半膜肌总腱 tendons of biceps femoris, semitendinous and semimembranousus
17. 坐骨 ischium
18. 肛提肌 levator ani
19. 阴道 vaginaa
20. 直肠 rectum
21. 坐骨肛门窝 ischioanal fossa
22. 阴部内动、静脉 internal pudendal artery and vein
23. 闭孔动、静脉和神经 obturator artery, vein and nerve
24. 臀下动、静脉 inferior gluteal artery and vein
25. 坐骨神经 sciatic nerve
26. 股方肌 quadratus femoris
27. 臀中肌 gluteus medius
28. 阔筋膜 fasciae lata
29. 阔筋膜张肌 tensor fasciae latae
30. 股直肌 rectus femoris
31. 缝匠肌 sartorius
32. 股神经 femoral nerve
33. 腹股沟浅淋巴结 superficial inguinal lymph nodes
34. 股深动脉 deep femoral artery

女性盆部与会阴连续横断层 63（FH.8130）

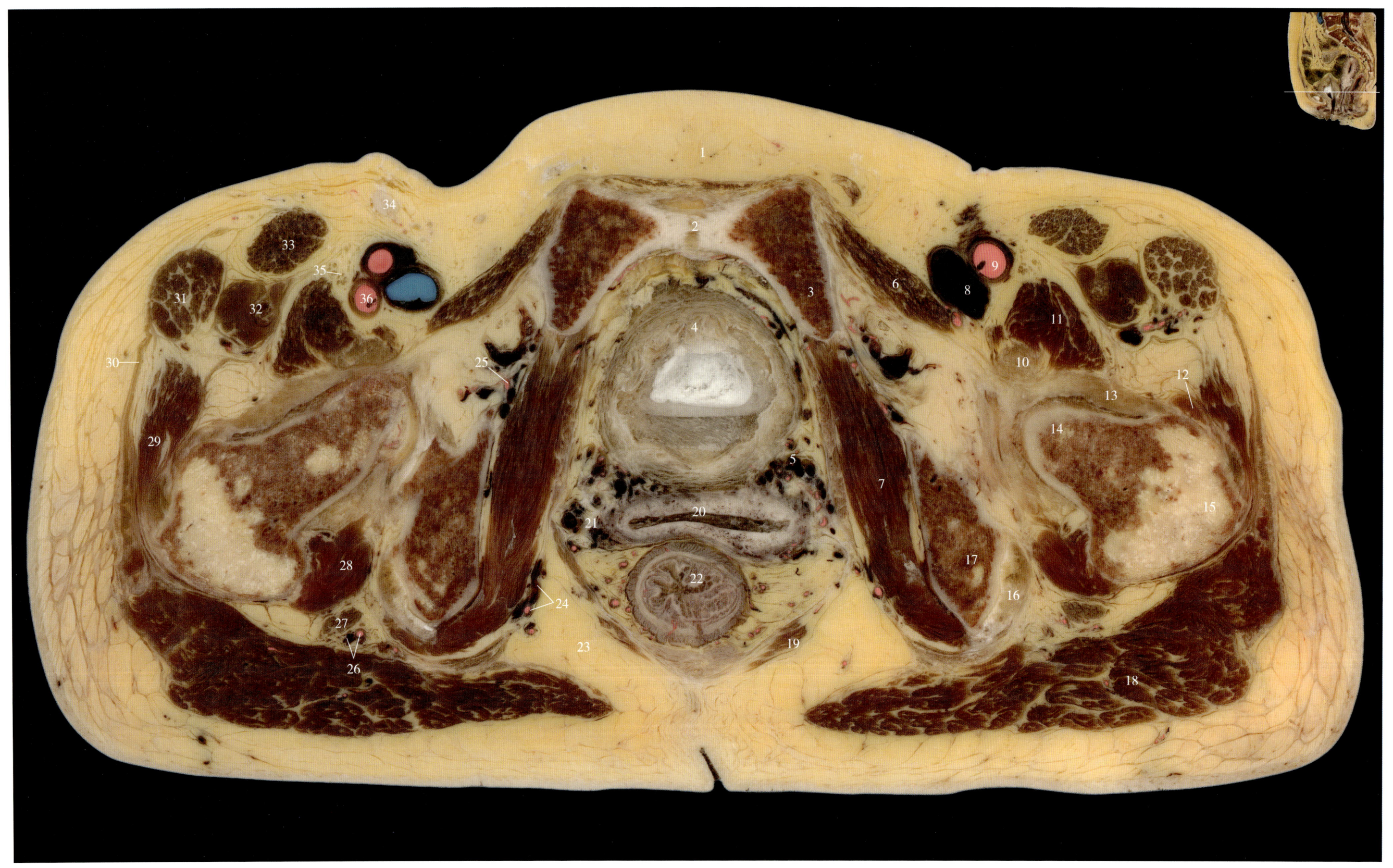

A. 断层标本图像

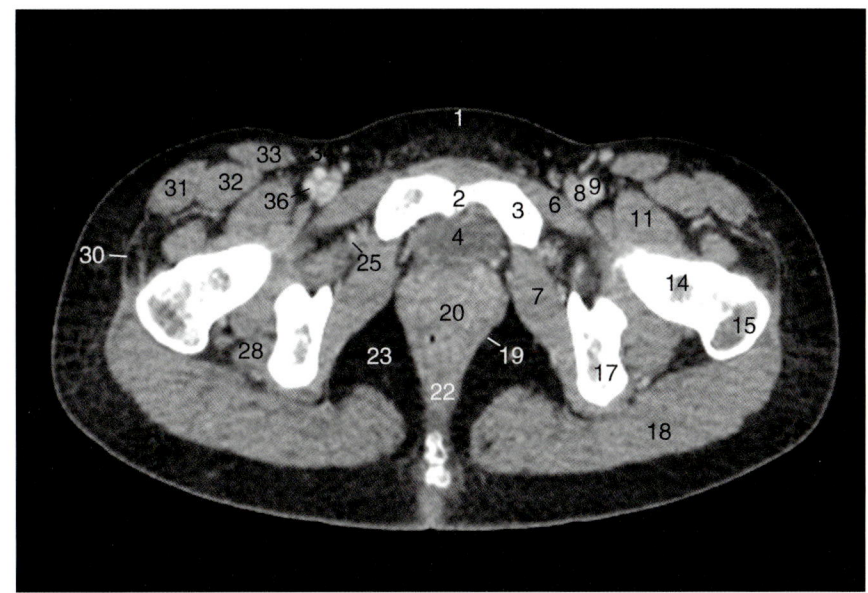
B. CT 增强图像

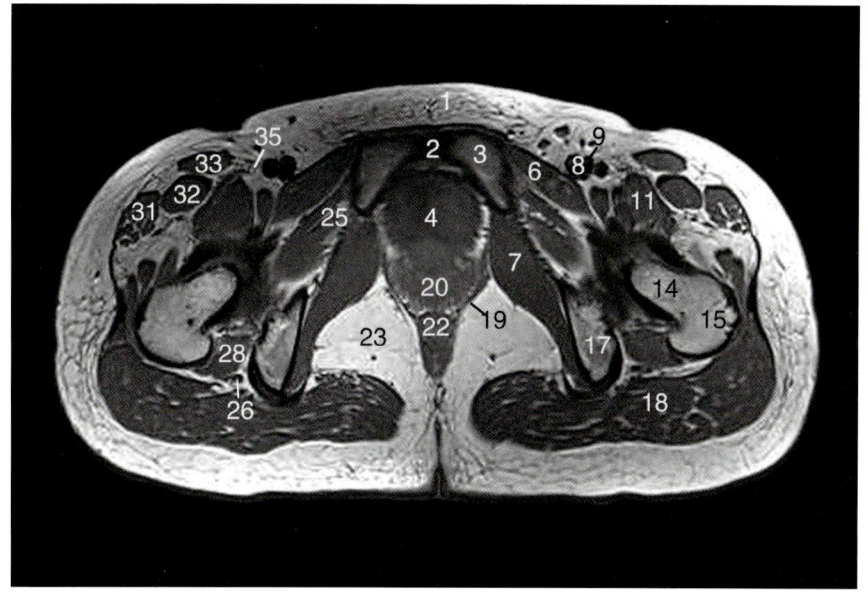
C. MR T1WI

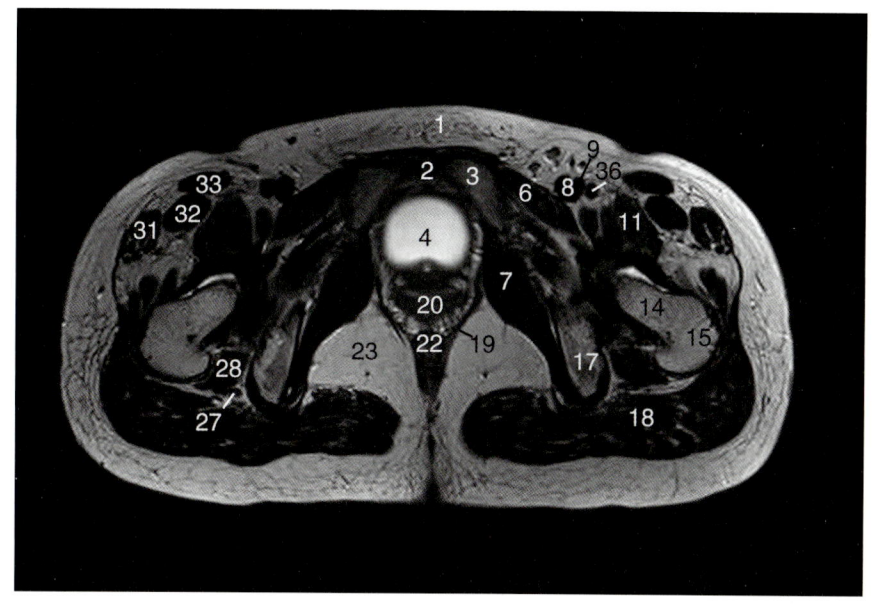
D. MR T2WI

1. 阴阜 mons pubis
2. 耻骨联合 pubic symphysis
3. 耻骨上支 superior ramus of pubis
4. 膀胱 urinary bladder
5. 膀胱静脉丛 vesical venous plexus
6. 耻骨肌 pectineus
7. 闭孔内肌 obturator internus 3
8. 股静脉 femoral vein
9. 股动脉 femoral artery
10. 髂腰肌肌腱 iliopsoas tendon
11. 髂腰肌 iliopsoas
12. 股外侧肌 vastus lateralis
13. 髂股韧带 iliofemoral ligament
14. 股骨颈 neck of femur
15. 股骨大转子 greater trochanter
16. 股二头肌、半腱肌和半膜肌总腱 tendons of biceps femoris, semitendinous and semimembranousus
17. 坐骨结节 ischial tuberosity
18. 臀大肌 gluteus maximus
19. 肛提肌 levator ani
20. 阴道 vaginaa
21. 阴道静脉丛 vaginaal venous plexus
22. 肛管 anal canal
23. 坐骨肛门窝 ischioanal fossa
24. 阴部内动、静脉 internal pudendal artery and vein
25. 闭孔动脉 obturator artery
26. 臀下动、静脉 inferior gluteal artery and vein
27. 坐骨神经 sciatic nerve
28. 股方肌 quadratus femoris
29. 臀中肌 gluteus medius
30. 阔筋膜 fasciae lata
31. 阔筋膜张肌 tensor fasciae latae
32. 股直肌 rectus femoris
33. 缝匠肌 sartorius
34. 腹股沟浅淋巴结 superficial inguinal lymph nodes
35. 股神经 femoral nerve
36. 股深动脉 deep femoral artery

关键结构：耻骨联合，肛管，膀胱，阴道。

此断层为女性盆腔第四段的开始。断面前方经耻骨联合上缘，耻骨联合正后方从前向后依次排列有膀胱、阴道和肛管，膀胱和阴道断面的周围，见许多膀胱静脉丛和阴道静脉丛的断面。直肠已移行为肛管，呈卵圆形管状结构。两侧肛提肌的条带状断面围成"V"形，绕于三脏器的后方和两侧。耻骨联合由两侧的耻骨联合面借耻骨间盘连接构成。耻骨间盘由纤维软骨构成，耻骨间盘中往往出现一矢状位的裂隙，女性较男性的厚，裂隙也较大，孕妇和经产妇尤为显著。在耻骨联合的上、下方分别有连接两侧耻骨的耻骨上韧带和耻骨弓状韧带。耻骨联合的活动甚微，但在分娩过程中，耻骨间盘中的裂隙增宽，以增大骨盆的径线。耻骨联合的血供来自闭孔动脉、阴部内动脉、腹壁下动脉和旋股内侧动脉的分支。其神经由阴部神经和生殖股神经分支支配[27]。

女性盆部与会阴连续横断层 64（FH.8110）

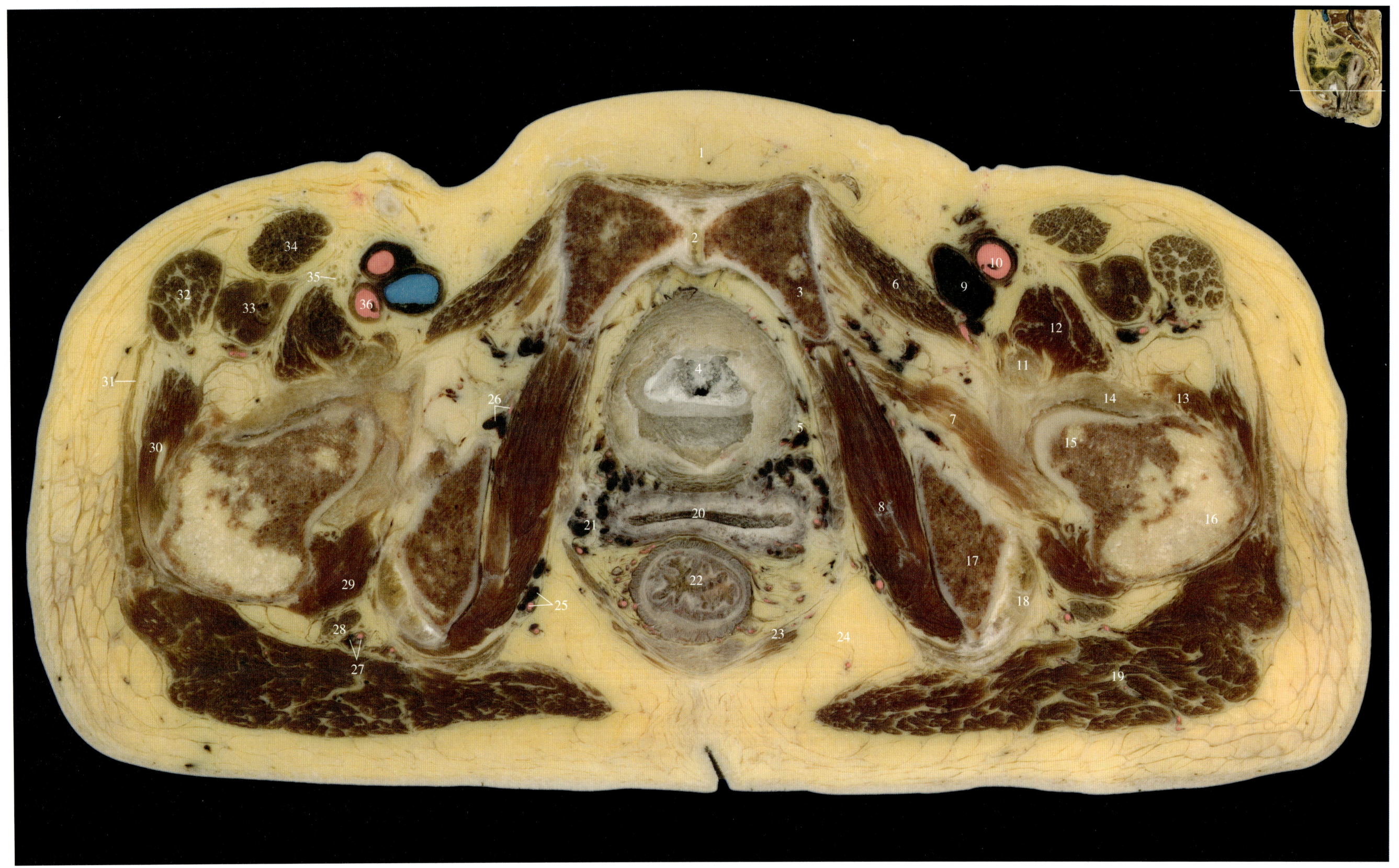

A. 断层标本图像

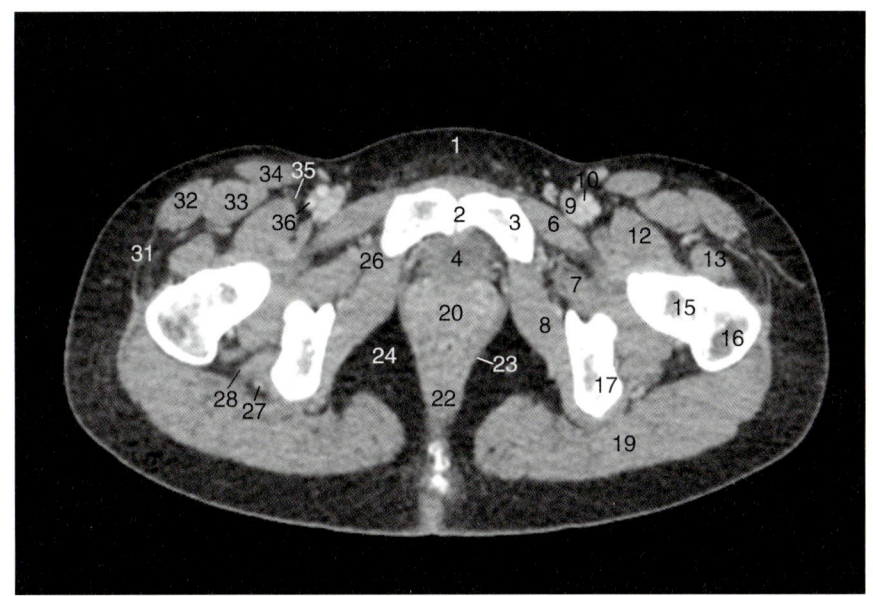
B. CT 增强图像

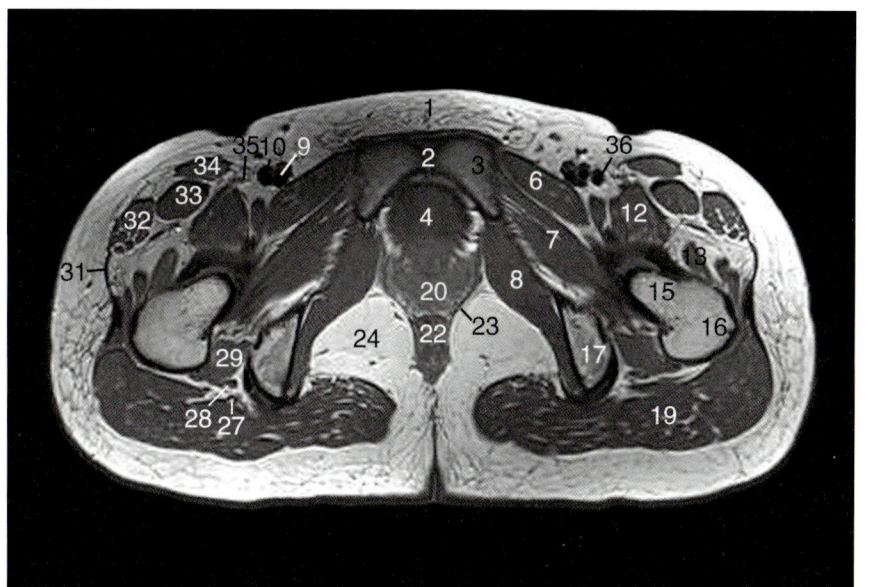
C. MR T1WI

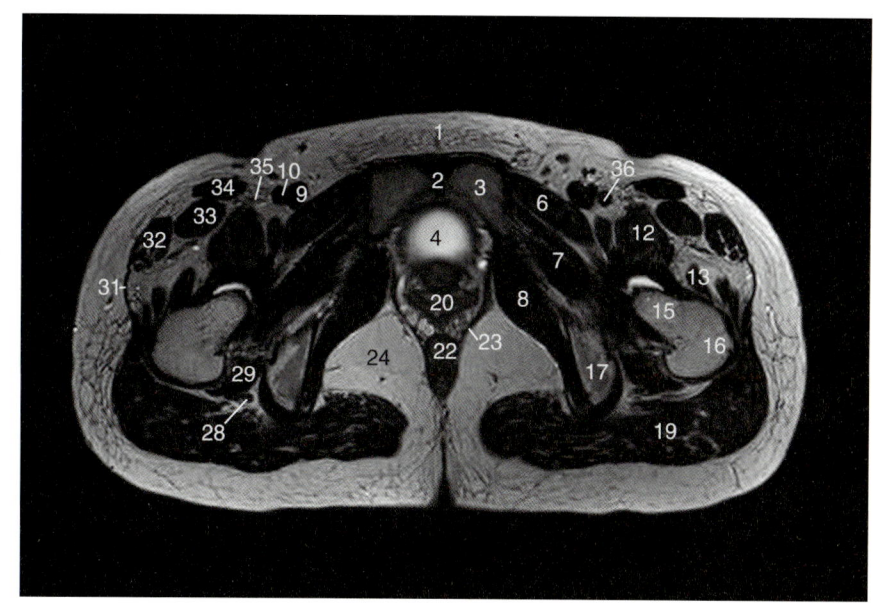
D. MR T2WI

1. 阴阜 mons pubis
2. 耻骨联合 pubic symphysis
3. 耻骨上支 superior ramus of pubis
4. 膀胱 urinary bladder
5. 膀胱静脉丛 vesical venous plexus
6. 耻骨肌 pectineus
7. 闭孔外肌 obturator externus
8. 闭孔内肌 obturator internus
9. 股静脉 femoral vein
10. 股动脉 femoral artery
11. 髂腰肌肌腱 iliopsoas tendon
12. 髂腰肌 iliopsoas
13. 股外侧肌 vastus lateralis
14. 髂股韧带 iliofemoral ligament
15. 股骨颈 neck of femur
16. 股骨大转子 greater trochanter
17. 坐骨结节 ischial tuberosity
18. 股二头肌、半腱肌和半膜肌总腱 tendons of biceps femoris, semitendinous and semimembranousus
19. 臀大肌 gluteus maximus
20. 阴道 vaginaa
21. 阴道静脉丛 vaginaal venous plexus
22. 肛管 anal canal
23. 肛提肌 levator ani
24. 坐骨肛门窝 ischioanal fossa
25. 阴部内动、静脉 internal pudendal artery and vein
26. 闭孔动、静脉 obturator artery and vein
27. 臀下动、静脉 inferior gluteal artery and vein
28. 坐骨神经 sciatic nerve
29. 股方肌 quadratus femoris
30. 臀中肌 gluteus medius
31. 阔筋膜 fasciae lata
32. 阔筋膜张肌 tensor fasciae latae
33. 股直肌 rectus femoris
34. 缝匠肌 sartorius
35. 股神经 femoral nerve
36. 股深动脉 deep femoral artery

关键结构：闭孔外肌，阴阜，膀胱，耻骨联合。

　　此断面经耻骨联合上份。耻骨联合位于盆前壁中央，其前方为阴阜，其后方的盆腔脏器依次排列有膀胱、阴道和肛管。两侧肛提肌呈"V"形，绕于三脏器的后方和两侧。盆腔侧壁由耻骨上支、坐骨结节及二者之间的闭孔膜构成，在闭孔膜的内侧有闭孔内肌附着，在闭孔膜的外侧开始出现闭孔外肌。闭孔外肌位于股方肌的深面，起自闭孔膜外面及其周围骨面，向后经股骨颈后方止于转子窝，收缩时使髋关节旋外。阴阜为耻骨联合前面的皮肤隆起，由大量富含皮下脂肪的结缔组织组成，青春期后生有阴毛，分布呈尖端向下的三角形。在该断面，膀胱位于盆腔内前部，周围见小动脉断面及静脉丛。膀胱主要由膀胱上动脉和膀胱下动脉供血，膀胱上动脉起自髂动脉近侧段，营养膀胱中上部；膀胱下动脉起自髂内动脉，分布于膀胱底、近端尿道及输尿管盆部下份。膀胱的静脉不与动脉伴行，在膀胱的两侧形成膀胱静脉丛汇入髂内静脉。膀胱前部的淋巴注入髂内淋巴结，膀胱三角和膀胱后部的淋巴大部分注入髂外淋巴结，少数注入髂内淋巴结或髂总淋巴结。支配膀胱的神经组成膀胱丛，包括交感和副交感神经，交感神经来自脊髓第11、12胸节和第1、2腰节，副交感神经来自脊髓第2~4骶节。膀胱的痛觉和膨胀感也可随交感和副交感神经传入[22]。

女性盆部与会阴连续横断层 65（FH.8090）

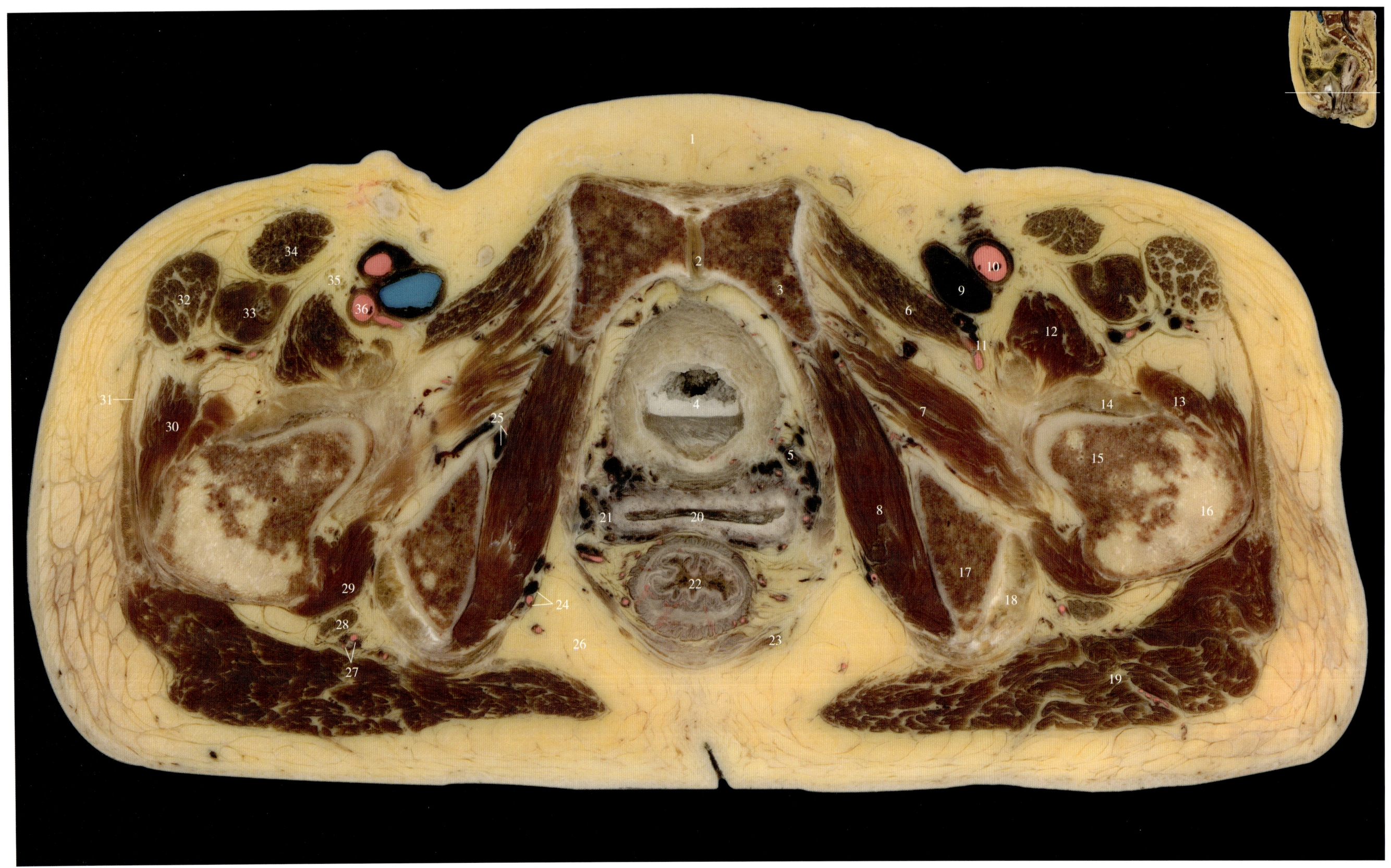

A. 断层标本图像

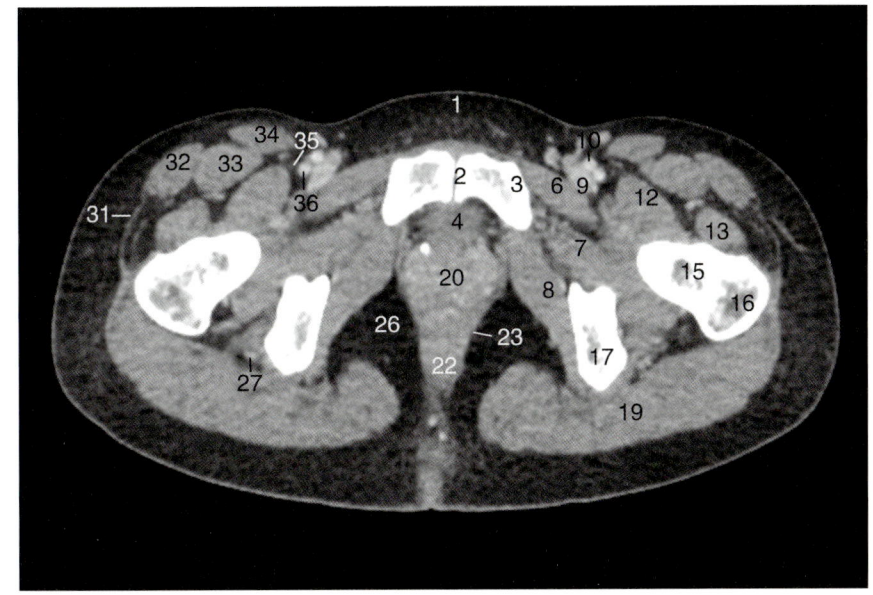

B. CT 增强图像

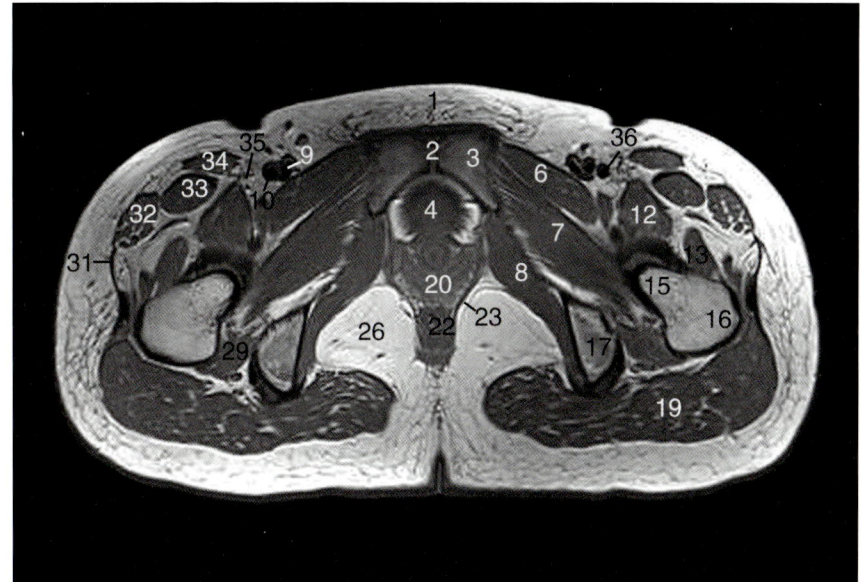

C. MR T1WI

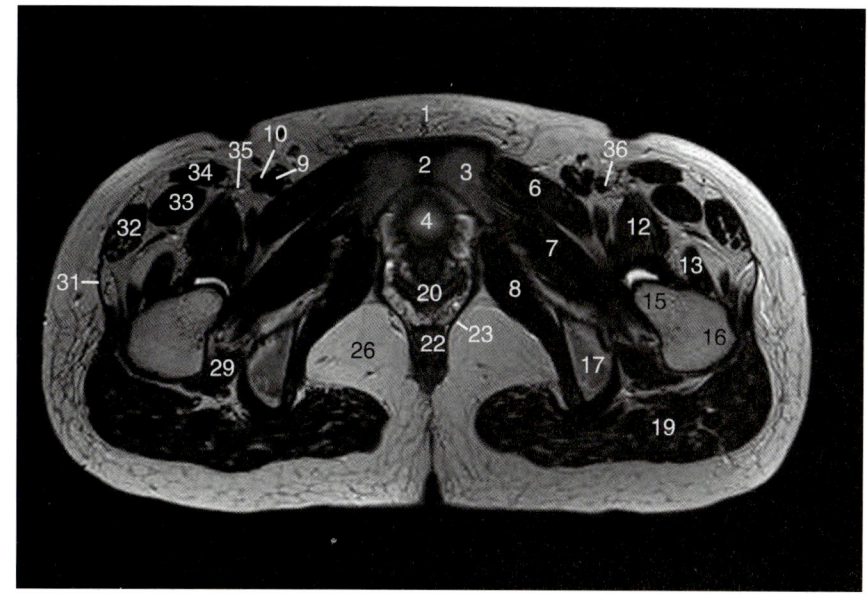

D. MR T2WI

1. 阴阜 mons pubis
2. 耻骨联合 pubic symphysis
3. 耻骨上支 superior ramus of pubis
4. 膀胱 urinary bladder
5. 膀胱静脉丛 vesical venous plexus
6. 耻骨肌 pectineus
7. 闭孔外肌 obturator externus
8. 闭孔内肌 obturator internus
9. 股静脉 femoral vein
10. 股动脉 femoral artery
11. 旋股内侧动脉 medial femoral circumflex artery
12. 髂腰肌 iliopsoas
13. 股外侧肌 vastus lateralis
14. 髂股韧带 iliofemoral ligament
15. 股骨颈 neck of femur
16. 股骨大转子 greater trochanter
17. 坐骨结节 ischial tuberosity
18. 股二头肌、半腱肌和半膜肌总腱 tendons of biceps femoris, semitendinous and semimembranosus
19. 臀大肌 gluteus maximus
20. 阴道 vaginaa
21. 阴道静脉丛 vaginaal venous plexus
22. 肛管 anal canal
23. 肛提肌 levator ani
24. 阴部内动、静脉 internal pudendal artery and vein
25. 闭孔动、静脉 obturator artery and vein
26. 坐骨肛门窝 ischioanal fossa
27. 臀下动、静脉和神经 inferior gluteal artery, vein and nerve
28. 坐骨神经 sciatic nerve
29. 股方肌 quadratus femoris
30. 臀中肌 gluteus medius
31. 阔筋膜 fasciae lata
32. 阔筋膜张肌 tensor fasciae latae
33. 股直肌 rectus femoris
34. 缝匠肌 sartorius
35. 股神经 femoral nerve
36. 股深动脉 deep femoral artery

关键结构：阴部管，坐骨肛门窝，肛提肌。

此断面前方经耻骨联合上份。耻骨联合位居盆腔前壁，耻骨上支与坐骨结节之间为闭孔上部，其内、外侧分别为闭孔内、外肌。盆腔内由前向后依次排列有膀胱、阴道和肛管，肛提肌包绕上述脏器，女性盆底和会阴肌包括闭孔肌、梨状肌、球底肌、闭孔肌、坐骨海绵体肌、肛门外括约肌、肛提肌（耻骨直肠肌、耻尾肌和髂尾肌）和尾骨肌。有学者对盆底和会阴肌进行了三维重建，并研究了其结构与功能[35]。在膀胱和阴道周围有膀胱静脉丛和阴道静脉丛。肛提肌、闭孔内肌和臀大肌之间为坐骨肛门窝，其内充满脂肪组织，在该窝的外侧壁上可见行于阴部管内的阴部神经和阴部内动、静脉。阴部神经由骶丛发出，与阴部内血管伴行出梨状肌下孔至臀部，随即绕坐骨棘经坐骨小孔至坐骨肛门窝。阴部神经主干沿坐骨肛门窝外侧壁上的阴部管向前走行，沿途分出肛神经、会阴神经及阴蒂背神经，分布至肛周、会阴肌、大阴唇、阴蒂等部位。由于阴部神经在行程中绕过坐骨棘，故在行会阴手术时，在坐骨结节与肛门连线的中点经皮刺向坐骨棘的下方，进行阴部神经阻滞麻醉。阴部内血管与神经伴行，分支分布与神经相同。在 CT 图像上，坐骨肛门窝脂肪组织显示为坐骨结节、肛管和臀大肌间的三角形低密度区域；在 MR T1WI 和 T2WI 呈高信号，在其外侧见低信号的阴部神经和阴部内血管[22]。

女性盆部与会阴连续横断层 66（FH.8070）

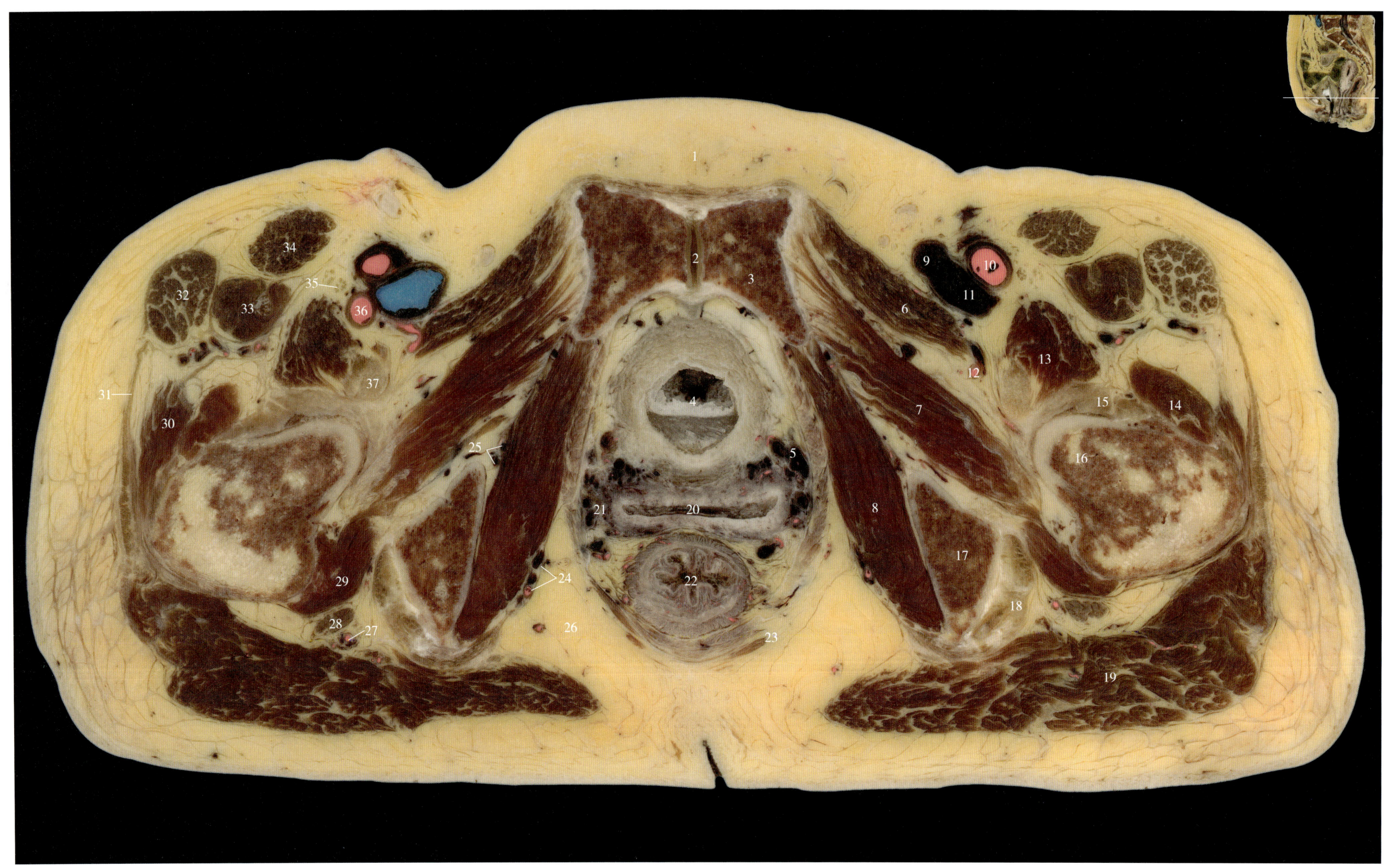

A. 断层标本图像

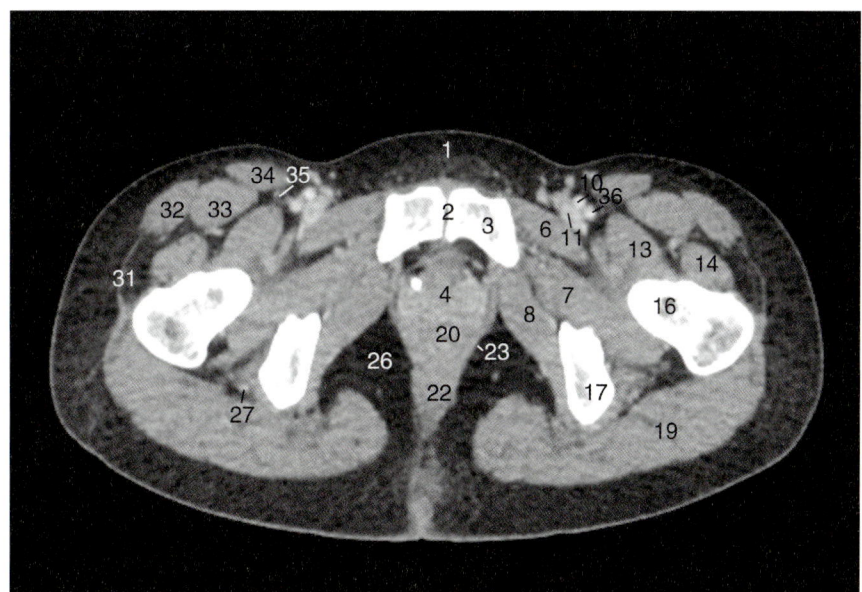
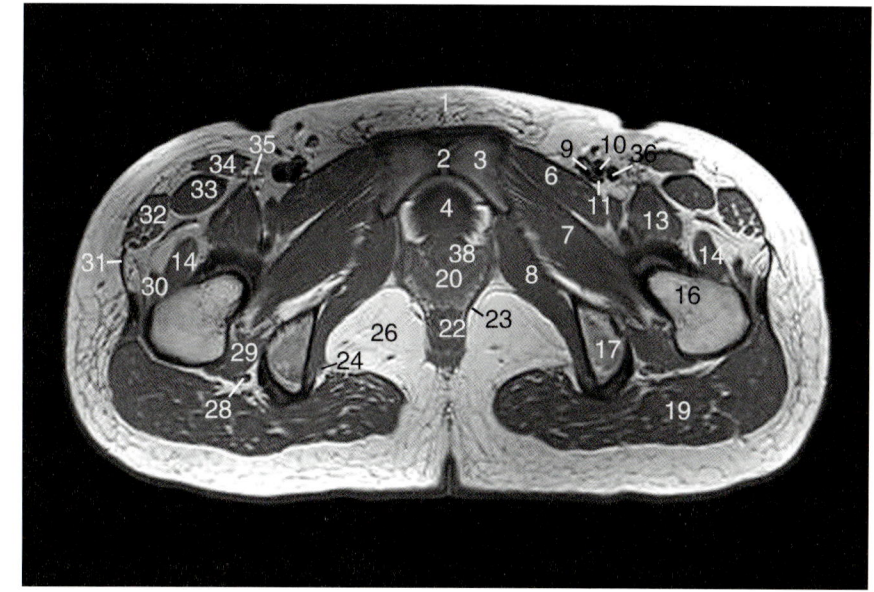
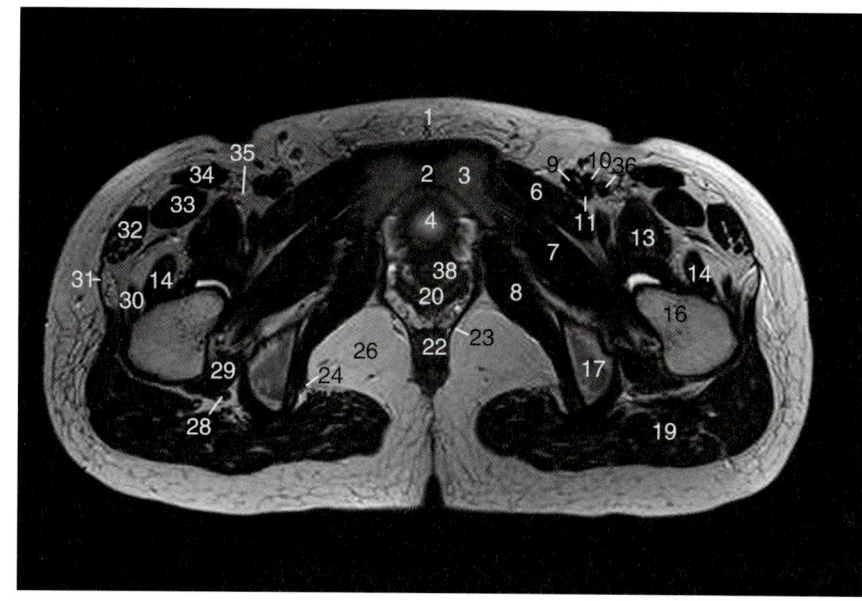

B. CT 增强图像　　　　　　　　　　C. MR T1WI　　　　　　　　　　D. MR T2WI

1. 阴阜 mons pubis
2. 耻骨联合 pubic symphysis
3. 耻骨上支 superior ramus of pubis
4. 膀胱 urinary bladder
5. 膀胱静脉丛 vesical venous plexus
6. 耻骨肌 pectineus
7. 闭孔外肌 obturator externus
8. 闭孔内肌 obturator internus
9. 大隐静脉 great saphenous vein
10. 股动脉 femoral artery
11. 股静脉 femoral vein
12. 旋股内侧动脉 medial femoral circumflex artery
13. 髂腰肌 iliopsoas
14. 股外侧肌 vastus lateralis
15. 髂股韧带 iliofemoral ligament
16. 股骨颈 neck of femur
17. 坐骨结节 ischial tuberosity
18. 股二头肌、半腱肌和半膜肌总腱 tendons of biceps femoris, semitendinous and semimembranousus
19. 臀大肌 gluteus maximus
20. 阴道 vaginaa
21. 阴道静脉丛 vaginaal venous plexus
22. 肛管 anal canal
23. 肛提肌 levator ani
24. 阴部内动、静脉 internal pudendal artery and vein
25. 闭孔动、静脉 obturator artery and vein
26. 坐骨肛门窝 ischioanal fossa
27. 臀下动脉 inferior gluteal artery
28. 坐骨神经 sciatic nerve
29. 股方肌 quadratus femoris
30. 臀中肌 gluteus medius
31. 阔筋膜 fasciae lata
32. 阔筋膜张肌 tensor fasciae latae
33. 股直肌 rectus femoris
34. 缝匠肌 sartorius
35. 股神经 femoral nerve
36. 股深动脉 deep femoral artery
37. 髂腰肌肌腱 iliopsoas tendon
38. 膀胱颈 neck of bladder

关键结构：臀大肌下间隙，膀胱，肛管。

此断面经耻骨联合上份。耻骨联合位居盆腔前壁，盆腔内由前向后依次排列有膀胱、阴道和肛管。在膀胱和阴道周围有膀胱静脉丛和阴道静脉丛，在肛管后方及上述三脏器的两侧有肛提肌包绕。耻骨上支与坐骨结节之间为闭孔上份，其内、外侧分别有闭孔内肌和闭孔外肌的粗大断面。坐骨结节外侧为股骨颈的外侧份和股骨体上份，二者之间为股方肌断面，二者后方为臀大肌断面。在臀大肌与股方肌之间可见臀大肌下间隙内的坐骨神经和臀下动、静脉。臀大肌下间隙是臀大肌与臀中肌、梨状肌、上孖肌、闭孔内肌、下孖肌和股方肌之间的疏松结缔组织间隙。此间隙向深面经梨状肌上、下孔与盆腔相通，向内经坐骨小孔与坐骨肛门窝相通，向下沿坐骨神经可达大腿后部，发生感染时可相互蔓延[22]。

女性盆部与会阴连续横断层 67（FH.8050）

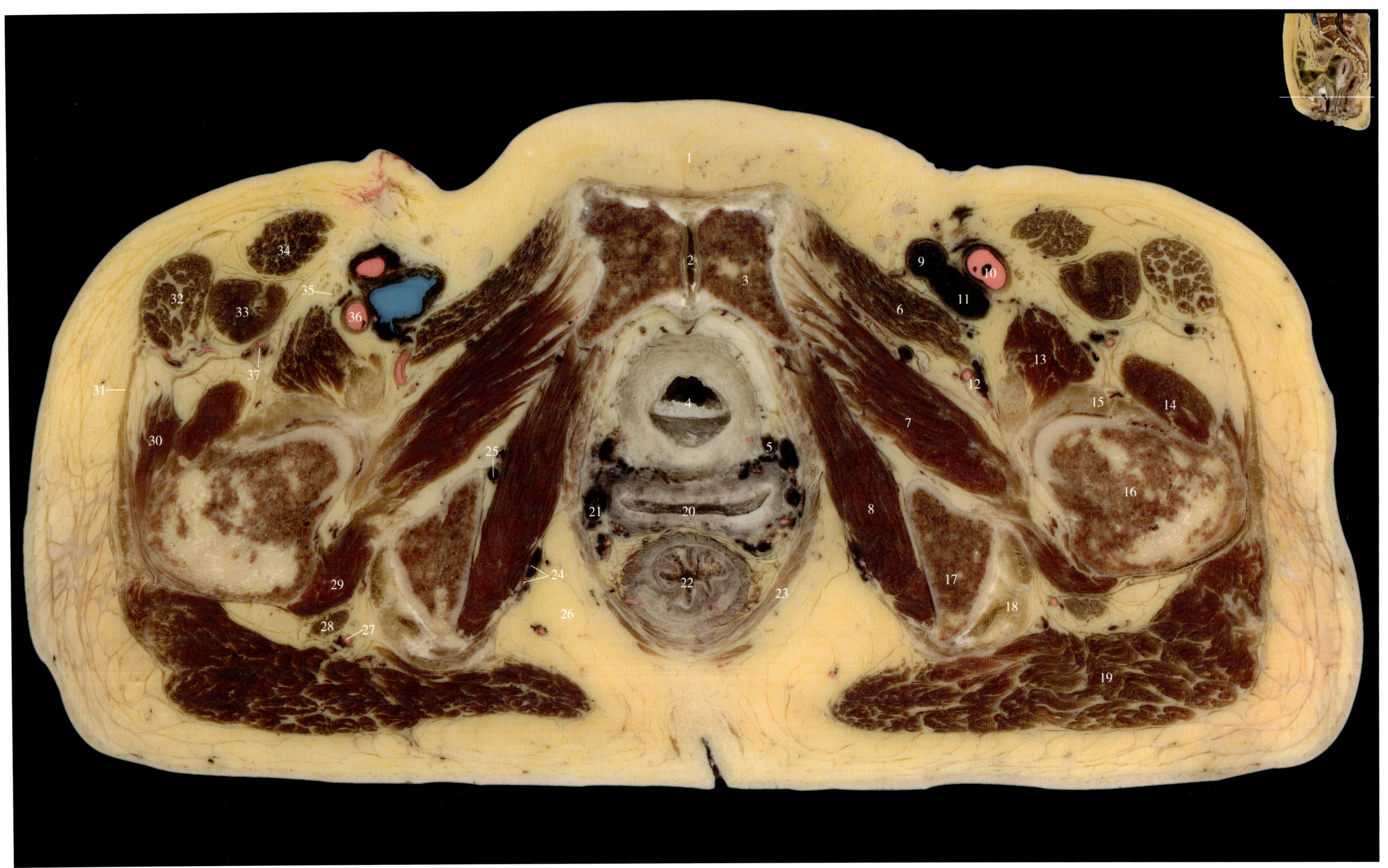

A. 断层标本图像

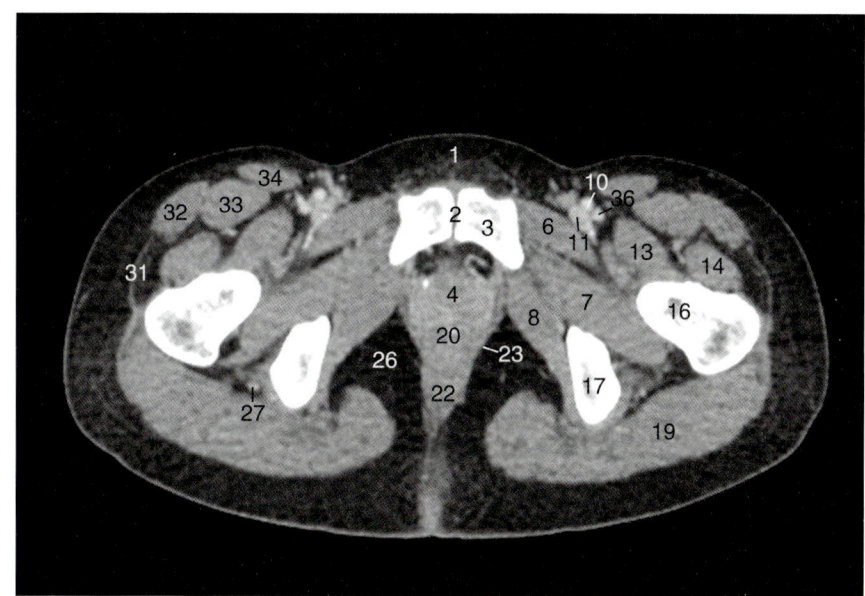

B. CT 增强图像

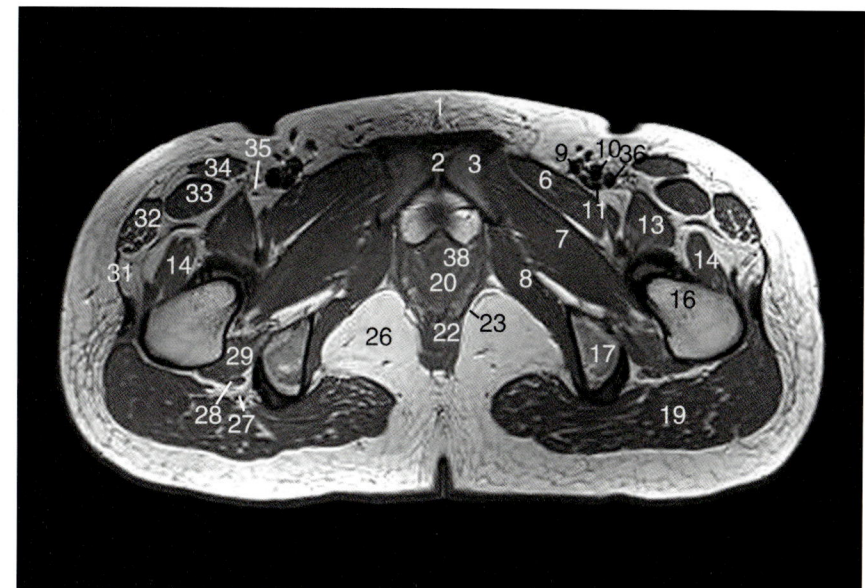

C. MR T1WI

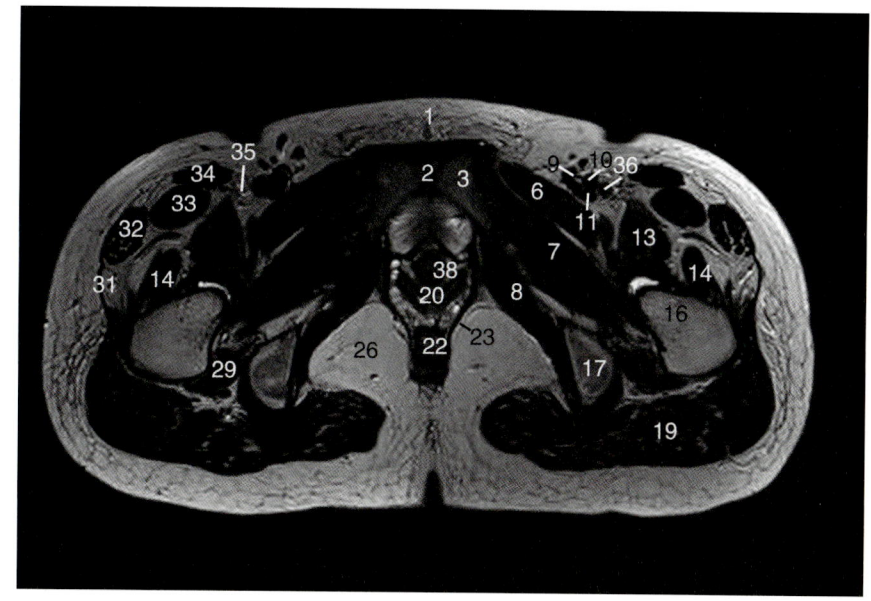

D. MR T2WI

1. 阴阜 mons pubis
2. 耻骨联合 pubic symphysis
3. 耻骨上支 superior ramus of pubis
4. 膀胱 urinary bladder
5. 膀胱静脉丛 vesical venous plexus
6. 耻骨肌 pectineus
7. 闭孔外肌 obturator externus
8. 闭孔内肌 obturator internus
9. 大隐静脉 great saphenous vein
10. 股动脉 femoral artery
11. 股静脉 femoral vein
12. 旋股内侧动脉 medial femoral circumflex artery
13. 髂腰肌 iliopsoas
14. 股外侧肌 vastus lateralis
15. 髂股韧带 iliofemoral ligament
16. 股骨 femur
17. 坐骨结节 ischial tuberosity
18. 股二头肌、半腱肌和半膜肌总腱 tendons of biceps femoris, semitendinous and semimembranousus
19. 臀大肌 gluteus maximus
20. 阴道 vaginaa
21. 阴道静脉丛 vaginaal venous plexus
22. 肛管 anal canal
23. 肛提肌 levator ani
24. 阴部内动、静脉 internal pudental artery and vein
25. 闭孔静脉 obturator vein
26. 坐骨肛门窝 ischioanal fossa
27. 臀下动脉 inferior gluteal artery
28. 坐骨神经 sciatic nerve
29. 股方肌 quadratus femoris
30. 臀中肌 gluteus medius
31. 阔筋膜 fasciae lata
32. 阔筋膜张肌 tensor fasciae latae
33. 股直肌 rectus femoris
34. 缝匠肌 sartorius
35. 股神经 femoral nerve
36. 股深动脉 deep femoral artery
37. 旋股外侧动脉升支 ascending branch of lateral femoral circumflex artery
38. 膀胱颈 neck of bladder

关键结构：耻骨联合，膀胱，阴道。

此断面经耻骨联合上份。耻骨联合构成盆腔前壁，其前方为阴阜，后方依次排列有膀胱、阴道和肛管。在膀胱和阴道周围有膀胱静脉丛和阴道静脉丛。肛提肌呈"U"形绕于脏器的两侧和后方。耻骨支与坐骨之间为闭孔中份，其内、外侧分别有闭孔内肌和闭孔外肌附着。在臀大肌与股方肌之间可见坐骨神经和臀下动、静脉。在股三角区内，大隐静脉在前，股静脉在后，二者居于股三角区内侧，股动脉（和股深动脉）居中，股神经居外侧。在阴道与直肠之间有直肠阴道隔，上端起自直肠子宫陷凹，下到盆底，两侧附于盆侧壁的筋膜，并与子宫和阴道上端两侧的筋膜连接，后方与直肠系膜筋膜相延续。在膀胱底与子宫颈和阴道上部之间还有膀胱阴道隔[22]。

女性盆部与会阴连续横断层 68（FH.8030）

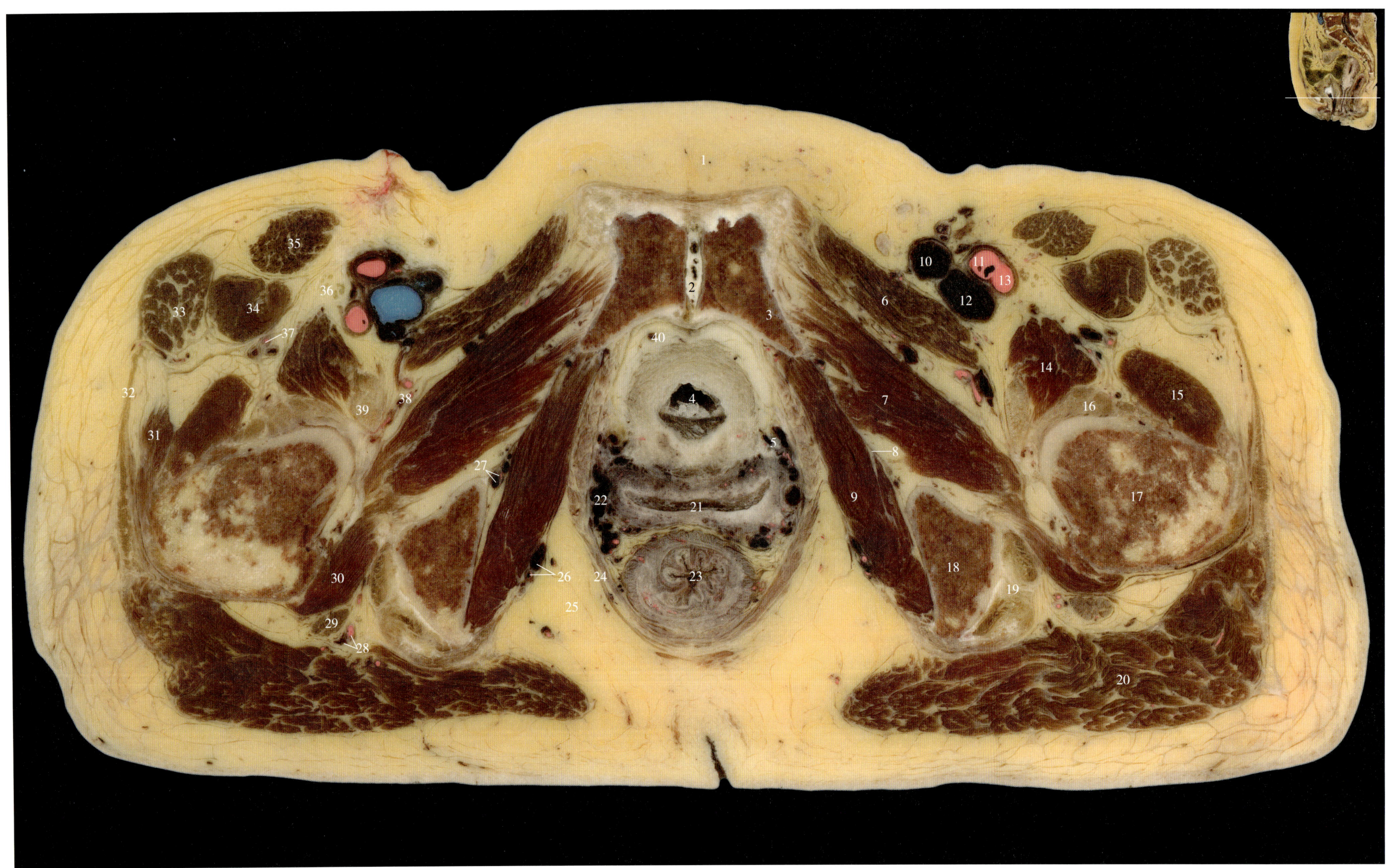

A. 断层标本图像

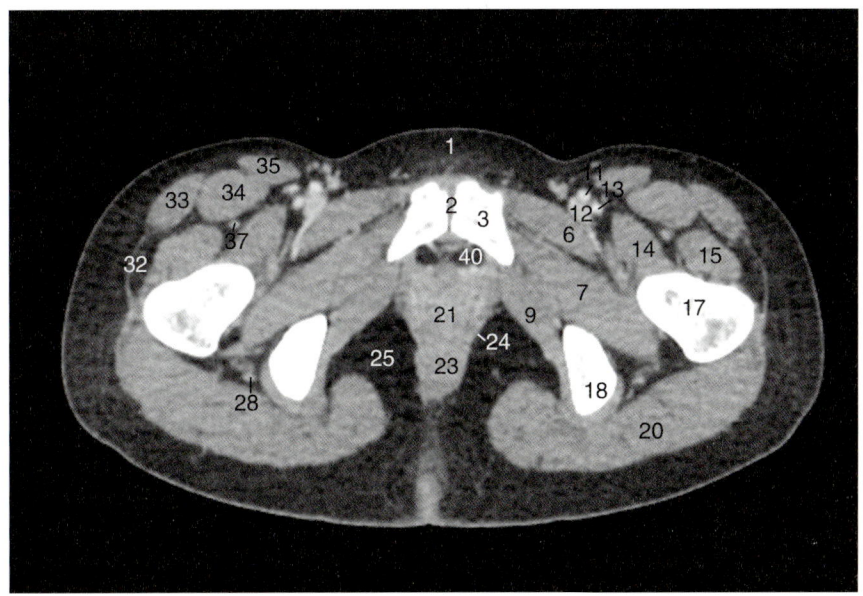

B. CT 增强图像

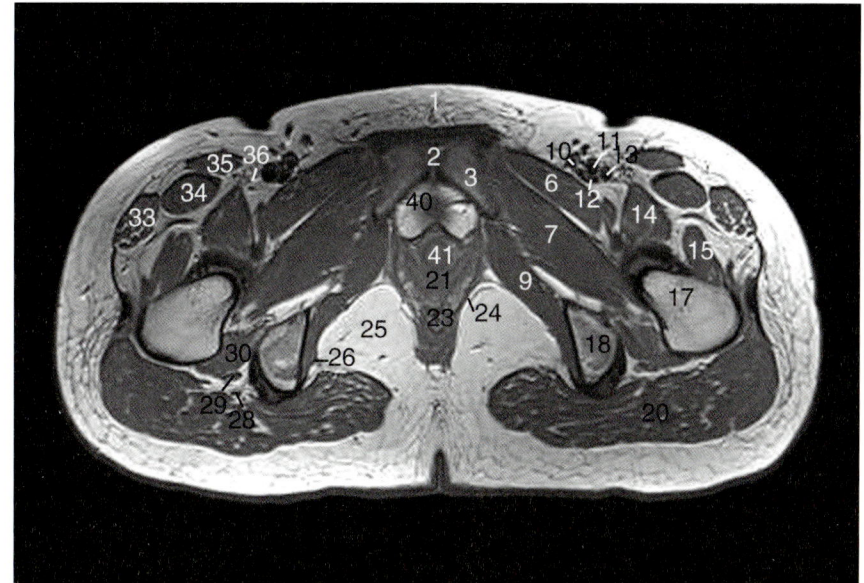

C. MR T1WI

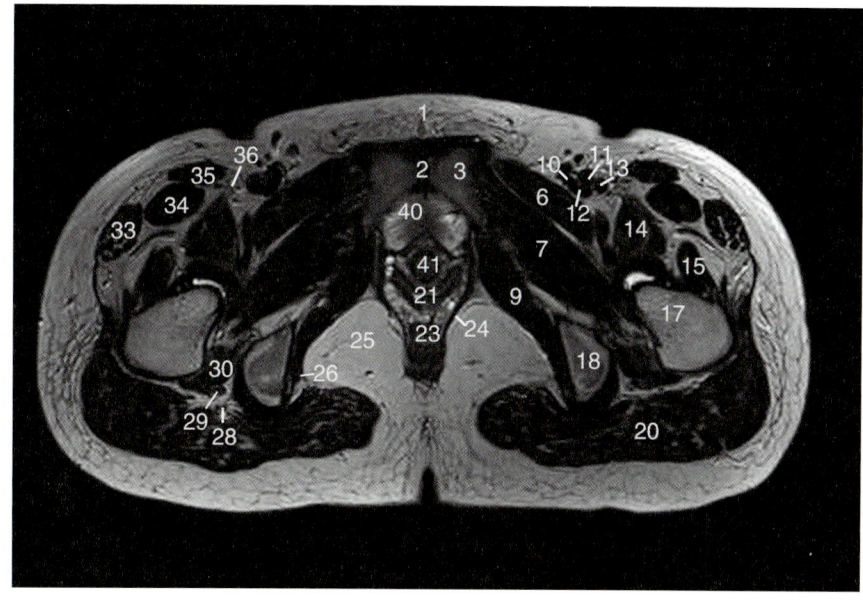

D. MR T2WI

1. 阴阜 mons pubis
2. 耻骨联合 pubic symphysis
3. 耻骨上支 superior ramus of pubis
4. 膀胱 urinary bladder
5. 膀胱静脉丛 vesical venous plexus
6. 耻骨肌 pectineus
7. 闭孔外肌 obturator externus
8. 闭孔膜 obturator membrane
9. 闭孔内肌 obturator internus
10. 大隐静脉 great saphenous vein
11. 股动脉 femoral artery
12. 股静脉 femoral vein
13. 股深动脉 deep femoral artery
14. 髂腰肌 iliopsoas
15. 股外侧肌 vastus lateralis
16. 髂股韧带 iliofemoral ligament
17. 股骨 femur
18. 坐骨结节 ischial tuberosity
19. 股二头肌、半腱肌和半膜肌总腱 tendons of biceps femoris, semitendinous and semimembranousus
20. 臀大肌 gluteus maximus
21. 阴道 vaginaa
22. 阴道静脉丛 vaginaal venous plexus
23. 肛管 anal canal
24. 肛提肌 levator ani
25. 坐骨肛门窝 ischioanal fossa
26. 阴部内动、静脉 internal pudendal artery and vein
27. 闭孔动、静脉 obturator artery and vein
28. 臀下动、静脉 inferior gluteal artery and vein
29. 坐骨神经 sciatic nerve
30. 股方肌 quadratus femoris
31. 臀中肌 gluteus medius
32. 阔筋膜 fasciae lata
33. 阔筋膜张肌 tensor fasciae latae
34. 股直肌 rectus femoris
35. 缝匠肌 sartorius
36. 股神经 femoral nerve
37. 旋股外侧动脉升支 ascending branch of lateral femoral circumflex artery
38. 旋股内侧动脉 medial femoral circumflex artery
39. 髂腰肌肌腱 iliopsoas tendon
40. 耻骨后间隙 retropubic space
41. 膀胱颈 neck of bladder

关键结构：耻骨联合，耻骨后间隙，膀胱。

此断面经耻骨联合中份。耻骨联合构成盆腔前壁，盆腔侧壁为闭孔及其内外侧的闭孔内肌与闭孔外肌，耻骨两侧见耻骨肌，与闭孔外肌大致呈"八"形平行排列，耻骨肌与髂腰肌之间见股血管及神经。臀部见臀大肌，臀大肌下间隙见臀下血管及坐骨神经断面，臀大肌、肛提肌与闭孔内肌间为坐骨肛门窝。盆腔内脏器从前向后依次排列有膀胱、阴道和肛管。在膀胱和阴道周围有膀胱静脉丛和阴道静脉丛。耻骨联合与膀胱之间为耻骨后间隙（膀胱前隙），在女性其前界为耻骨联合、耻骨上支及闭孔内肌筋膜，后界为膀胱，两侧界为脐内侧韧带，上界为壁腹膜至膀胱上面的反折部，下界为盆膈和耻骨膀胱韧带。耻骨骨折引起的血肿和膀胱前壁损伤的尿外渗常潴留于此间隙[22]。正常情况下耻骨后间隙内富含脂肪，在 CT 上呈低密度，在 MR T1WI 和 T2WI 呈高信号。

女性盆部与会阴连续横断层 69（FH.8010）

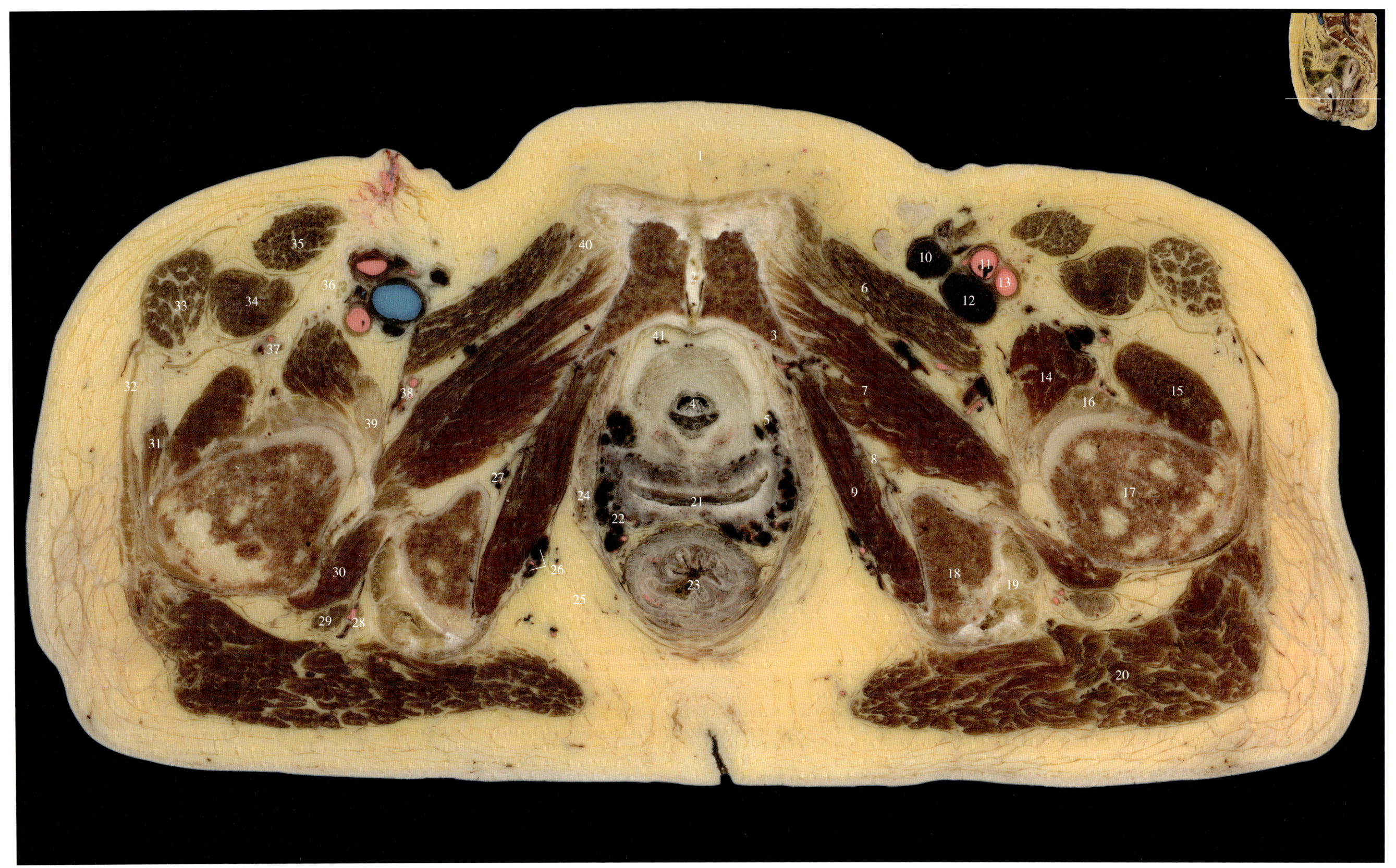

A. 断层标本图像

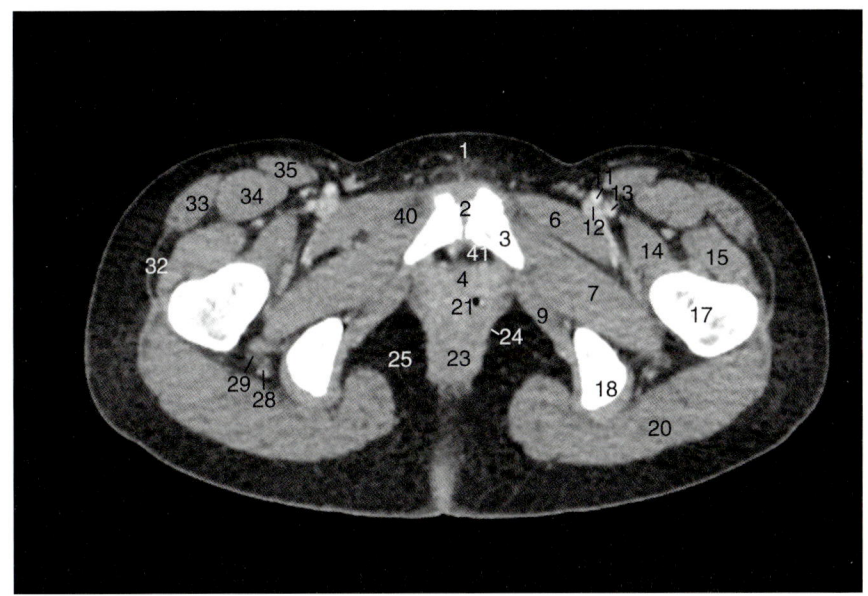

B. CT 增强图像

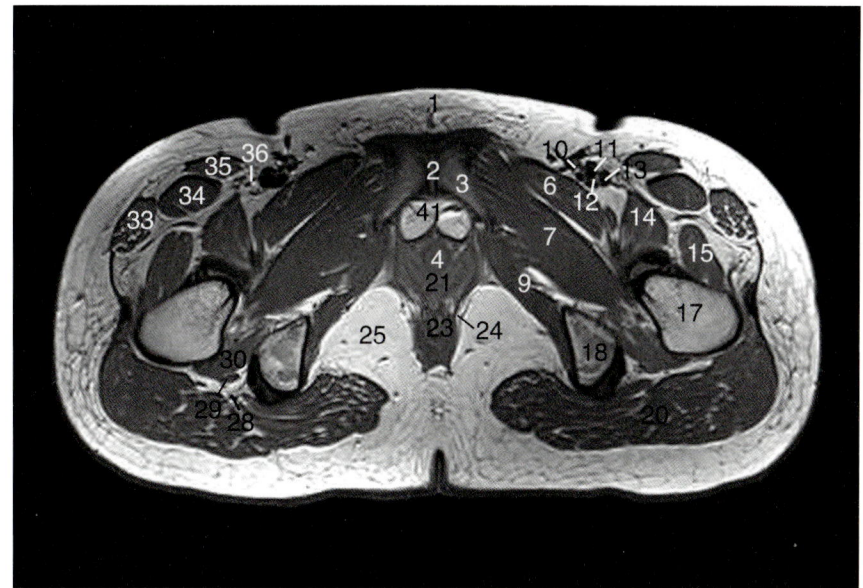

C. MR T1WI

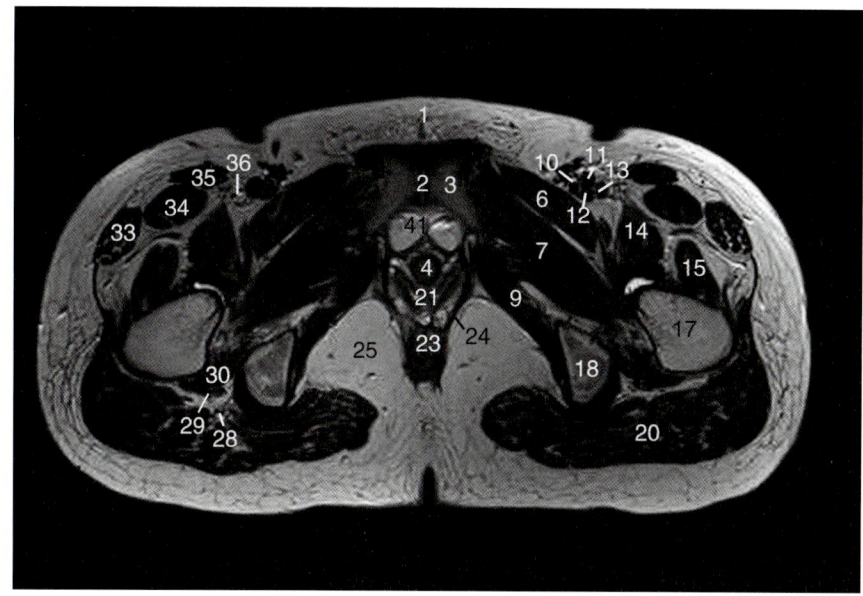

D. MR T2WI

1. 阴阜 mons pubis
2. 耻骨联合 pubic symphysis
3. 耻骨上支 superior ramus of pubis
4. 膀胱颈 neck of bladder
5. 膀胱静脉丛 vesical venous plexus
6. 耻骨肌 pectineus
7. 闭孔外肌 obturator externus
8. 闭孔膜 obturator membrance
9. 闭孔内肌 obturator internus
10. 大隐静脉 great saphenous vein
11. 股动脉 femoral artery
12. 股静脉 femoral vein
13. 股深动脉 deep femoral artery
14. 髂腰肌 iliopsoas
15. 股外侧肌 vastus lateralis
16. 髂股韧带 iliofemoral ligament
17. 股骨 femur
18. 坐骨结节 ischial tuberosity
19. 股二头肌、半腱肌和半膜肌总腱 tendons of biceps femoris, semitendinous and semimembranousus
20. 臀大肌 gluteus maximus
21. 阴道 vaginaa
22. 阴道静脉丛 vaginaal venous plexus
23. 肛管 anal canal
24. 肛提肌 levator ani
25. 坐骨肛门窝 ischioanal fossa
26. 阴部内动、静脉 internal pudendal artery and vein
27. 闭孔动、静脉 obturator artery and vein
28. 臀下动、静脉 inferior gluteal artery and vein
29. 坐骨神经 sciatic nerve
30. 股方肌 quadratus femoris
31. 臀中肌 gluteus medius
32. 阔筋膜 fasciae lata
33. 阔筋膜张肌 tensor fasciae latae
34. 股直肌 rectus femoris
35. 缝匠肌 sartorius
36. 股神经 femoral nerve
37. 旋股外侧血管升支 lateral femoral circumflex vessel ascending branch
38. 旋股内侧动脉 medial femoral circumflex artery
39. 髂腰肌肌腱 iliopsoas tendon
40. 短收肌 adductor brevis
41. 耻骨后间隙 retropubic space

关键结构：膀胱颈，阴道，肛管。

此断面经耻骨联合中份。在断面中央从前向后依次为阴阜、耻骨联合、耻骨后间隙、膀胱颈、阴道、肛管、肛提肌及其两侧的坐骨肛门窝。在大腿内侧和盆壁上，可见耻骨肌、闭孔外肌和闭孔内肌从前向后有 3 组呈 "八" 形排列。此断层膀胱体接近消失，移行为膀胱颈。男性中膀胱颈下面是前列腺；女性中其直接位于短尿道周围的盆腔筋膜上，阴道位于后面[36]。膀胱颈部的平滑肌在组织学、药理学等方面与固有逼尿肌不同，因此膀胱颈应该被看作是一个独立的功能单位。膀胱颈平滑肌的排列方式在男女之间有明显的差别。男性膀胱颈的平滑肌细胞形成一个完整的领状结构，该结构一直向下延伸并环绕在尿道的前列腺前部。根据其位置和肌纤维的排列方式，称其为尿道近端内括约肌或尿道前列腺前部括约肌。在远侧部，膀胱颈的肌肉与前列腺基质和被膜中的肌肉相互混合，而且它们在结构上并无差异。女性膀胱颈也由形态学独特的平滑肌构成，在该处逼尿肌粗大的肌束已不存在，代之以较细小的肌束。但这些肌束不像男性前列腺前部的平滑肌那样呈环形，而是倾向于呈斜行或纵行并穿入尿道壁。所以在女性的膀胱颈部并不存在一个平滑肌性括约肌，而且这一部位的主动收缩似乎并不具有明显的排尿节制功能。女性膀胱颈平滑肌只接受很少地去甲肾上腺素能（交感）神经的支配，但富有胆碱能（副交感）神经的支配，而男性则相反[5]。

女性盆部与会阴连续横断层 70（FH.7990）

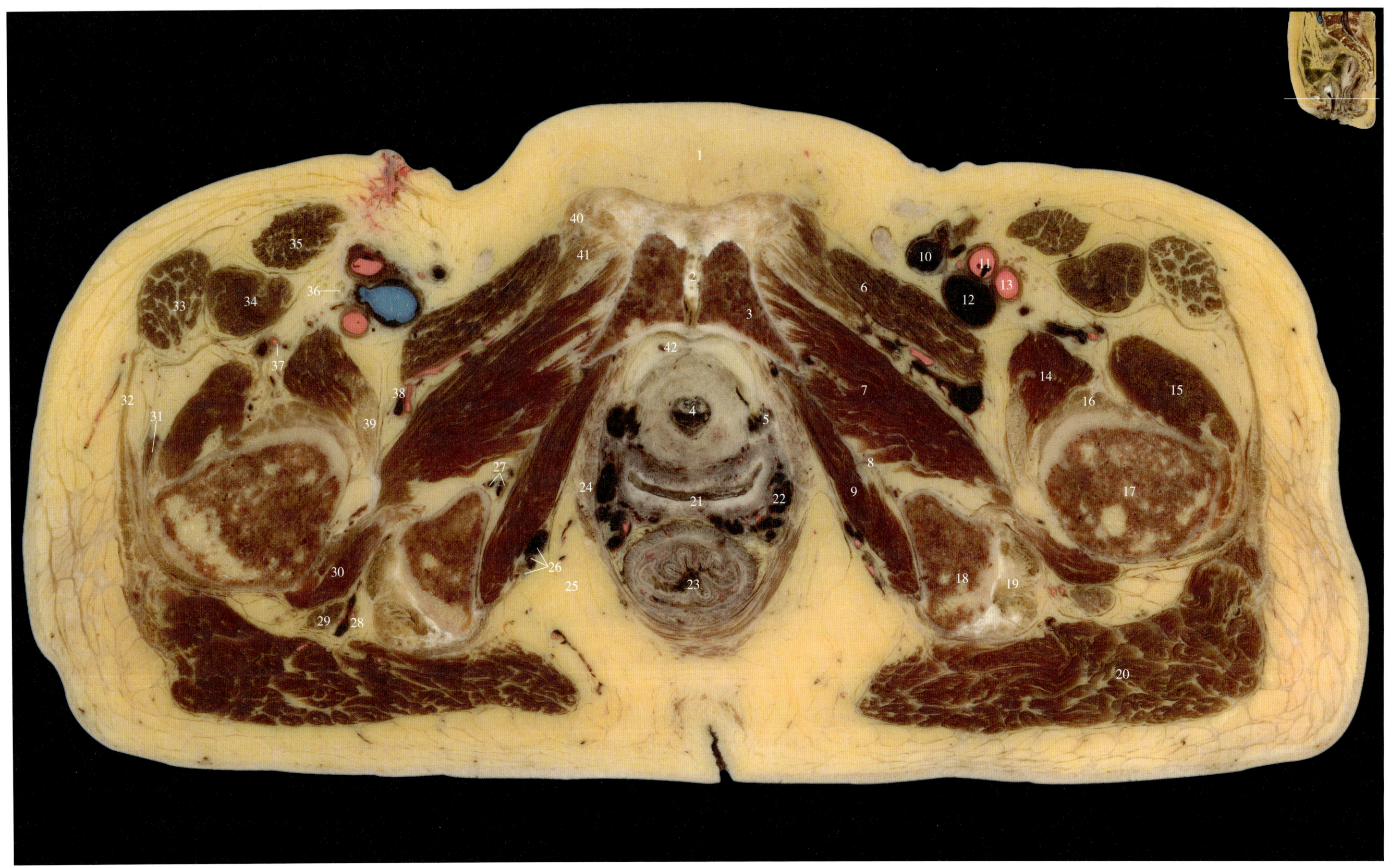

A. 断层标本图像

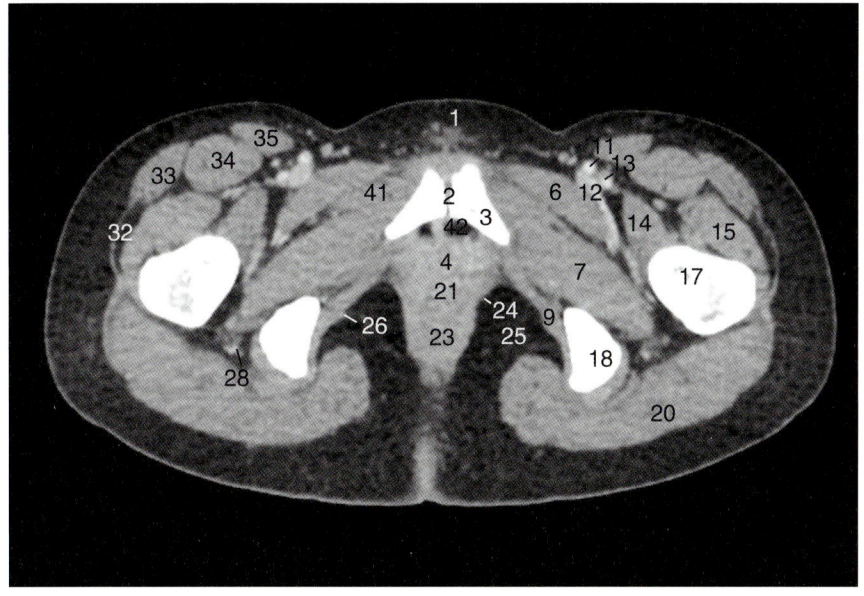
B. CT 增强图像

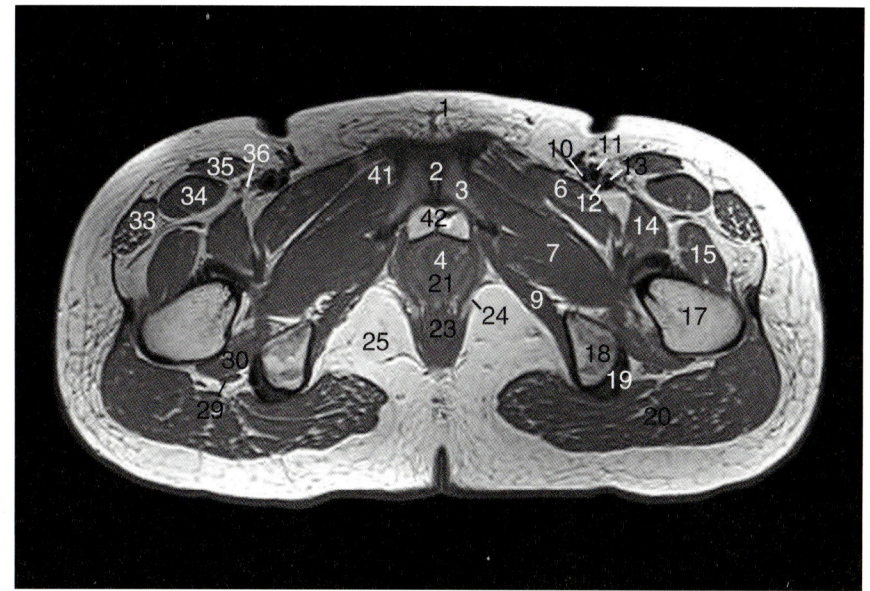
C. MR T1WI

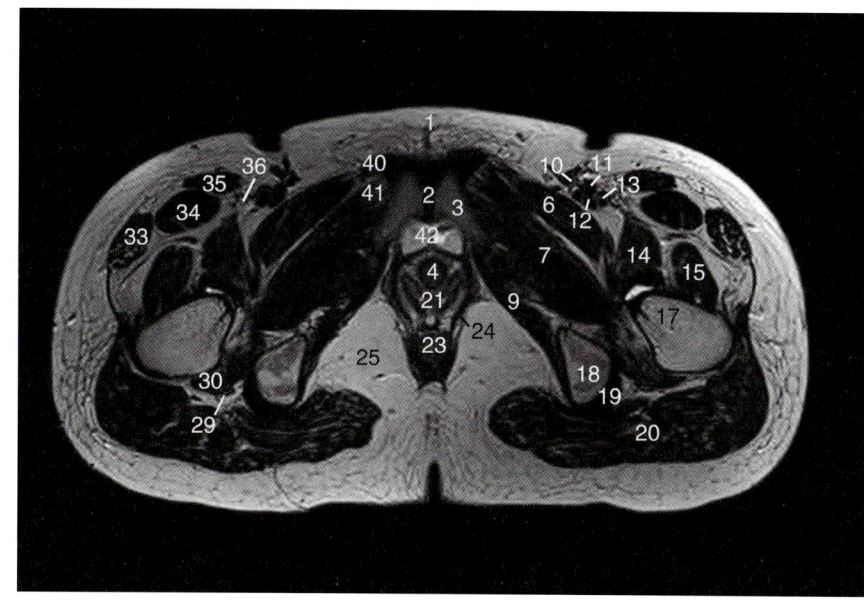
D. MR T2WI

1. 阴阜 mons pubis
2. 耻骨联合 pubic symphysis
3. 耻骨上支 superior ramus of pubis
4. 尿道 urethra
5. 膀胱静脉丛 vesical venous plexus
6. 耻骨肌 pectineus
7. 闭孔外肌 obturator externus
8. 闭孔膜 obturator membrane
9. 闭孔内肌 obturator internus
10. 大隐静脉 great saphenous vein
11. 股动脉 femoral artery
12. 股静脉 femoral vein
13. 股深动脉 deep femoral artery
14. 髂腰肌 iliopsoas
15. 股外侧肌 vastus lateralis
16. 髂股韧带 iliofemoral ligament
17. 股骨 femur
18. 坐骨结节 ischial tuberosity
19. 股二头肌、半腱肌和半膜肌总腱 tendons of biceps femoris, semitendinous and semimembranousus
20. 臀大肌 gluteus maximus
21. 阴道 vaginaa
22. 阴道静脉丛 vaginaal venous plexus
23. 肛管 anal canal
24. 肛提肌 levator ani
25. 坐骨肛门窝 ischioanal fossa
26. 阴部内动、静脉和阴部神经 internal pudendal artery and vein & pudendal nerve
27. 闭孔动、静脉 obturator artery and vein
28. 臀下动、静脉 inferior gluteal artery and vein
29. 坐骨神经 sciatic nerve
30. 股方肌 quadratus femoris
31. 臀中肌 gluteus medius
32. 阔筋膜 fasciae lata
33. 阔筋膜张肌 tensor fasciae latae
34. 股直肌 rectus femoris
35. 缝匠肌 sartorius
36. 股神经 femoral nerve
37. 旋股外侧动脉升支 ascending branch of lateral femoral circumflex artery
38. 旋股内侧动、静脉 medial femoral circumflex artery and vein
39. 髂腰肌腱 iliopsoas tendon
40. 长收肌肌腱 tendon of adductor longus
41. 短收肌 adductor brevis
42. 耻骨后间隙 retropubic space

关键结构：女性尿道，耻骨后间隙，坐骨肛门窝。

此断面经耻骨联合中份。在断面中央从前向后依次为阴阜、耻骨联合、耻骨后间隙、尿道、阴道、肛管、肛提肌和坐骨肛门窝。耻骨后间隙和坐骨肛门窝内有大量脂肪填充，在T1WI和T2WI上均呈高信号。紧贴盆腔内侧壁的闭孔内肌断面逐渐缩小。此断面膀胱颈消失，开始出现尿道。女性尿道较男性尿道宽、短、直，其平均长3~5 cm，直径约0.6 cm，绝经与否、有无性生活史、累计性生活史的时间、生育与否及生育方式对尿道长度均有影响[37]。尿道内口约平耻骨联合后面中央或下部，女性低于男性。尿道内口的周围为平滑肌组成的膀胱括约肌所环绕。尿道向前下方走行，穿过尿生殖膈，开口于阴道前庭的尿道外口。在穿尿生殖膈被由横纹肌组成的尿道阴道括约肌所环绕。女性尿道血供丰富，尿道上段由膀胱下动脉供血，中段由阴道中动脉供血，下段由阴部内动脉的分支供血，上述血管彼此吻合。静脉汇入膀胱静脉丛和阴道静脉丛，最后流入髂内静脉。Hennigan和Dubose研究了正常女性尿道的超声解剖，在膀胱颈正下方，尿道的前后径为1~1.5 cm，横径稍大，经此点的超声横断影像上，成年女性尿道若呈卵圆形，尿道常常突入膀胱，会被误诊为膀胱肿瘤[38]。

女性盆部与会阴连续横断层 71（FH.7970）

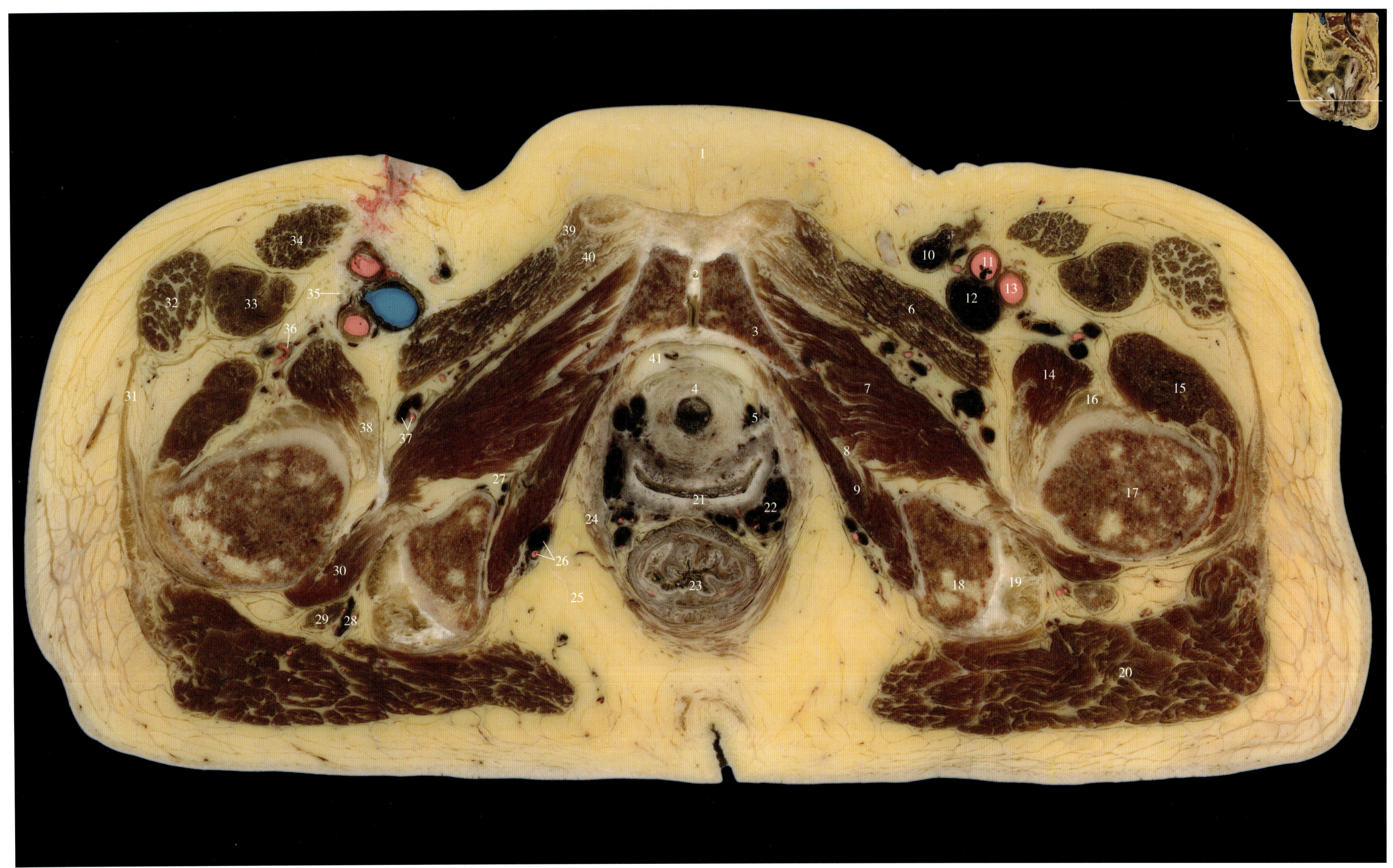

A. 断层标本图像

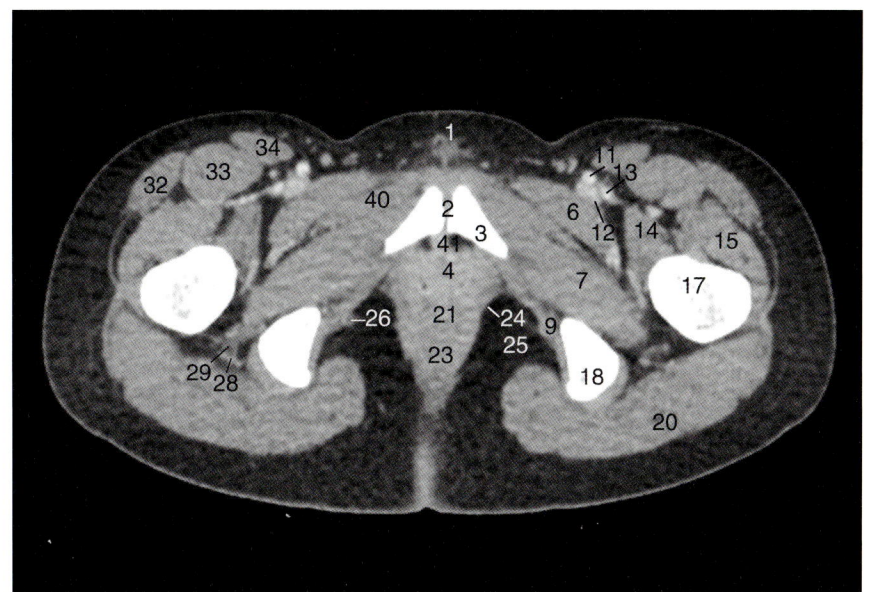
B. CT 增强图像

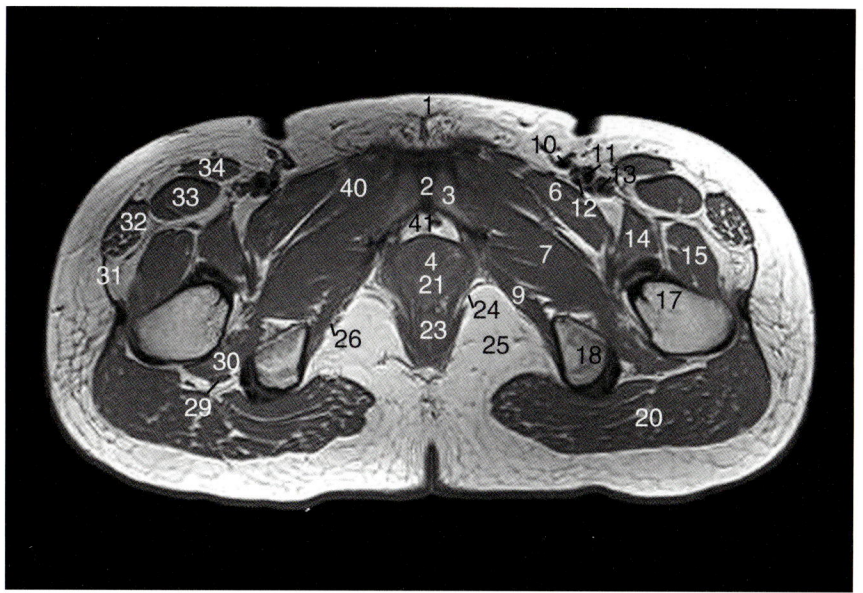
C. MR T1WI

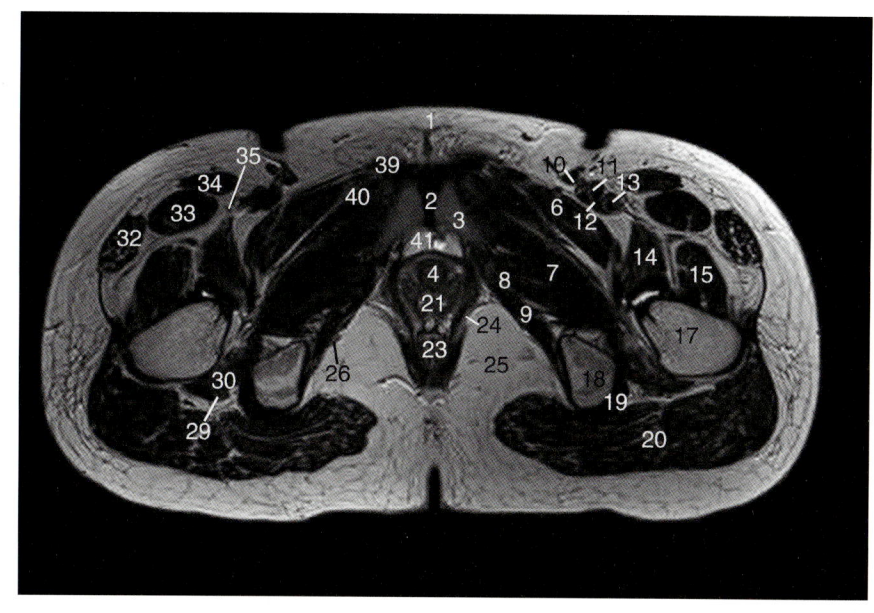
D. MR T2WI

1. 阴阜 mons pubis
2. 耻骨联合 pubic symphysis
3. 耻骨下支 inferior ramus of pubis
4. 尿道 urethra
5. 膀胱静脉丛 vesical venous plexus
6. 耻骨肌 pectineus
7. 闭孔外肌 obturator externus
8. 闭孔膜 obturator membrance
9. 闭孔内肌 obturator internus
10. 大隐静脉 great saphenous vein
11. 股动脉 femoral artery
12. 股静脉 femoral vein
13. 股深动脉 deep femoral artery
14. 髂腰肌 iliopsoas
15. 股外侧肌 vastus lateralis
16. 髂股韧带 iliofemoral ligament
17. 股骨 femur
18. 坐骨结节 ischial tuberosity
19. 股二头肌、半腱肌和半膜肌总腱 tendons of biceps femoris, semitendinous and semimembranousus
20. 臀大肌 gluteus maximus
21. 阴道 vaginaa
22. 阴道静脉丛 vaginaal venous plexus
23. 肛管 anal canal
24. 肛提肌 levator ani
25. 坐骨肛门窝 ischioanal fossa
26. 阴部内动、静脉 internal pudental artery and vein
27. 闭孔静脉 obturator vein
28. 臀下动、静脉 inferior gluteal artery and vein
29. 坐骨神经 sciatic nerve
30. 股方肌 quadratus femoris
31. 阔筋膜 fasciae lata
32. 阔筋膜张肌 tensor fasciae latae
33. 股直肌 rectus femoris
34. 缝匠肌 sartorius
35. 股神经 femoral nerve
36. 旋股外侧动脉升支 ascending branch of lateral femoral circumflex artery
37. 旋股内侧动、静脉 medial femoral circumflex artery and vein
38. 髂腰肌腱 iliopsoas tendon
39. 长收肌 adductor longus
40. 短收肌 adductor brevis
41. 耻骨后间隙 retropubic space

关键结构：阴道，尿道，肛管。

此断面经耻骨联合中份。在断面中央从前向后依次为阴阜、耻骨联合、耻骨后间隙、尿道、阴道、肛管、肛提肌和坐骨肛门窝。在尿道和阴道周围有静脉丛的断面。耻骨后间隙和坐骨肛门窝内有大量脂肪填充，在 T1WI 和 T2WI 上均呈高信号。紧贴盆腔内侧壁的闭孔内肌断面逐渐缩小。在耻骨支前方，开始出现长收肌和短收肌。在后方的臀大肌下间隙内，股方肌与臀大肌之间的粗大神经为坐骨神经，其内侧为臀下动、静脉和神经。此断面为阴道下段断面。阴道横径由上而下逐渐变窄，阴道中部断面为"一"形横裂，至此断面，逐渐过渡到开口向前的半"H"形，再向下的断面，形成完整的"H"形，末端断面为纵裂隙形。

女性盆部与会阴连续横断层 72（FH.7950）

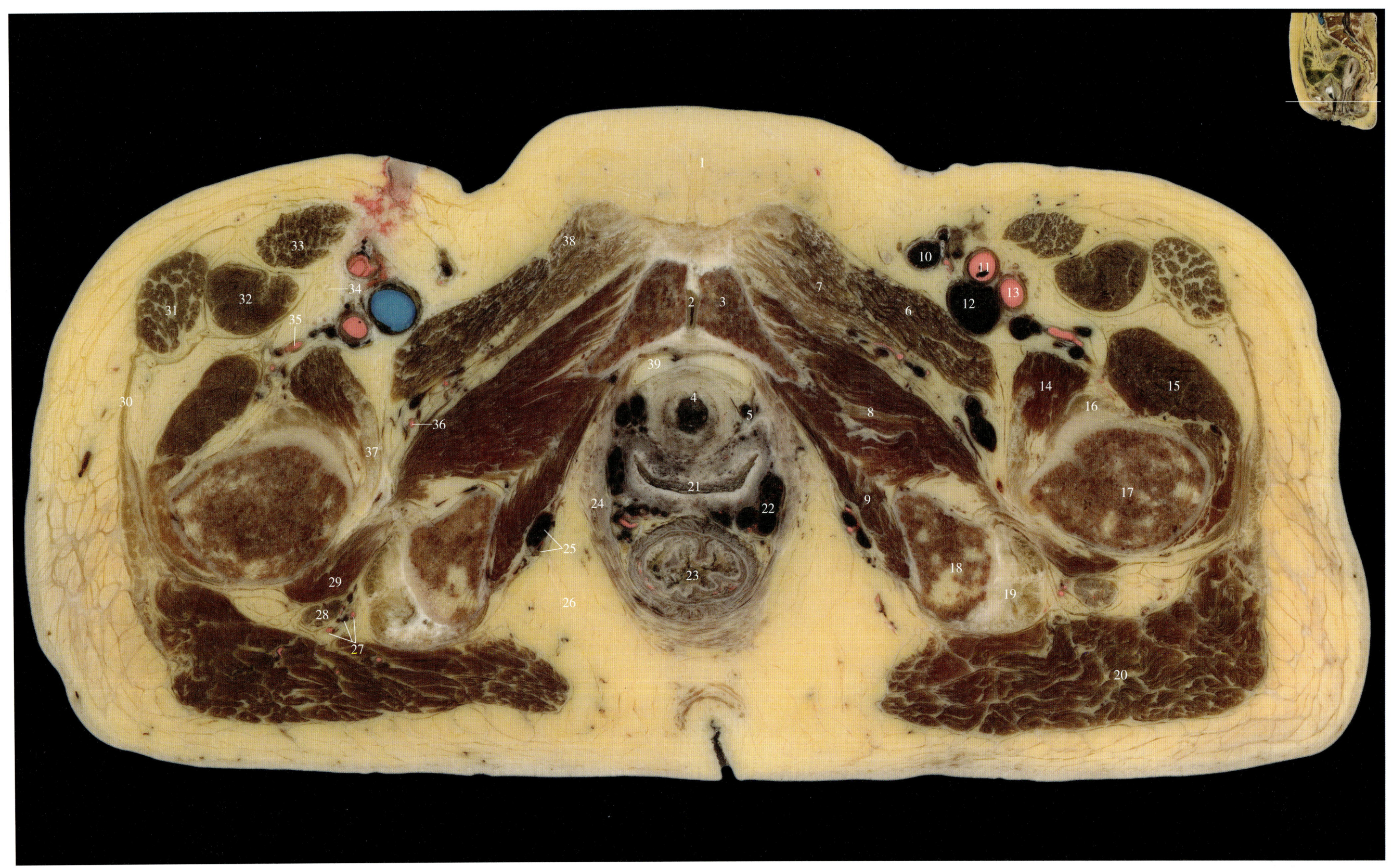

A. 断层标本图像

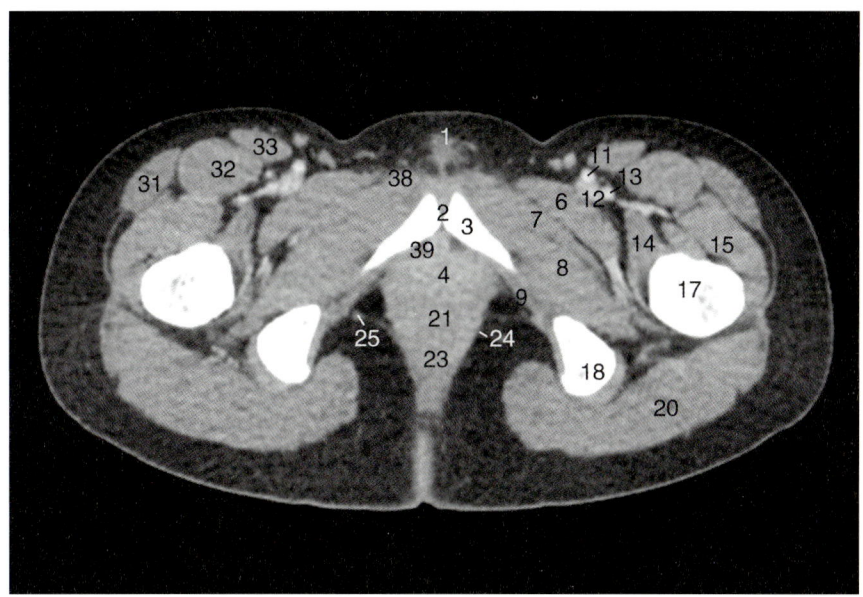

B. CT 增强图像

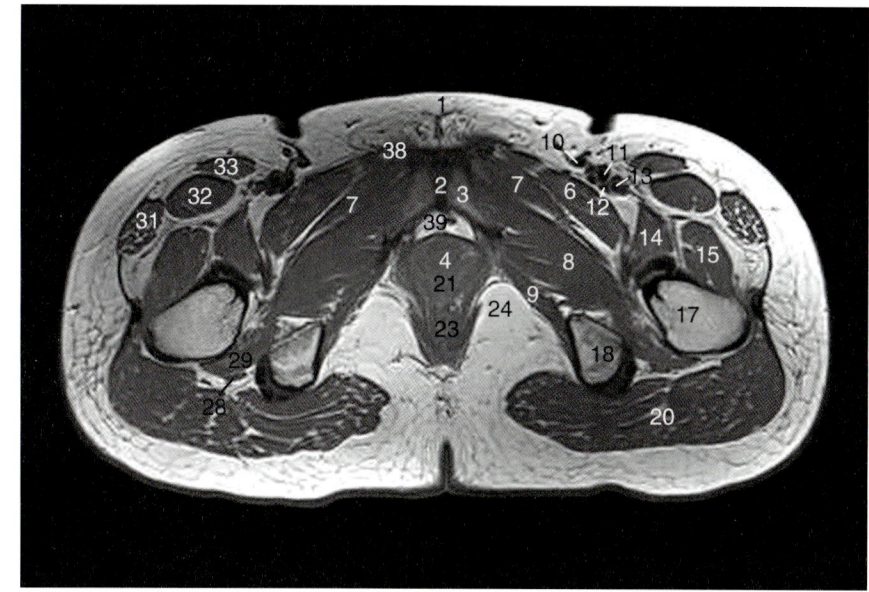

C. MR T1WI

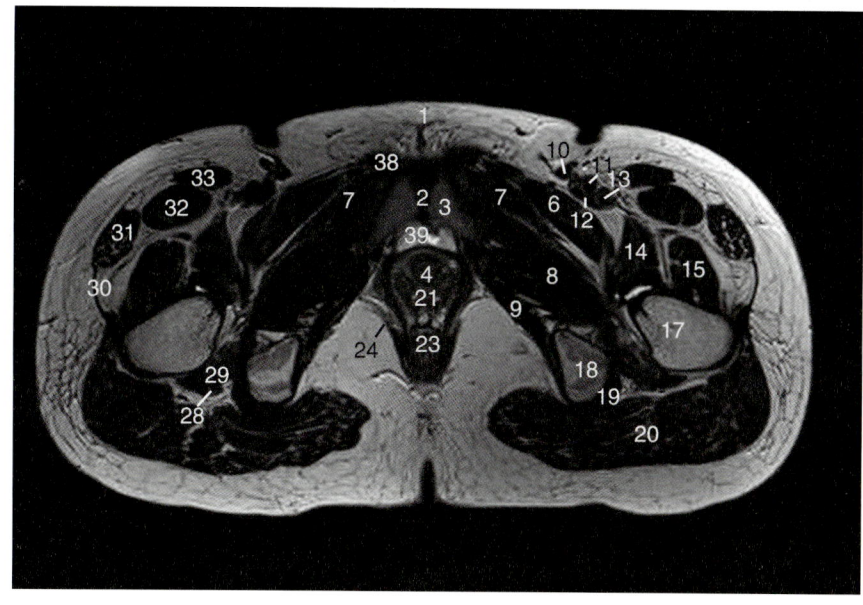

D. MR T2WI

1. 阴阜 mons pubis
2. 耻骨联合 pubic symphysis
3. 耻骨下支 inferior ramus of pubis
4. 尿道 urethra
5. 膀胱静脉丛 vesical venous plexus
6. 耻骨肌 pectineus
7. 短收肌 adductor brevis
8. 闭孔外肌 obturator externus
9. 闭孔内肌 obturator internus
10. 大隐静脉 great saphenous vein
11. 股动脉 femoral artery
12. 股静脉 femoral vein
13. 股深动脉 deep femoral artery
14. 髂腰肌 iliopsoas
15. 股外侧肌 vastus lateralis
16. 髂股韧带 iliofemoral ligament
17. 股骨体与小转子 shaft and lesser trochanter of femur
18. 坐骨结节 ischial tuberosity
19. 股二头肌、半腱肌和半膜肌总腱 tendons of biceps femoris, semitendinous and semimembranousus
20. 臀大肌 gluteus maximus
21. 阴道 vaginaa
22. 阴道静脉丛 vaginaal venous plexus
23. 肛管 anal canal
24. 肛提肌 levator ani
25. 阴部内动、静脉 internal pudendal artery and vein
26. 坐骨肛门窝 ischioanal fossa
27. 臀下动、静脉 inferior gluteal artery and vein
28. 坐骨神经 sciatic nerve
29. 股方肌 quadratus femoris
30. 阔筋膜 fasciae lata
31. 阔筋膜张肌 tensor fasciae latae
32. 股直肌 rectus femoris
33. 缝匠肌 sartorius
34. 股神经 femoral nerve
35. 旋股外侧动脉升支 ascending branch of lateral femoral circumflex artery
36. 旋股内侧动脉 medial femoral circumflex artery
37. 髂腰肌肌腱 iliopsoas tendon
38. 长收肌 adductor longus
39. 耻骨后间隙 retropubic space

关键结构：肛管，尿道，阴道。

此断面经耻骨联合下份。耻骨联合正后方，由前至后有尿道、阴道和肛管排列。在尿道和阴道周围见大量阴部静脉丛及阴道静脉丛的断面。在肛管内可见突入腔内的肛柱。肛柱一般有 6~10 条，与肛管长轴平行，肛柱上端连线称为肛直肠线，肛柱下端与各肛瓣边缘的锯齿状连线称齿状线。齿状线下方约 1 cm 处有一环形线称白线，由于此线位于肛门外括约肌皮下部与肛门内括约肌下缘之间的水平，因此在活体肛诊时可触知此处为一环形浅沟（括约肌浅沟）。肛管的最末端称肛缘线或者肛门缘。以肛直肠线、齿状线、白线和肛缘线为界可将肛管分为三部分：①柱带部：位于肛直肠线与齿状线之间，成人长约为 2.41 cm，儿童长约为 1.32 cm，新生儿长约为 0.5 cm；②痔带部（肛梳）：位于齿状线与白线之间，成人长约为 1.02 cm，儿童长约为 0.94 cm，新生儿长约为 0.3 cm；③皮带部：位于白线与肛缘线之间，成人与儿童长约为 1.0 cm，新生儿长约为 0.6 cm[16]。

女性盆部与会阴连续横断层 73（FH.7930）

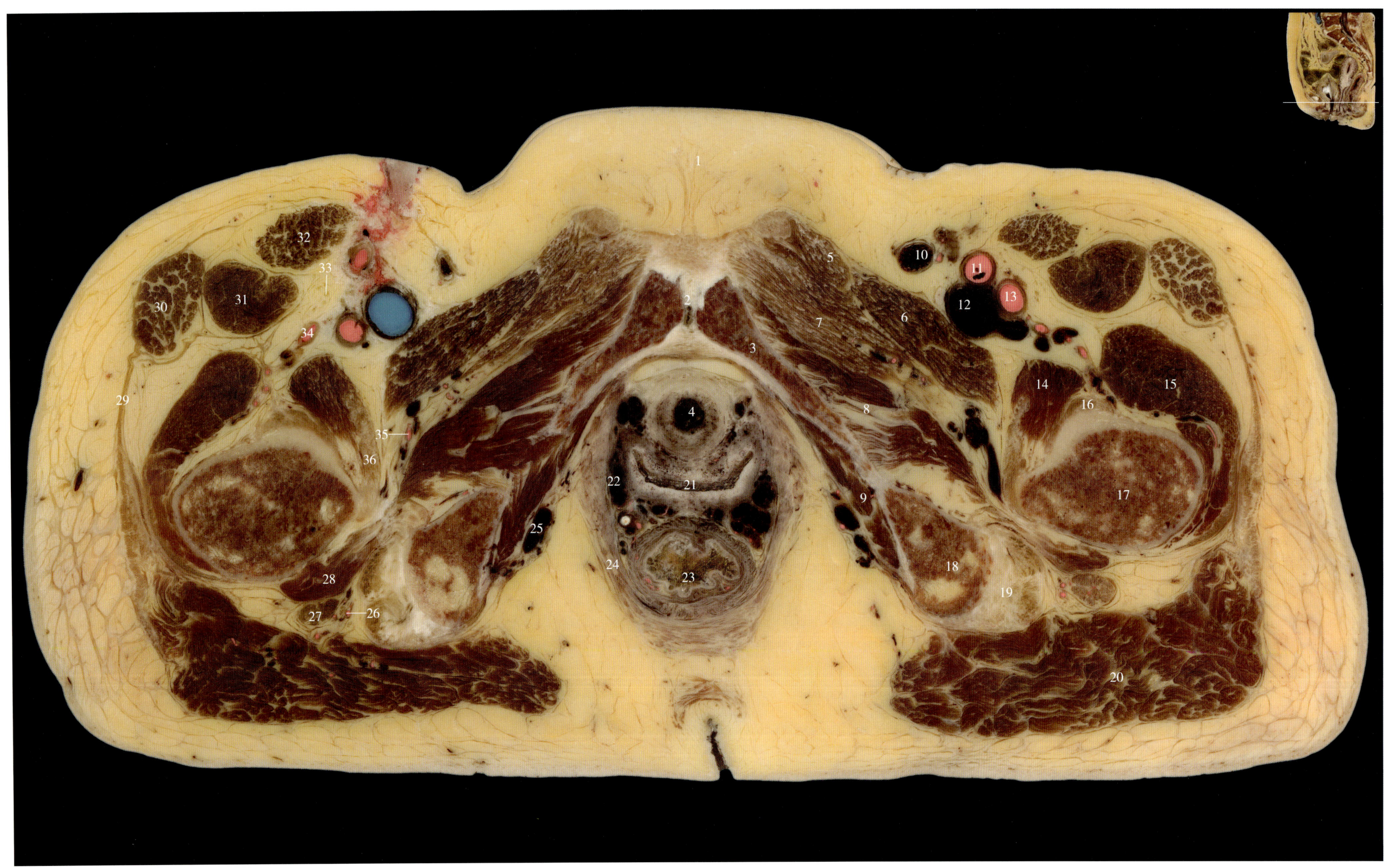

A. 断层标本图像

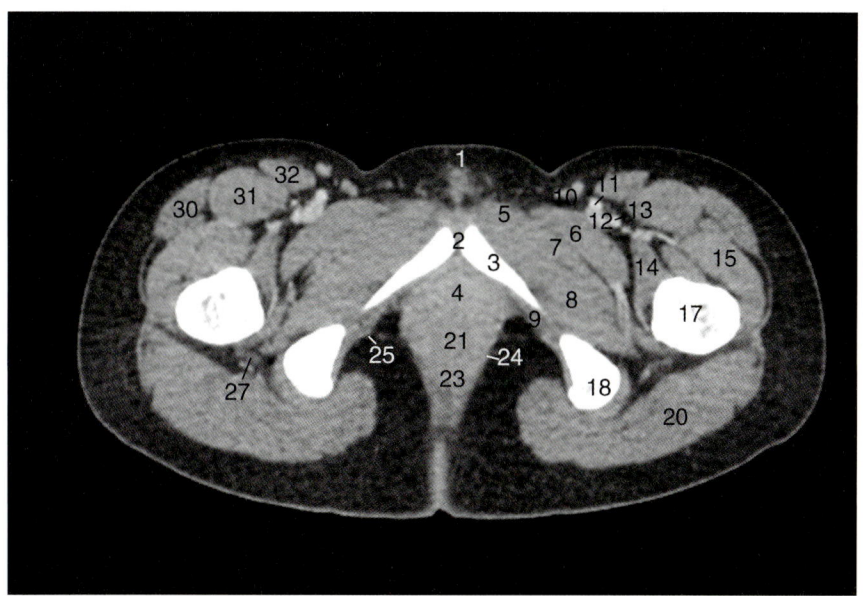
B. CT 增强图像

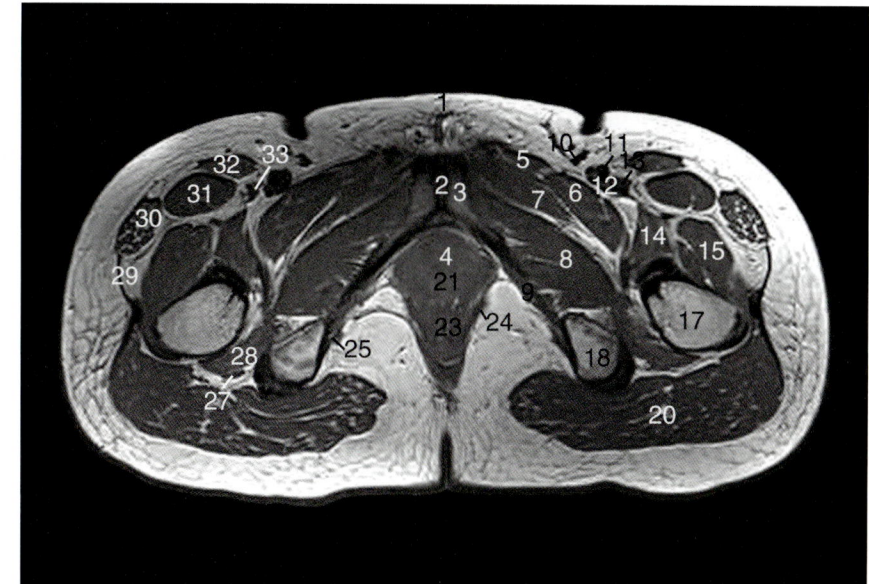
C. MR T1WI

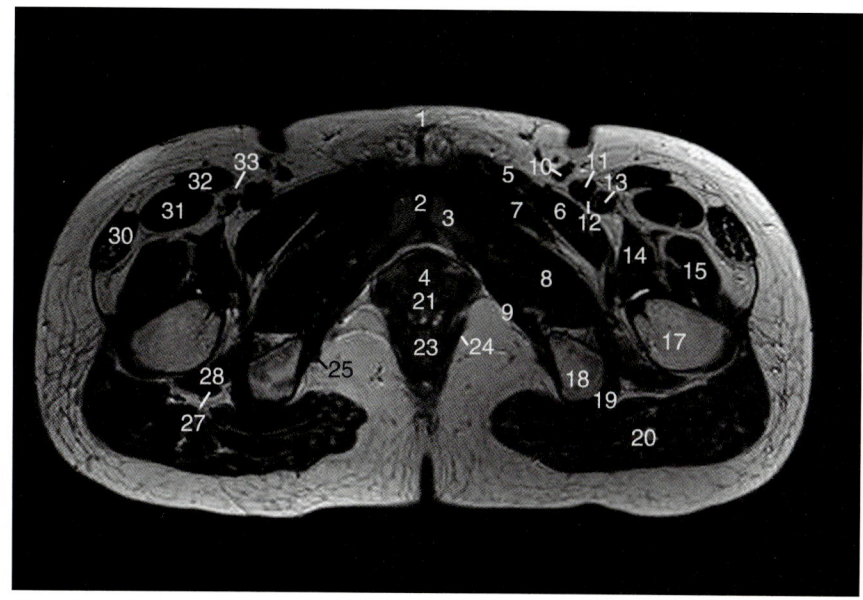
D. MR T2WI

1. 阴阜 mons pubis
2. 耻骨联合 pubic symphysis
3. 耻骨下支 inferior ramus of pubis
4. 尿道 urethra
5. 长收肌 adductor longus
6. 耻骨肌 pectineus
7. 短收肌 adductor brevis
8. 闭孔外肌 obturator externus
9. 闭孔内肌 obturator internus
10. 大隐静脉 great saphenous vein
11. 股动脉 femoral artery
12. 股静脉 femoral vein
13. 股深动脉 deep femoral artery
14. 髂腰肌 iliopsoas
15. 股外侧肌 vastus lateralis
16. 髂股韧带 iliofemoral ligament
17. 股骨体与小转子 shaft and lesser trochanter of femur
18. 坐骨结节 ischial tuberosity
19. 股二头肌、半腱肌和半膜肌总腱 tendons of biceps femoris, semitendinous and semimembranousus
20. 臀大肌 gluteus maximus
21. 阴道 vaginaa
22. 阴道静脉丛 vaginaal venous plexus
23. 肛管 anal canal
24. 肛提肌 levator ani
25. 阴部内静脉 internal pudendal vein
26. 臀下动脉 inferior gluteal artery
27. 坐骨神经 sciatic nerve
28. 股方肌 quadratus femoris
29. 阔筋膜 fasciae lata
30. 阔筋膜张肌 tensor fasciae latae
31. 股直肌 rectus femoris
32. 缝匠肌 sartorius
33. 股神经 femoral nerve
34. 旋股外侧动脉升支 ascending branch of lateral femoral circumflex artery
35. 旋股内侧动脉 medial femoral circumflex artery
36. 髂腰肌肌腱 iliopsoas tendon

关键结构：肛管，阴道，肛提肌。

此断面经耻骨联合下份。左侧断面耻骨下支已与坐骨支连接，闭孔消失。右侧断面耻骨下支与坐骨支逐渐靠近，闭孔内侧附着的闭孔内肌断面显著减小。在耻骨下支的前外侧，两侧有三组呈"八"形排列的肌肉，它们从前向后依次分别是长收肌、短收肌和闭孔外肌。在长收肌、短收肌外侧有耻骨肌。耻骨联合后方依次为尿道、阴道和肛管。肛管在齿状线上下的胚胎来源不同，因此其血管、淋巴管和神经等的来源、分布与回流不一致。齿状线以上的肛管由内胚层的泄殖腔演化而来，其内表面为黏膜，黏膜上皮为单层柱状上皮，癌变时为腺癌；齿状线以下肛管由外胚层的原肛演化而来，其内表面为皮肤，被覆上皮为复层扁平上皮，癌变时为鳞状细胞癌。齿状线以上肛管的神经支配来自盆丛，由于内脏感觉神经对刺激的敏感性差，所以患内痔时常无痛感；在齿状线以下，肛门及其附近皮肤、肛门外括约肌则由躯体神经分布，主要来自第 3、4 骶神经前支组成的肛门神经，通常躯体神经对刺激很敏感，所以外痔常有痛感。由于肛门和膀胱的神经均来自第 4 骶神经，故一个器官患病，可能出现牵涉性症状，即反射性的影响其他器官的功能，如肛门疾患，疼痛可能向会阴、臀部和股部放射，有时可发生反射性的尿闭。相反膀胱颈部疾患，也可反射性地引起里急后重等症状[30]。

147

女性盆部与会阴连续横断层 74（FH.7910）

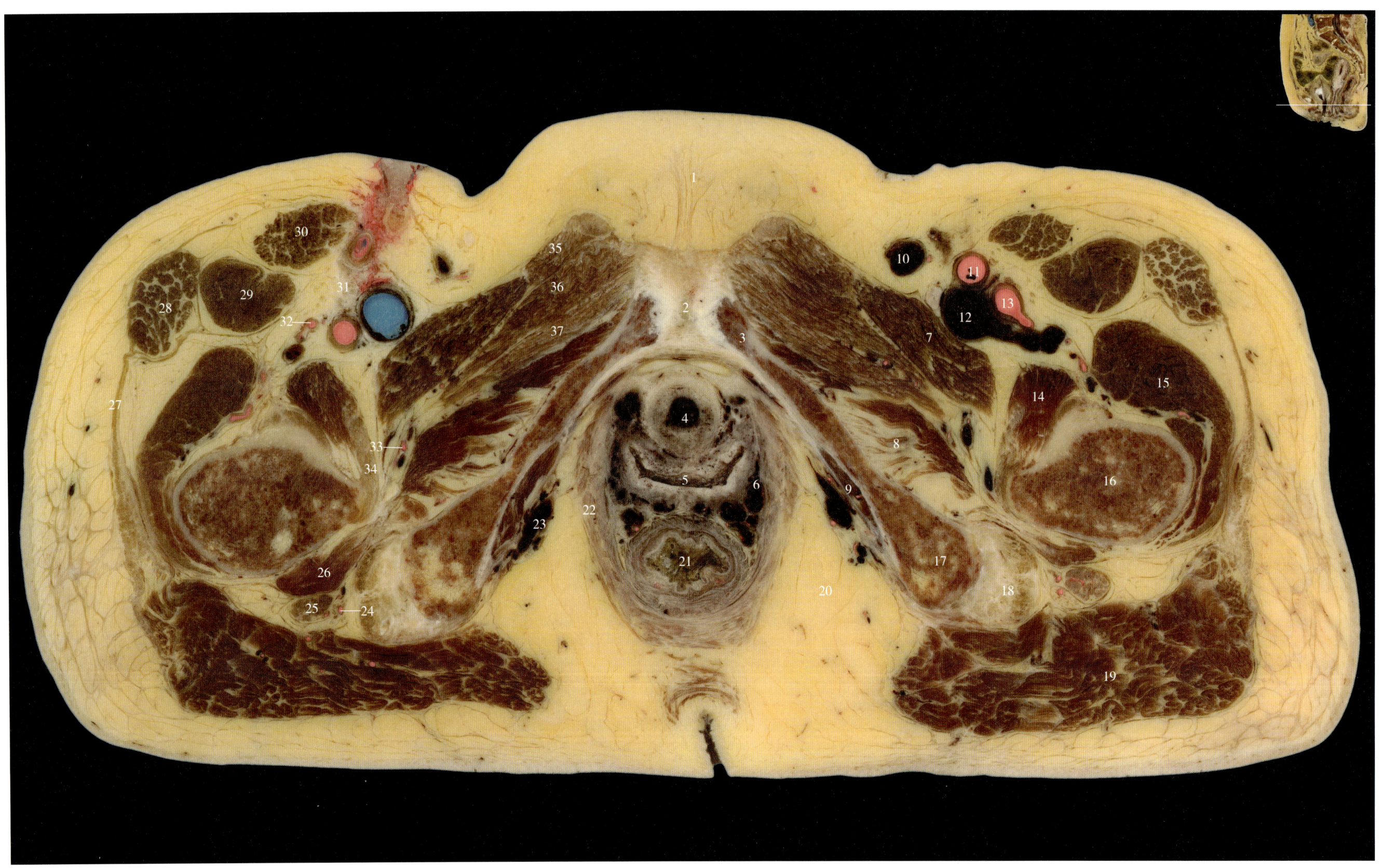

A. 断层标本图像

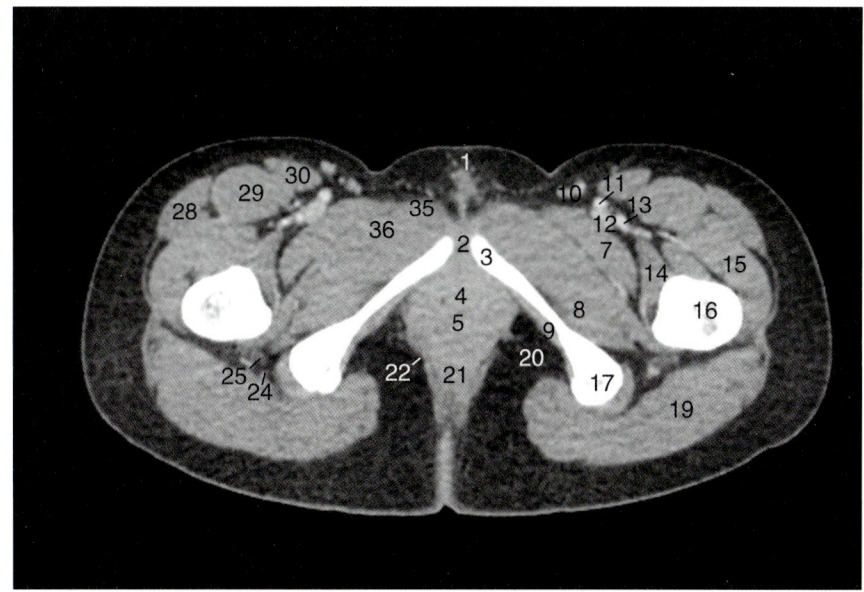

B. CT 增强图像

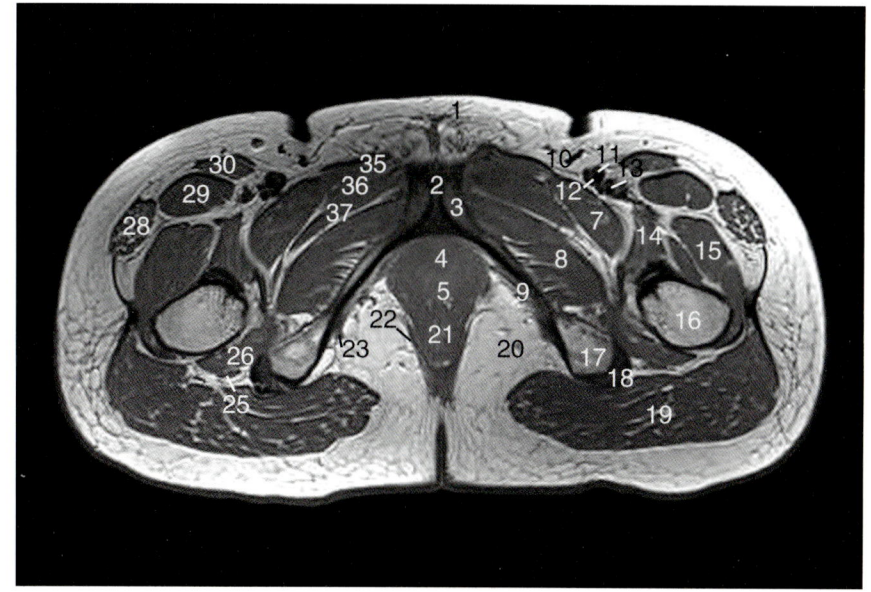

C. MR T1WI

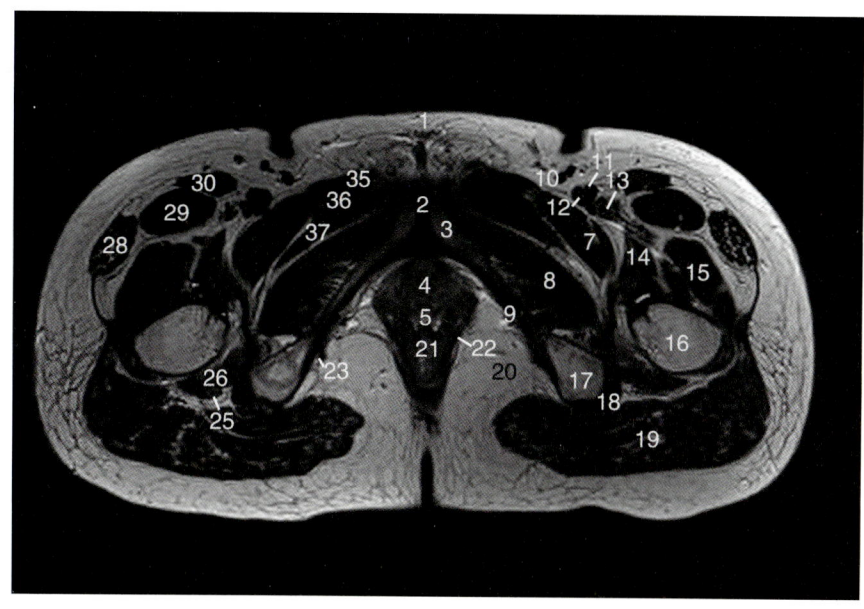

D. MR T2WI

1. 阴阜 mons pubis
2. 耻骨联合 pubic symphysis
3. 耻骨下支 inferior ramus of pubis
4. 尿道 urethra
5. 阴道 vaginaa
6. 阴道静脉丛 vaginaal venous plexus
7. 耻骨肌 pectineus
8. 闭孔外肌 obturator externus
9. 闭孔内肌 obturator internus
10. 大隐静脉 great saphenous vein
11. 股动脉 femoral artery
12. 股静脉 femoral vein
13. 股深动脉 deep femoral artery
14. 髂腰肌 iliopsoas
15. 股外侧肌 vastus lateralis
16. 股骨体与小转子 shaft and lesser trochanter of femur
17. 坐骨结节 ischial tuberosity
18. 股二头肌、半腱肌和半膜肌总腱 tendons of biceps femoris, semitendinous and semimembranousus
19. 臀大肌 gluteus maximus
20. 坐骨肛门窝 ischioanal fossa
21. 肛管 anal canal
22. 肛提肌 levator ani
23. 阴部内静脉 internal pudendal vein
24. 臀下动脉 inferior gluteal artery
25. 坐骨神经 sciatic nerve
26. 股方肌 quadratus femoris
27. 阔筋膜 fasciae lata
28. 阔筋膜张肌 tensor fasciae latae
29. 股直肌 rectus femoris
30. 缝匠肌 sartorius
31. 股神经 femoral nerve
32. 旋股外侧动脉升支 ascending branch of lateral femoral circumflex artery
33. 旋股内侧动脉 medial femoral circumflex artery
34. 髂腰肌肌腱 iliopsoas tendon
35. 长收肌 adductor longus
36. 短收肌 adductor brevis
37. 大收肌 adductor magnus

关键结构：耻骨下支，阴道静脉丛，尿道。

此断面经耻骨联合下缘。耻骨联合后方为尿道、阴道和肛管，肛提肌断面已由尾骨尖断面的典型 "V" 形逐渐过渡到 "U" 形，包绕在尿道、阴道和肛管的后方和两侧。尿道和阴道周围有静脉丛。此断面闭孔消失。耻骨下支与坐骨支相连，与耻骨联合下缘构成耻骨弓。耻骨弓为骨盆的一条约束弓，可约束坐骶弓不致散开。另一条约束弓在耻骨联合上部连接两侧耻骨上支，可防止股骶弓被挤压。坐骶弓和股骶弓是骨盆传递重力的两条重力弓。人体直立时，体重自第 5 腰椎、骶骨经两侧的骶髂关节、髋臼传至股骨头，再由股骨头往下传导至下肢，这种弓形力传递线称为股骶弓。当人体呈坐位时，重力由骶髂关节传至两侧坐骨结节，这种弓形力传递称为坐骶弓。由于约束弓不如重力弓坚强有力，所以当发生外伤导致骨盆损伤时，约束弓的耻骨上支较下支更易发生骨折[30]。

女性盆部与会阴连续横断层 75（FH.7890）

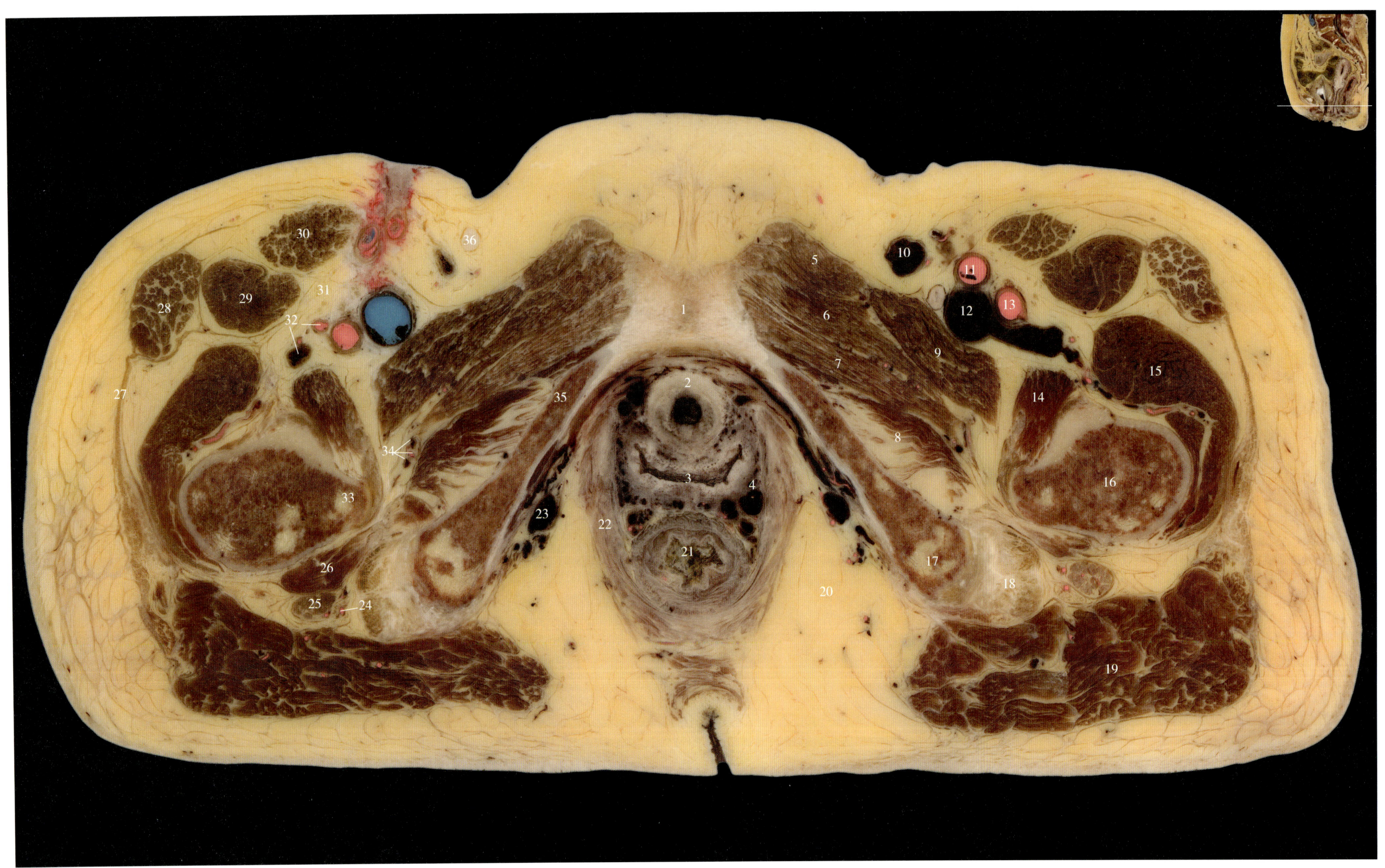

A. 断层标本图像

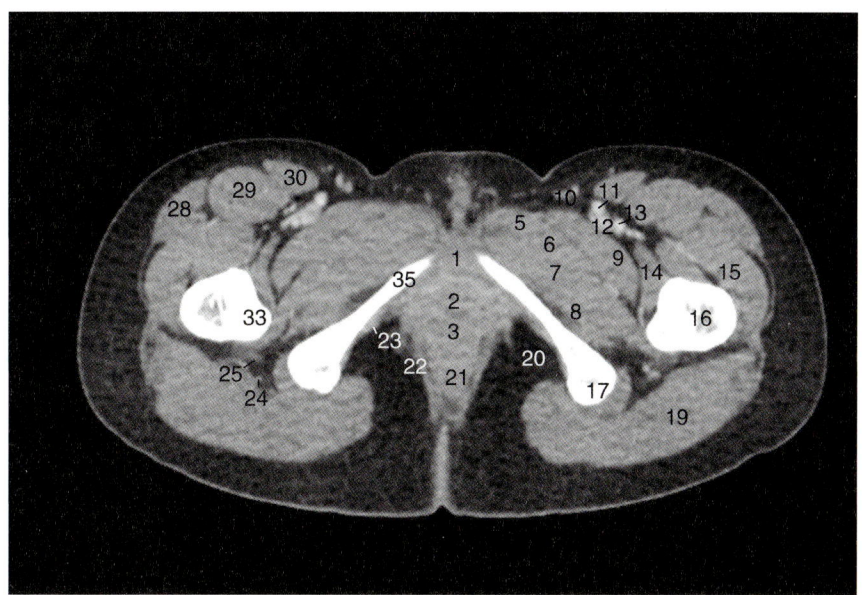
B. CT 增强图像

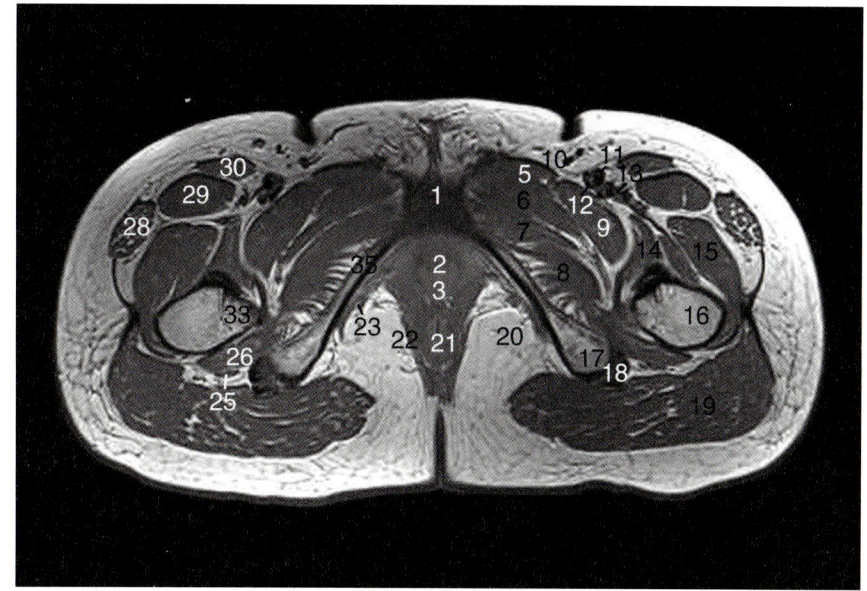
C. MR T1WI

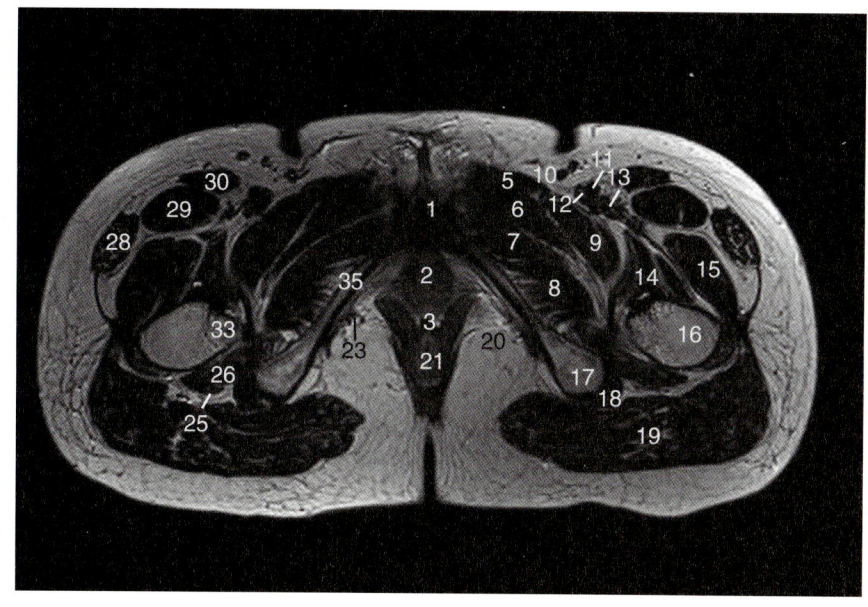
D. MR T2WI

1. 耻骨弓状韧带 arcuate pubic ligament
2. 尿道 urethra
3. 阴道 vaginaa
4. 阴道静脉丛 vaginaal venous plexus
5. 长收肌 adductor longus
6. 短收肌 adductor brevis
7. 大收肌 adductor magnus
8. 闭孔外肌 obturator externus
9. 耻骨肌 pectineus
10. 大隐静脉 great saphenous vein
11. 股动脉 femoral artery
12. 股静脉 femoral vein
13. 股深动脉 deep femoral artery
14. 髂腰肌 iliopsoas
15. 股外侧肌 vastus lateralis
16. 股骨体 shaft of femur
17. 坐骨结节 ischial tuberosity
18. 股二头肌、半腱肌和半膜肌总腱 tendons of biceps femoris, semitendinous and semimembranousus
19. 臀大肌 gluteus maximus
20. 坐骨肛门窝 ischioanal fossa
21. 肛管 anal canal
22. 肛提肌 levator ani
23. 阴部内静脉 internal pudendal vein
24. 臀下动脉 inferior gluteal artery
25. 坐骨神经 sciatic nerve
26. 股方肌 quadratus femoris
27. 阔筋膜 fasciae lata
28. 阔筋膜张肌 tensor fasciae latae
29. 股直肌 rectus femoris
30. 缝匠肌 sartorius
31. 股神经 femoral nerve
32. 旋股外侧动、静脉 lateral femoral circumflex artery and vein
33. 股骨小转子 lesser trochanter of femur
34. 旋股内侧动、静脉 medial femoral circumflex artery and vein
35. 耻骨下支 inferior ramus of pubis
36. 腹股沟浅淋巴结 superficial inguinal lymph nodes

关键结构：耻骨弓状韧带，耻骨下支，阴道。

在此断面，耻骨联合已到最下端，切及耻骨弓状韧带。耻骨弓状韧带呈弓状跨过耻骨联合的下方，连接两侧耻骨下支之间。此韧带较厚，上面与耻骨间纤维软骨板相愈着，下面游离，与尿生殖膈膜间有裂隙，有血管通过。耻骨联合的韧带除了耻骨弓状韧带外，还有耻骨上韧带和耻骨前韧带。耻骨上韧带连接左、右耻骨，其中部与纤维软骨板愈合；耻骨前韧带位于联合的前面，厚而强，由相互交错的纤维构成。盆腔内侧壁的闭孔内肌消失，外侧壁的闭孔外肌断面显著减小。耻骨下支与坐骨支相连，两侧呈"八"形排列。两侧耻骨下支之间的夹角称为耻骨下角。耻骨下角有显著的性别差异。这种差异在胚胎时期就开始出现，成年女性的耻骨下角可达90°~100°，男性则为70°~75°[21]。盆腔内脏器从前向后依次为尿道、阴道和肛管。

女性盆部与会阴连续横断层 76（FH.7870）

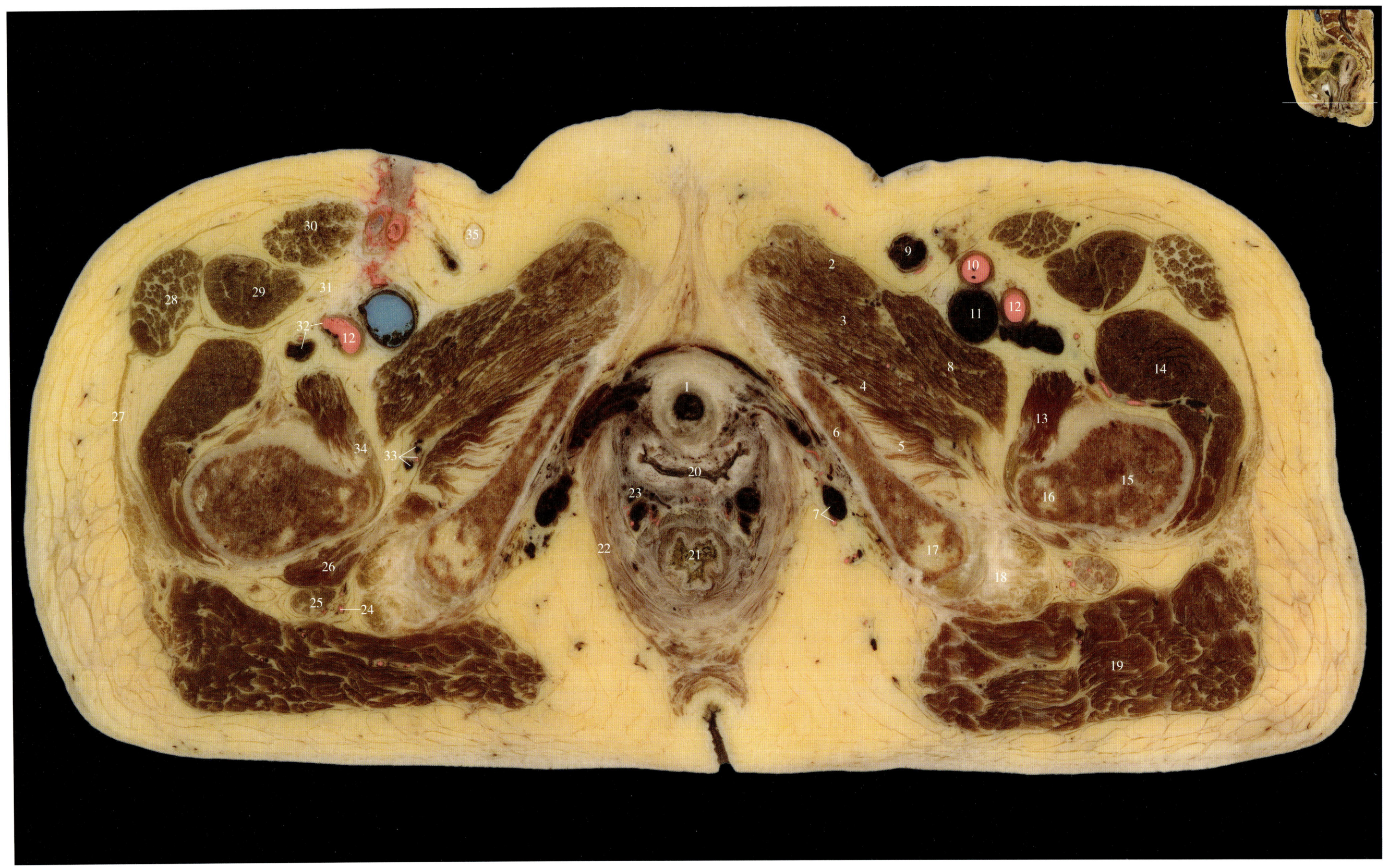

A. 断层标本图像

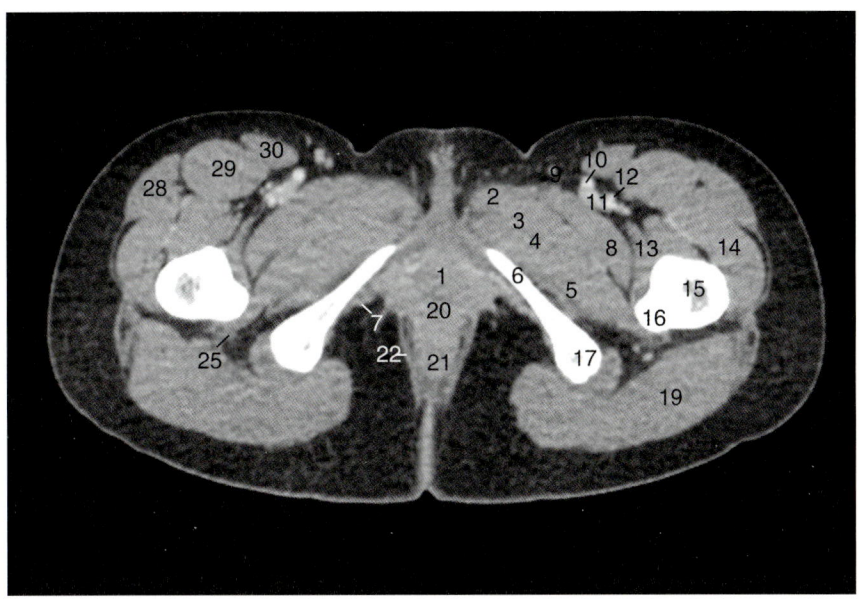

B. CT 增强图像

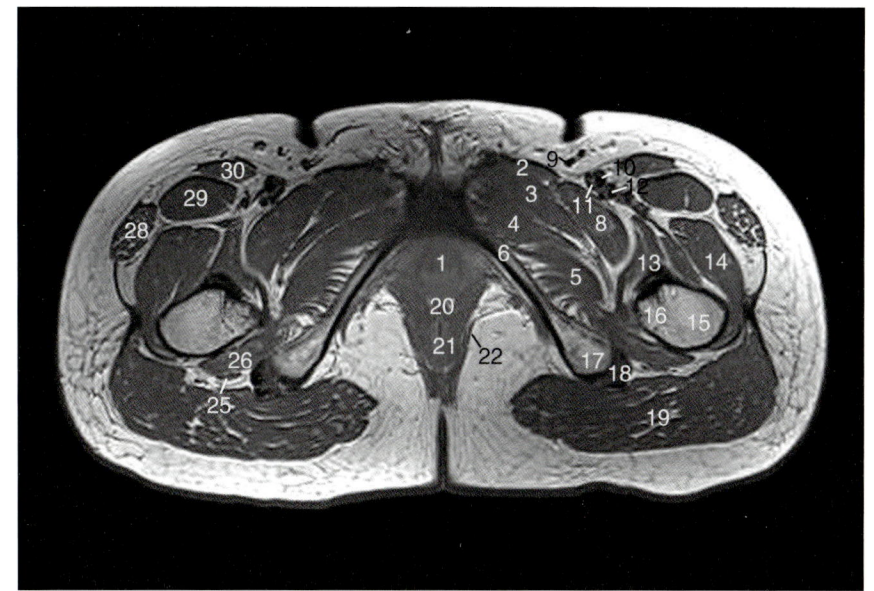

C. MR T1WI

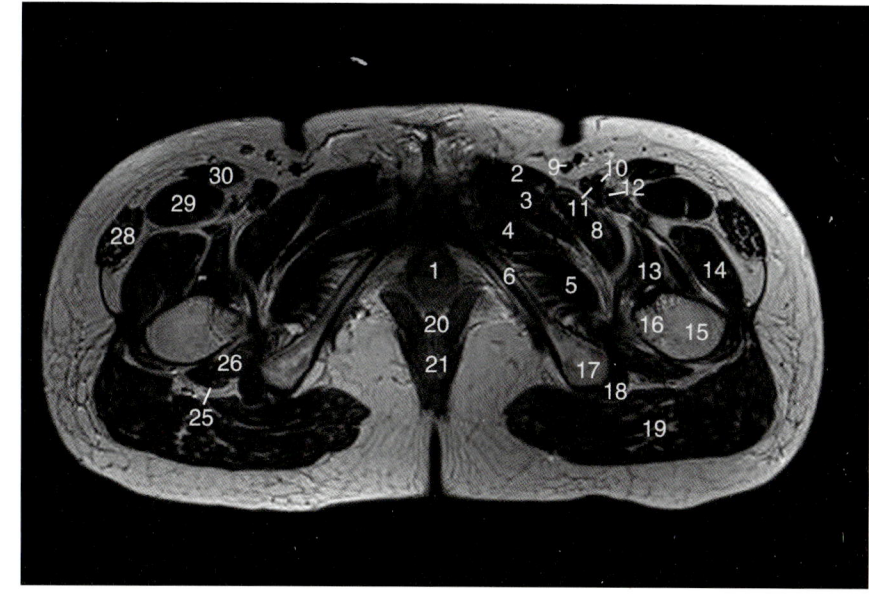

D. MR T2WI

1. 尿道 urethra
2. 长收肌 adductor longus
3. 短收肌 adductor brevis
4. 大收肌 adductor magnus
5. 闭孔外肌 obturator externus
6. 耻骨下支 inferior ramus of pubis
7. 阴部内动、静脉 internal pudendal artery and vein
8. 耻骨肌 pectineus
9. 大隐静脉 great saphenous vein
10. 股动脉 femoral artery
11. 股静脉 femoral vein
12. 股深动脉 deep femoral artery
13. 髂腰肌 iliopsoas
14. 股外侧肌 vastus lateralis
15. 股骨体 shaft of femur
16. 股骨小转子 femur, lesser trochanter
17. 坐骨结节 ischial tuberosity
18. 股二头肌、半腱肌和半膜肌总腱 tendons of biceps femoris, semitendinous and semimembranousus
19. 臀大肌 gluteus maximus
20. 阴道 vaginaa
21. 肛管 anal canal
22. 肛提肌 levator ani
23. 阴道静脉丛 vaginaal venous plexus
24. 臀下动脉 inferior gluteal artery
25. 坐骨神经 sciatic nerve
26. 股方肌 quadratus femoris
27. 阔筋膜 fasciae lata
28. 阔筋膜张肌 tensor fasciae latae
29. 股直肌 rectus femoris
30. 缝匠肌 sartorius
31. 股神经 femoral nerve
32. 旋股外侧动、静脉 lateral femoral circumflex artery and vein
33. 旋股内侧动、静脉 medial femoral circumflex artery and vein
34. 髂腰肌肌腱 iliopsoas tendon
35. 腹股沟浅淋巴结 superficial inguinal lymph nodes

关键结构：耻骨下支，坐骨支。

此断面为耻骨弓上份层面。耻骨下支与坐骨支相连，呈"八"形排列。其内侧从前向后依次为尿道、阴道和肛管，其外侧依次排列长收肌、短收肌、大收肌和闭孔外肌。耻骨下支与坐骨支参与围成骨盆的下口。骨盆的性别差异在全身骨骼中是最明显的。在婴儿期，男婴整个骨盆的尺寸（如髂嵴间径）大于女婴，但是女婴的骨盆腔体积仍大于男婴。这种差别在儿童时期普遍存在，但在22个月时差别最大。成年时期，女性的骨盆，尤其是小骨盆，要适应分娩，从而导致骨盆在比例和形状上发生适应性改变。男性的骨盆腔更长，呈圆锥形；女性的骨盆腔更短，呈圆柱形。骨盆下口的差异比边缘更大。骨盆下口的径线测量方法包括：①前后径，为尾骨尖至耻骨联合下缘中点之间的距离，男性约为 8 cm，女性约为 12.5 cm；②横径，为两侧坐骨结节内侧面下缘的距离，男性约为 8.5 cm，女性约为 11.8 cm；③斜径，为一侧骶结节韧带中间点至对侧坐耻骨结合处的距离，男性约为 10 cm，女性约为 11.8 cm。径线数值存在个体和种族差异[5]。

女性盆部与会阴连续横断层 77（FH.7850）

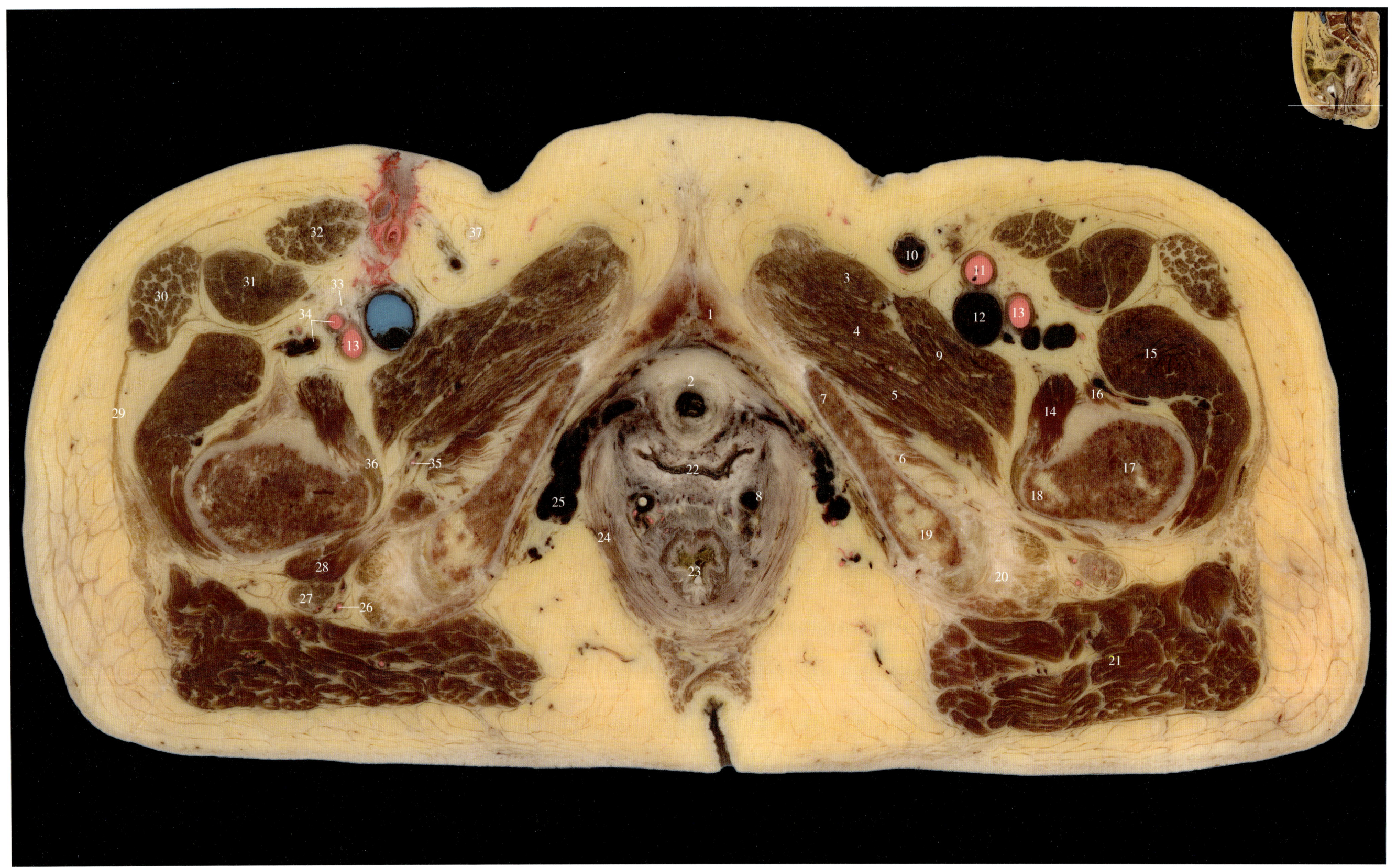

A. 断层标本图像

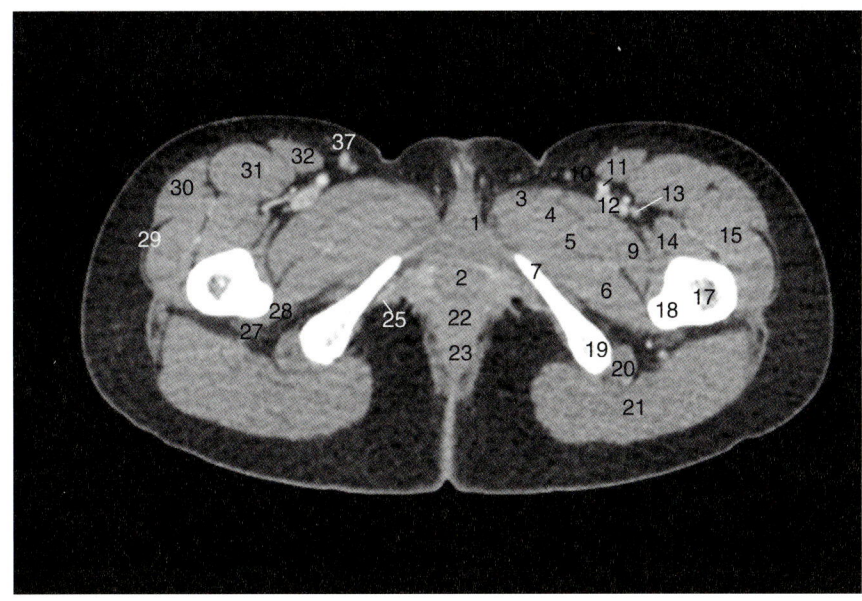
B. CT 增强图像

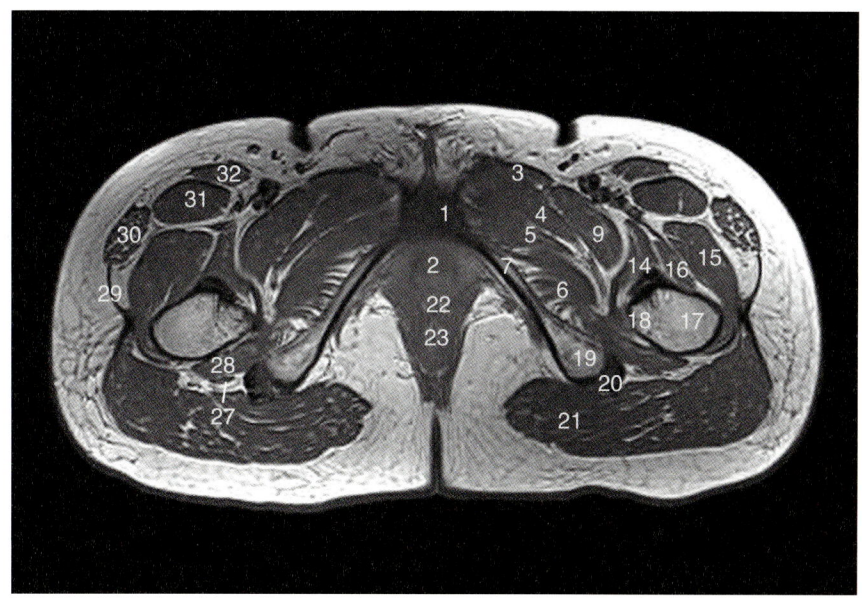
C. MR T1WI

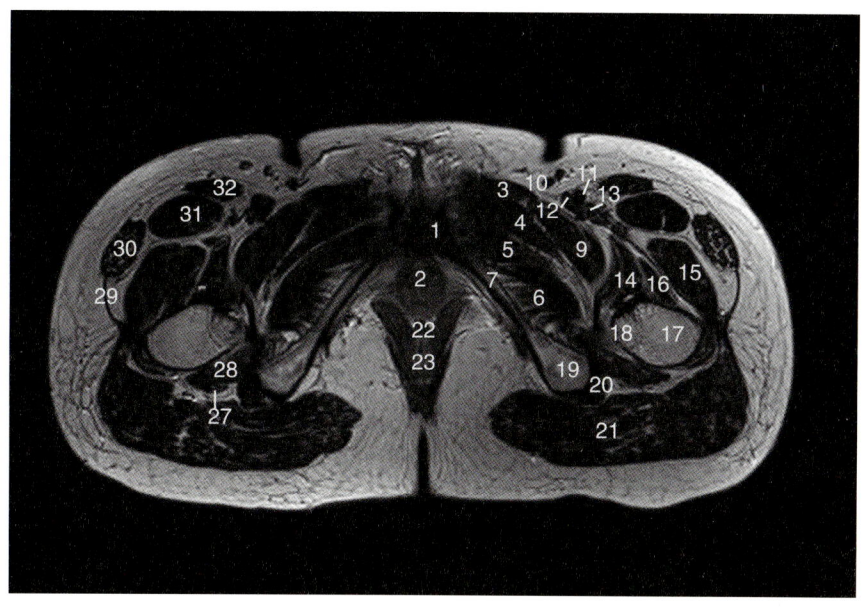
D. MR T2WI

1. 前庭球 bulb of vestibule
2. 尿道 urethra
3. 长收肌 adductor longus
4. 短收肌 adductor brevis
5. 大收肌 adductor magnus
6. 闭孔外肌 obturator externus
7. 耻骨下支 inferior ramus of pubis
8. 阴道静脉丛 vaginaal venous plexus
9. 耻骨肌 pectineus
10. 大隐静脉 great saphenous vein
11. 股动脉 femoral artery
12. 股静脉 femoral vein
13. 股深动脉 deep femoral artery
14. 髂腰肌 iliopsoas
15. 股外侧肌 vastus lateralis
16. 股中间肌 vastus intermedius
17. 股骨体 shaft of femur
18. 股骨小转子 lesser trochanter of femur
19. 坐骨结节 ischial tuberosity
20. 股二头肌、半腱肌和半膜肌总腱 tendons of biceps femoris, semitendinous and semimembranousus
21. 臀大肌 gluteus maximus
22. 阴道 vaginaa
23. 肛管 anal canal
24. 肛提肌 levator ani
25. 阴部内静脉 internal pudendal vein
26. 臀下动脉 inferior gluteal artery
27. 坐骨神经 sciatic nerve
28. 股方肌 quadratus femoris
29. 阔筋膜 fasciae lata
30. 阔筋膜张肌 tensor fasciae latae
31. 股直肌 rectus femoris
32. 缝匠肌 sartorius
33. 股神经 femoral nerve
34. 旋股外侧动、静脉 lateral femoral circumflex artery and vein
35. 旋股内侧动脉 medial femoral circumflex artery
36. 髂腰肌肌腱 iliopsoas tendon
37. 腹股沟浅淋巴结 superficial inguinal lymph nodes

关键结构：前庭球，阴道，肛管。

此断面经前庭球的前端。两侧前庭球在阴阜的深面中线处相连，居于断面中央部的前份。前庭球由具有勃起性的静脉丛构成，是男性尿道海绵体的同源体，呈蹄铁形，其中位于阴道两侧者，称为前庭球外侧部，长约为 1 cm，宽约为 1 cm。其后端钝圆，与前庭大腺相邻；其前端狭窄，与对侧连合，此连合部称前庭球中间部，位于阴蒂和尿道之间，并借两条细弱的勃起组织束与阴蒂头密接。前庭球主要由静脉丛构成。静脉极度迂曲，互相吻合成海绵体样结构，具有一定的勃起性。其静脉与阴蒂的静脉吻合。前庭球深部与尿生殖膈下筋膜相接，浅面后部被球海绵体肌覆盖[5, 30]。

女性盆部与会阴连续横断层 78（FH.7830）

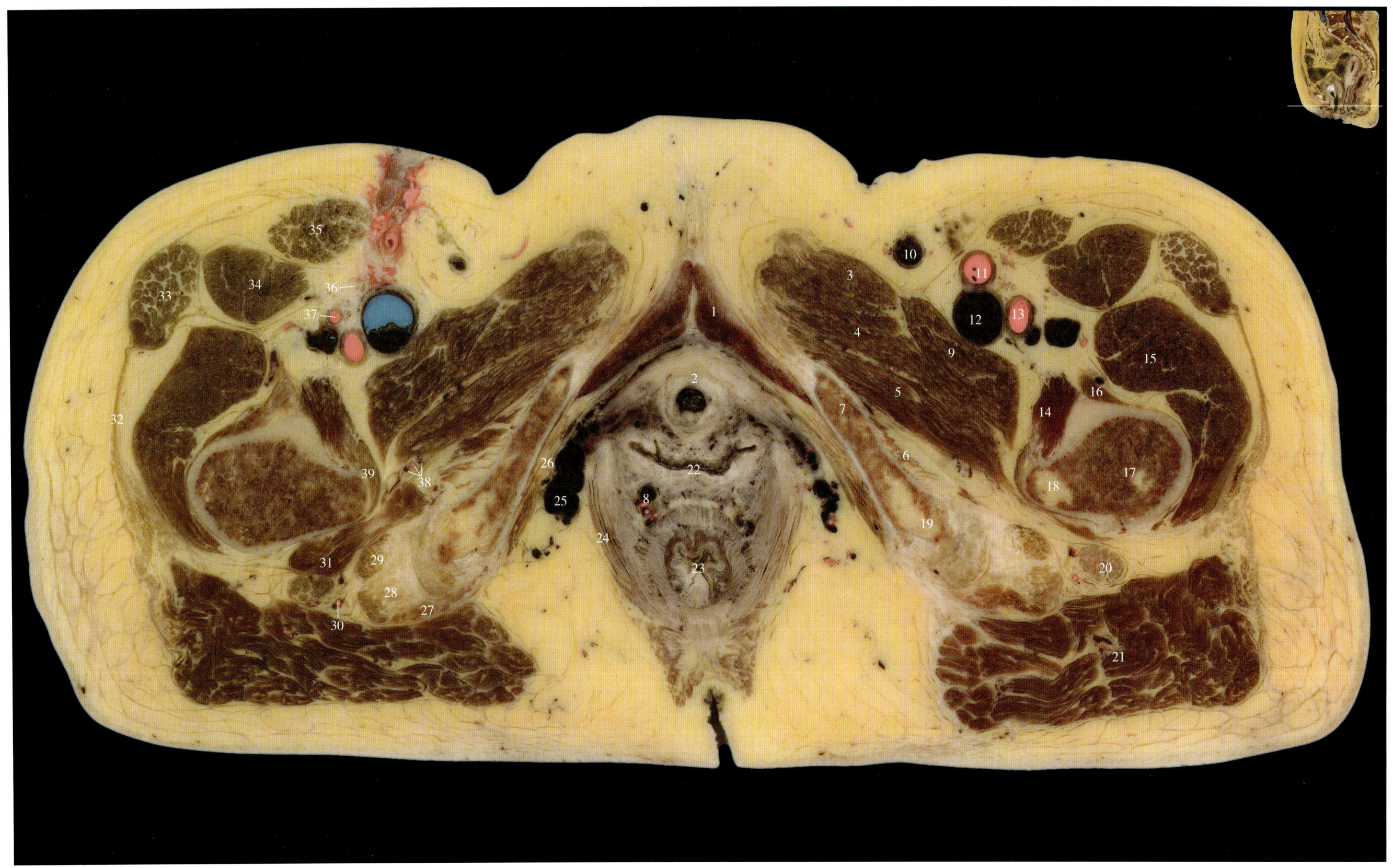

A. 断层标本图像

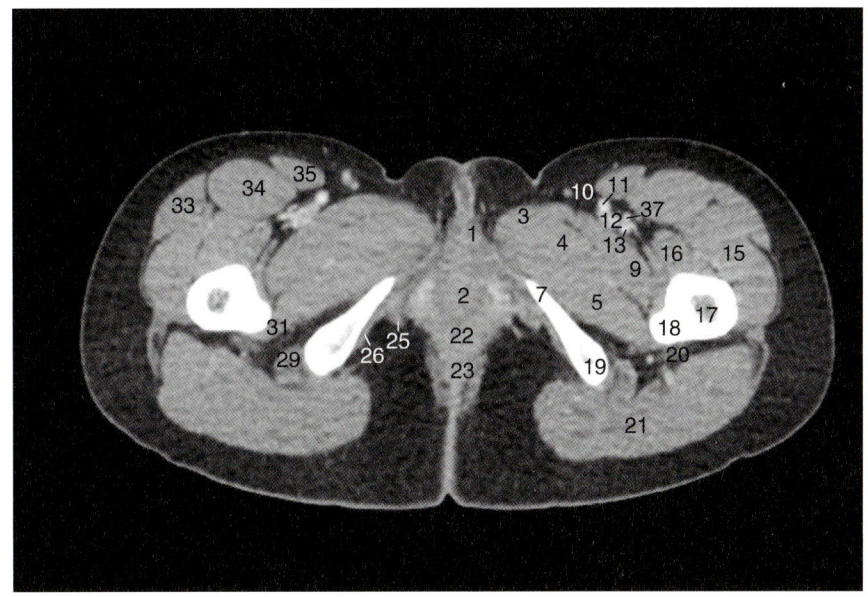
B. CT 增强图像

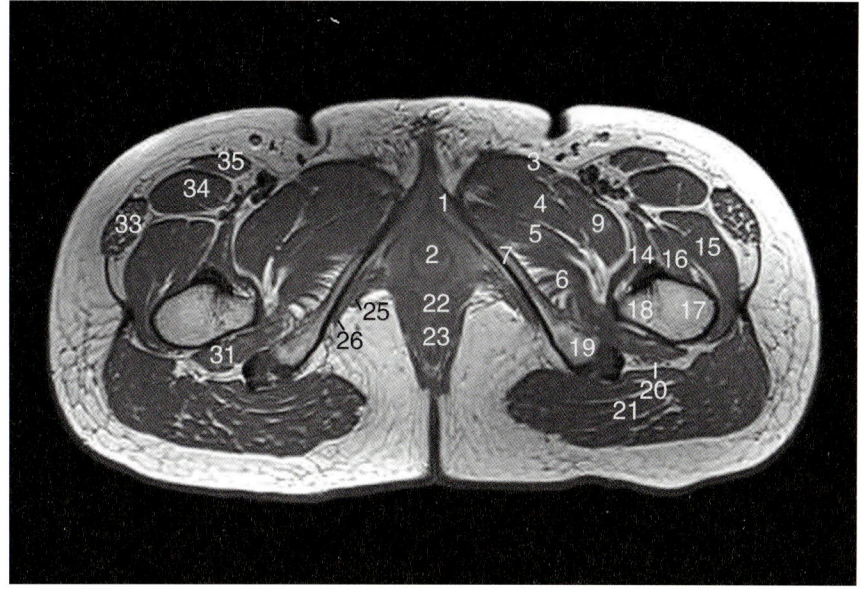
C. MR T1WI

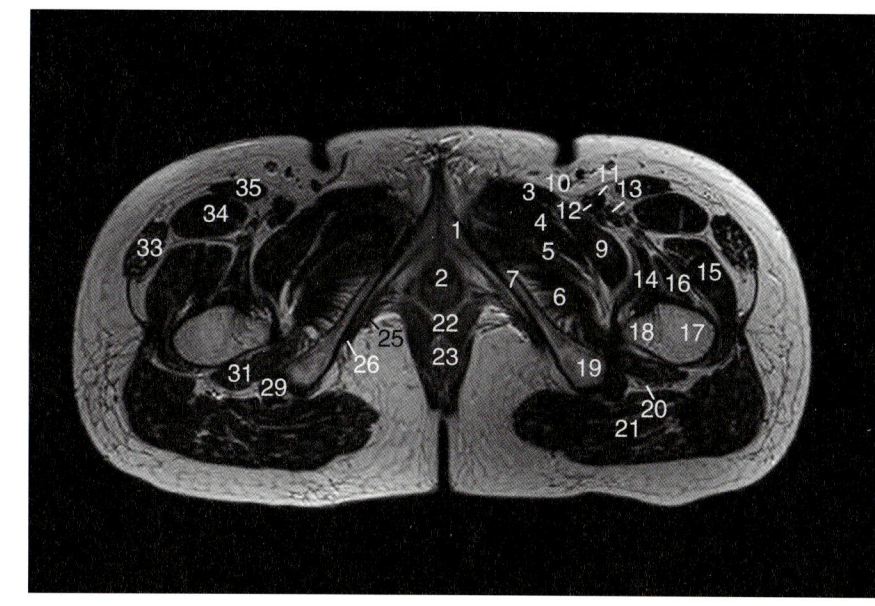
D. MR T2WI

1. 前庭球 bulb of vestibule
2. 尿道 urethra
3. 长收肌 adductor longus
4. 短收肌 adductor brevis
5. 大收肌 adductor magnus
6. 闭孔外肌 obturator externus
7. 耻骨下支 inferior ramus of pubis
8. 阴道静脉丛 vaginaal venous plexus
9. 耻骨肌 pectineus
10. 大隐静脉 great saphenous vein
11. 股动脉 femoral artery
12. 股静脉 femoral vein
13. 股深动脉 deep femoral artery
14. 髂腰肌 iliopsoas
15. 股外侧肌 vastus lateralis
16. 股中间肌 vastus intermedius
17. 股骨体 shaft of femur
18. 股骨小转子 lesser trochanter of femur
19. 坐骨结节 ischial tuberosity
20. 坐骨神经 sciatic nerve

21. 臀大肌 gluteus maximus
22. 阴道 vaginaa
23. 肛管 anal canal
24. 肛提肌 levator ani
25. 阴部内静脉 internal pudendal vein
26. 坐骨海绵体肌 ischiocavernosus
27. 半腱肌 semitendinosus
28. 股二头肌长头肌肌腱 tendon of long head of biceps femoris
29. 半膜肌肌腱 tendon of semimembranosus
30. 臀下动脉 inferior gluteal artery
31. 股方肌 quadratus femoris
32. 阔筋膜 fasciae lata
33. 阔筋膜张肌 tensor fasciae latae
34. 股直肌 rectus femoris
35. 缝匠肌 sartorius
36. 股神经 femoral nerve
37. 旋股外侧动脉 lateral femoral circumflex artery
38. 旋股内侧动、静脉 medial femoral circumflex artery and vein
39. 髂腰肌肌腱 iliopsoas tendon

关键结构：坐骨海绵体肌，前庭球，坐骨支。

此断面经前庭球上端。两侧前庭球呈"八"形排列，居于断面中央部的前份，其后方依次为尿道、阴道和肛管。阴道和尿道周围有丰富的静脉丛。肛管已接近末端，在肛管的后方和两侧有肛提肌包绕。耻骨下支与坐骨支相连，呈"八"形排列。在坐骨支与耻骨下支的外侧，从前向后依次排列长收肌、短收肌、大收肌和闭孔外肌，闭孔外肌接近消失。在坐骨支内侧可见坐骨海绵体肌的条索状断面，坐骨海绵体肌起自坐骨结节，覆盖于阴蒂脚表面，收缩时可压迫阴蒂脚，阻止阴蒂内静脉回流，使阴蒂勃起[12]。

女性盆部与会阴连续横断层 79（FH.7810）

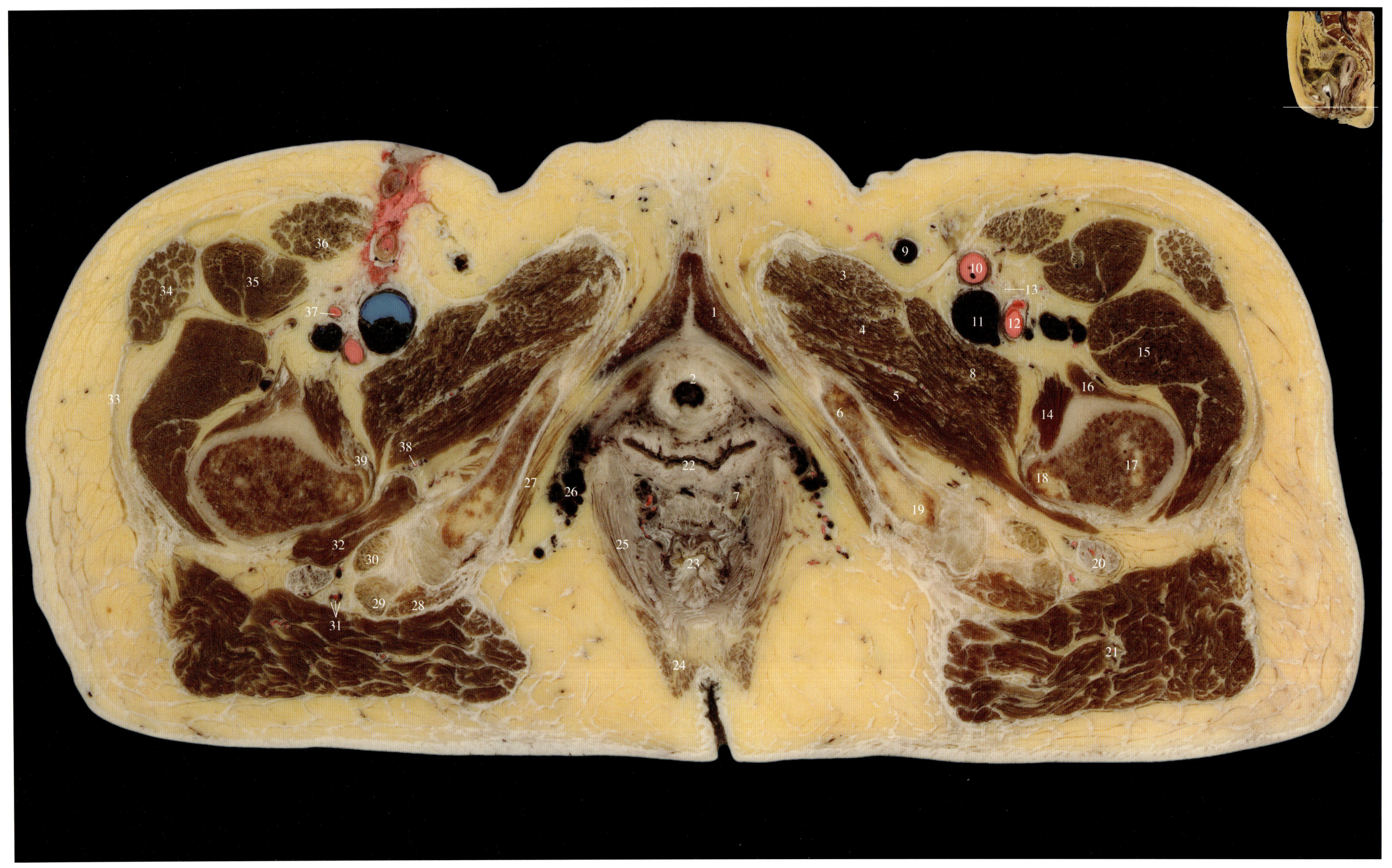

A. 断层标本图像

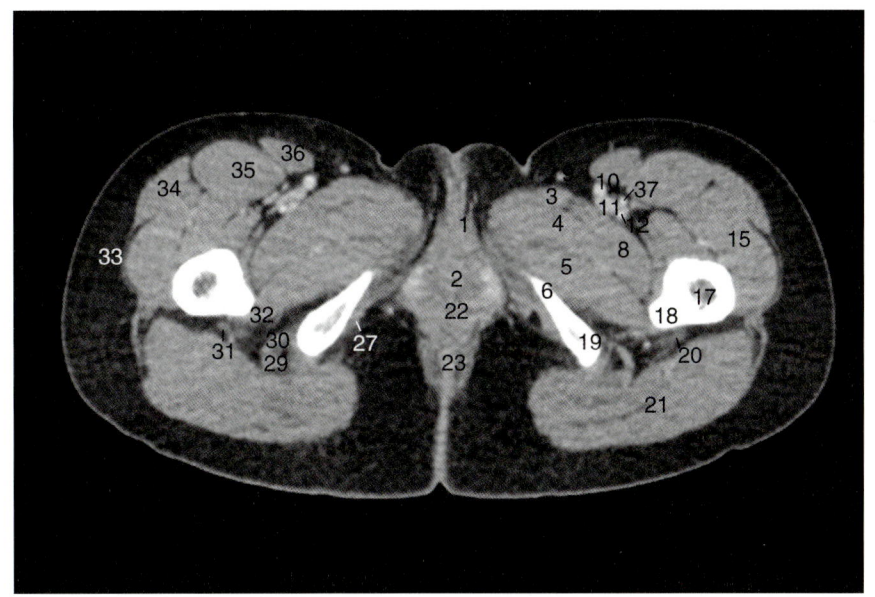
B. CT 增强图像

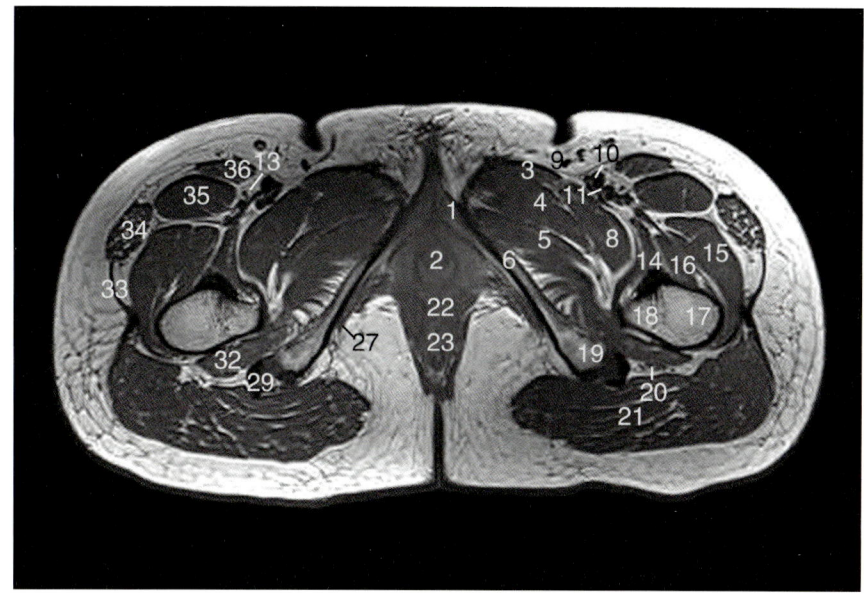
C. MR T1WI

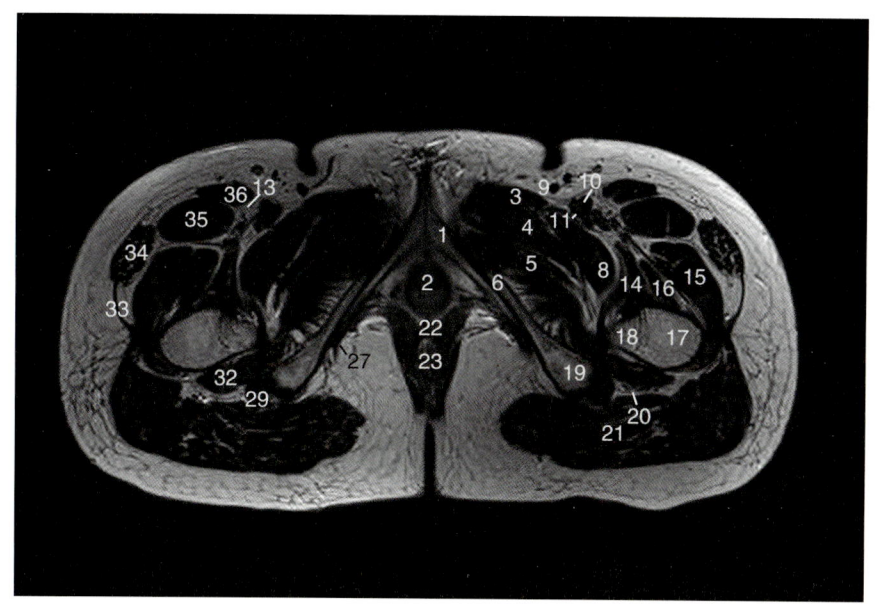
D. MR T2WI

关键结构：肛门外括约肌，前庭球，坐骨海绵体肌。

　　此断面经前庭球上端。在阴阜的深面，两侧前庭球呈"八"形排列，其后方依次为尿道、阴道和肛管。阴道和尿道周围有丰富的静脉丛。肛管已接近末端，在肛管的后方和两侧有肛提肌包绕，在肛管周围可见肛门外括约肌。肛门外括约肌按纤维所在部位分为皮下部、浅部和深部。皮下部位于肛管下端的皮下，肌束呈环形；浅部在皮下部之上，肌束围绕肛门内括约肌下部；深部肌束呈厚的环形带，围绕肛门内括约肌上部。肛门外括约肌的浅部和深部、肛门内括约肌、直肠下份的纵行肌及肛提肌等，共同构成肛直肠环，此环对肛管起着极其重要的括约作用，若手术损伤将导致大便失禁[5]。MRI可清晰显示肛管周围肌肉，冠状位T2WI显示最佳[39]。

1. 前庭球 bulb of vestibule
2. 尿道 urethra
3. 长收肌 adductor longus
4. 短收肌 adductor brevis
5. 大收肌 adductor magnus
6. 耻骨下支 inferior ramus of pubis
7. 阴道静脉丛 vaginaal venous plexus
8. 耻骨肌 pectineus
9. 大隐静脉 great saphenous vein
10. 股动脉 femoral artery
11. 股静脉 femoral vein
12. 股深动脉 deep femoral artery
13. 股神经 femoral nerve
14. 髂腰肌 iliopsoas
15. 股外侧肌 vastus lateralis
16. 股中间肌 vastus intermedius
17. 股骨 femur
18. 股骨小转子 femur, lesser trochanter
19. 坐骨支 ramus of ischium
20. 坐骨神经 sciatic nerve
21. 臀大肌 gluteus maximus
22. 阴道 vaginaa
23. 肛管 anal canal
24. 肛门外括约肌 sphincter ani externus
25. 肛提肌 levator ani
26. 阴部内静脉 internal pudendal vein
27. 坐骨海绵体肌 ischiocavernosus
28. 半腱肌 semitendinosus
29. 股二头肌长头 long head of biceps femoris
30. 半膜肌 semimembranosus
31. 臀下动、静脉 inferior gluteal artery and vein
32. 股方肌 quadratus femoris
33. 阔筋膜 fasciae lata
34. 阔筋膜张肌 tensor fasciae latae
35. 股直肌 rectus femoris
36. 缝匠肌 sartorius
37. 旋股外侧动脉 lateral femoral circumflex artery
38. 旋股内侧动脉 medial femoral circumflex artery
39. 髂腰肌肌腱 iliopsoas tendon

女性盆部与会阴连续横断层 80（FH.7790）

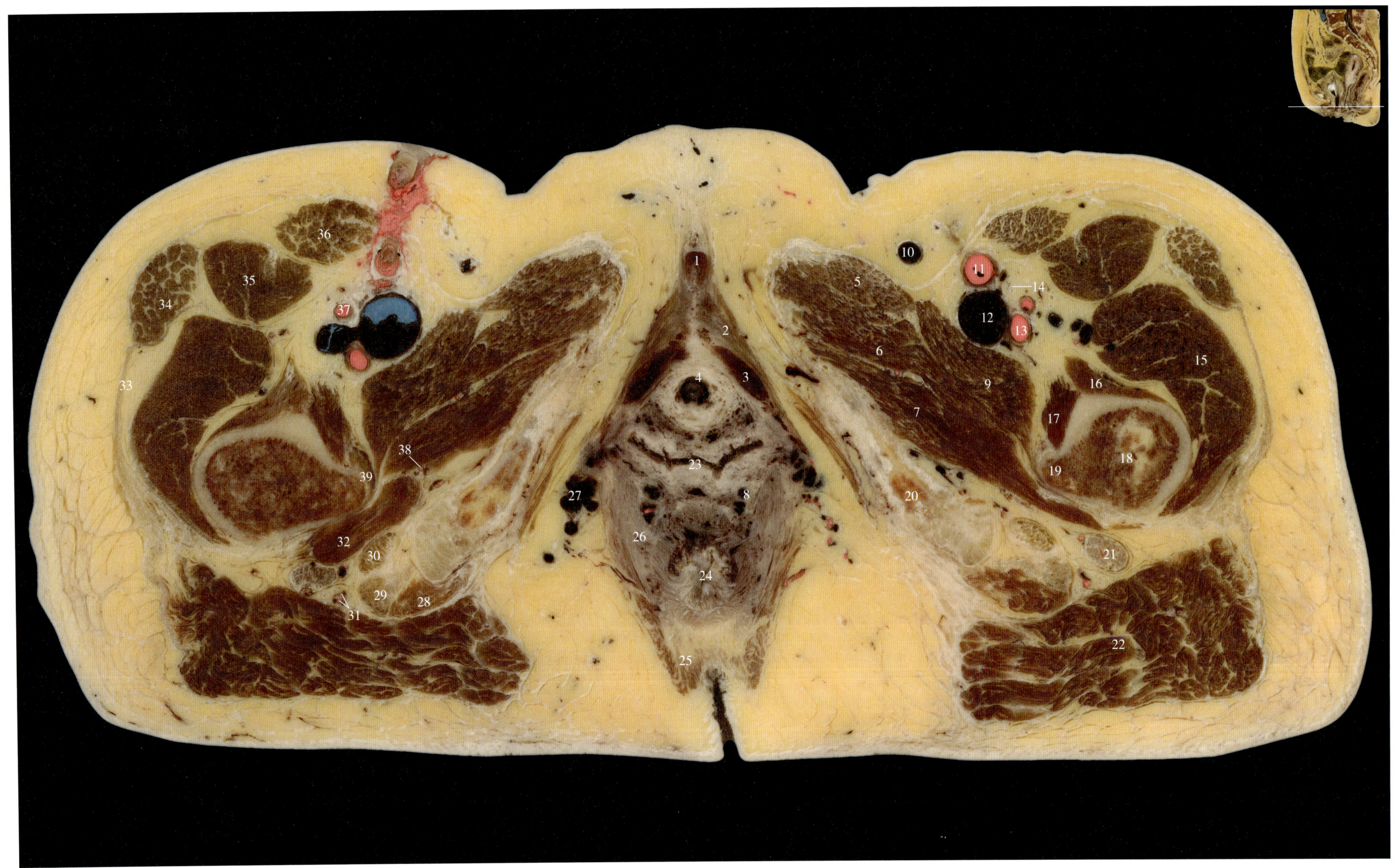

A. 断层标本图像

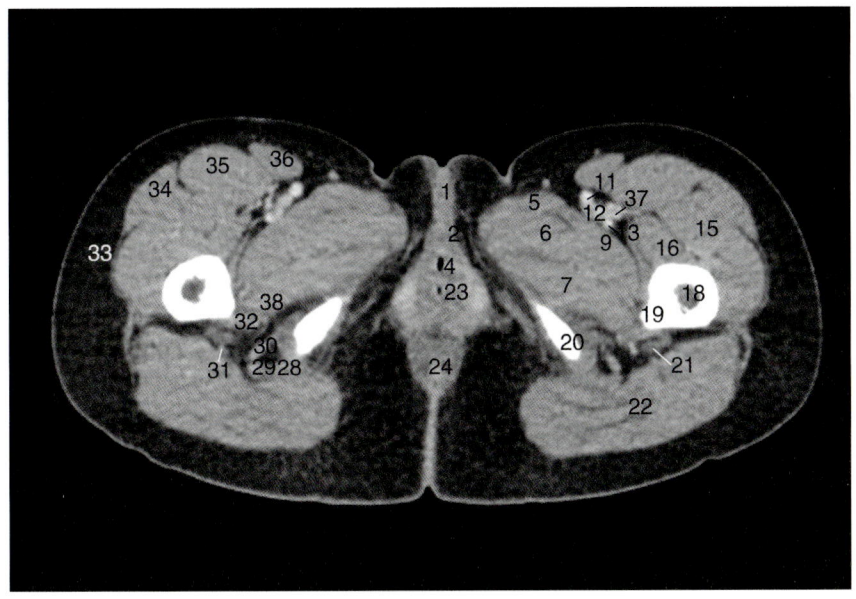
B. CT 增强图像

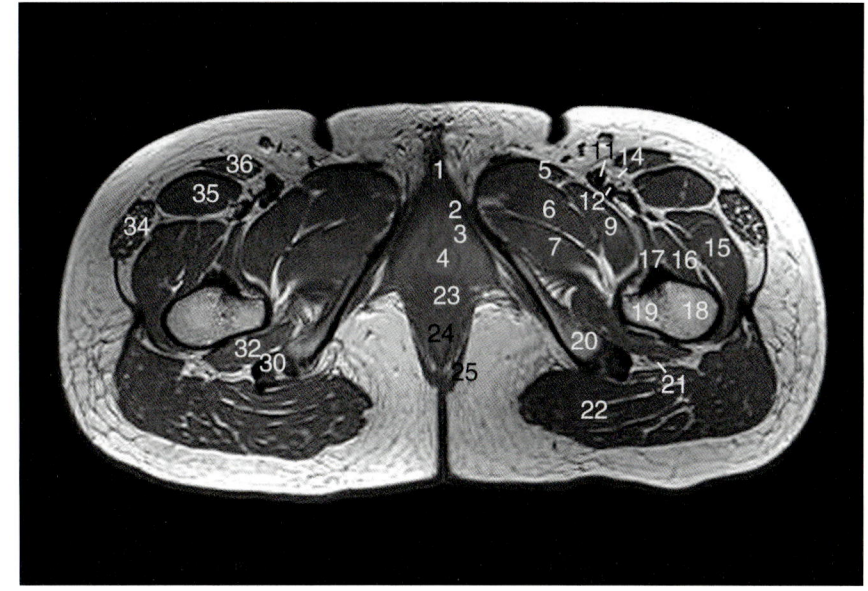
C. MR T1WI

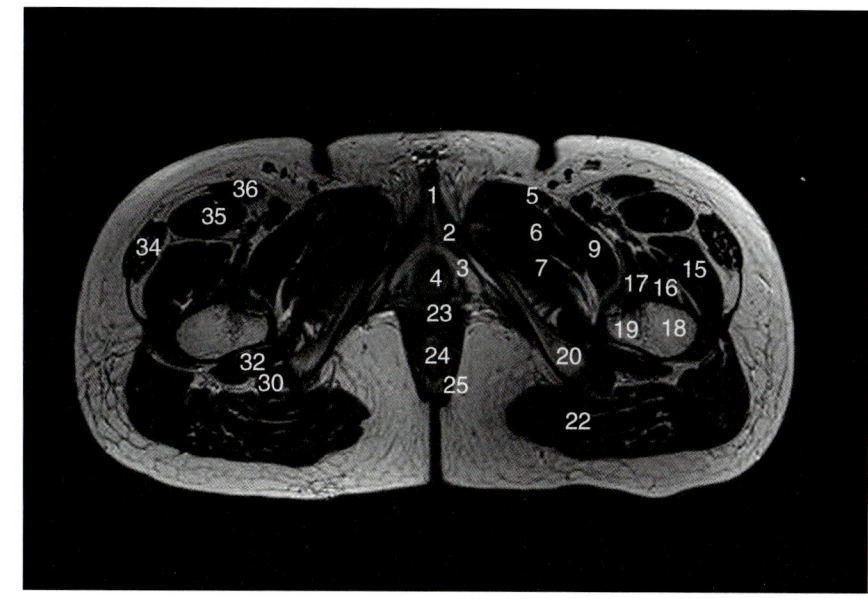
D. MR T2WI

1. 阴蒂 clitoris
2. 阴蒂脚 clitoral crura
3. 前庭球 bulb of vestibule
4. 尿道 urethra
5. 长收肌 adductor longus
6. 短收肌 adductor brevis
7. 大收肌 adductor magnus
8. 阴道静脉丛 vaginaal venous plexus
9. 耻骨肌 pectineus
10. 大隐静脉 great saphenous vein
11. 股动脉 femoral artery
12. 股静脉 femoral vein
13. 股深动脉 deep femoral artery
14. 股神经 femoral nerve
15. 股外侧肌 vastus lateralis
16. 股中间肌 vastus intermedius
17. 髂腰肌 iliopsoas
18. 股骨体 shaft of femur
19. 股骨小转子 femur, lesser trochanter
20. 坐骨支 ramus of ischium

21. 坐骨神经 sciatic nerve
22. 臀大肌 gluteus maximus
23. 阴道 vaginaa
24. 肛管 anal canal
25. 肛门外括约肌 sphincter ani externus
26. 肛提肌 levator ani
27. 阴部内静脉 internal pudental vein
28. 半腱肌 semitendinosus
29. 股二头肌长头 long head of biceps femoris
30. 半膜肌 semimembranosus
31. 臀下动脉 inferior gluteal artery
32. 股方肌 quadratus femoris
33. 阔筋膜 fasciae lata
34. 阔筋膜张肌 tensor fasciae latae
35. 股直肌 rectus femoris
36. 缝匠肌 sartorius
37. 旋股外侧动脉 lateral femoral circumflex artery
38. 旋股内侧动脉 medial femoral circumflex artery
39. 髂腰肌肌腱 iliopsoas tendon

关键结构：阴蒂，阴蒂脚，前庭球。

　　此断面开始出现阴蒂。断面中部前份为阴蒂体和阴蒂脚，其深面为前庭球。前庭球向后依次为尿道、阴道和肛管，在阴道周围有阴道静脉丛，在肛管周围有肛门外括约肌。骨盆两侧壁的骨性结构为坐骨支和耻骨下支，附于其内面的为坐骨海绵体肌。闭孔内肌和闭孔外肌均消失。在坐骨肛门窝内阴部内动、静脉逐渐沿其侧壁向前走行，到达阴部管的前端。此断面开始出现阴蒂。阴蒂由两条阴蒂海绵体构成，阴蒂海绵体的构造与男性阴茎海绵体类似，具有勃起功能。阴蒂后端称阴蒂脚，呈圆柱形，起于耻骨下支和坐骨下支的骨膜，向内上方至耻骨联合下缘附近，左、右阴蒂海绵体在中线处连合成阴蒂体，其间亦有不完全的结缔组织中隔，称为海绵体中隔或梳状隔。阴蒂体几成直角折转向前下方，其游离端称阴蒂头，为圆形小结节，突出于阴蒂包皮下面。阴蒂头下面以阴蒂系带连于小阴唇。阴蒂海绵体外面，也包有白膜，但较男性阴茎海绵体白膜稍薄，白膜外面包有阴蒂筋膜，阴蒂体背侧与耻骨联合前面下部之间有带弹性的浅、深两条结缔组织索。浅者为阴蒂系韧带；深者为阴蒂悬韧带。阴蒂头主要由海绵状勃起组织构成。阴蒂头和阴蒂皮肤富有血管及神经末梢（环层小体和触觉小体），感觉敏锐，易于勃起[30]。

女性盆部与会阴连续横断层 81（FH.7770）

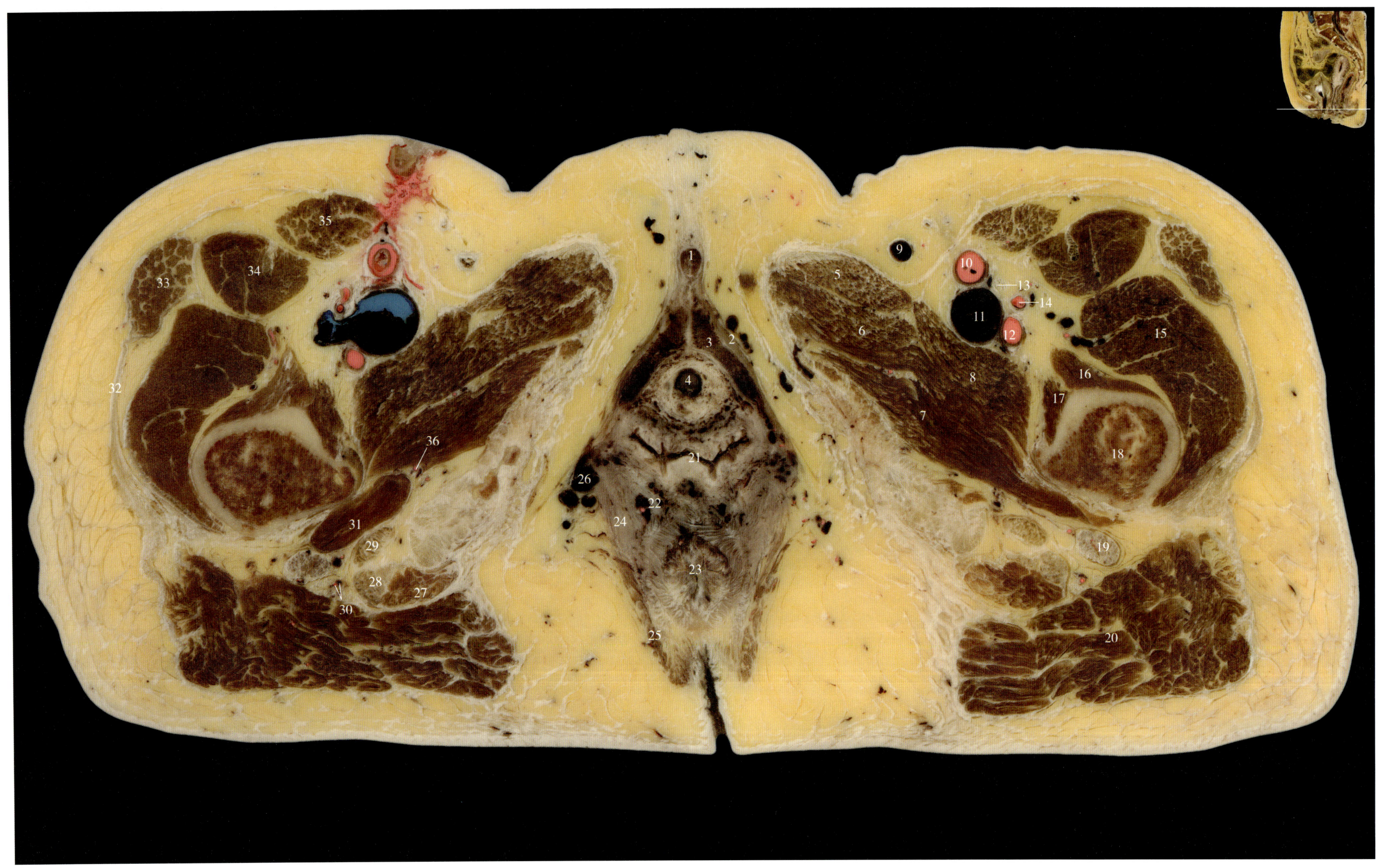

A. 断层标本图像

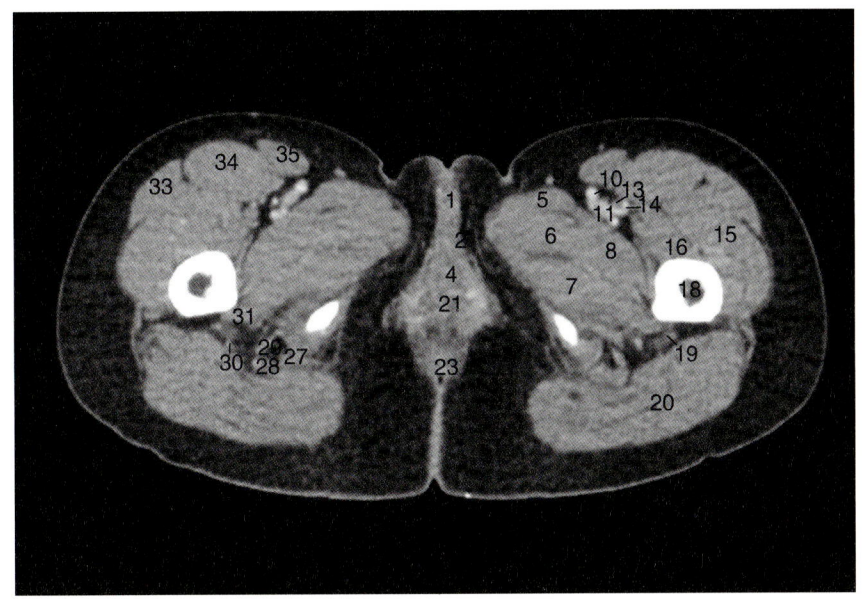
B. CT 增强图像

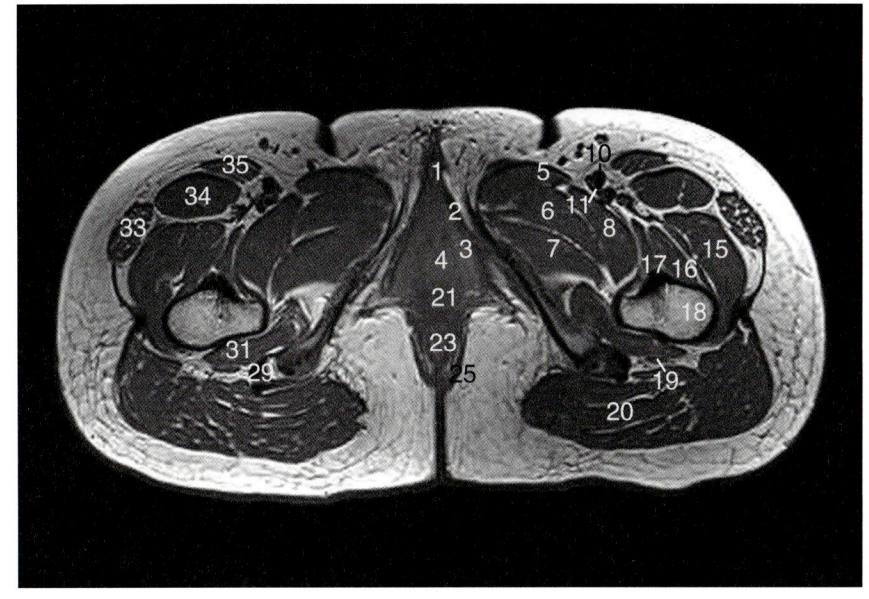
C. MR T1WI

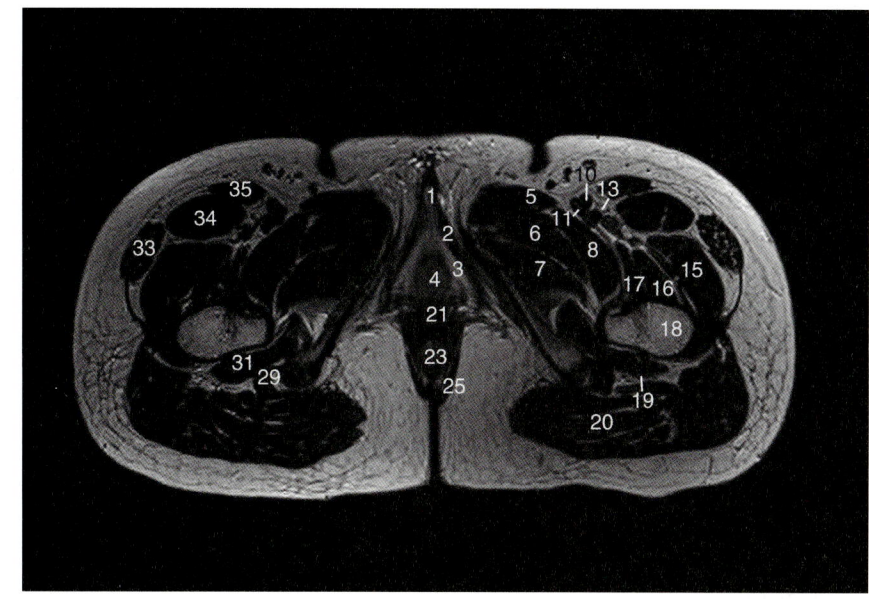
D. MR T2WI

1. 阴蒂 clitoris
2. 阴蒂脚 clitoral crura
3. 前庭球 bulb of vestibule
4. 尿道 urethra
5. 长收肌 adductor longus
6. 短收肌 adductor brevis
7. 大收肌 adductor magnus
8. 耻骨肌 pectineus
9. 大隐静脉 great saphenous vein
10. 股动脉 femoral artery
11. 股静脉 femoral vein
12. 股深动脉 deep femoral artery
13. 股神经 femoral nerve
14. 旋股外侧动脉 lateral femoral circumflex artery
15. 股外侧肌 vastus lateralis
16. 股中间肌 vastus intermedius
17. 髂腰肌 iliopsoas
18. 股骨 femur
19. 坐骨神经 sciatic nerve
20. 臀大肌 gluteus maximus
21. 阴道 vaginaa
22. 阴道静脉丛 vaginaal venous plexus
23. 肛门 anus
24. 肛提肌 levator ani
25. 肛门外括约肌 sphincter ani externus
26. 阴部内静脉 internal pudendal vein
27. 半腱肌 semitendinosus
28. 股二头肌长头 long head of biceps femoris
29. 半膜肌 semimembranosus
30. 臀下动、静脉 inferior gluteal artery and vein
31. 股方肌 quadratus femoris
32. 阔筋膜 fasciae lata
33. 阔筋膜张肌 tensor fasciae latae
34. 股直肌 rectus femoris
35. 缝匠肌 sartorius
36. 旋股内侧动脉 medial femoral circumflex artery

关键结构：前庭球，阴蒂，肛门。

此断面经阴蒂和前庭球上部。断面中部前份为阴蒂体和阴蒂脚，其深面为前庭球。前庭球又称球海绵体，位于前庭两侧，由具有勃起性的静脉丛组成，表面覆有球海绵体肌。前庭球包绕尿道，其后的阴道断面呈"H"形。阴道后方为肛门。在肛门和外生殖器之间有会阴中心腱又称"会阴体"，为一纤维性中隔，长约为1.3 cm。其位于会阴缝深部、两侧会阴肌间，有肛门外括约肌、球海绵体肌及成对的会阴浅横肌、会阴深横肌和肛提肌等附于此，直肠壶腹和肛管的纵肌层亦参与其组成。此腱有加固盆底的作用。女性会阴中心腱较大，有韧性和弹性，对阴道后壁有支持作用[21]，分娩时要加以保护。

女性盆部与会阴连续横断层 82（FH.7750）

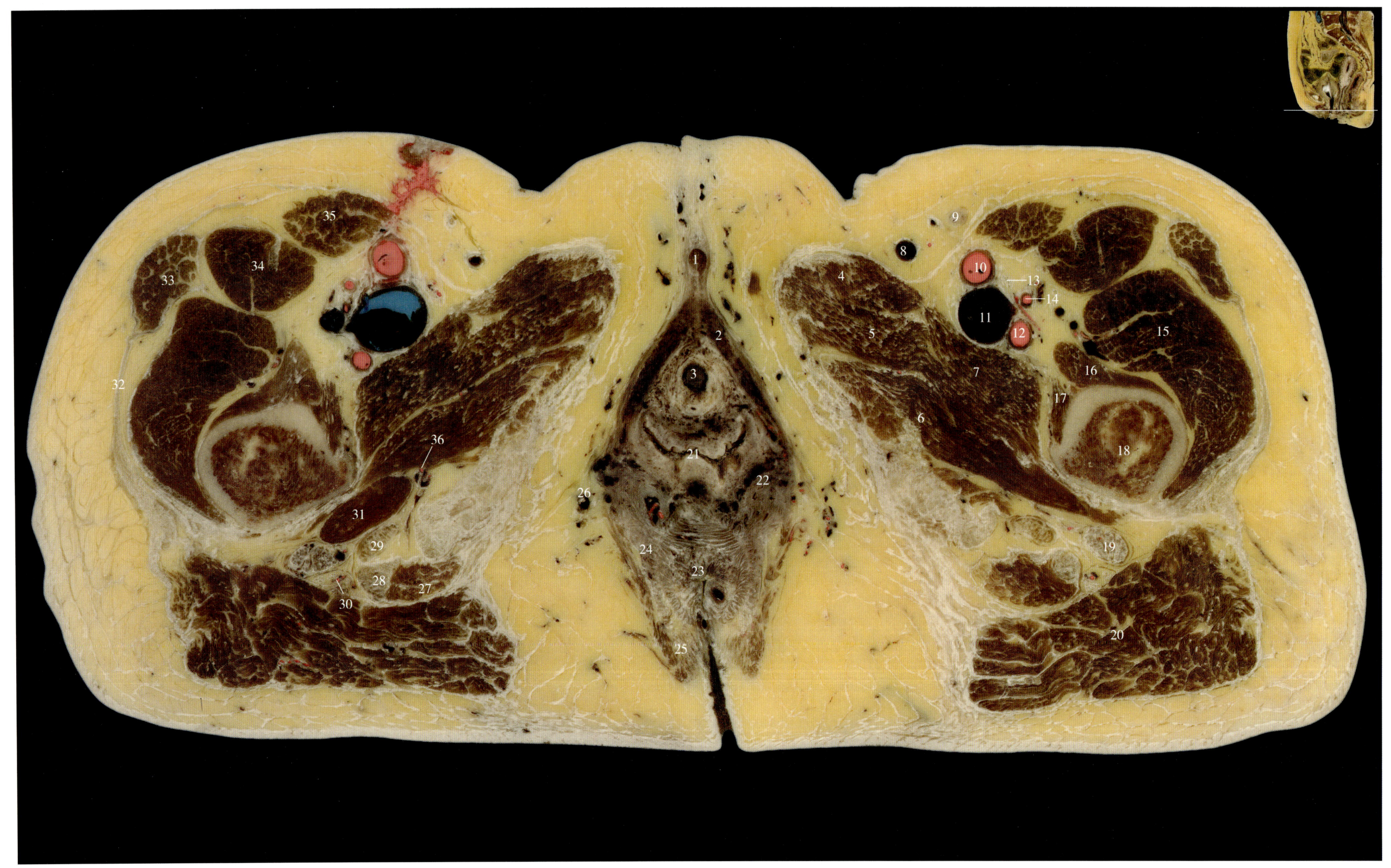

A. 断层标本图像

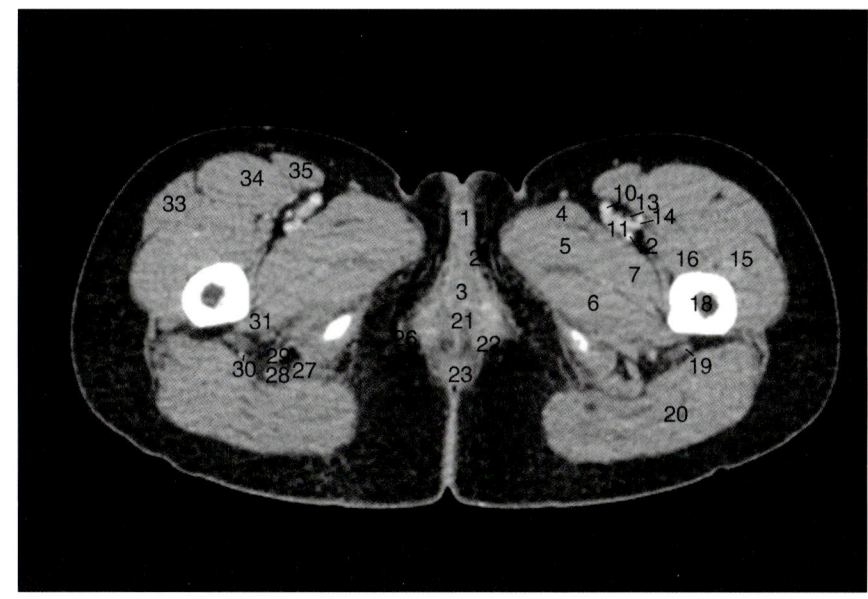

B. CT 增强图像

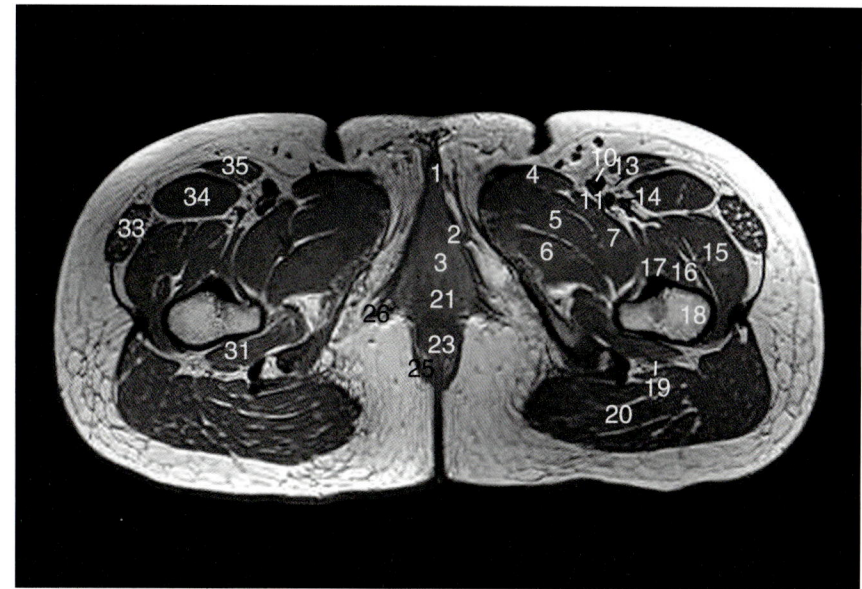

C. MR T1WI

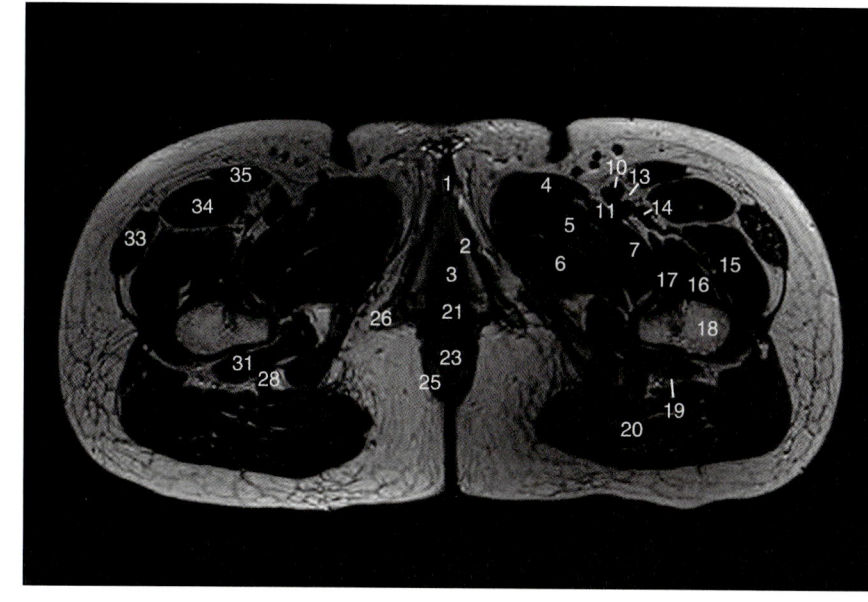

D. MR T2WI

1. 阴蒂 clitoris
2. 前庭球 bulb of vestibule
3. 尿道 urethra
4. 长收肌 adductor longus
5. 短收肌 adductor brevis
6. 大收肌 adductor magnus
7. 耻骨肌 pectineus
8. 大隐静脉 great saphenous vein
9. 腹股沟浅淋巴结 superficial inguinal lymph nodes
10. 股动脉 femoral artery
11. 股静脉 femoral vein
12. 股深动脉 deep femoral artery
13. 股神经 femoral nerve
14. 旋股外侧动脉 lateral femoral circumflex artery
15. 股外侧肌 vastus lateralis
16. 股中间肌 vastus intermedius
17. 髂腰肌 iliopsoas
18. 股骨 femur
19. 坐骨神经 sciatic nerve
20. 臀大肌 gluteus maximus
21. 阴道 vaginaa
22. 阴道静脉丛 vaginaal venous plexus
23. 肛门 anus
24. 肛提肌 levator ani
25. 肛门外括约肌 sphincter ani externus
26. 阴部内静脉 internal pudendal vein
27. 半腱肌 semitendinosus
28. 股二头肌长头 long head of biceps femoris
29. 半膜肌 semimembranosus
30. 臀下动脉 inferior gluteal artery
31. 股方肌 quadratus femoris
32. 阔筋膜 fasciae lata
33. 阔筋膜张肌 tensor fasciae latae
34. 股直肌 rectus femoris
35. 缝匠肌 sartorius
36. 旋股内侧动脉 medial femoral circumflex artery

关键结构：阴道，阴道静脉丛，阴蒂。

此断面经过阴蒂和前庭球上部。断面中部最前端为大阴唇，其深面有阴蒂和前庭球。前庭球位于尿道和阴道两侧，阴道后方为肛门，在阴道周围有阴道静脉丛。此丛与子宫静脉丛合成子宫阴道静脉丛，并与邻近的膀胱静脉丛和直肠静脉丛相吻合。阴道的静脉血经子宫静脉丛汇入髂内静脉。阴道上部主要由子宫动脉的子宫颈支和阴道支分布；中部由膀胱动脉阴道支分布；下部由直肠下动脉和阴部内动脉的分支分布。以上各支均彼此互相吻合。阴道壁有致密的淋巴管网。阴道上部的淋巴管与子宫动脉伴行，入髂内淋巴结；中部淋巴管与阴道动脉伴行入髂外淋巴结。下部淋巴管入腹股沟下浅淋巴结。阴道后壁的淋巴管，还可入肛门直肠淋巴结；子宫由子宫阴道丛和盆内脏神经的分支分布。在外膜的神经丛中，可见到神经节细胞。其中交感神经来自髂内神经丛；副交感神经来自脊髓第3~4骶节。在阴道下部还有阴部神经的小分支分布[30]。

女性盆部与会阴连续横断层 83（FH.7730）

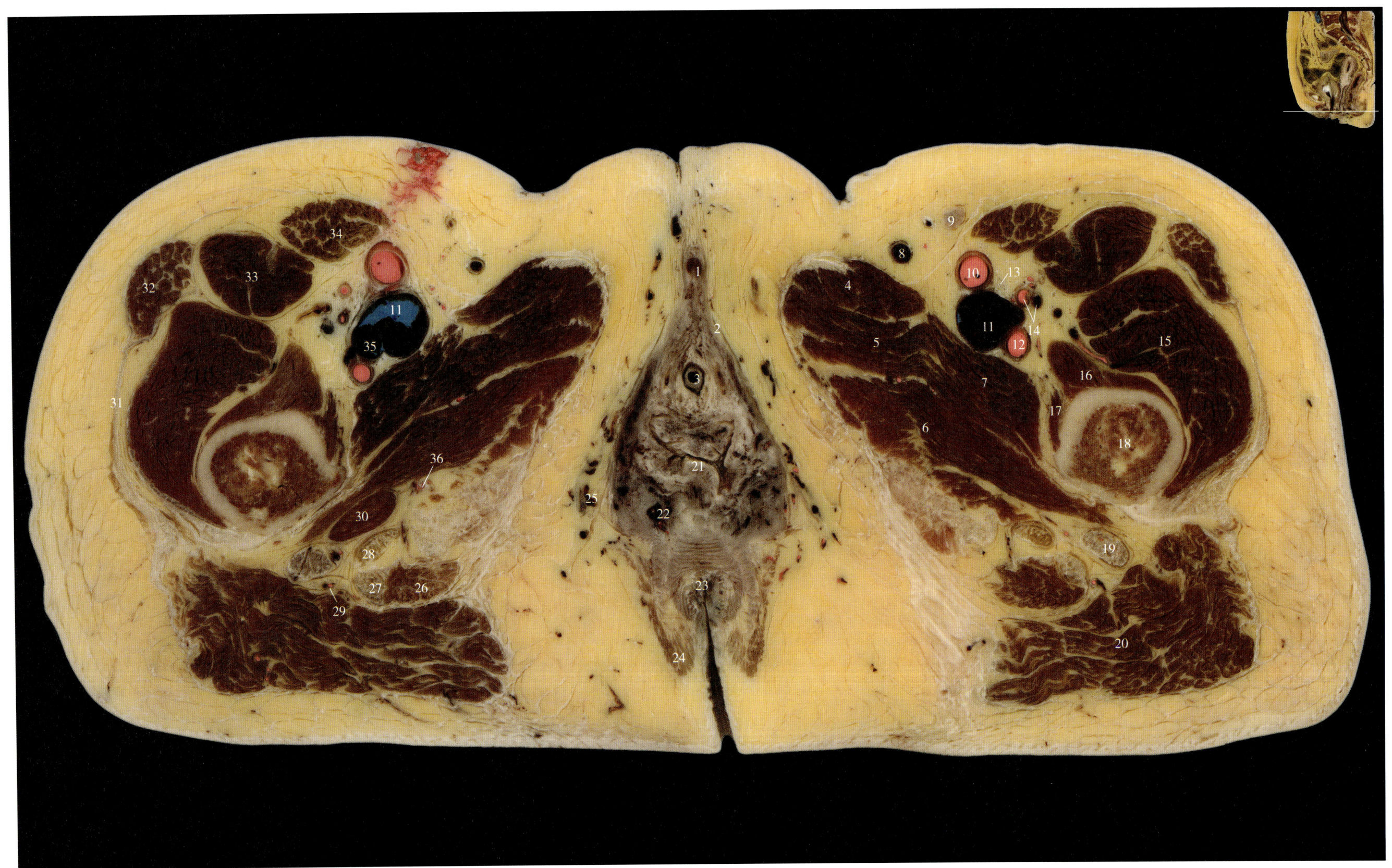

A. 断层标本图像

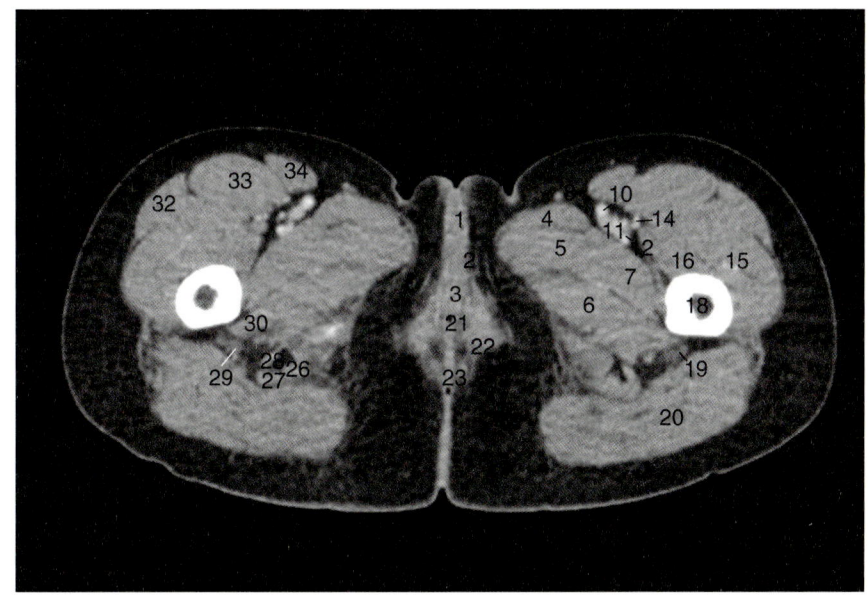
B. CT 增强图像

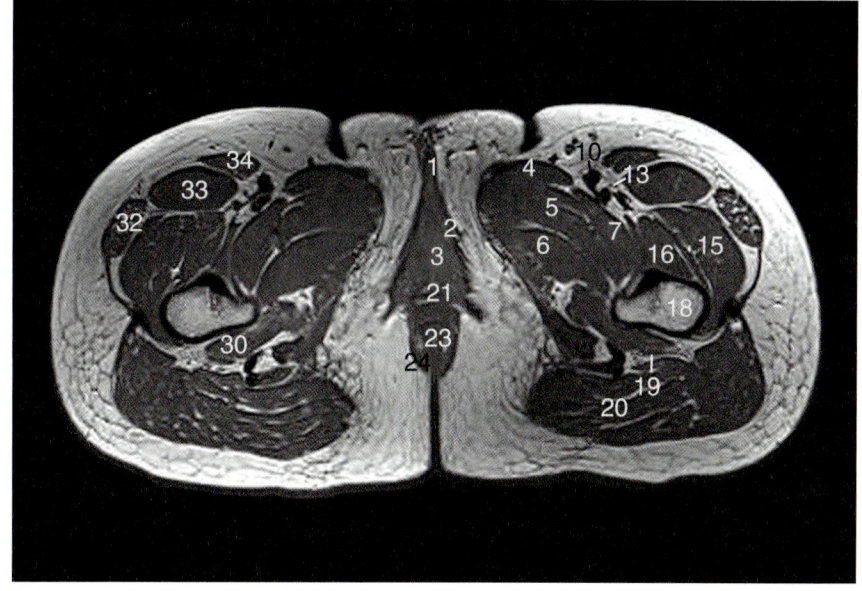
C. MR T1WI

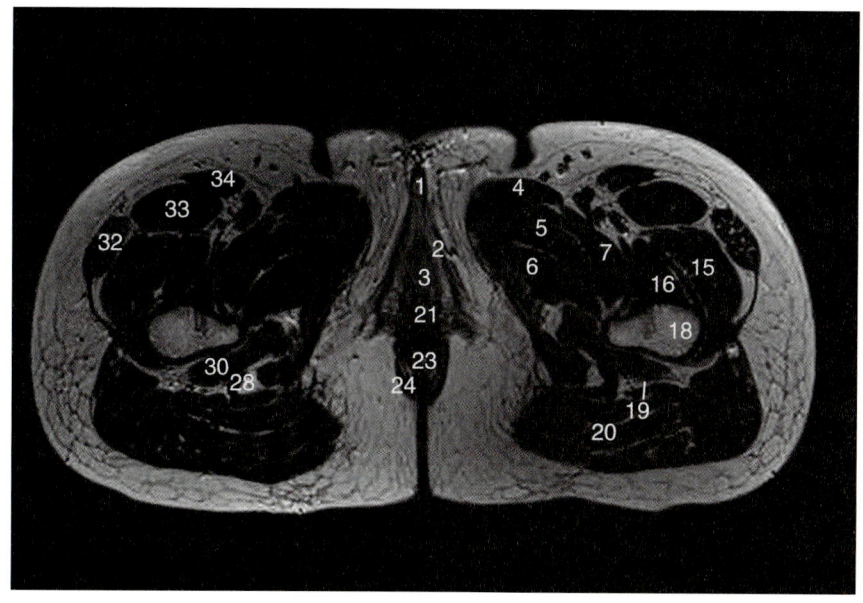
D. MR T2WI

关键结构：阴蒂，阴道，肛门，前庭大腺。

　　此断面经阴蒂上部。断面中部最前端为大阴唇，其深面有阴蒂、阴蒂脚和前庭球。再向后依次为尿道、阴道和肛门，在阴道周围有阴道静脉丛，在肛门周围有肛门外括约肌。前庭大腺与男性的尿道球腺同源，为两个似豌豆或黄豆大小的圆形或卵圆形小体，呈红黄色，位于阴道口两侧，前庭球的后内侧，与前庭球相接，并往往与其重叠在一起。其深部依附于会阴深横肌，其表面盖以球海绵体肌。前庭大腺属于复泡管状腺，质较坚硬，于唇后连合附近隔以皮肤即可触知，其排泄管长 1.5~2 cm，向内前方斜行，开口于阴道前庭的阴道口两侧，在处女膜或处女膜痕附着部与小阴唇后部之间的沟内。其分泌物黏稠，有滑润阴道前庭的作用[30]。

1. 阴蒂 clitoris
2. 阴蒂脚 clitoral crura
3. 尿道 urethra
4. 长收肌 adductor longus
5. 短收肌 adductor brevis
6. 大收肌 adductor magnus
7. 耻骨肌 pectineus
8. 大隐静脉 great saphenous vein
9. 腹股沟浅淋巴结 superficial inguinal lymph nodes
10. 股动脉 femoral artery
11. 股静脉 femoral vein
12. 股深动脉 deep femoral artery
13. 股神经 femoral nerve
14. 旋股外侧动、静脉 lateral femoral circumflex artery and vein
15. 股外侧肌 vastus lateralis
16. 股中间肌 vastus intermedius
17. 髂腰肌 iliopsoas
18. 股骨 femur
19. 坐骨神经 sciatic nerve
20. 臀大肌 gluteus maximus
21. 阴道 vaginaa
22. 阴道静脉丛 vaginaal venous plexus
23. 肛门 anus
24. 肛门外括约肌 sphincter ani externus
25. 阴部内静脉 internal pudendal vein
26. 半腱肌 semitendinosus
27. 股二头肌长头 long head of biceps femoris
28. 半膜肌 semimembranosus
29. 臀下动脉 inferior gluteal artery
30. 股方肌 quadratus femoris
31. 阔筋膜 fasciae lata
32. 阔筋膜张肌 tensor fasciae latae
33. 股直肌 rectus femoris
34. 缝匠肌 sartorius
35. 股深静脉 deep femoral vein
36. 旋股内侧动脉 medial femoral circumflex artery

女性盆部与会阴连续横断层 84（FH.7710）

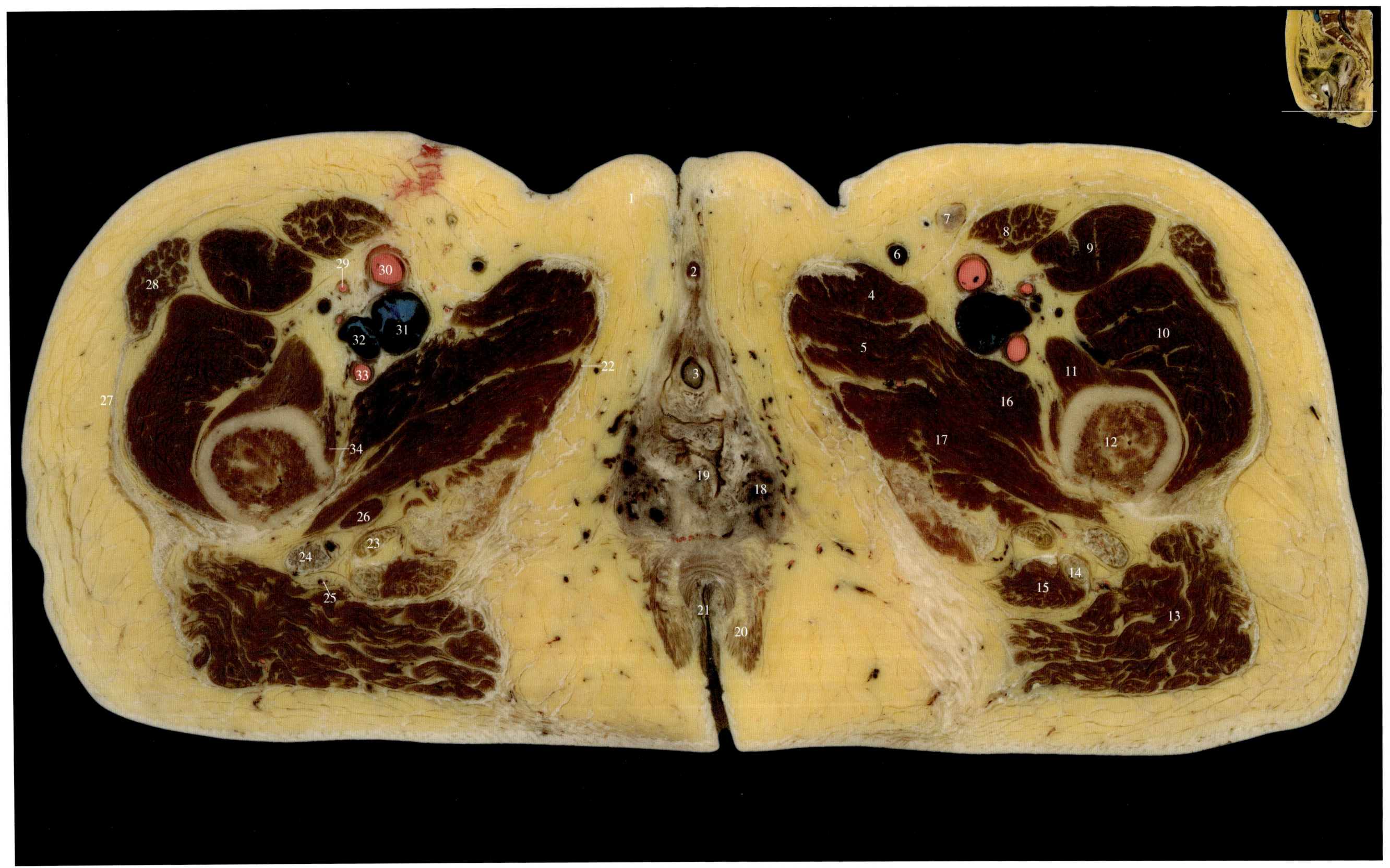

A. 断层标本图像

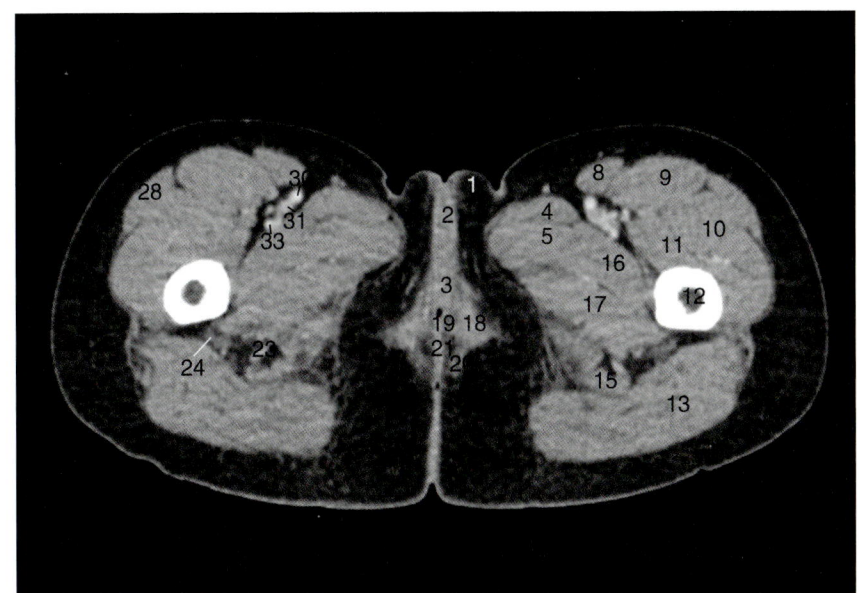

B. CT 增强图像

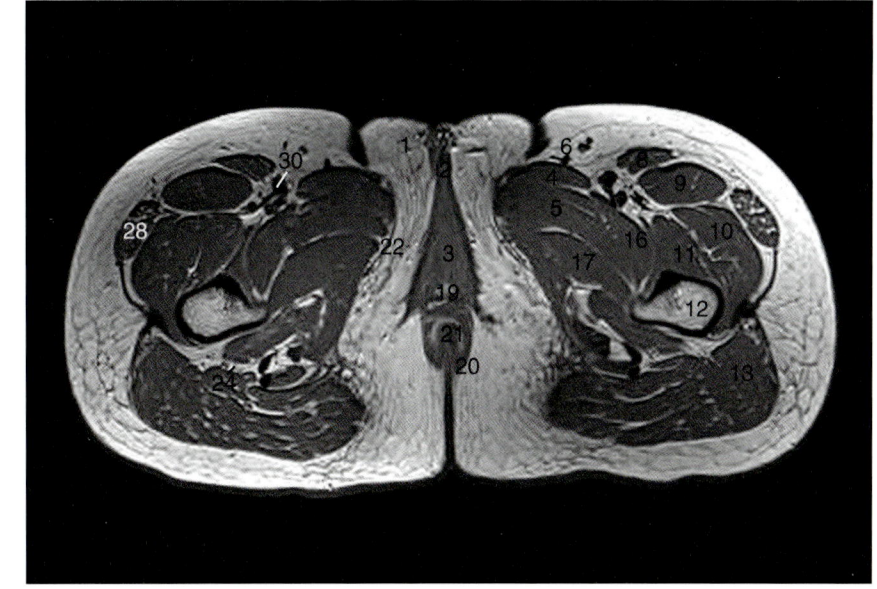

C. MR T1WI

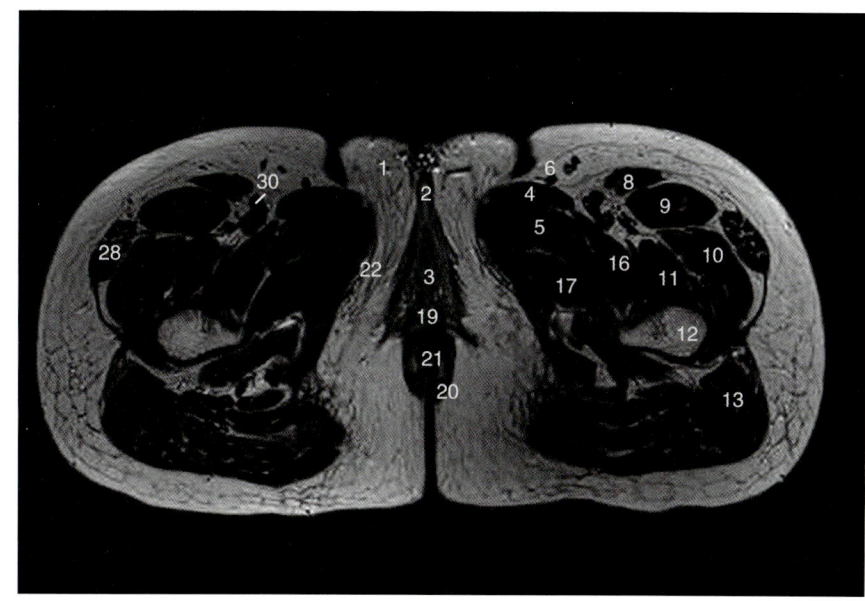

D. MR T2WI

关键结构：大阴唇，阴蒂，肛门括约肌。

此断面经阴蒂上部。断面中部最前端为大阴唇，其深面有阴蒂，再向后依次为尿道、阴道和肛门，在阴道周围有阴道静脉丛，在肛门周围有肛门外括约肌。两侧为大腿上部。在股骨体的前内侧从前向后依次排列着长收肌、短收肌、大收肌，三者外侧为耻骨肌，内侧开始出现股薄肌的断面。大阴唇是两片突出的纵行皮肤皱襞，从阴阜向后伸展到会阴。它们形成外阴的外侧缘。在发生学上，与男性阴囊相当。大阴唇的外面有色素和卷曲的阴毛，内面光滑呈粉红色，有大量的皮脂腺。内、外面之间是许多疏松结缔组织和脂肪组织，之间混有与阴囊肉膜相似的平滑肌、血管、神经和腺体。皮下层由两层组成，浅层为脂肪层（与 Camper 筋膜相似），深层为膜性层，又称 Colles 筋膜，是腹前壁 Scarpa 筋膜的延续。子宫圆韧带终止于大阴唇前部的脂肪组织和皮肤。大阴唇前部形成唇前连合，后部并不结合，几乎平行，止于邻近皮肤。它们中间的皮肤形成较低的崎称唇后连合，覆盖着会阴体，是外阴的后界，它与肛门相距 2.5~3 cm，称"产科"会阴。当腹膜鞘突存在时，先天性腹股沟斜疝可下降到大阴唇内[5, 30]。

1. 大阴唇 greater lip of pudendum
2. 阴蒂 clitoris
3. 尿道 urethra
4. 长收肌 adductor longus
5. 短收肌 adductor brevis
6. 大隐静脉 great saphenous vein
7. 腹股沟浅淋巴结 superficial inguinal lymph nodes
8. 缝匠肌 sartorius
9. 股直肌 rectus femoris
10. 股外侧肌 vastus lateralis
11. 股中间肌 vastus intermedius
12. 股骨 femur
13. 臀大肌 gluteus maximus
14. 股二头肌长头 long head of biceps femoris
15. 半腱肌 semitendinosus
16. 耻骨肌 pectineus
17. 大收肌 adductor magnus
18. 阴道静脉丛 vaginaal venous plexus
19. 阴道 vaginaa
20. 肛门外括约肌 sphincter ani externus
21. 肛门 anus
22. 股薄肌 gracilis
23. 半膜肌肌腱 tendon of semimembranosus
24. 坐骨神经 sciatic nerve
25. 臀下动脉 inferior gluteal artery
26. 股方肌 quadratus femoris
27. 阔筋膜 fasciae lata
28. 阔筋膜张肌 tensor fasciae latae
29. 旋股外侧动脉 lateral femoral circumflex artery
30. 股动脉 femoral artery
31. 股静脉 femoral vein
32. 股深静脉 deep femoral vein
33. 股深动脉 deep femoral artery
34. 髂腰肌 iliopsoas

女性盆部与会阴连续横断层 85（FH.7690）

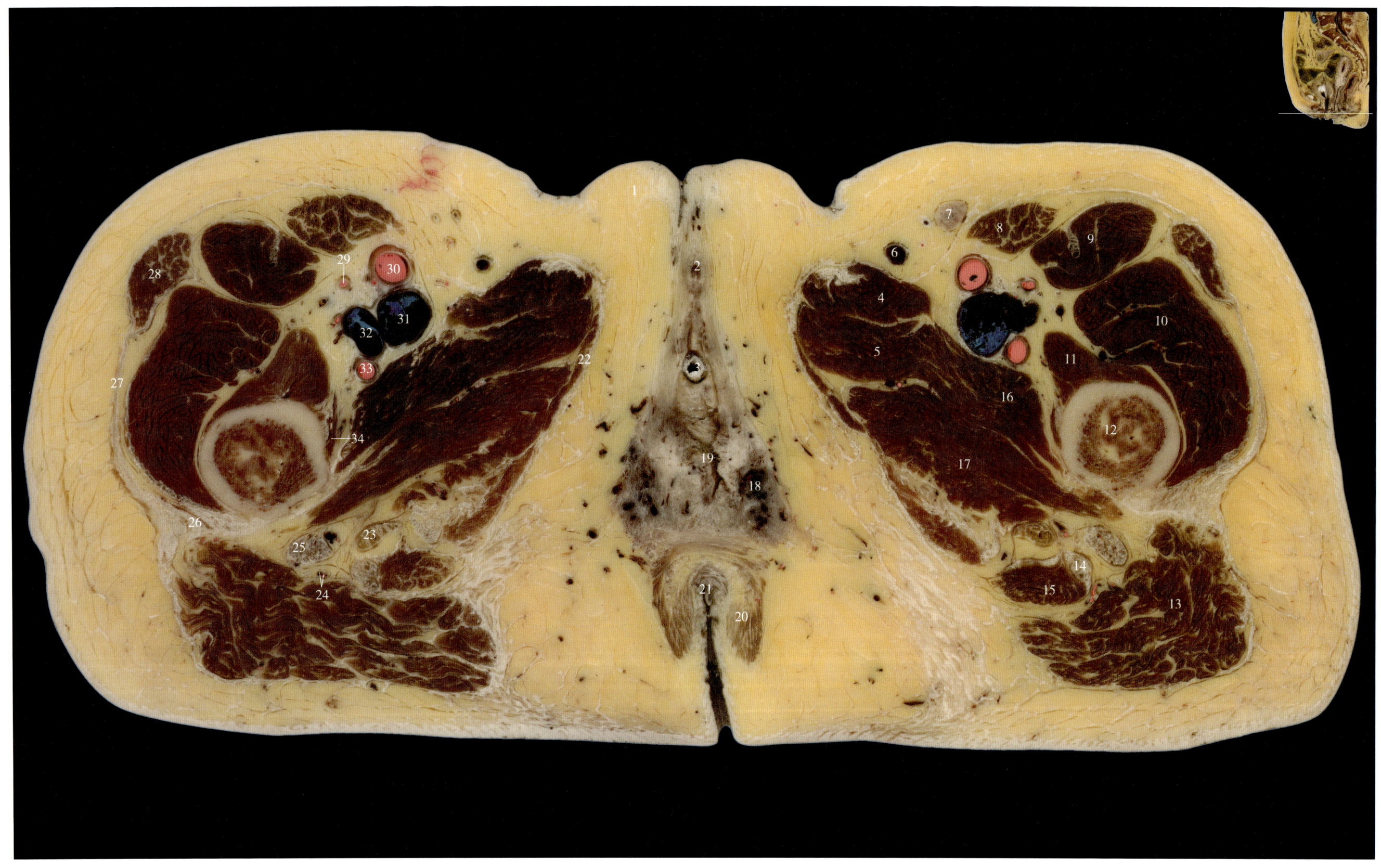

A. 断层标本图像

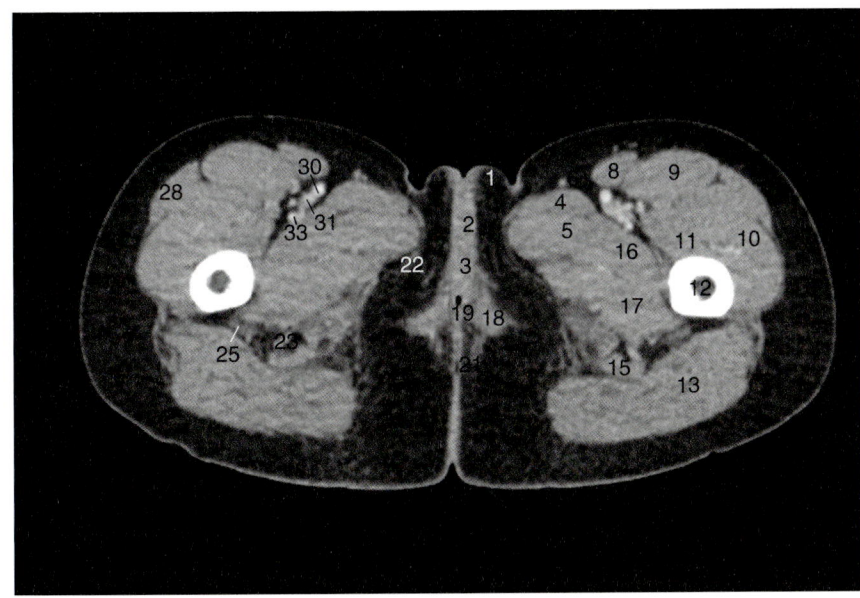
B. CT 增强图像

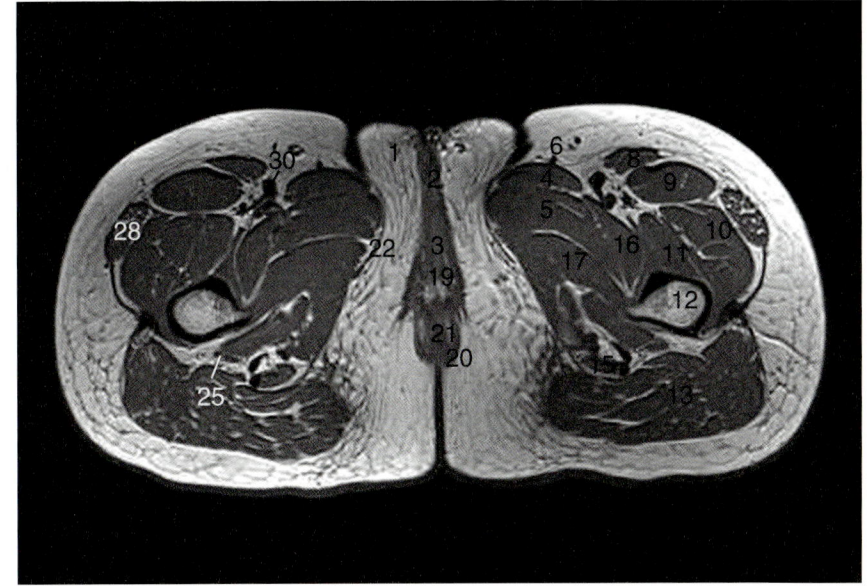
C. MR T1WI

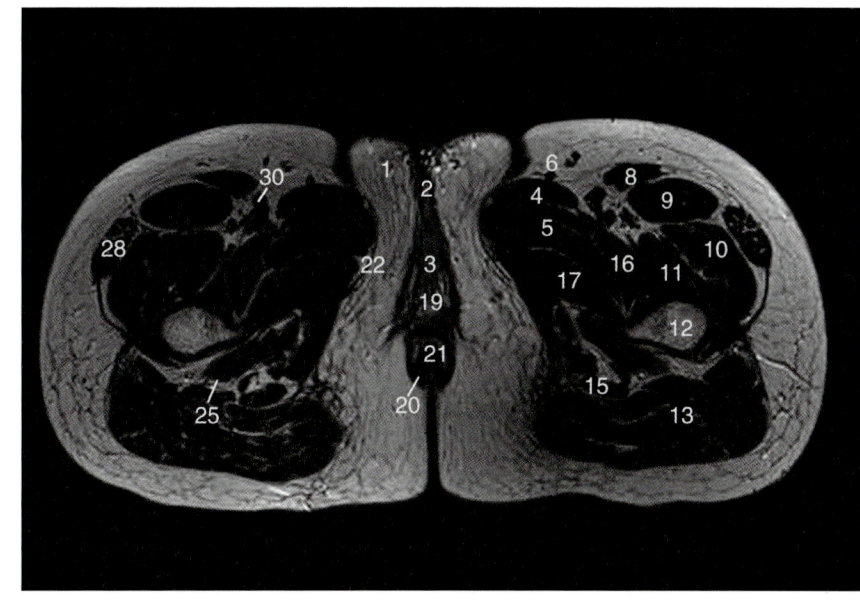
D. MR T2WI

1. 大阴唇 greater lip of pudendum
2. 阴蒂 clitoris
3. 尿道 urethra
4. 长收肌 adductor longus
5. 短收肌 adductor brevis
6. 大隐静脉 great saphenous vein
7. 腹股沟浅淋巴结 superficial inguinal lymph nodes
8. 缝匠肌 sartorius
9. 股直肌 rectus femoris
10. 股外侧肌 vastus lateralis
11. 股中间肌 vastus intermedius
12. 股骨 femur
13. 臀大肌 gluteus maximus
14. 股二头肌长头 long head of biceps femoris
15. 半腱肌 semitendinosus
16. 耻骨肌 pectineus
17. 大收肌 adductor magnus
18. 阴道静脉丛 vaginaal venous plexus
19. 阴道 vaginaa
20. 肛门外括约肌 sphincter ani externus
21. 肛门 anus
22. 股薄肌 gracilis
23. 半膜肌肌腱 tendon of semimembranosus
24. 臀下动、静脉 inferior gluteal artery and vein
25. 坐骨神经 sciatic nerve
26. 股外侧肌间隔 lateral femoral intermuscular septum
27. 阔筋膜 fasciae lata
28. 阔筋膜张肌 tensor fasciae latae
29. 旋股外侧动脉降支 descending branch of lateral femoral circumflex artery
30. 股动脉 femoral artery
31. 股静脉 femoral vein
32. 股深静脉 deep femoral vein
33. 股深动脉 deep femoral artery
34. 髂腰肌 iliopsoas

关键结构：阴道，大阴唇，阴蒂。

此断面经阴蒂中部。

断面中部最前份为大阴唇，中份有阴蒂、尿道和阴道。此断面阴道呈纵裂状，已接近末端。阴道常见的疾病有先天性异常、瘤样病变、良性肿瘤和恶性肿瘤。阴道恶性肿瘤转移途径有[21]：①淋巴转移，阴道上 1/3 淋巴转移途径与宫颈癌相似，主要经闭孔和髂内淋巴结向盆腔外侧和后侧淋巴结转移。阴道中段肿瘤向盆腔外侧淋巴结转移，阴道下 1/3 和远侧端，则向股部和腹股沟淋巴结转移。以上淋巴引流网络间存在吻合网和交通支。②直接浸润，阴道癌经局部浸润可扩散至阴道旁、膀胱旁和子宫旁组织，或经直肠阴道隔扩散至直肠和肛门。向上则浸润至宫颈，向下则浸润至外阴部。当肿瘤扩散至邻近器官组织或肛门时，临床则很难确定其原发癌灶。③血行转移，发生于晚期病例，可转移至远处器官。

女性盆部与会阴连续横断层 86（FH.7670）

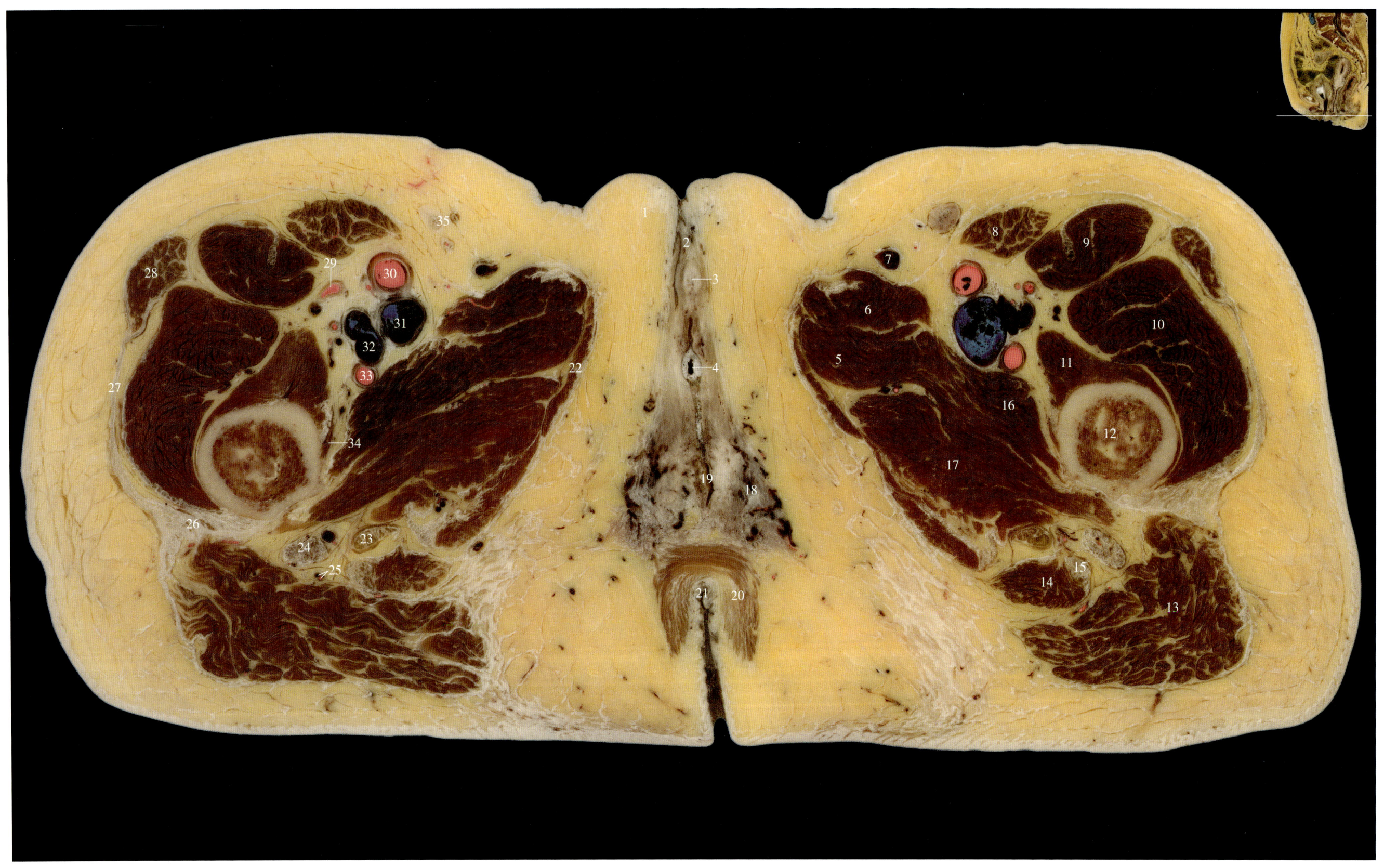

A. 断层标本图像

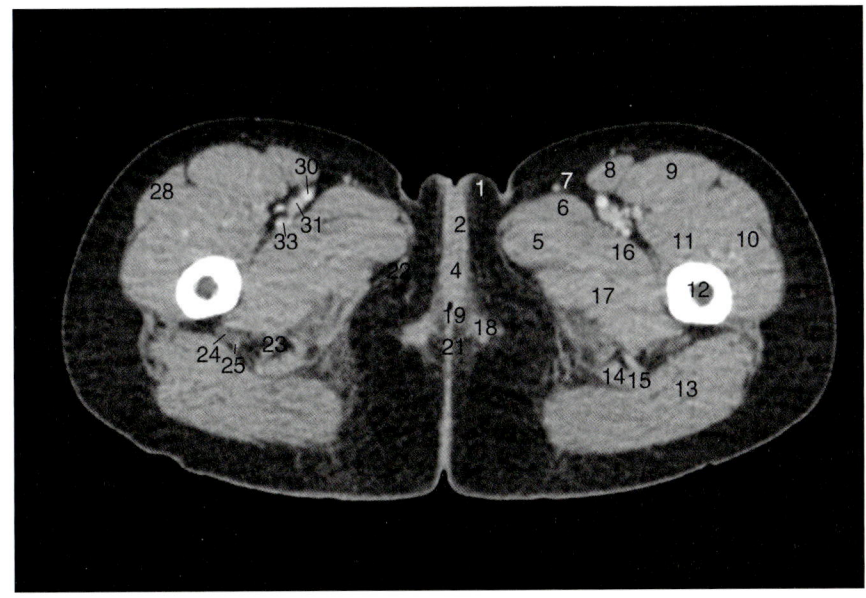

B. CT 增强图像

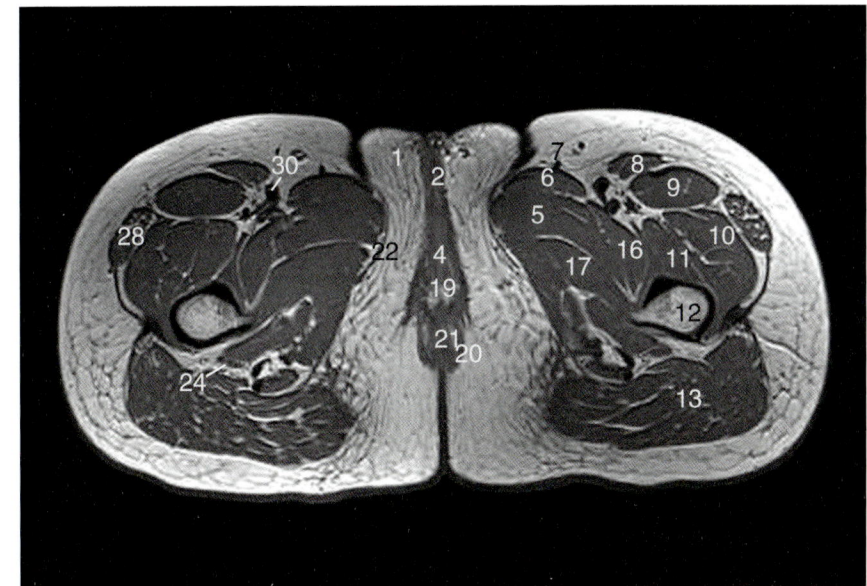

C. MR T1WI

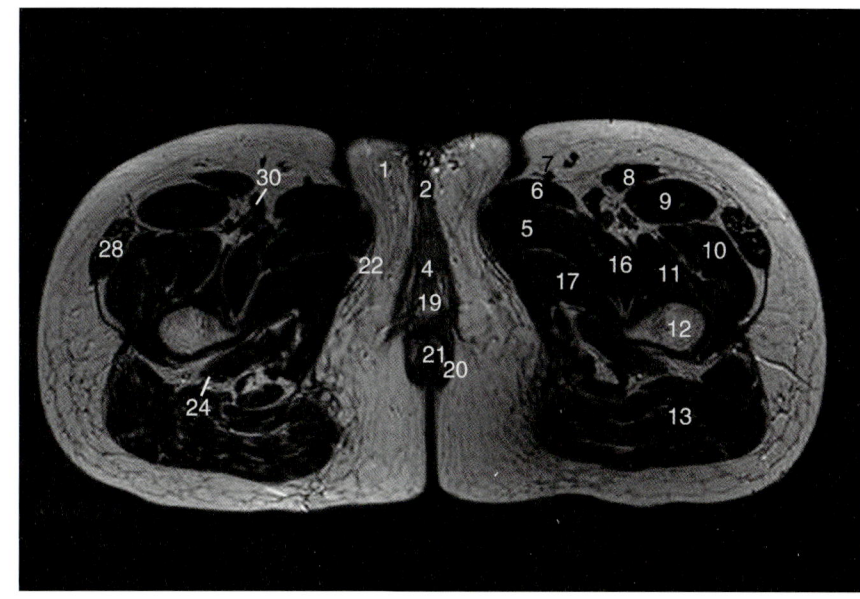

D. MR T2WI

1. 大阴唇 greater lip of pudendum
2. 阴蒂 clitoris
3. 阴蒂海绵体 cavernous body of clitoris
4. 尿道 urethra
5. 短收肌 adductor brevis
6. 长收肌 adductor longus
7. 大隐静脉 great saphenous vein
8. 缝匠肌 sartorius
9. 股直肌 rectus femoris
10. 股外侧肌 vastus lateralis
11. 股中间肌 vastus intermedius
12. 股骨 femur
13. 臀大肌 gluteus maximus
14. 半腱肌 semitendinosus
15. 股二头肌长头 long head of biceps femoris
16. 耻骨肌 pectineus
17. 大收肌 adductor magnus
18. 阴道静脉丛 vaginaal venous plexus
19. 阴道口 vaginaal orifice
20. 肛门外括约肌 sphincter ani externus
21. 肛门 anus
22. 股薄肌 gracilis
23. 半膜肌肌腱 tendon of semimembranosus
24. 坐骨神经 sciatic nerve
25. 臀下动、静脉 inferior gluteal artery and vein
26. 股外侧肌间隔 lateral femoral intermuscular septum
27. 阔筋膜 fasciae lata
28. 阔筋膜张肌 tensor fasciae latae
29. 旋股外侧动脉降支 descending branch of lateral femoral circumflex artery
30. 股动脉 femoral artery
31. 股静脉 femoral vein
32. 股深静脉 deep femoral vein
33. 股深动脉 deep femoral artery
34. 髂腰肌 iliopsoas
35. 腹股沟浅淋巴结 superficial inguinal lymph nodes

关键结构：阴道，阴蒂，肛门括约肌。

　　此断面经阴蒂中份。断面中部最前方为大阴唇，两侧大阴唇间的阴裂内可见阴蒂。向后依次有尿道、阴道和肛门。阴道壁由黏膜、肌层和纤维组织外膜构成。阴道黏膜覆盖复层鳞状上皮细胞，无腺体。阴道疾病分类有：阴道瘤样病变、阴道良性肿瘤、阴道恶性肿瘤及阴道先天性异常。阴道上部两侧有丰富的静脉丛、神经丛、子宫动脉的阴道支和输尿管，及阴道旁结缔组织。前壁的上 2/3 与膀胱壁之间隔以疏松的膀胱阴道隔，隔内有静脉丛和结缔组织。阴道后壁中部借一薄层与直肠壶腹相贴。因此肿瘤如位于阴道穹隆上部或前后壁，手术时应预防损伤周围的输尿管、膀胱及直肠。由于阴道前为尿道、膀胱、输尿管，后为直肠，毗邻关系密切，其间隔厚度不超过 5 mm，器官之间无疏松组织，因而发生阴道癌后，其相邻组织器官极易受到浸润。因此术前要考虑到可能切除部分邻近器官，以达到彻底切除病灶的目的。阴道与尿道、膀胱之间的界限不明显，分离时可用剪刀锐性分离并注意创面止血。尿道外口允许切除 2 cm，但要注意避免损伤尿道内口及三角区，以免产生尿失禁或尿道瘘。由于阴道与直肠之间组织较疏松，易于分离，若损伤直肠也容易成功修补[21]。

女性盆部与会阴连续横断层 87（FH.7650）

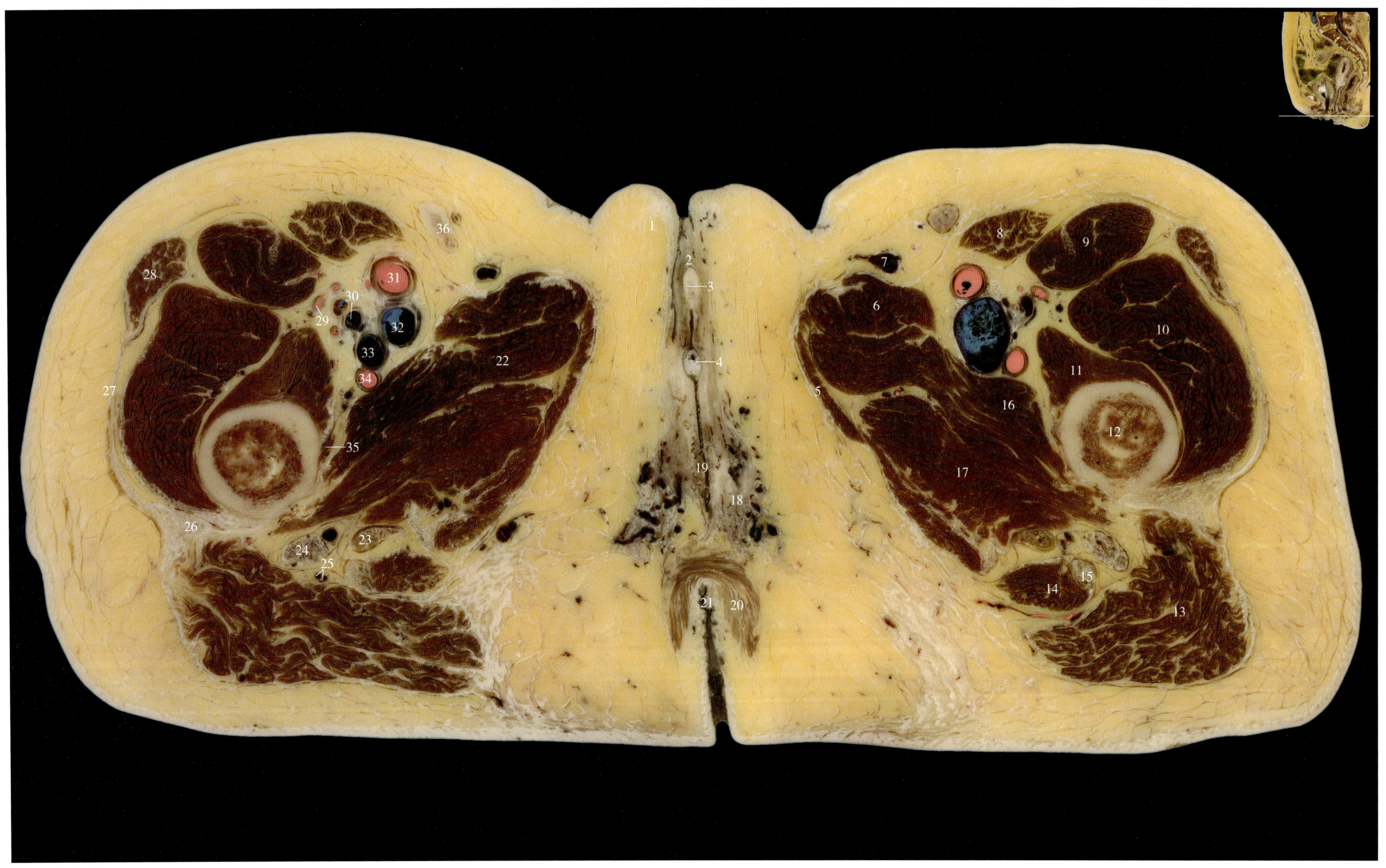

A. 断层标本图像

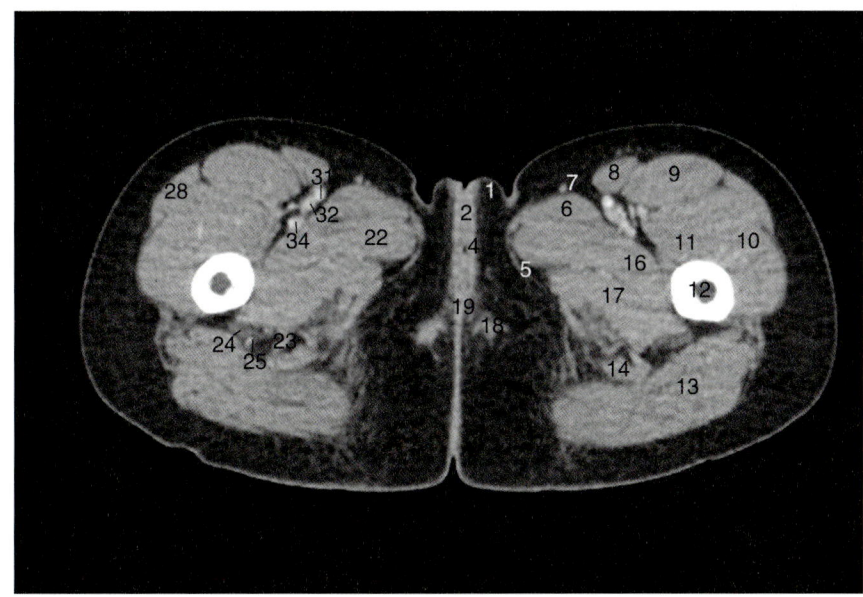
B. CT 增强图像

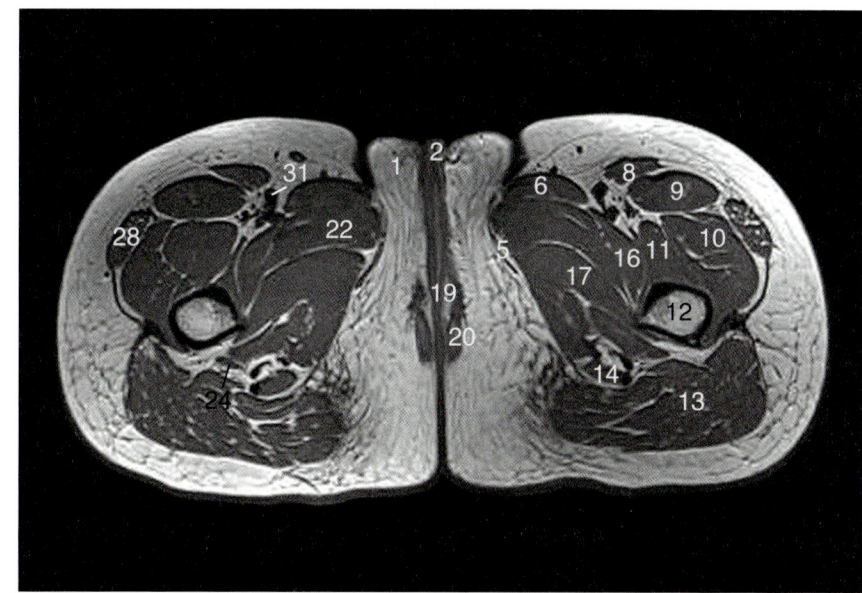
C. MR T1WI

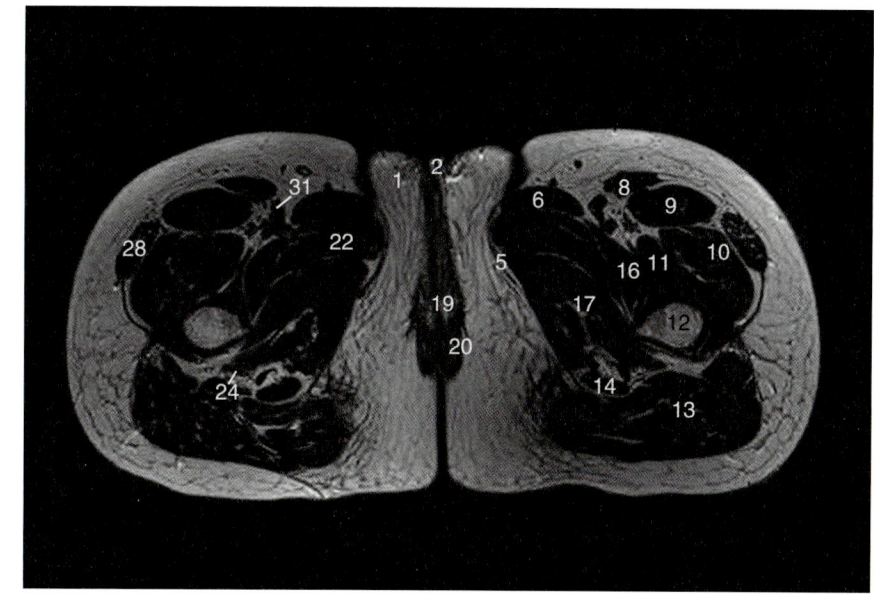
D. MR T2WI

1. 大阴唇 greater lip of pudendum
2. 阴蒂 clitoris
3. 阴蒂海绵体 cavernous body of clitoris
4. 尿道 urethra
5. 股薄肌 gracilis
6. 长收肌 adductor longus
7. 大隐静脉 great saphenous vein
8. 缝匠肌 sartorius
9. 股直肌 rectus femoris
10. 股外侧肌 vastus lateralis
11. 股中间肌 vastus intermedius
12. 股骨 femur
13. 臀大肌 gluteus maximus
14. 半腱肌 semitendinosus
15. 股二头肌长头 long head of biceps femoris
16. 耻骨肌 pectineus
17. 大收肌 adductor magnus
18. 阴道静脉丛 vaginaal venous plexus
19. 阴道口 vaginaal orifice
20. 肛门外括约肌 sphincter ani externus
21. 肛门 anus
22. 短收肌 adductor brevis
23. 半膜肌肌腱 tendon of semimembranosus
24. 坐骨神经 sciatic nerve
25. 臀下动、静脉 inferior gluteal artery and vein
26. 股外侧肌间隔 lateral femoral intermuscular septum
27. 阔筋膜 fasciae lata
28. 阔筋膜张肌 tensor fasciae latae
29. 旋股外侧动脉降支 descending branch of lateral femoral circumflex artery
30. 旋股外侧静脉降支 descending tributary of lateral femoral circumflex vein
31. 股动脉 femoral artery
32. 股静脉 femoral vein
33. 股深静脉 deep femoral vein
34. 股深动脉 deep femoral artery
35. 髂腰肌 iliopsoas
36. 腹股沟浅淋巴结 superficial inguinal lymph nodes

关键结构：尿道，阴道，阴道前庭。

此断面经阴蒂中份。断面中部最前方为大阴唇，两侧大阴唇间的阴裂内可见阴蒂。阴道前庭呈纵裂隙状位于断面中央。阴道前庭是位于两侧小阴唇之间的裂隙，前后两端狭窄，中部宽大。前端较尖锐达阴蒂，后端较钝圆，后界为阴唇系带。阴道前庭的中央有阴道口，阴道口周围有处女膜或处女膜痕。尿道外口较小，位于阴道口的前方、阴蒂的后下方，距阴蒂头约 2.5 cm，一般为短的矢状裂隙，周缘隆起呈乳头状。尿道外口后外侧，往往有小的开口，为尿道旁腺管口。此外，在阴道口的后外侧，左、右各有一个前庭大腺排泄管的开口。前庭小腺的开口位于尿道外口及阴道口附近。阴道口后端与阴唇系带间有一小陷窝，名舟状窝。此窝在未产妇显著，经产妇多不明显。阴道前庭后部是直肠瘘管常见的开口部位，可以在先天性直肠闭锁的女性中见到[5, 30]。

女性盆部与会阴连续横断层 88（FH.7630）

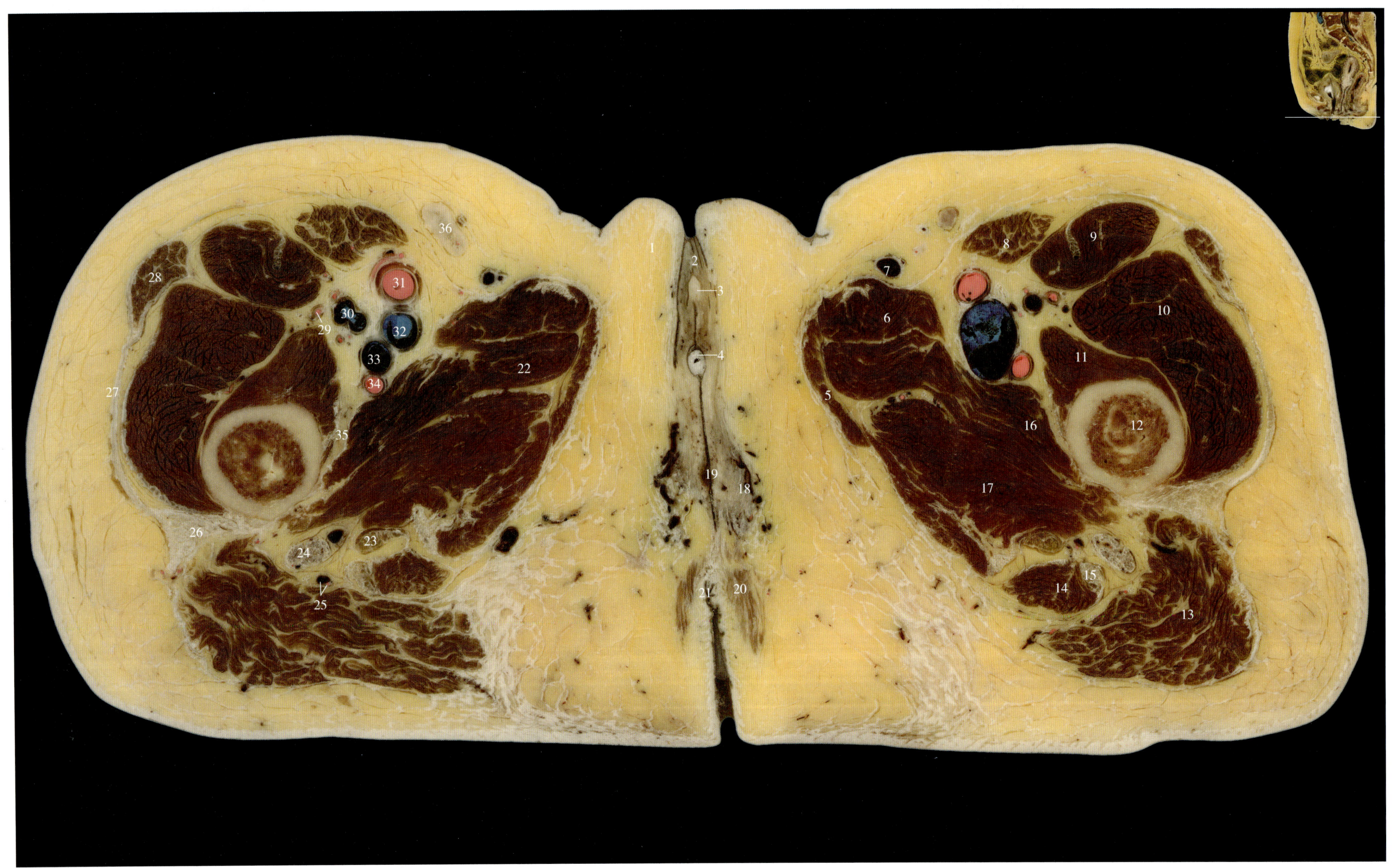

A. 断层标本图像

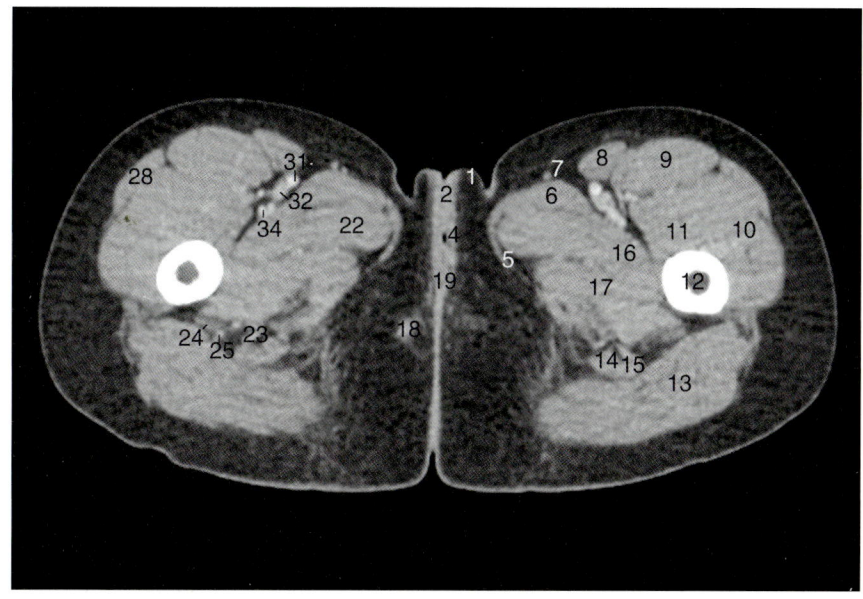

B. CT 增强图像

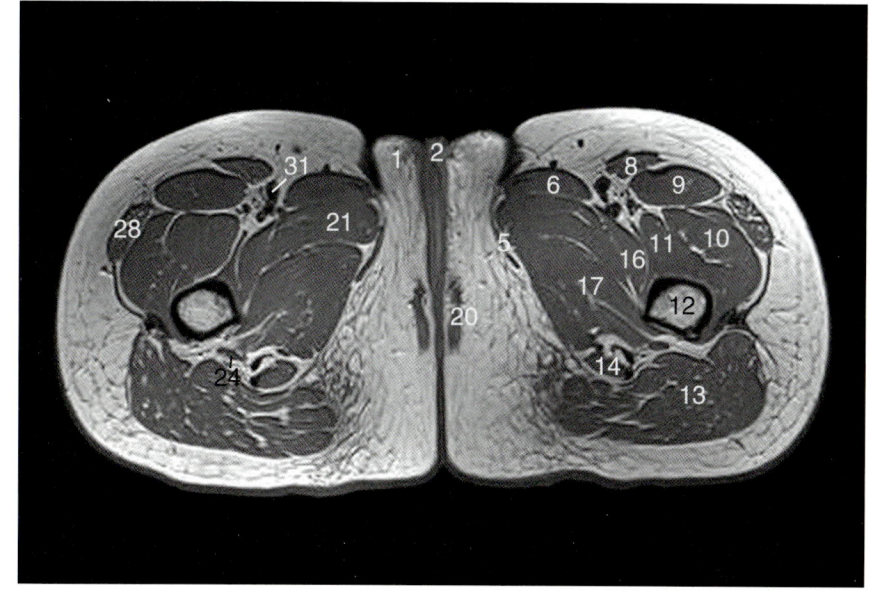

C. MR T1WI

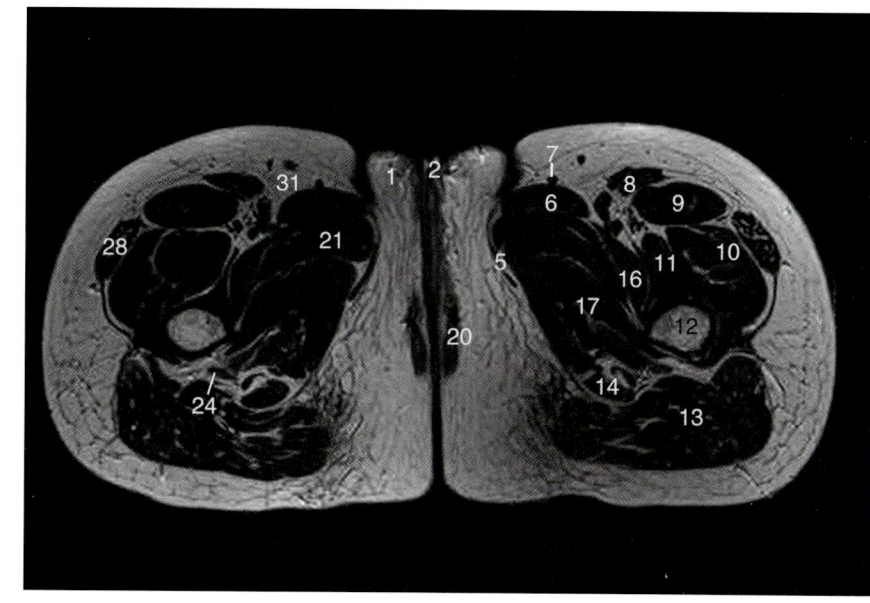

D. MR T2WI

1. 大阴唇 greater lip of pudendum
2. 阴蒂 clitoris
3. 阴蒂海绵体 cavernous body of clitoris
4. 尿道 urethra
5. 股薄肌 gracilis
6. 长收肌 adductor longus
7. 大隐静脉 great saphenous vein
8. 缝匠肌 sartorius
9. 股直肌 rectus femoris
10. 股外侧肌 vastus lateralis
11. 股中间肌 vastus intermedius
12. 股骨 femur
13. 臀大肌 gluteus maximus
14. 半腱肌 semitendinosus
15. 股二头肌长头 long head of biceps femoris
16. 耻骨肌 pectineus
17. 大收肌 adductor magnus
18. 阴道静脉丛 vaginaal venous plexus
19. 阴道前庭 vaginaal vestibule
20. 肛门外括约肌 sphincter ani externus
21. 肛门 anus
22. 短收肌 adductor brevis
23. 半膜肌肌腱 tendon of semimembranosus
24. 坐骨神经 sciatic nerve
25. 臀下动、静脉 inferior gluteal artery and vein
26. 股外侧肌间隔 lateral femoral intermuscular septum
27. 阔筋膜 fasciae lata
28. 阔筋膜张肌 tensor fasciae latae
29. 旋股外侧动脉降支 descending branch of lateral femoral circumflex artery
30. 旋股外侧静脉降支 descending tributary of lateral femoral circumflex vein
31. 股动脉 femoral artery
32. 股静脉 femoral vein
33. 股深静脉 deep femoral vein
34. 股深动脉 deep femoral artery
35. 股内侧肌间隔 medial femoral intermuscular septum
36. 腹股沟浅淋巴结 superficial inguinal lymph nodes

关键结构：大阴唇，阴蒂，阴道口。

此断面经阴蒂下份。断面两侧为经股骨体上份断面结构。中部为女阴的结构：最前方仍旧为大阴唇，中间为阴道前庭，在阴蒂的后方有尿道外口和阴道口。后方有肛门和肛门外括约肌。在股前肌群中，在股中间肌的内侧开始出现股内侧肌的细小截面，在下方的断面中截面逐渐增大。生殖器官的发育约始于胚胎第 5 周，此时泄殖腔两侧形成皱褶，向前汇合于中线形成生殖结节。随着泄殖腔被尿直肠隔及随后形成的会阴所分隔，前方的泄殖腔褶称为泌尿生殖褶，而后方的称为肛门褶。胚胎第 7 周，发育开始出现性别差异，在女性胚胎中，生殖结节生长缓慢，成为阴蒂；泌尿生殖褶形成小阴唇。在男性胚胎中，生殖结节持续生长，形成阴茎；泌尿生殖褶相互融合，包绕阴茎尿道。在泌尿生殖褶外侧，形成另外一对隆起，在未分化期称为阴唇阴囊突。在没有雄激素的情况下，这对隆突不融合，形成大阴唇。泌尿生殖窦最终发育为阴道前庭，尿道、阴道和前庭大腺开口于此[21, 40]。

177

女性盆部与会阴连续横断层 89（FH.7610）

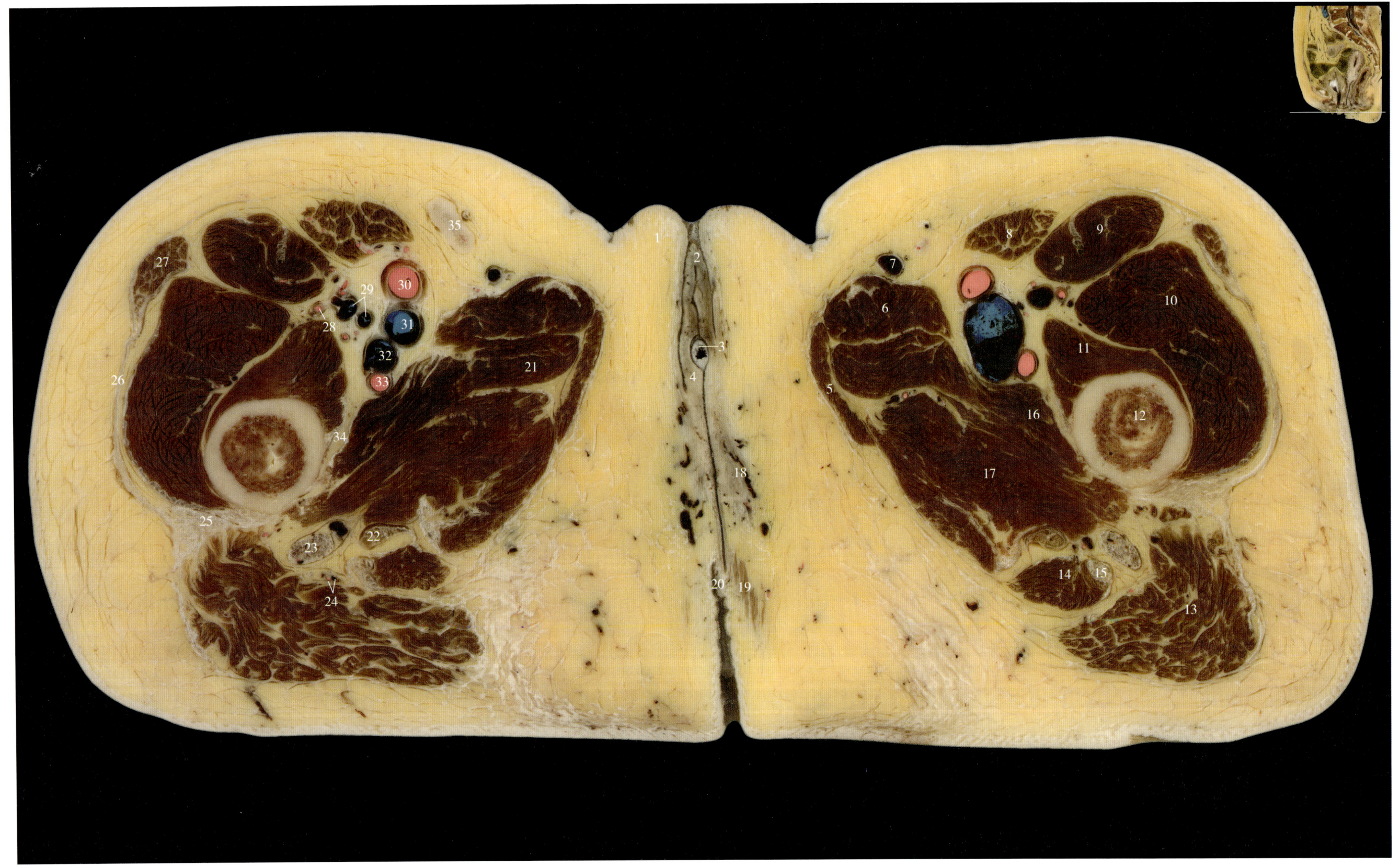

A. 断层标本图像

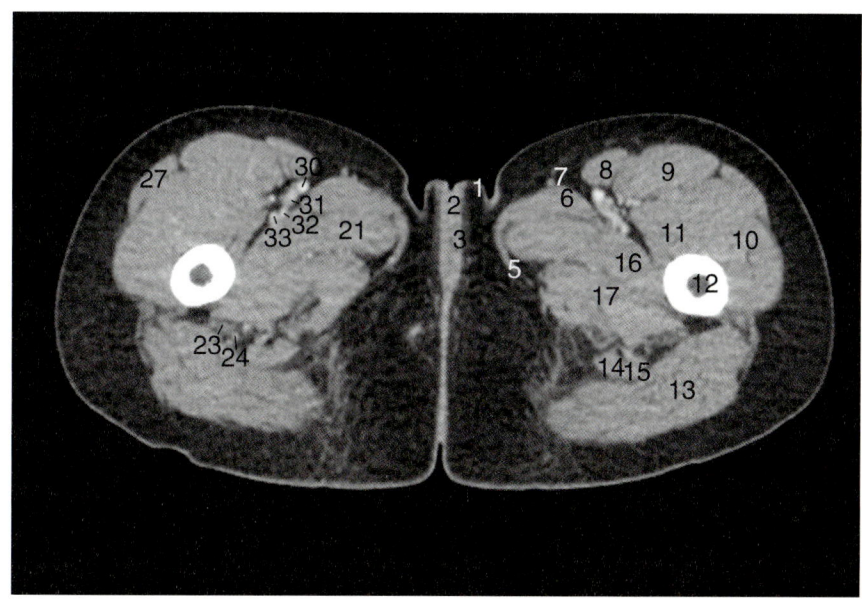
B. CT 增强图像

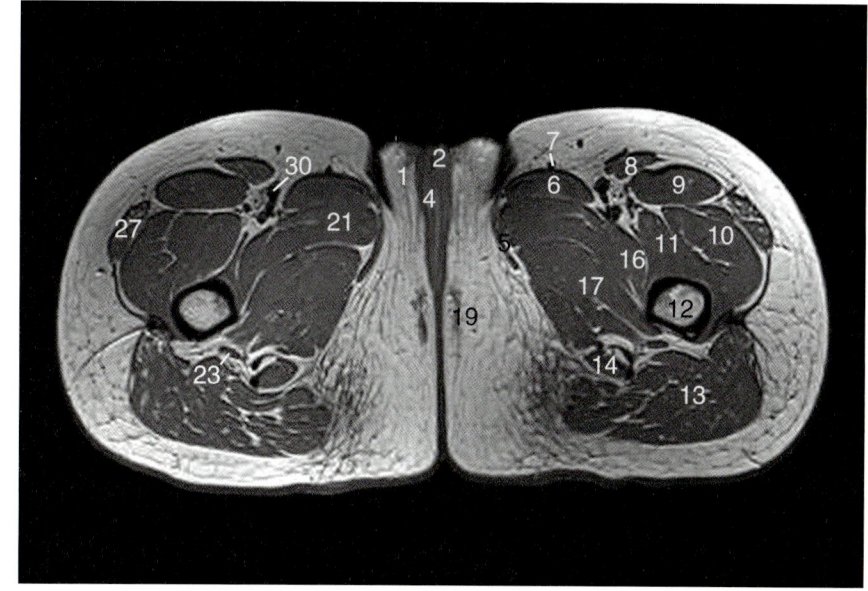
C. MR T1WI

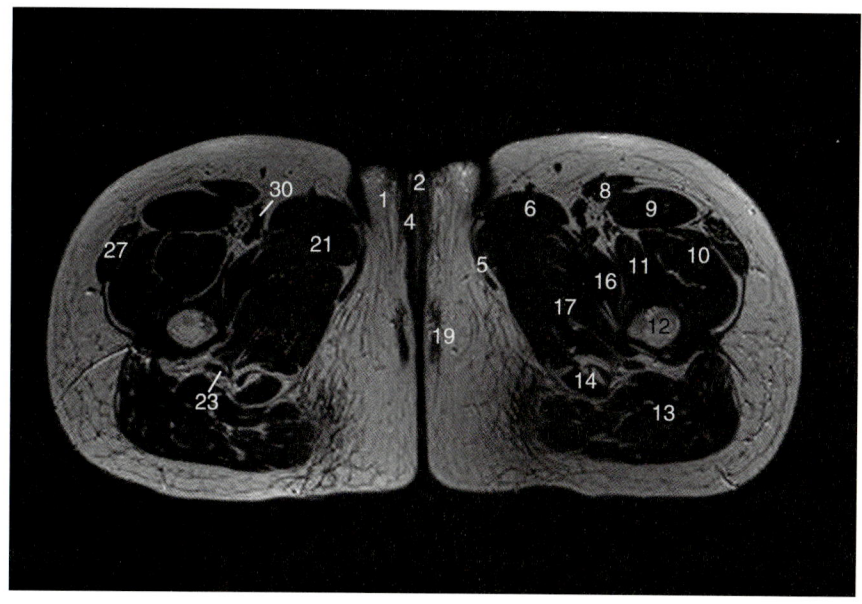
D. MR T2WI

1. 大阴唇 greater lip of pudendum
2. 阴蒂 clitoris
3. 尿道外口 external orifice of urethra
4. 小阴唇 lesser lip of pudendum
5. 股薄肌 gracilis
6. 长收肌 adductor longus
7. 大隐静脉 great saphenous vein
8. 缝匠肌 sartorius
9. 股直肌 rectus femoris
10. 股外侧肌 vastus lateralis
11. 股中间肌 vastus intermedius
12. 股骨 femur
13. 臀大肌 gluteus maximus
14. 半腱肌 semitendinosus
15. 股二头肌长头 long head of biceps femoris
16. 耻骨肌 pectineus
17. 大收肌 adductor magnus
18. 阴道静脉丛 vaginaal venous plexus
19. 肛门外括约肌 sphincter ani externus
20. 肛门 anus
21. 短收肌 adductor brevis
22. 半膜肌肌腱 tendon of semimembranosus
23. 坐骨神经 sciatic nerve
24. 臀下动、静脉 inferior gluteal artery and vein
25. 股外侧肌间隔 lateral femoral intermuscular septum
26. 阔筋膜 fasciae lata
27. 阔筋膜张肌 tensor fasciae latae
28. 旋股外侧动脉降支 descending branch of lateral femoral circumflex artery
29. 旋股外侧静脉降支 descending tributaries of lateral femoral circumflex vein
30. 股动脉 femoral artery
31. 股静脉 femoral vein
32. 股深静脉 deep femoral vein
33. 股深动脉 deep femoral artery
34. 股内侧肌间隔 medial femoral intermuscular septum
35. 腹股沟浅淋巴结 superficial inguinal lymph nodes

关键结构：小阴唇，大阴唇，尿道外口。

此断面经阴蒂下份。在断面中央前份可见大、小阴唇和阴蒂，小阴唇位于大阴唇内侧，是一对纵长隆起的皮肤皱襞，环绕阴道口左右，呈唇状。在前方小阴唇分叉，其上层行于阴蒂上方，与对侧相连形成的皱襞称阴蒂包皮，悬于阴蒂的上方；其下层在阴蒂下方与对侧一起形成阴蒂系带。后端两侧互相汇合形成阴唇系带。小阴唇相对面的皮脂腺数目较多，有时在一侧或两侧小阴唇和大阴唇之间可发现额外的阴唇皱襞（第三阴唇）。小阴唇之间粘连在青春期前的女性很常见，可能诱发泌尿系统感染[5]。

女性盆部与会阴连续横断层 90（FH.7590）

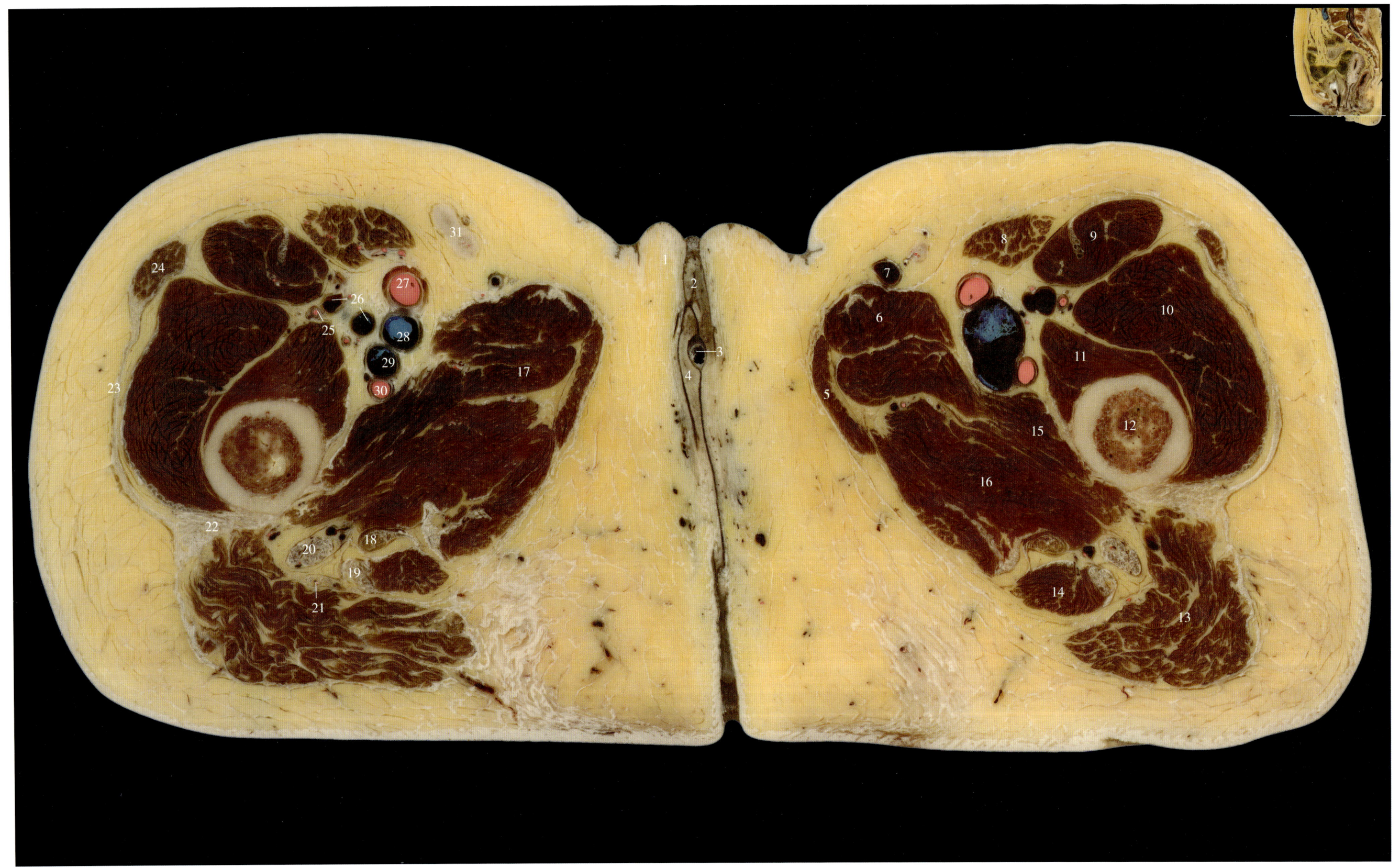

A. 断层标本图像

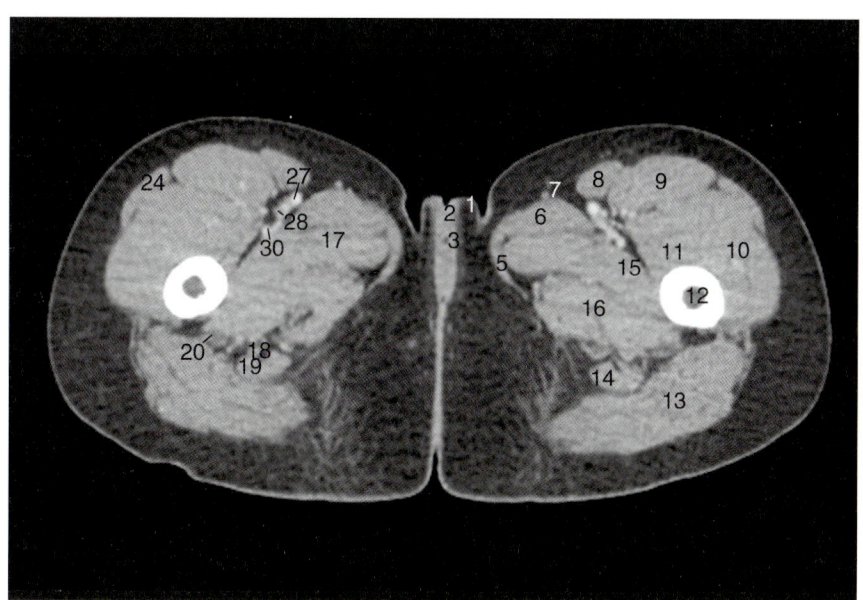

B. CT 增强图像

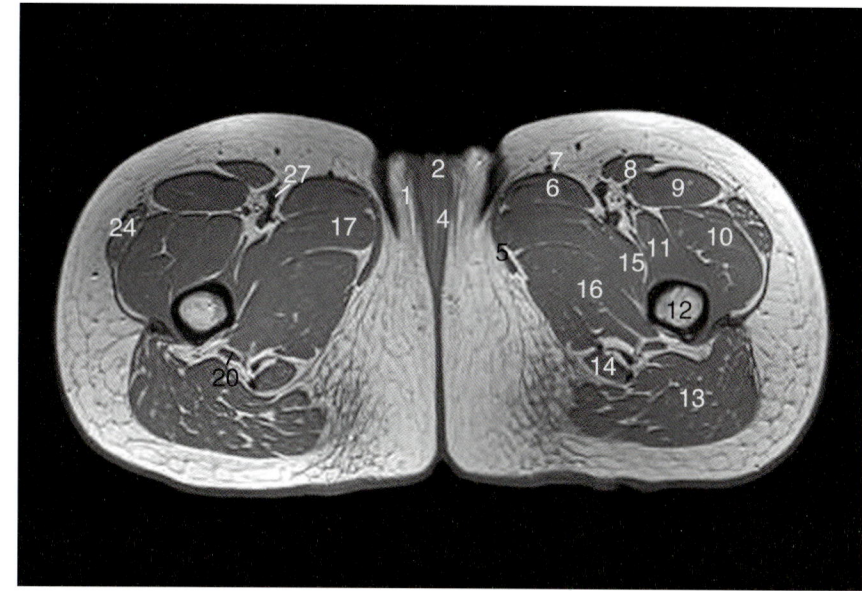

C. MR T1WI

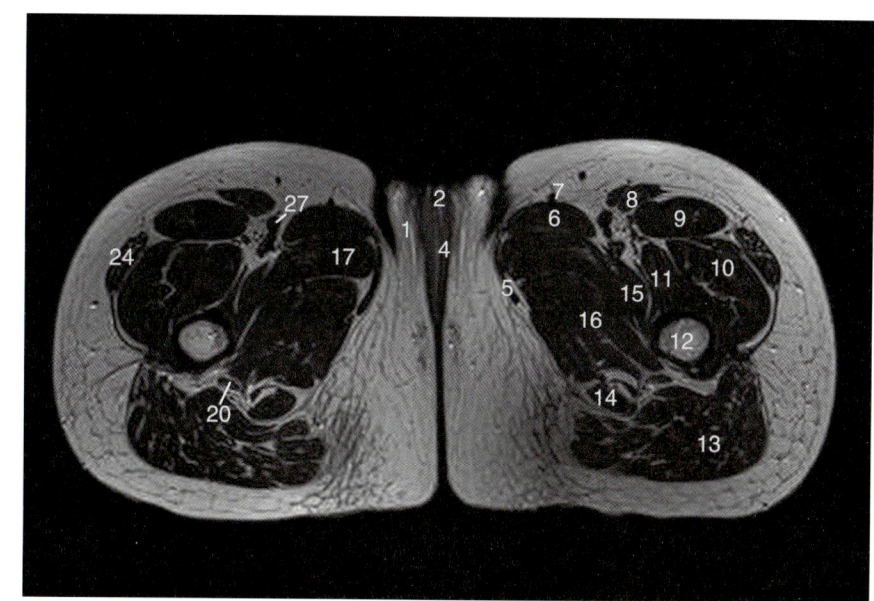

D. MR T2WI

1. 大阴唇 greater lip of pudendum
2. 阴蒂 clitoris
3. 尿道外口 external orifice of urethra
4. 小阴唇 lesser lip of pudendum
5. 股薄肌 gracilis
6. 长收肌 adductor longus
7. 大隐静脉 great saphenous vein
8. 缝匠肌 sartorius
9. 股直肌 rectus femoris
10. 股外侧肌 vastus lateralis
11. 股中间肌 vastus intermedius
12. 股骨 femur
13. 臀大肌 gluteus maximus
14. 半腱肌 semitendinosus
15. 耻骨肌 pectineus
16. 大收肌 adductor magnus
17. 短收肌 adductor brevis
18. 半膜肌肌腱 tendon of semimembranosus
19. 股二头肌长头 long head of biceps femoris
20. 坐骨神经 sciatic nerve
21. 臀下动脉 inferior gluteal artery
22. 股外侧肌间隔 lateral femoral intermuscular septum
23. 阔筋膜 fasciae lata
24. 阔筋膜张肌 tensor fasciae latae
25. 旋股外侧动脉降支 descending branch of lateral femoral circumflex artery
26. 旋股外侧静脉降支 descending tributary of lateral femoral circumflex vein
27. 股动脉 femoral artery
28. 股静脉 femoral vein
29. 股深静脉 deep femoral vein
30. 股深动脉 deep femoral artery
31. 腹股沟浅淋巴结 superficial inguinal lymph nodes

关键结构：大阴唇，小阴唇，阴蒂。

此断面经阴蒂下份。在断面中央前份可见大、小阴唇和阴蒂，两侧小阴唇间的阴道前庭内仍可见尿道外口。女性外生殖器各器官形态随年龄而变化。胎儿大阴唇不发达，阴裂敞开，其内可见阴蒂、小阴唇及阴道前庭等结构。新生儿大阴唇已较发达。成年未婚女子的左、右大阴唇密接，阴裂闭合；小阴唇呈暗蓝色，较发达，阴道口狭小，处女膜清楚可见。婚后尤其是经产妇，处女膜破裂，形成处女膜痕，阴道口扩大，大阴唇失去弹力而变松弛，阴裂开大，阴道前后壁可突出于阴道前庭，以前壁突出较为显著。阴唇后连合和阴唇系带由于分娩受损，常出现瘢痕。老年妇女，大阴唇、小阴唇、阴蒂海绵体及前庭腺逐渐萎缩[30]。

女性盆部与会阴连续横断层 91（FH.7570）

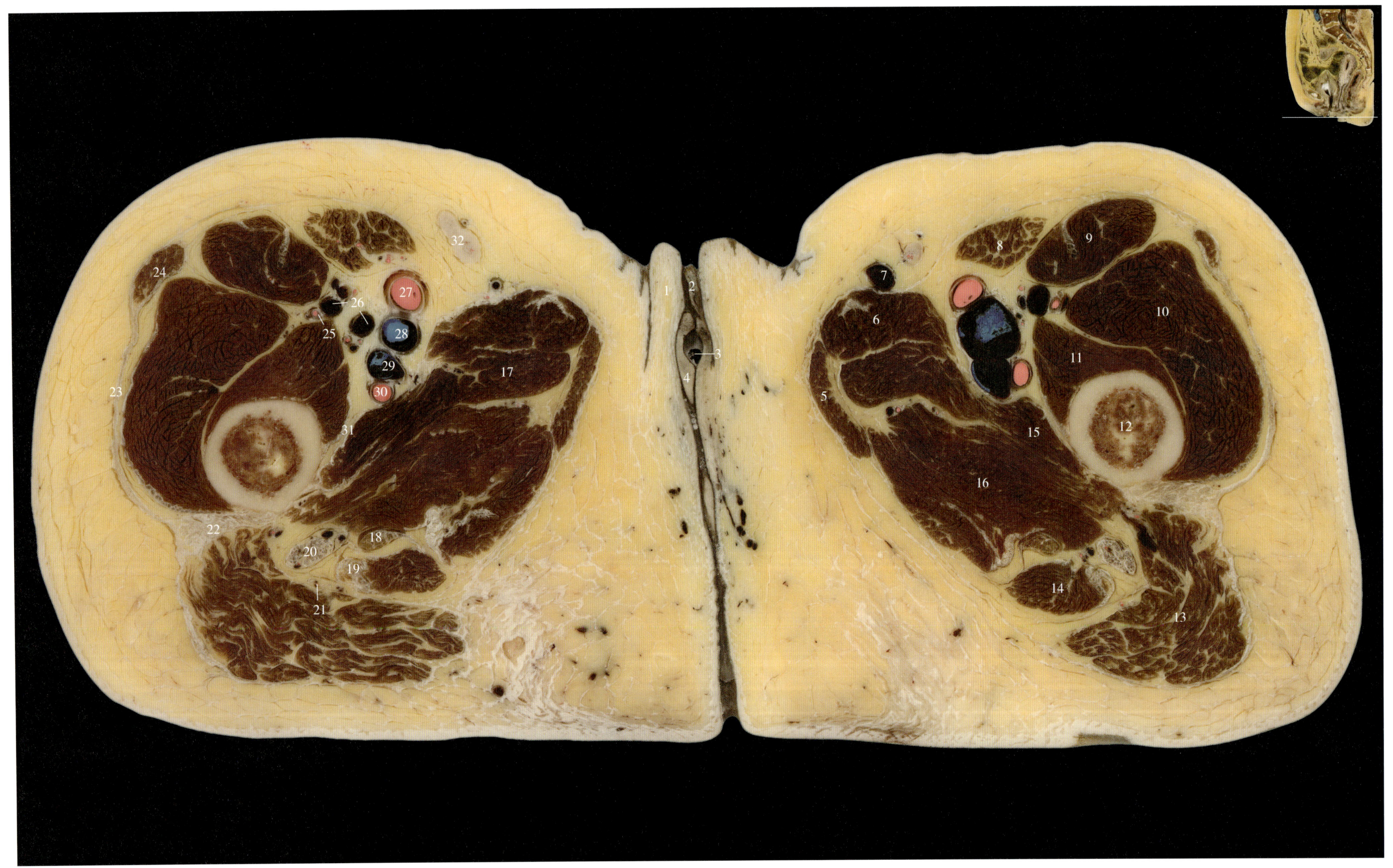

A. 断层标本图像

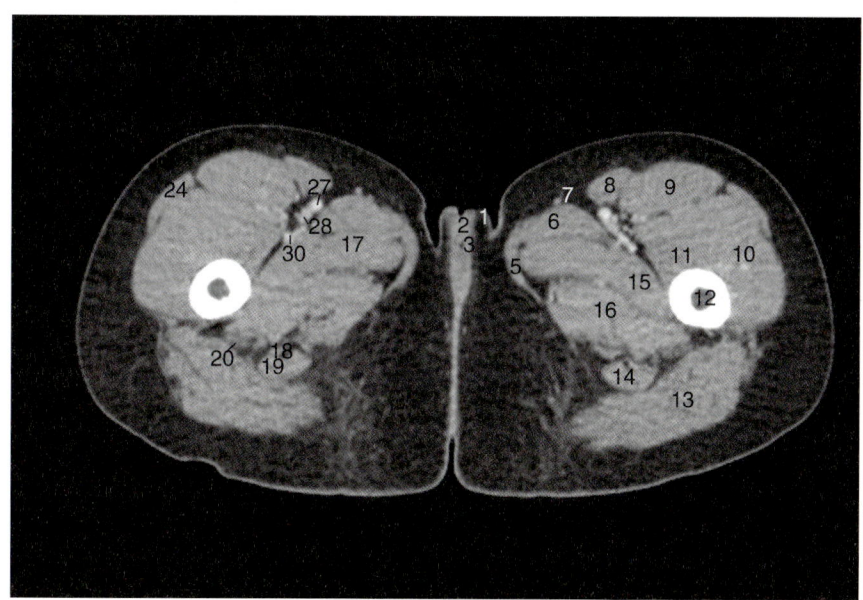

B. CT 增强图像

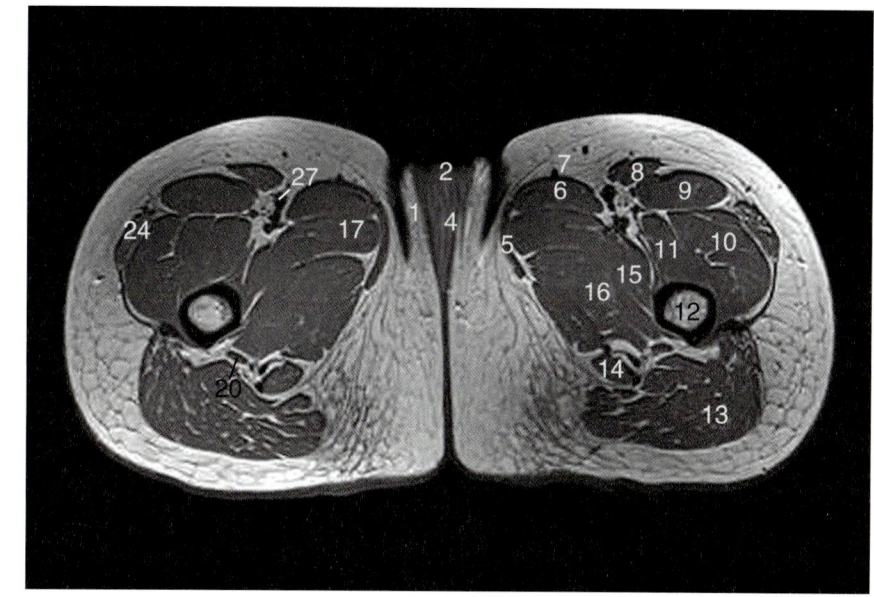

C. MR T1WI

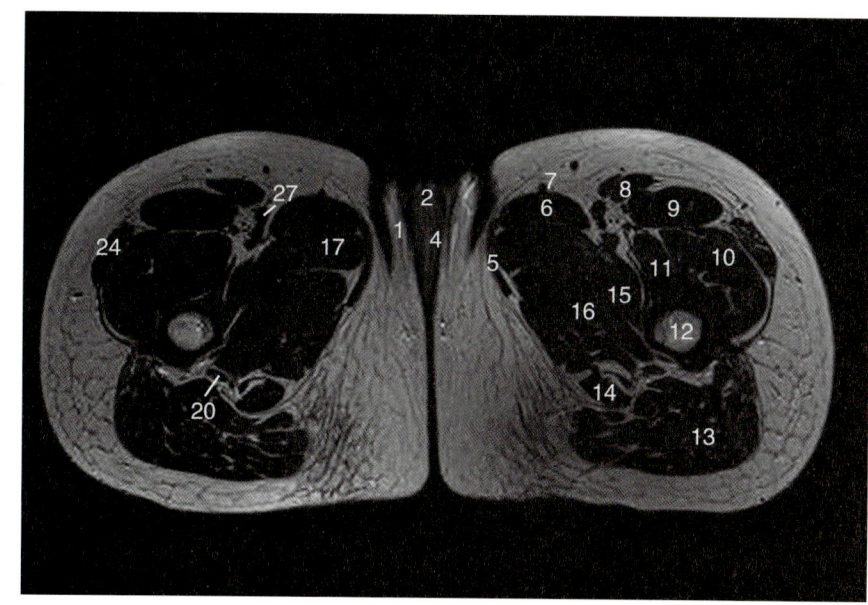

D. MR T2WI

1. 大阴唇 greater lip of pudendum
2. 阴蒂 clitoris
3. 尿道外口 external orifice of urethra
4. 小阴唇 lesser lip of pudendum
5. 股薄肌 gracilis
6. 长收肌 adductor longus
7. 大隐静脉 great saphenous vein
8. 缝匠肌 sartorius
9. 股直肌 rectus femoris
10. 股外侧肌 vastus lateralis
11. 股中间肌 vastus intermedius
12. 股骨 femur
13. 臀大肌 gluteus maximus
14. 半腱肌 semitendinosus
15. 耻骨肌 pectineus
16. 大收肌 adductor magnus
17. 短收肌 adductor brevis
18. 半膜肌肌腱 tendon of semimembranosus
19. 股二头肌长头 long head of biceps femoris
20. 坐骨神经 sciatic nerve
21. 臀下动脉 inferior gluteal artery
22. 股外侧肌间隔 lateral femoral intermuscular septum
23. 阔筋膜 fasciae lata
24. 阔筋膜张肌 tensor fasciae latae
25. 旋股外侧动脉降支 descending branch of lateral femoral circumflex artery
26. 旋股外侧静脉降支 descending tributary of lateral femoral circumflex vein
27. 股动脉 femoral artery
28. 股静脉 femoral vein
29. 股深静脉 deep femoral vein
30. 股深动脉 deep femoral artery
31. 股内侧肌间隔 medial femoral intermuscular septum
32. 腹股沟浅淋巴结 superficial inguinal lymph nodes

关键结构：大阴唇，小阴唇，阴蒂。

此断面经大、小阴唇下份。断面的中央前份为大、小阴唇和阴蒂的断面，两侧为经股骨体上份的大腿横断面。在股直肌、股外侧肌和股中间肌之间有旋股外侧动脉降支，其向下走行并发出分支营养股四头肌和膝关节。女性外生殖器由阴部内动脉的阴唇后动脉、前庭球动脉、阴蒂深动脉及阴蒂背动脉和股动脉发出的阴部外动脉的分支供血。女阴的静脉大部分入阴部内静脉，一部分入阴部外静脉。会阴部皮肤的静脉引流是通过阴部外静脉汇入大隐静脉的。前庭球的静脉汇入阴部内静脉、闭孔静脉及髂内静脉。阴蒂背浅静脉入阴部静脉丛。阴蒂背深静脉汇入阴部内静脉[5, 30]。

女性盆部与会阴连续横断层 92（FH.7550）

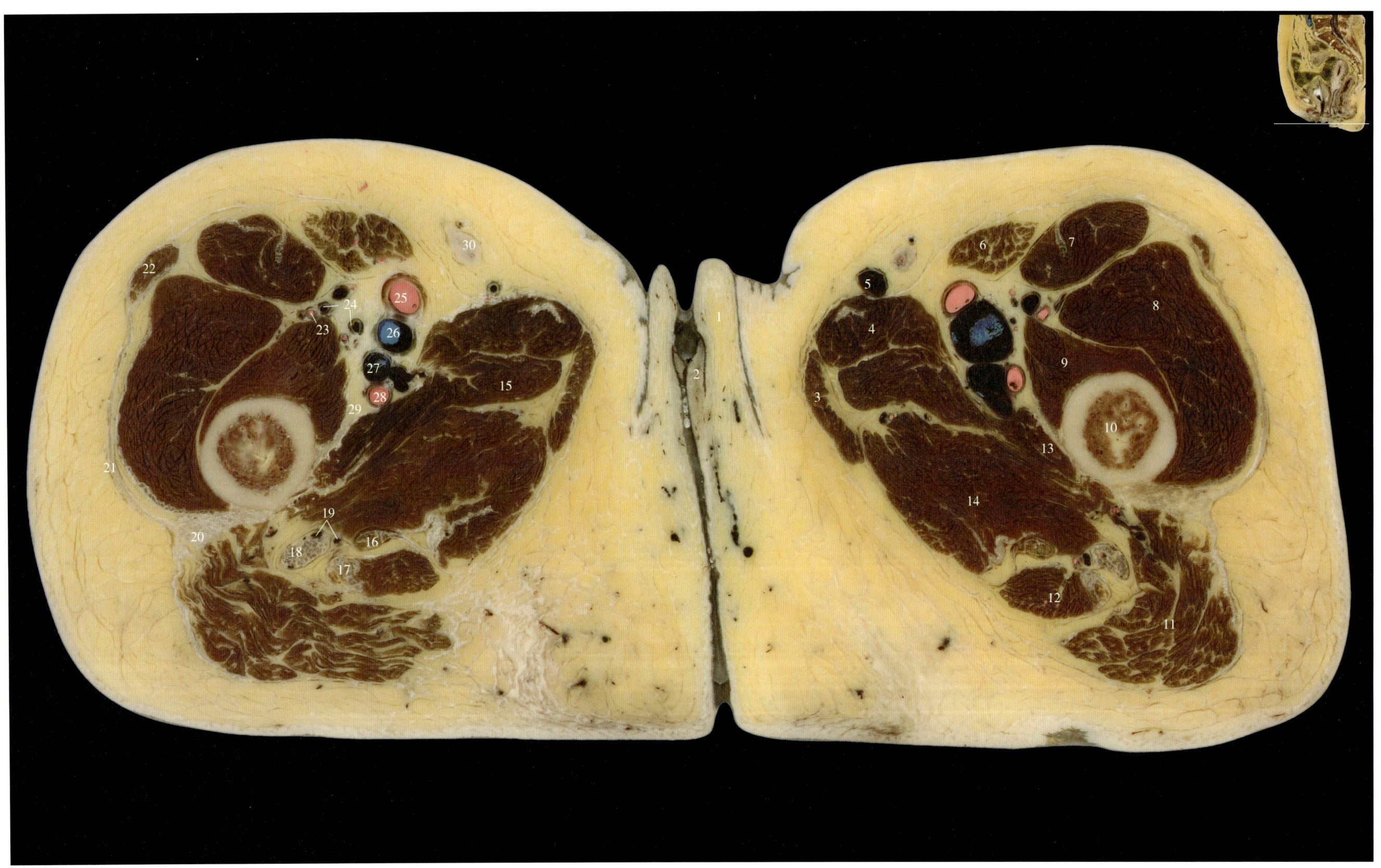

A. 断层标本图像

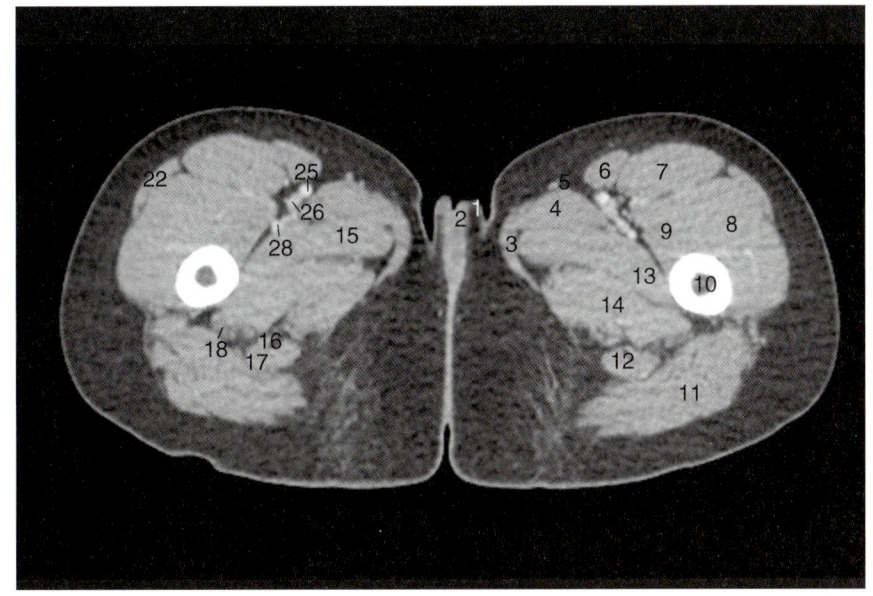

B. CT 增强图像

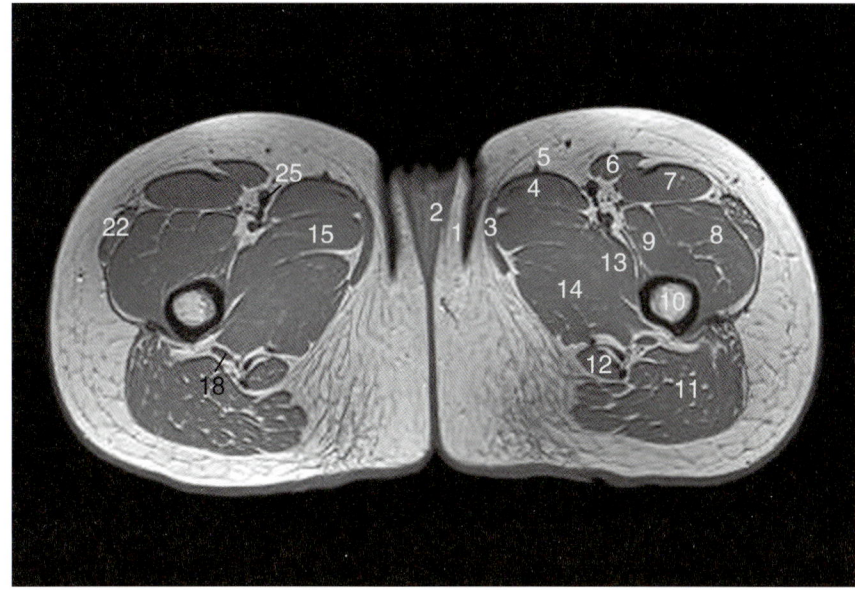

C. MR T1WI

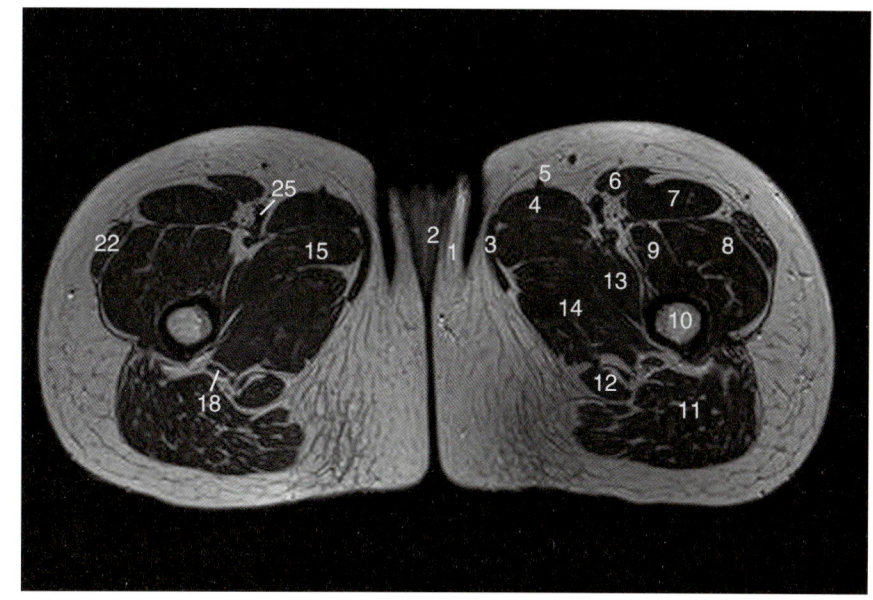

D. MR T2WI

关键结构：大阴唇，小阴唇。

此断面经大、小阴唇下部。整个断面可明显分为三部分，中央为大、小阴唇。两侧为渐成圆形的大腿上部横切面，中央为股骨，周围包绕股部各肌群。阴唇、阴蒂和会阴部的淋巴管交织成网，最后汇集成3~4条淋巴管，汇入腹股沟浅淋巴结（覆盖在股动脉、股静脉表面的筛筋膜上），这些淋巴结的输出淋巴管穿过筛状筋膜进入股静脉内侧的腹股沟深淋巴结。这些腹股沟深淋巴结通过股管引流至盆腔淋巴结。最末的腹股沟深淋巴结位于股管内居于腹股沟韧带下面，经常被称Cloquet淋巴结。阴蒂的淋巴管可直接引流到腹股沟深淋巴结，也可以直接引流到髂内淋巴结。会阴和大阴唇下部的淋巴管引流到直肠淋巴丛[5]。

1. 大阴唇 greater lip of pudendum
2. 小阴唇 lesser lip of pudendum
3. 股薄肌 gracilis
4. 长收肌 adductor longus
5. 大隐静脉 great saphenous vein
6. 缝匠肌 sartorius
7. 股直肌 rectus femoris
8. 股外侧肌 vastus lateralis
9. 股中间肌 vastus intermedius
10. 股骨 femur
11. 臀大肌 gluteus maximus
12. 半腱肌 semitendinosus
13. 耻骨肌 pectineus
14. 大收肌 adductor magnus
15. 短收肌 adductor brevis
16. 半膜肌肌腱 tendon of semimembranosus
17. 股二头肌长头 long head of biceps femoris
18. 坐骨神经 sciatic nerve
19. 坐骨神经滋养静脉 veins of sciatic nerve
20. 股外侧肌间隔 lateral femoral intermuscular septum
21. 阔筋膜 fasciae lata
22. 阔筋膜张肌 tensor fasciae latae
23. 旋股外动脉降支 descending branch of lateral femoral circumflex artery
24. 旋股外侧静脉降支 descending tributaries of lateral femoral circumflex vein
25. 股动脉 femoral artery
26. 股静脉 femoral vein
27. 股深静脉 deep femoral vein
28. 股深动脉 deep femoral artery
29. 股内侧肌间隔 medial femoral intermuscular septum
30. 腹股沟浅淋巴结 superficial inguinal lymph nodes

女性盆部与会阴连续横断层 93（FH.7530）

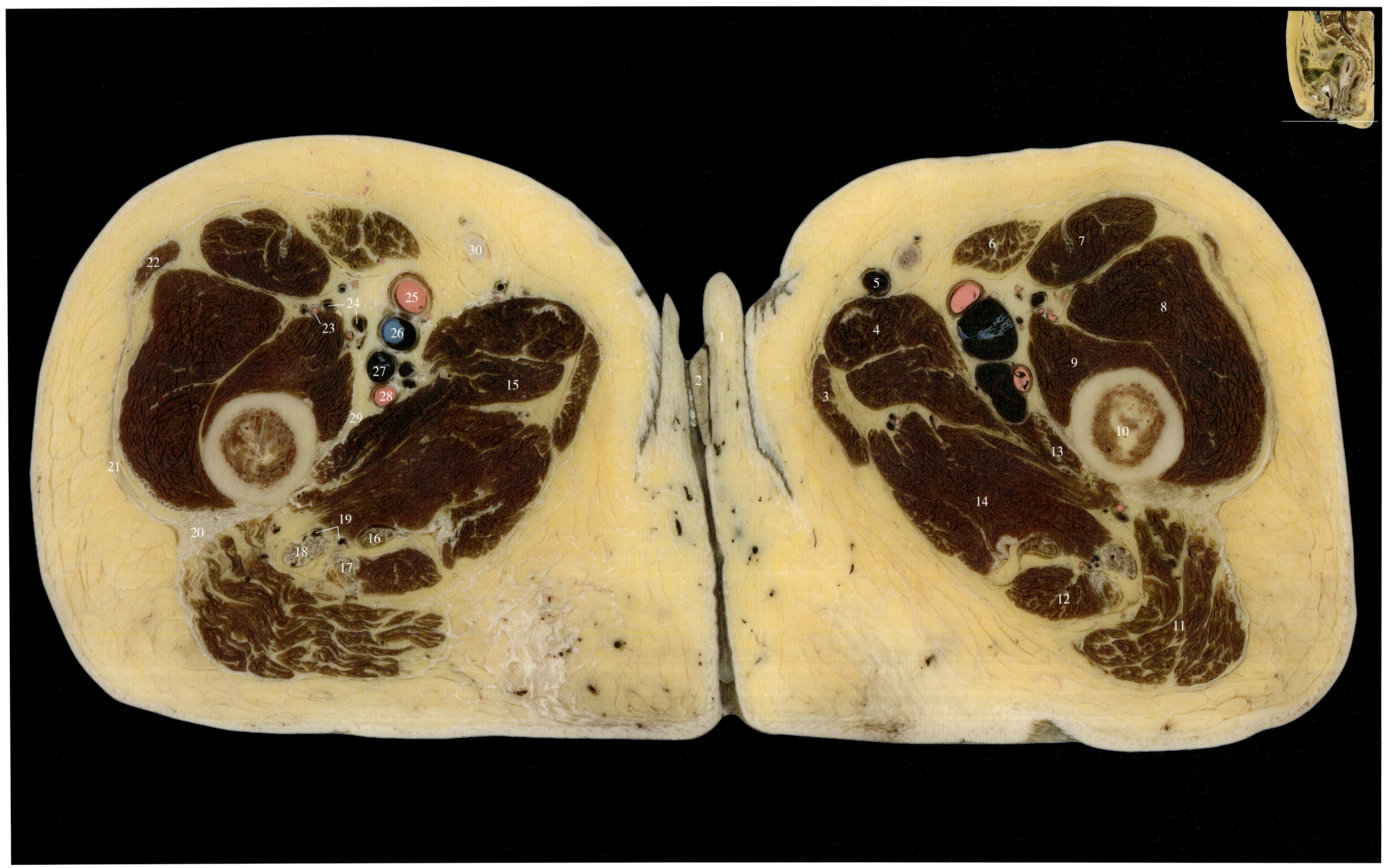

A. 断层标本图像

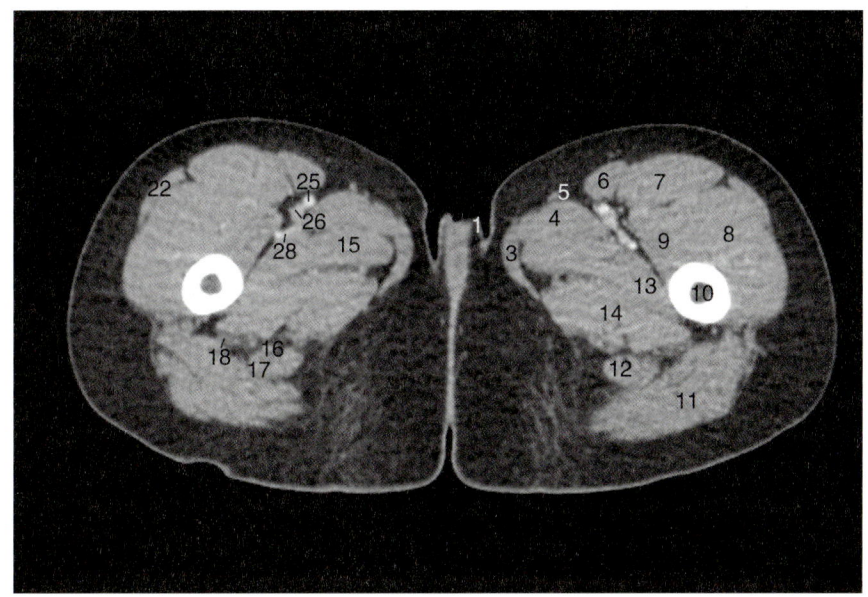

B. CT 增强图像

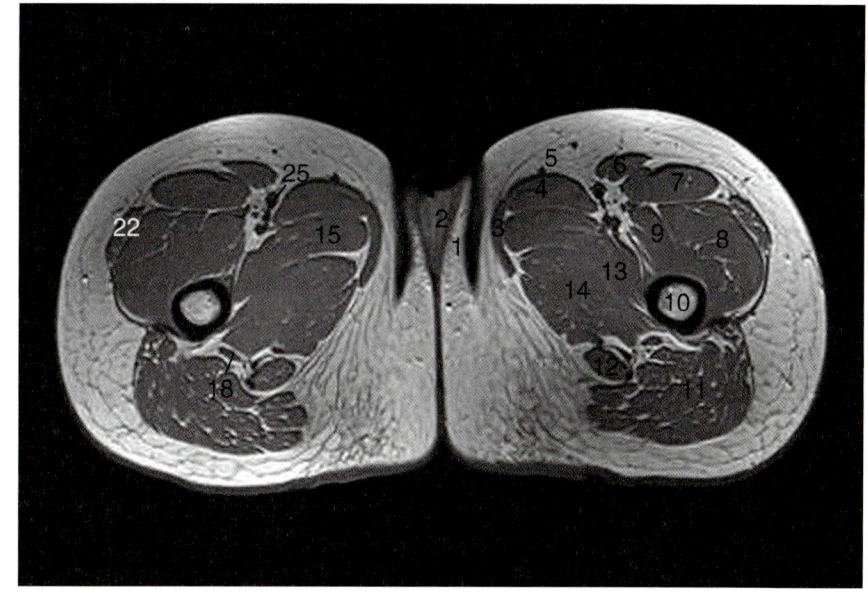

C. MR T1WI

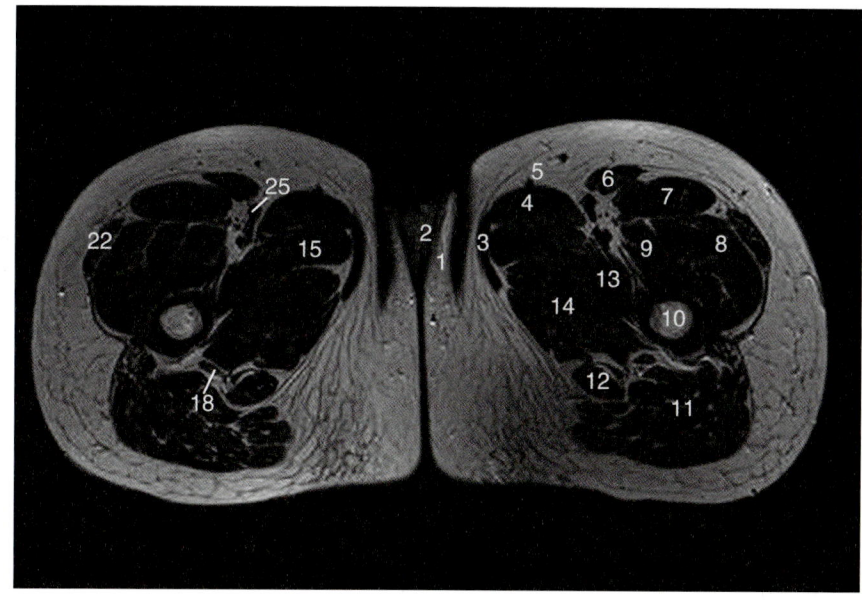

D. MR T2WI

关键结构：大阴唇，小阴唇。

  本断面为女性盆部的最后一个断面。断面的中央为大、小阴唇，两侧为股部的断面。在左侧断面，阔筋膜张肌的肌纤维消失，向下移行为髂胫束。外阴的神经为腰骶丛及盆神经丛的分支。大阴唇的前部由髂腹股沟神经的阴唇前神经分布；大阴唇后部由阴部神经通过会阴神经的阴唇后支分布。此外，生殖股神经的生殖支也分布于阴唇皮肤。阴蒂由阴部神经的阴蒂背神经（属躯体神经）和来自盆神经丛的阴蒂海绵体神经（属交感神经）分布。外阴的神经容易被外伤和炎症损伤，导致外阴疼痛综合征[5, 30]。

1. 大阴唇 greater lip of pudendum
2. 小阴唇 lesser lip of pudendum
3. 股薄肌 gracilis
4. 长收肌 adductor longus
5. 大隐静脉 great saphenous vein
6. 缝匠肌 sartorius
7. 股直肌 rectus femoris
8. 股外侧肌 vastus lateralis
9. 股中间肌 vastus intermedius
10. 股骨 femur
11. 臀大肌 gluteus maximus
12. 半腱肌 semitendinosus
13. 耻骨肌 pectineus
14. 大收肌 adductor magnus
15. 短收肌 adductor brevis
16. 半膜肌肌腱 tendon of semimembranosus
17. 股二头肌长头 long head of biceps femoris
18. 坐骨神经 sciatic nerve
19. 坐骨神经滋养静脉 veins of sciatic nerve
20. 股外侧肌间隔 lateral femoral intermuscular septum
21. 阔筋膜 fasciae lata
22. 阔筋膜张肌 tensor fasciae latae
23. 旋股外动脉降支 descending branch of lateral femoral circumflex artery
24. 旋股外侧静脉降支 descending tributaries of lateral femoral circumflex vein
25. 股动脉 femoral artery
26. 股静脉 femoral vein
27. 股深静脉 deep femoral vein
28. 股深动脉 deep femoral artery
29. 股内侧肌间隔 medial femoral intermuscular septum
30. 腹股沟浅淋巴结 superficial inguinal lymph nodes

男性盆部与会阴连续横断层解剖

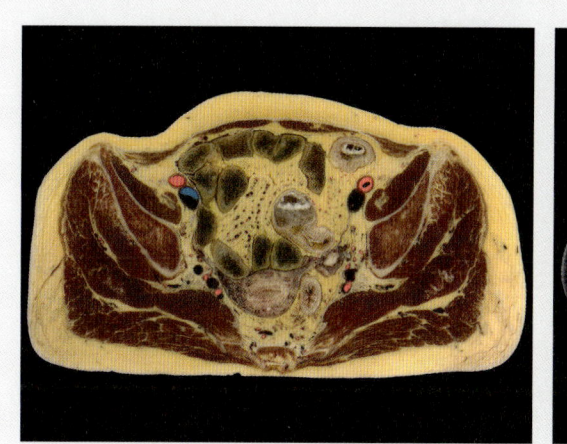
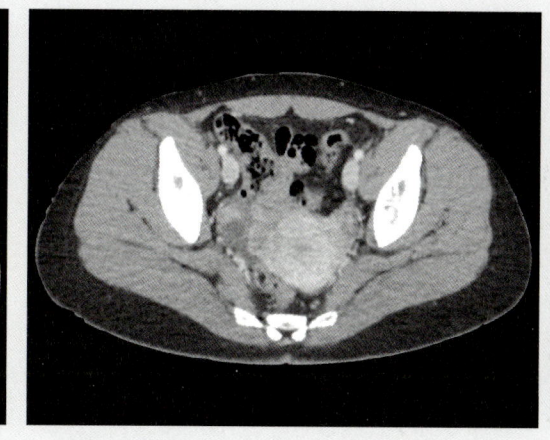
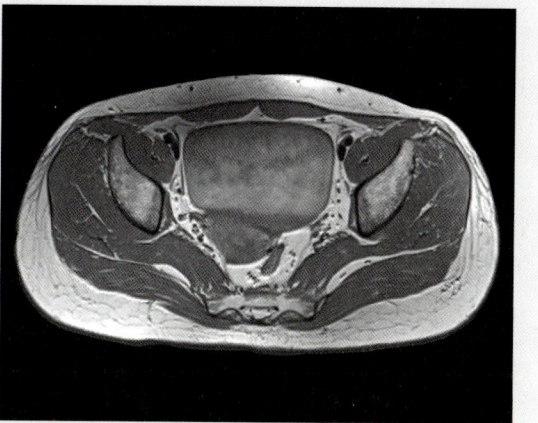

男性盆部连续横断层 1（MH.6580）

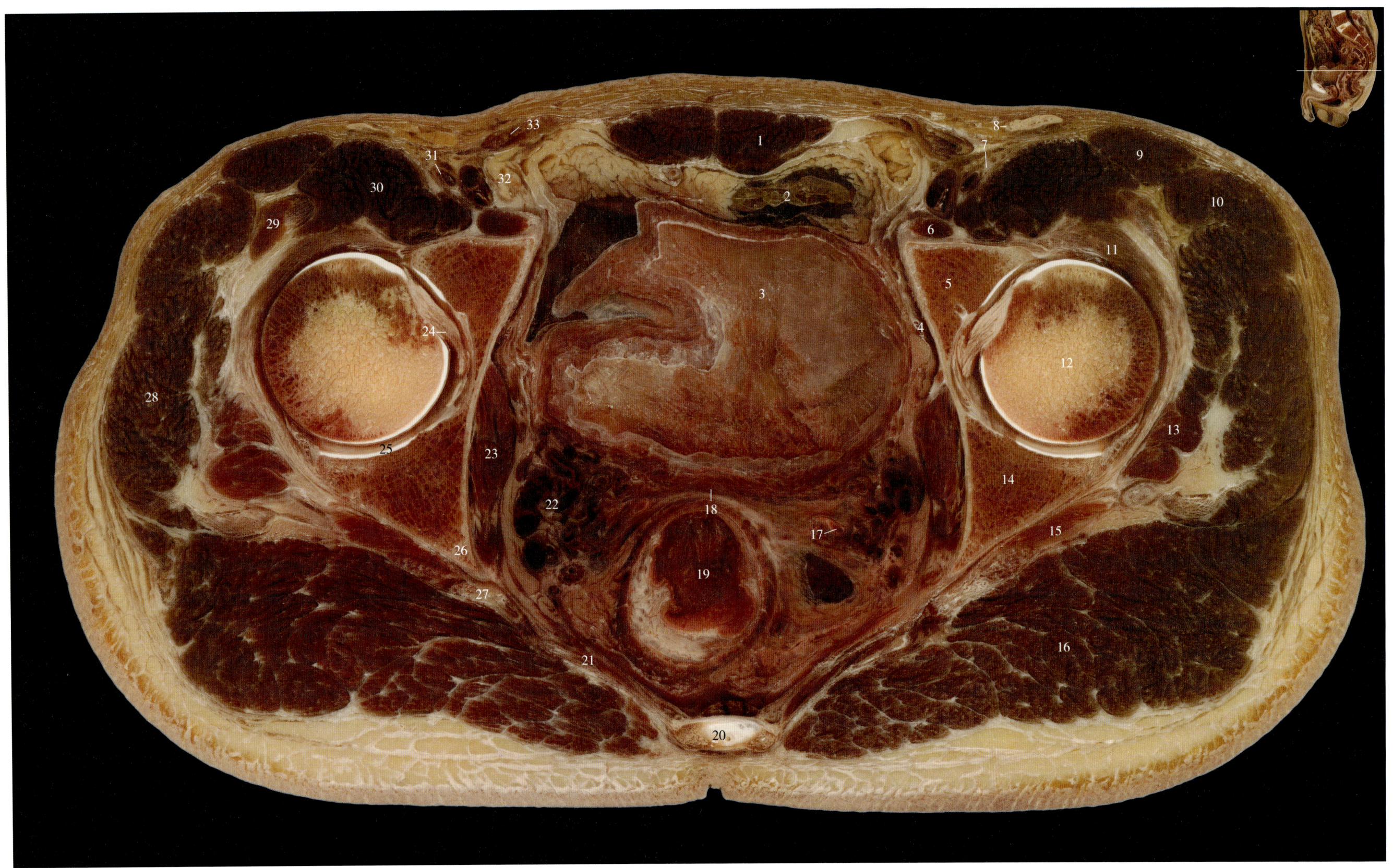

A. 断层标本图像

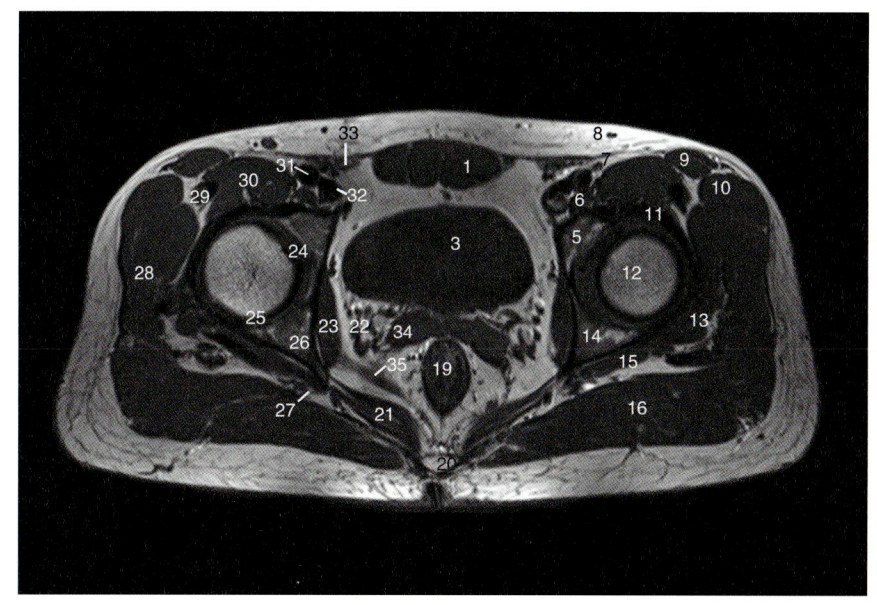
B. MR T1WI

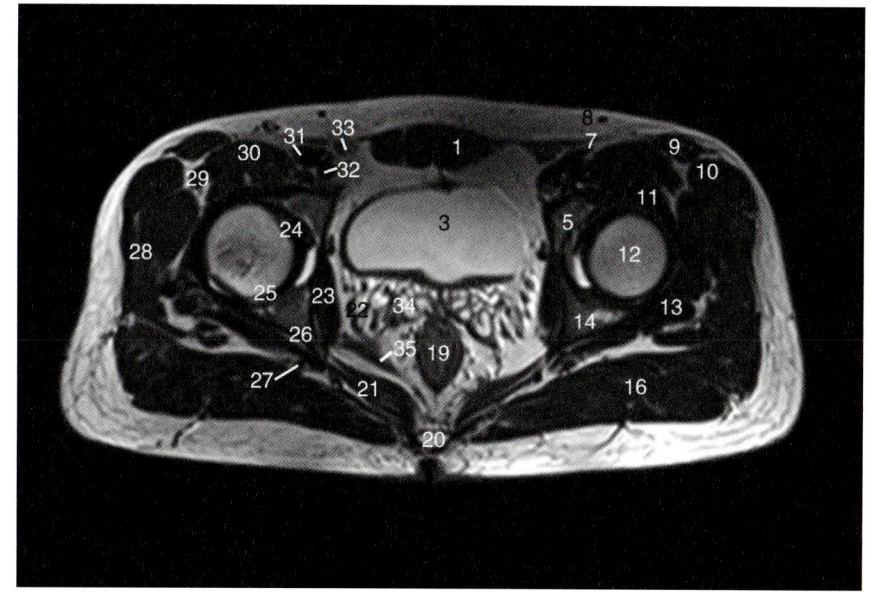
C. MR T2WI

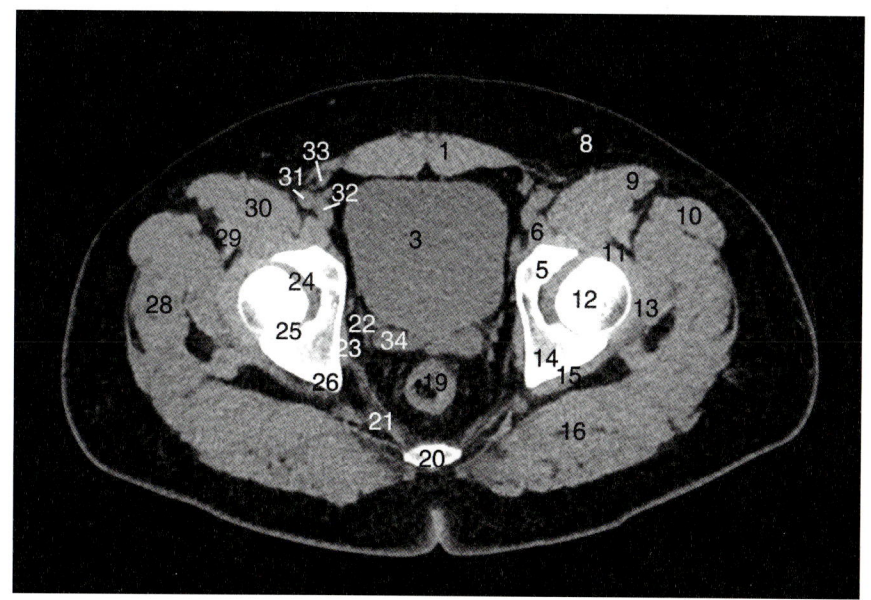
D. CT 平扫图像

关键结构：膀胱，髋关节，直肠。

此断面经过股骨头中份及股骨头韧带。小骨盆腔断面近似圆形，占据体腔大部分，其侧壁由耻骨体和坐骨体构成。髋臼与股骨头形成的髋关节明显增大。髂骨向后伸出锥状的坐骨棘，与尾骨之间有尾骨肌和骶棘韧带相连，构成盆腔后外侧壁。盆腔内膀胱占据前份大部，膀胱左前方与腹壁见管腔呈绿色管状断面为回肠，直肠位于尾骨前方，膀胱与直肠间有输精管和精囊。直肠的两侧及后方与盆壁之间的结缔组织区间分别为直肠旁隙和骶前间隙。腹前壁腹直肌外侧可见精索。空虚膀胱呈三面锥体形，尖端借膀胱脐正中韧带（胚胎时为脐尿管）连于脐部，下方连接尿道处为膀胱颈，膀胱底呈三角形，朝向后下方，膀胱尖与底之间为膀胱体。膀胱最下部的膀胱颈与前列腺底相接。膀胱壁由黏膜、肌层及外膜组成。黏膜是由变移上皮和固有层结缔组织构成；肌层由平滑肌构成，可分为内纵、中环和外纵3层；外膜除膀胱顶部有浆膜覆盖外，其余均为纤维膜，属于腹膜间位器官[41]。新生儿盆腔浅小，膀胱颈上移至耻骨联合上缘，膀胱成为腹腔内器官。当充盈时膀胱上界可上升超过脐部。随着年龄的增长，膀胱逐渐下移，到6岁左右降至盆腔内，约在青春期才达成人位置[31]。活体脏器形态、位置、大小等与标本差异较大，该断面CT图像出现了精囊，MR图像出现了肛提肌。

1. 腹直肌 rectus abdominis
2. 回肠 ileum
3. 膀胱 urinary bladder
4. 闭孔神经 obturator nerve
5. 耻骨体 body of pubis
6. 耻骨肌 pectineus
7. 股神经 femoral nerve
8. 腹股沟浅淋巴结 superficial inguinal lymph nodes
9. 缝匠肌 sartorius
10. 阔筋膜张肌 tensor fasciae latae
11. 髂股韧带 iliofemoral ligament
12. 股骨头 femoral head
13. 臀小肌 gluteus minimuss
14. 坐骨体 body of ischium
15. 梨状肌 piriformis
16. 臀大肌 gluteus maximus
17. 输精管 ductus deferens
18. 直肠膀胱陷凹 rectovesical pouch
19. 直肠 rectum
20. 尾骨 coccyx
21. 尾骨肌 coccygeus
22. 膀胱静脉丛 vesical venous plexus
23. 闭孔内肌 obturator internus
24. 股骨头韧带 ligament of head of femur
25. 髋关节 hip joint
26. 坐骨棘 ischial spine
27. 坐骨神经 sciatic nerve
28. 臀中肌 gluteus medius
29. 股直肌 rectus femoris
30. 髂腰肌 iliopsoas
31. 股动脉 femoral artery
32. 股静脉 femoral vein
33. 精索 spermatic cord
34. 精囊 seminal vesicle
35. 肛提肌 levator ani

男性盆部连续横断层 2（MH.6570）

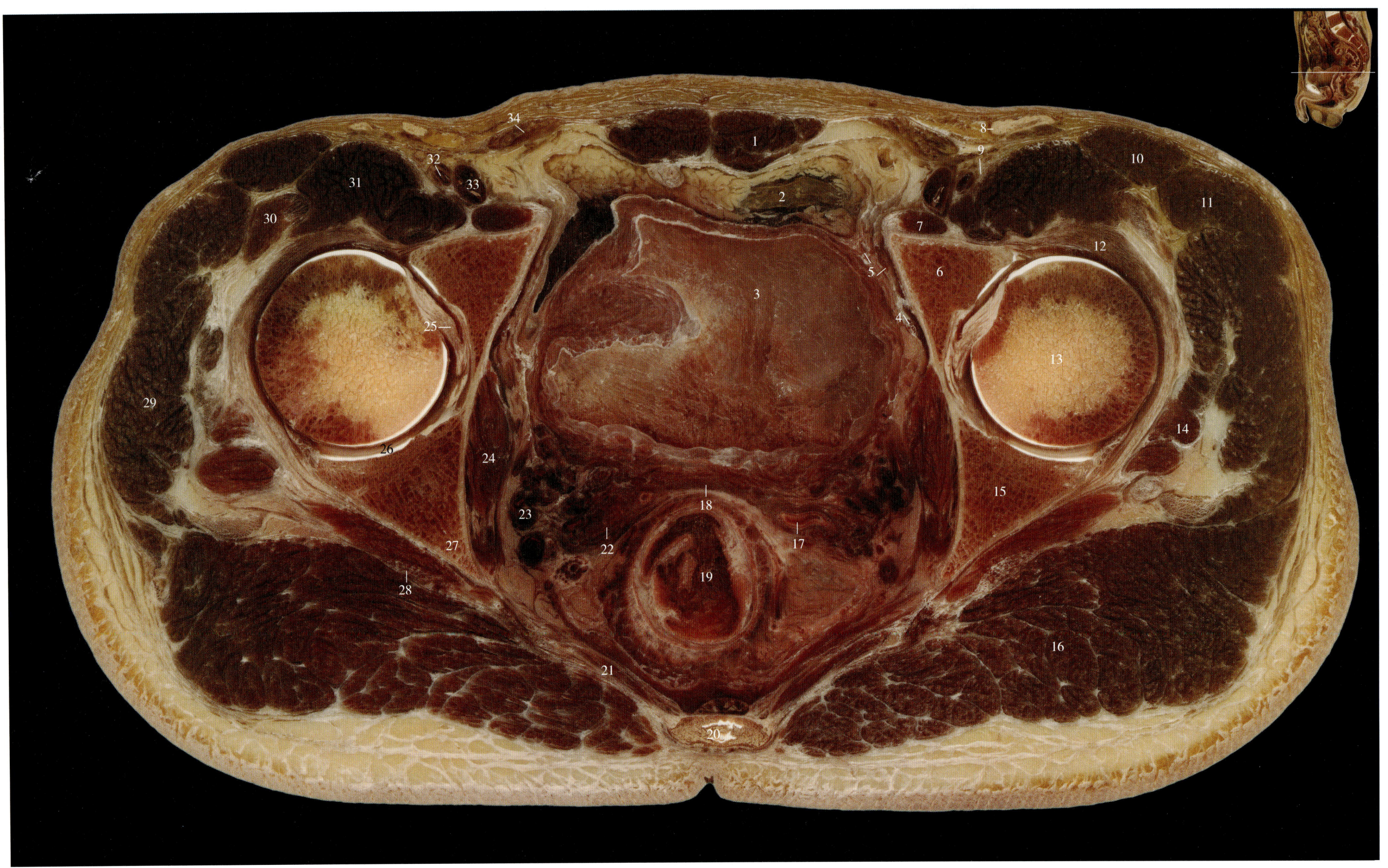

A. 断层标本图像

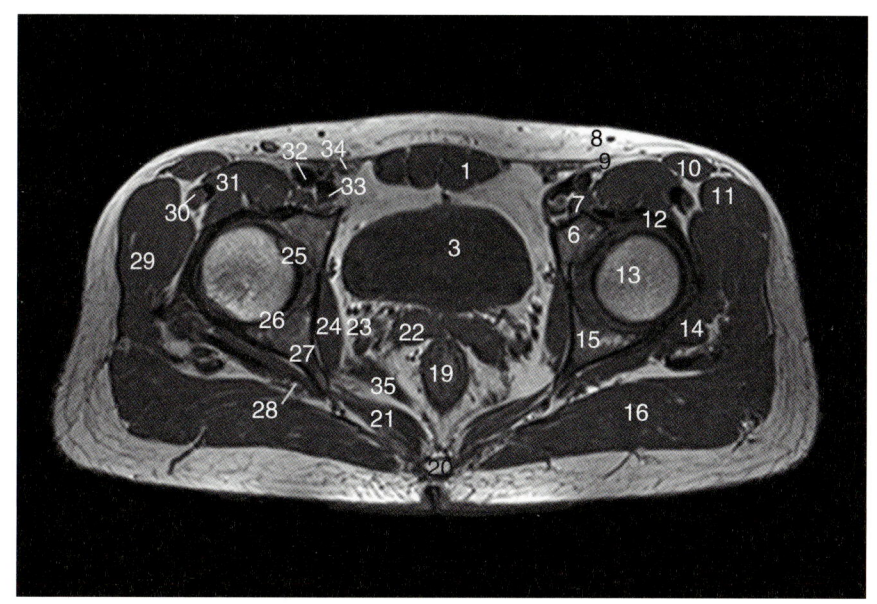
B. MR T1WI

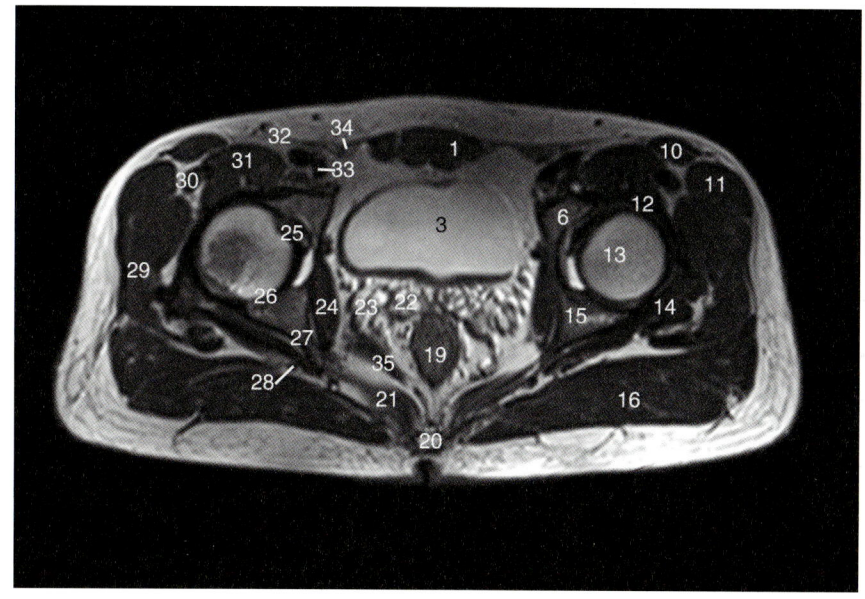
C. MR T2WI

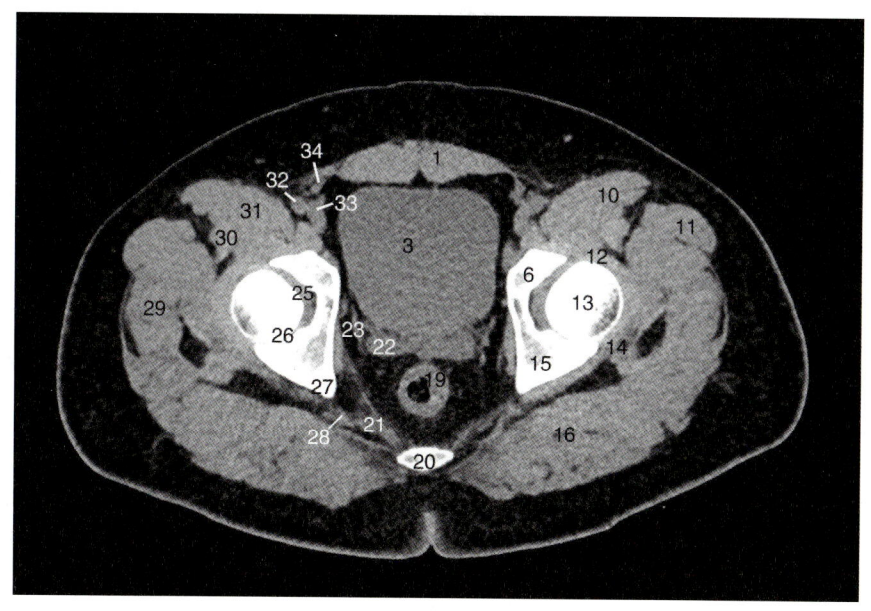
D. CT 平扫图像

关键结构：膀胱，直肠膀胱陷凹，直肠。

此断面经过股骨头中份。骨盆的侧壁由髋关节、耻骨体和坐骨体构成，股骨头韧带附于股骨头凹。髋臼内侧为闭孔内肌，该肌前缘可见由脂肪组织充填的闭膜管，其内可见闭孔血管和闭孔神经。前壁正中为两块腹直肌，其外侧、股血管的前内侧见腹股沟管内的精索。盆腔内脏器由前往后分别见回肠、膀胱和直肠。膀胱和直肠间是直肠膀胱陷凹，该处为男性直立时腹膜腔的最低点[41]。膀胱后方出现精囊，其内侧为输精管。膀胱适度充盈时，膀胱尖、体和底的上部可升至耻骨联合的上方，因而腹前壁到膀胱的腹膜反折线也随之上移，使膀胱前壁直接与腹前壁相贴。临床上利用这种解剖关系，在耻骨联合上方做膀胱的腹膜外手术或穿刺，以免伤及腹膜。直肠淋巴结位于直肠筋膜和肌层之间的直肠后外侧肛提肌上方，并位于直肠上动脉分支形成的夹角内。直肠上部的淋巴管注入直肠壁外的直肠旁淋巴结，其输出管注入直肠上淋巴结和肠系膜下淋巴结。直肠下部的淋巴管注入髂内淋巴结和骶淋巴结，直肠系膜淋巴结短径不超过 4 mm[42]。

1. 腹直肌 rectus abdominis
2. 回肠 ileum
3. 膀胱 urinary bladder
4. 闭孔神经 obturator nerve
5. 闭孔血管 obturator blood vessels
6. 耻骨体 body of pubis
7. 耻骨肌 pectineus
8. 腹股沟浅淋巴结 superficial inguinal lymph nodes
9. 股神经 femoral nerve
10. 缝匠肌 sartorius
11. 阔筋膜张肌 tensor fasciae latae
12. 髂股韧带 iliofemoral ligament
13. 股骨头 femoral head
14. 臀小肌 gluteus minimuss
15. 坐骨体 body of ischium
16. 臀大肌 gluteus maximus
17. 输精管 ductus deferens
18. 直肠膀胱陷凹 rectovesical pouch
19. 直肠 rectum
20. 尾骨 coccyx
21. 尾骨肌 coccygeus
22. 精囊 seminal vesicle
23. 膀胱静脉丛 vesical venous plexus
24. 闭孔内肌 obturator internus
25. 股骨头韧带 ligament of head of femur
26. 髋关节 hip joint
27. 坐骨棘 ischial spine
28. 坐骨神经 sciatic nerve
29. 臀中肌 gluteus medius
30. 股直肌 rectus femoris
31. 髂腰肌 iliopsoas
32. 股动脉 femoral artery
33. 股静脉 femoral vein
34. 精索 spermatic cord
35. 肛提肌 levator ani

男性盆部连续横断层 3（MH.6560）

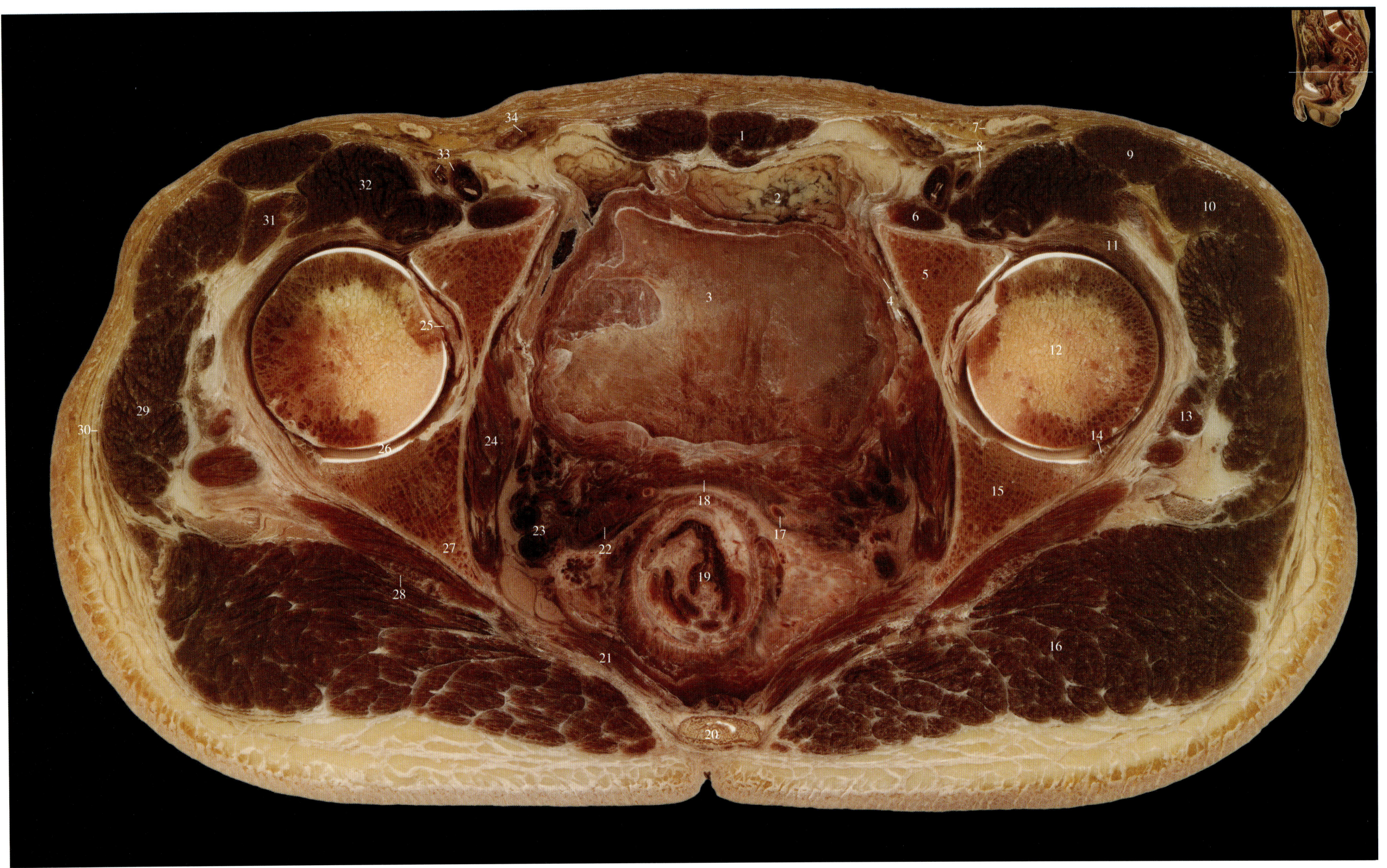

A. 断层标本图像

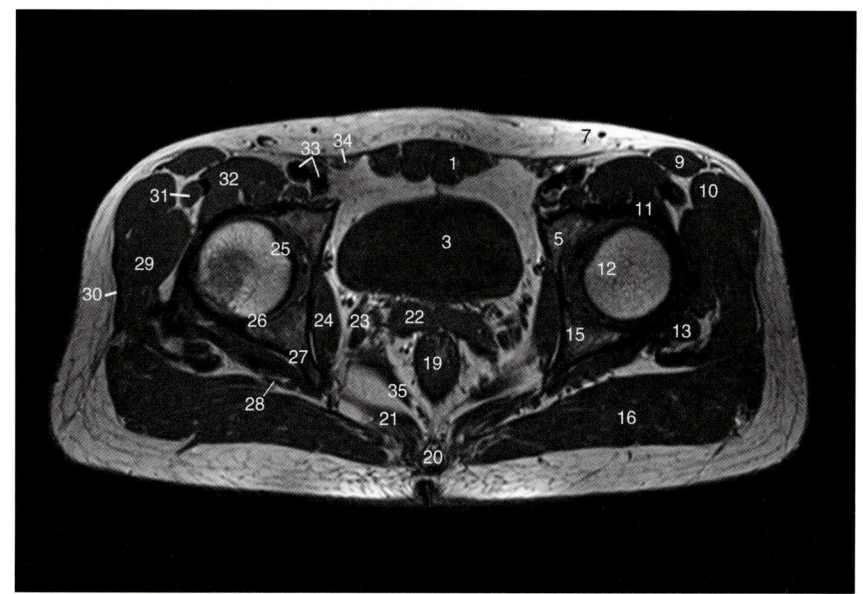

B. MR T1WI

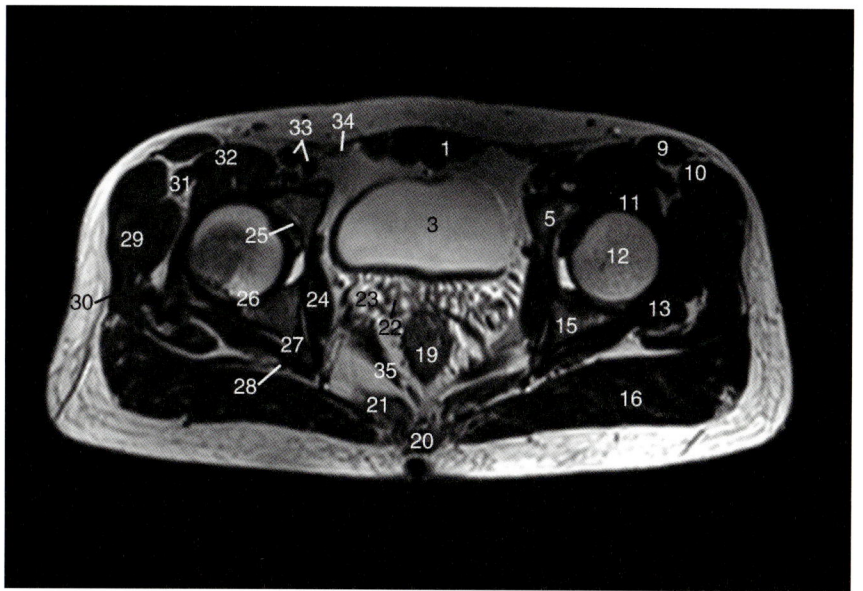

C. MR T2WI

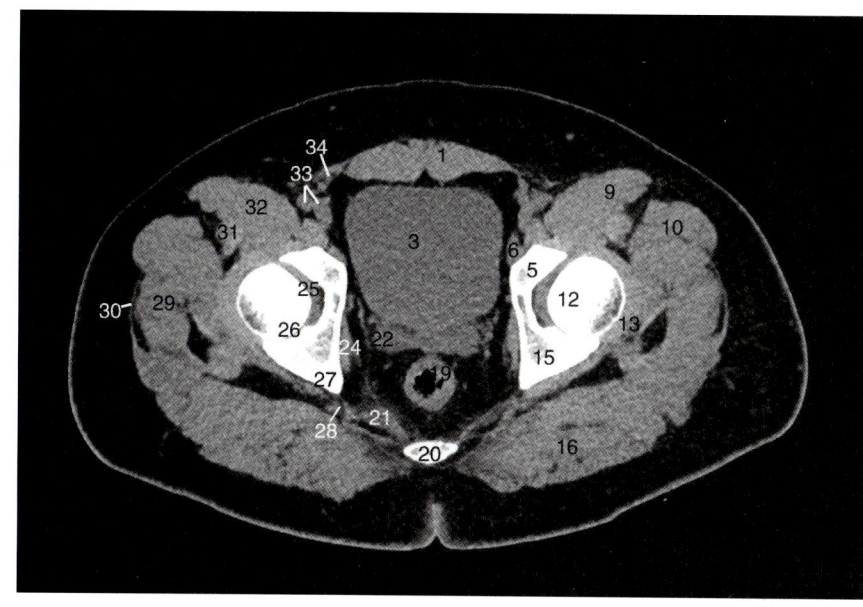

D. CT 平扫图像

1. 腹直肌 rectus abdominis
2. 回肠 ileum
3. 膀胱 urinary bladder
4. 闭孔血管和神经 obturator blood vessels and nerve
5. 耻骨体 body of pubis
6. 耻骨肌 pectineus
7. 腹股沟浅淋巴结 superficial inguinal lymph nodes
8. 股神经 femoral nerve
9. 缝匠肌 sartorius
10. 阔筋膜张肌 tensor fasciae latae
11. 髂股韧带 iliofemoral ligament
12. 股骨头 femoral head
13. 臀小肌 gluteus minimuss
14. 髋臼唇 acetabular labrum
15. 坐骨体 body of ischium
16. 臀大肌 gluteus maximus
17. 输精管 ductus deferens
18. 直肠膀胱陷凹 rectovesical pouch
19. 直肠 rectum
20. 尾骨 coccyx
21. 尾骨肌 coccygeus
22. 精囊 seminal vesicle
23. 膀胱静脉丛 vesical venous plexus
24. 闭孔内肌 obturator internus
25. 股骨头韧带 ligament of head of femur
26. 髋关节 hip joint
27. 坐骨棘 ischial spine
28. 坐骨神经 sciatic nerve
29. 臀中肌 gluteus medius
30. 阔筋膜 fasciae lata
31. 股直肌 rectus femoris
32. 髂腰肌 iliopsoas
33. 股动、静脉 femoral artery and vein
34. 精索 spermatic cord
35. 肛提肌 levator ani

关键结构：髋臼，精索。

骨盆侧壁由髋臼构成。髋臼内侧为闭孔内肌，该肌前缘可见由脂肪组织充填的闭膜管（由闭孔膜的上缘与耻骨的闭孔沟围成），其内可见闭孔血管和闭孔神经。髋臼前、后缘和同侧股骨头中心点的连线与双侧股骨头中心点的连线的内侧夹角，分别称髋臼前断面角和髋臼后断面角，二者之和称髋臼水平断面角。髋臼断面角在临床上是用于衡量髋臼发育情况的重要指标，成年男性正常值：前角平均为61.56°~83.56°，后角平均为89.33°~111.91°[43]。盆后壁正中见尾骨及其两侧的尾骨肌。盆前壁见腹直肌及两侧皮下的腹股沟管及精索。精索内结构的配布是：输精管位于下方，输精管静脉及蔓状静脉丛位于前方，动脉居诸静脉中间偏上方。蔓状静脉丛是由10~12条静脉组成，最终汇成睾丸静脉。精索静脉曲张较常见，93%的患者发生在左侧[44]。一般认为这是由于左侧静脉较右侧长，并以直角注入左肾静脉，血液回流较困难所致。盆腔内脏器排列与上一断面基本相同：前为膀胱，后为直肠，膀胱及直肠间两侧分别见输精管、精囊及静脉丛。

男性盆部连续横断层 4（MH.6550）

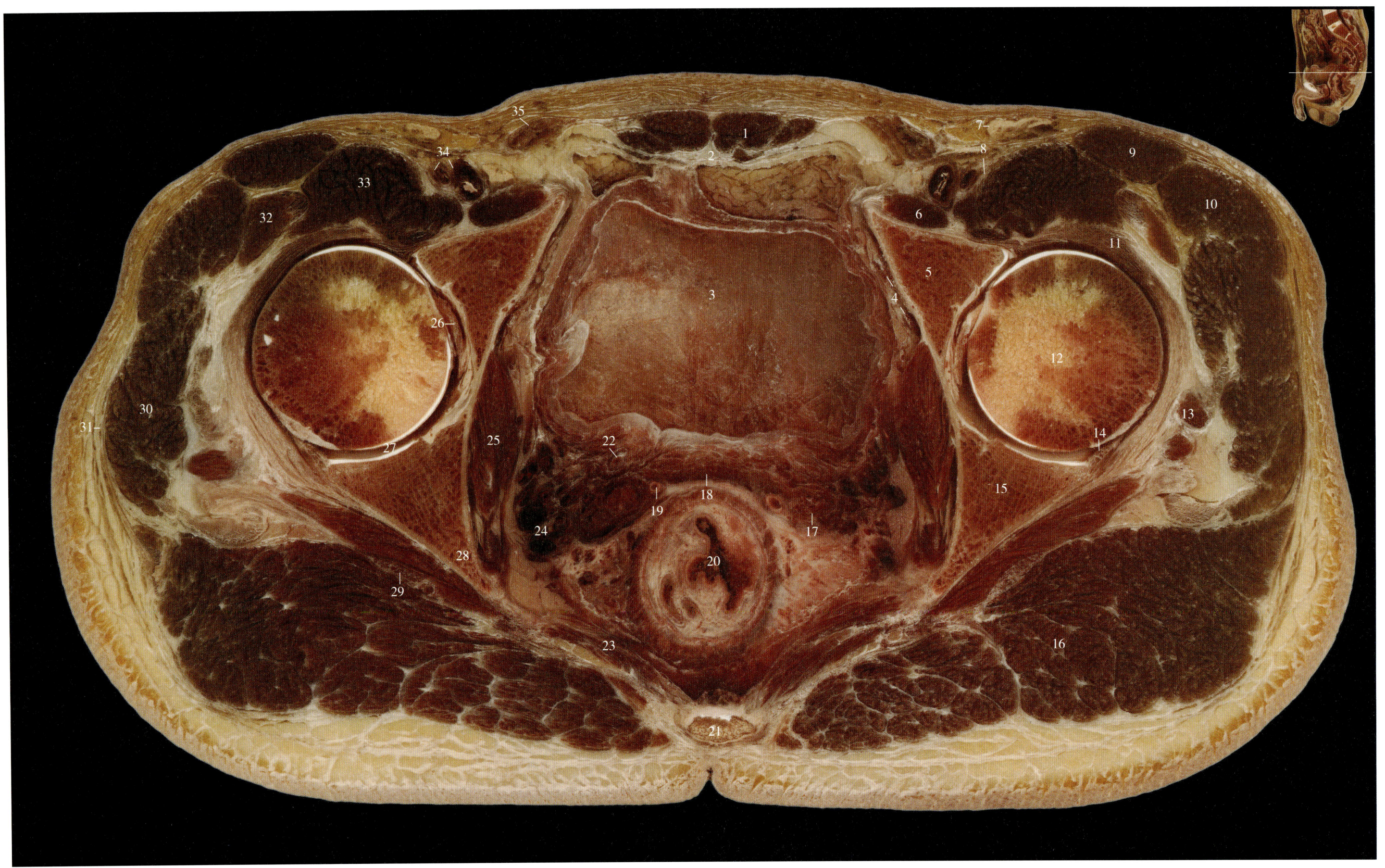

A. 断层标本图像

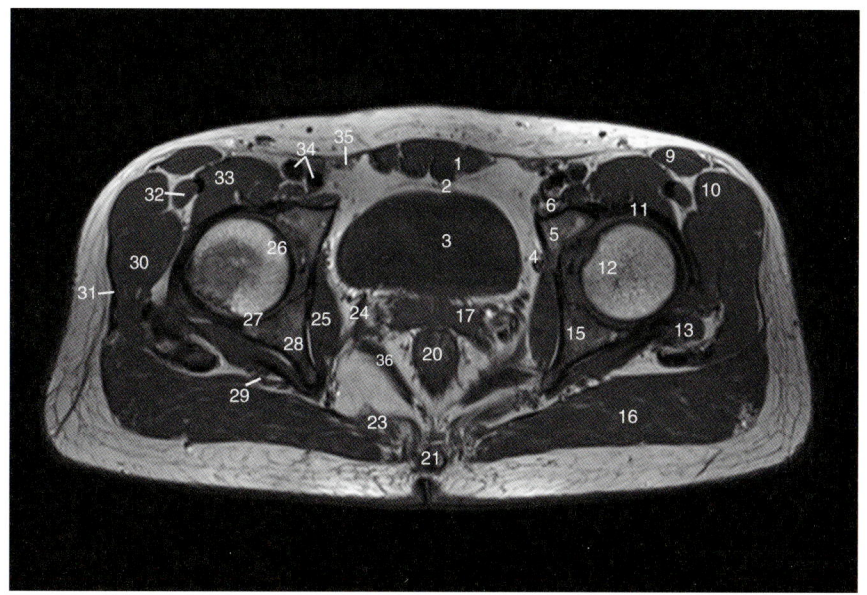
B. MR T1WI

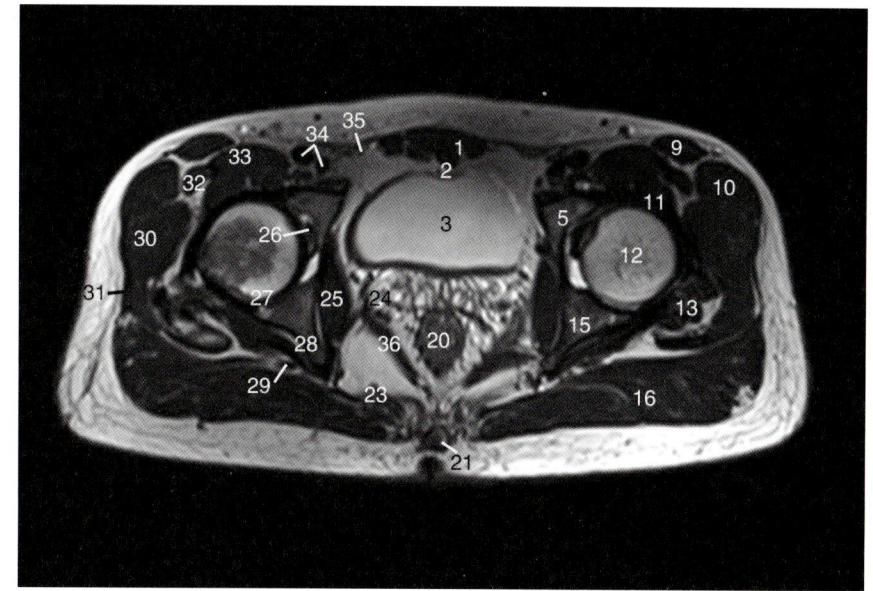
C. MR T2WI

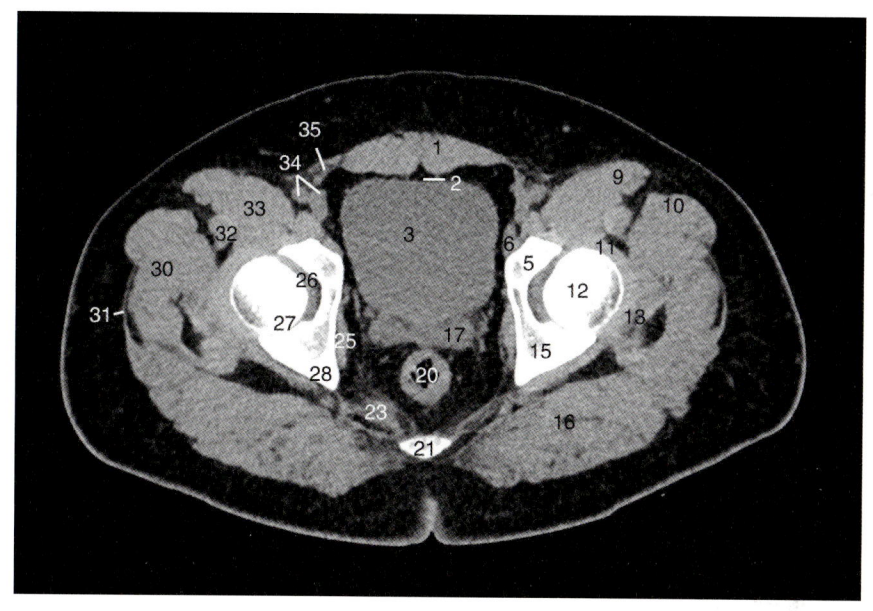
D. CT 平扫图像

1. 腹直肌 rectus abdominis
2. 膀胱前间隙 prevesical space
3. 膀胱 urinary bladder
4. 闭孔血管和神经 obturator blood vessels and nerve
5. 耻骨体 body of pubis
6. 耻骨肌 pectineus
7. 腹股沟浅淋巴结 superficial inguinal lymph nodes
8. 股神经 femoral nerve
9. 缝匠肌 sartorius
10. 阔筋膜张肌 tensor fasciae latae
11. 髂股韧带 iliofemoral ligament
12. 股骨头 femoral head
13. 臀小肌 gluteus minimuss
14. 髋臼唇 acetabular labrum
15. 坐骨体 body of ischium
16. 臀大肌 gluteus maximus
17. 精囊 seminal vesicle
18. 直肠膀胱陷凹 rectovesical pouch
19. 输精管 ductus deferens
20. 直肠 rectum
21. 尾骨 coccyx
22. 输尿管 ureter
23. 尾骨肌 coccygeus
24. 膀胱静脉丛 vesical venous plexus
25. 闭孔内肌 obturator internus
26. 股骨头韧带 ligament of head of femur
27. 髋关节 hip joint
28. 坐骨棘 ischial spine
29. 坐骨神经 sciatic nerve
30. 臀中肌 gluteus medius
31. 阔筋膜 fasciae lata
32. 股直肌 rectus femoris
33. 髂腰肌 iliopsoas
34. 股动、静脉 femoral artery and vein
35. 精索 spermatic cord
36. 肛提肌 levator ani

关键结构：输尿管，膀胱，股骨头。

此断面经过股骨头中份及股骨头韧带。构成骨盆侧壁的股骨头骨松质内可见浅黄色的黄骨髓和暗红色的红骨髓，红、黄骨髓可以因骨髓造血状态发生转换。两种骨髓在 T1WI 图像上信号不同，黄骨髓呈脂肪样高信号，红骨髓呈水样低信号。盆腔脏器从前往后分别是膀胱体和直肠，膀胱前见回肠肠壁，膀胱、直肠间从中心向两侧可见直肠膀胱陷凹、输精管、精囊腺和静脉丛。输尿管在此平面开始离开盆壁行向膀胱。左侧输尿管越过左侧髂总动脉末端，右侧输尿管越过右侧髂外动脉始段入盆腔，即为输尿管盆部。输尿管盆部在腹膜深面沿着盆腔侧壁下行，于盆侧壁腹膜外结缔组织内，经髂血管、腰骶干和骶髂关节前方，在脐动脉起始部、闭孔神经和闭孔血管的内侧跨过，达坐骨棘水平，转向前内方，移行为壁内部；男性输尿管向前下内经直肠前外侧壁与膀胱底之间，输精管的后外侧，并呈直角与之交叉，然后至输精管的内下方，经精囊顶上方，向内下斜穿膀胱壁，最后开口于膀胱三角的外侧角。膀胱空虚时，两侧输尿管口相距约 2.5 cm，膀胱充盈较满时，可增至 5 cm[1]。在 CT 检查中，输尿管内无造影剂时，不易显示。

男性盆部连续横断层 5（MH.6540）

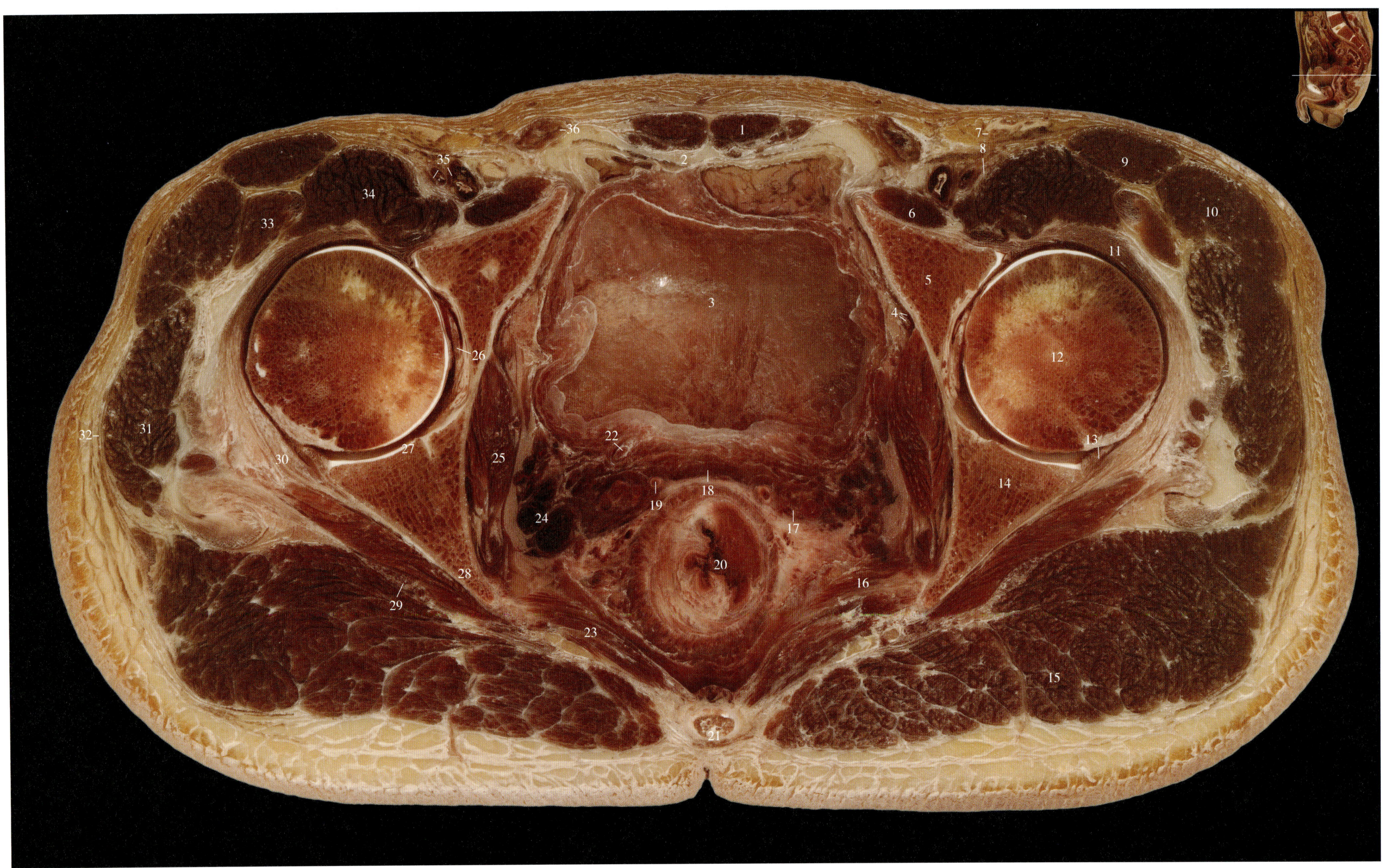

A. 断层标本图像

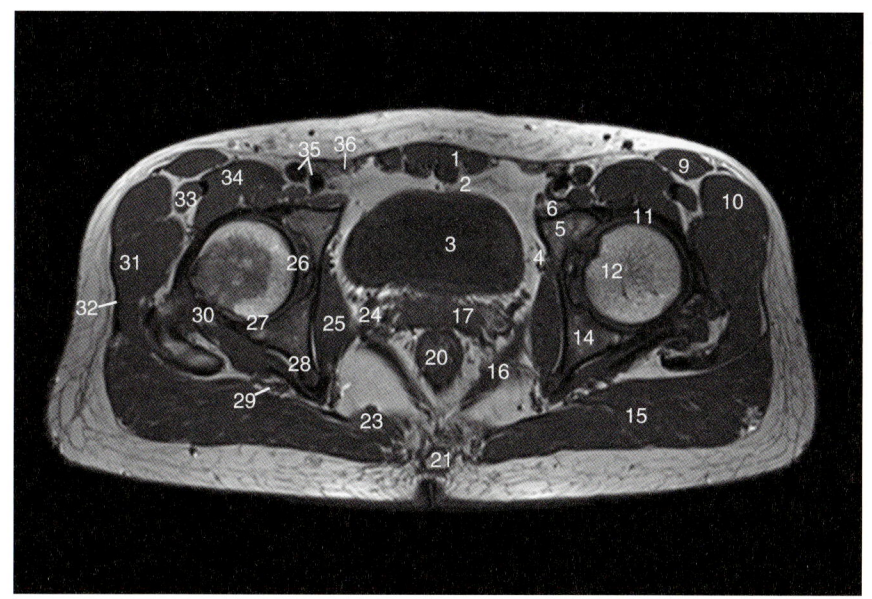

B. MR T1WI

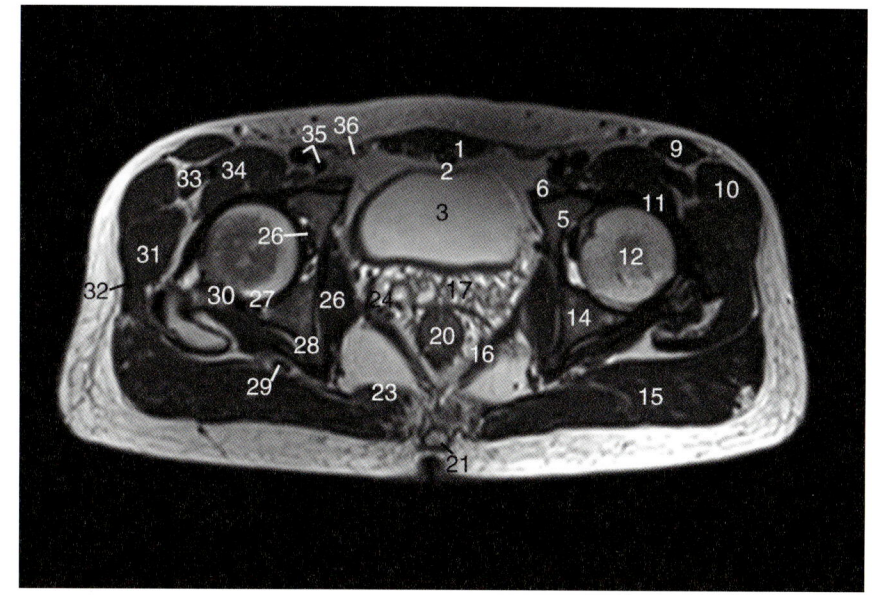

C. MR T2WI

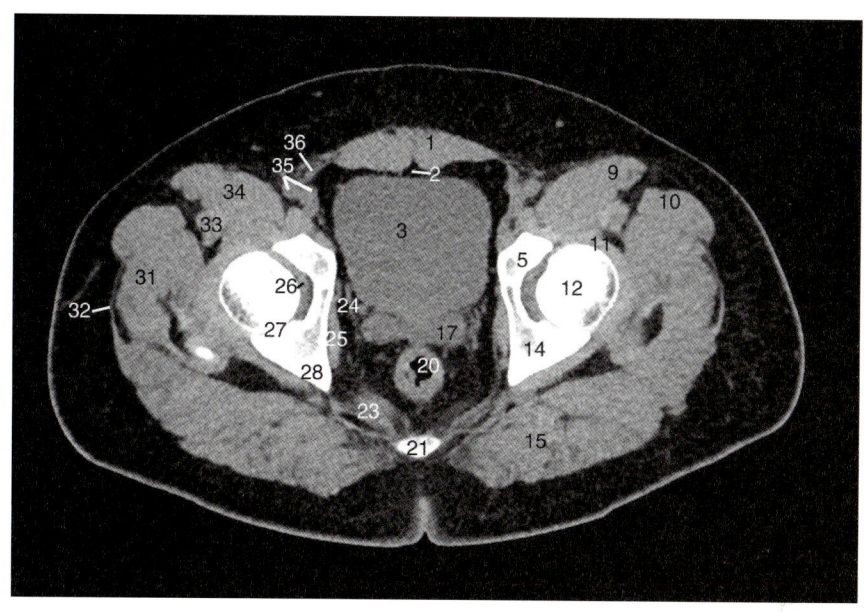

D. CT 平扫图像

1. 腹直肌 rectus abdominis
2. 膀胱前间隙 prevesical space
3. 膀胱 urinary bladder
4. 闭孔血管和神经 obturator blood vessels and nerve
5. 耻骨体 body of pubis
6. 耻骨肌 pectineus
7. 腹股沟浅淋巴结 superficial inguinal lymph nodes
8. 股神经 femoral nerve
9. 缝匠肌 sartorius
10. 阔筋膜张肌 tensor fasciae latae
11. 髂股韧带 iliofemoral ligament
12. 股骨头 femoral head
13. 髋臼唇 acetabular labrum
14. 坐骨体 body of ischium
15. 臀大肌 gluteus maximus
16. 肛提肌 levator ani
17. 精囊 seminal vesicle
18. 直肠膀胱陷凹 rectovesical pouch
19. 输精管 ductus deferens
20. 直肠 rectum
21. 尾骨 coccyx
22. 输尿管 ureter
23. 尾骨肌 coccygeus
24. 膀胱静脉丛 vesical venous plexus
25. 闭孔内肌 obturator internus
26. 股骨头韧带 ligament of head of femur
27. 髋关节 hip joint
28. 坐骨棘 ischial spine
29. 坐骨神经 sciatic nerve
30. 坐股韧带 ischiofemoral ligament
31. 臀中肌 gluteus medius
32. 阔筋膜 fasciae lata
33. 股直肌 rectus femoris
34. 髂腰肌 iliopsoas
35. 股动、静脉 femoral artery and vein
36. 精索 spermatic cord

关键结构：膀胱三角，输尿管，输精管。

　　此断面经过股骨头中份及股骨头韧带。盆腔内脏器排列是：前部为膀胱，后部为直肠，二者之间可见直肠膀胱陷凹及其两侧的输精管、精囊与膀胱静脉丛。膀胱内面被覆黏膜，膀胱壁收缩时，黏膜聚集成皱襞称膀胱襞。在膀胱底内面，左、右输尿管口和尿道内口之间有一个三角形的区域，称膀胱三角，此处缺少黏膜下层组织，黏膜与肌层紧密连接，无论膀胱扩张或收缩，始终保持平滑。膀胱三角是肿瘤、结核、炎症的好发位置。膀胱镜检查时应该特别注意。两个输尿管口之间的皱襞称输尿管间襞，膀胱下所见为一苍白带，该处是临床寻找输尿管口的标志。在男性尿道内后方的膀胱三角处，受前列腺中叶推挤形成纵嵴状隆起称膀胱垂。在膀胱后壁两侧的壁内见由外侧向内侧斜行的输尿管。输尿管向内下斜穿膀胱壁，开口在膀胱三角的外上角，这一段成为壁内段，长约1.5 cm[41]。当膀胱充盈时，膀胱内压增加将输尿管内壁压扁，阻止膀胱内的尿液反流。输尿管壁内部、输尿管与肾盂移行处和输尿管跨越髂血管处是输尿管3个生理性狭窄的部位，常是结石滞留处。

男性盆部连续横断层 6（MH.6530）

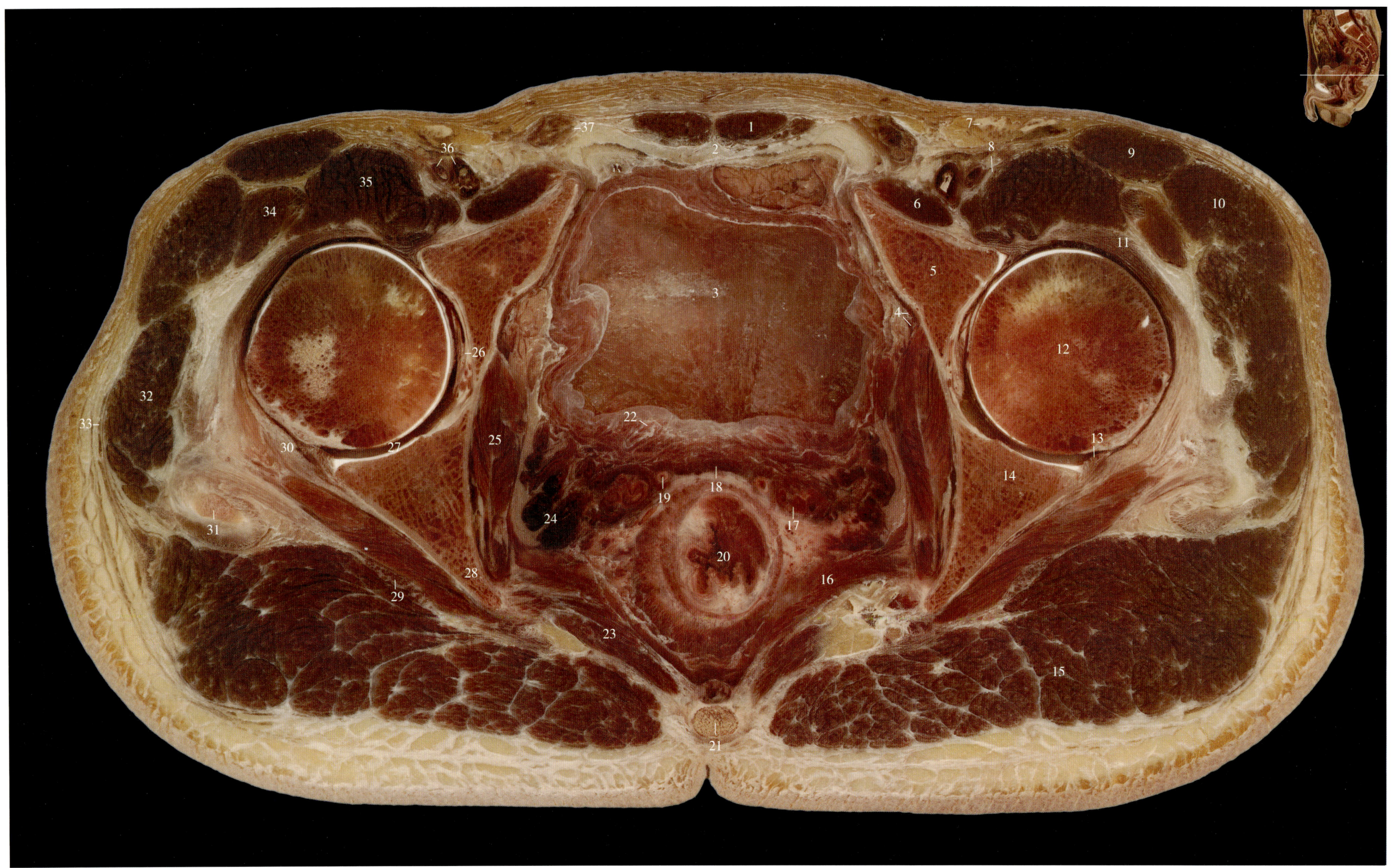

A. 断层标本图像

1. 腹直肌 rectus abdominis
2. 膀胱前间隙 prevesical space
3. 膀胱 urinary bladder
4. 闭孔血管和神经 obturator blood vessels and nerve
5. 耻骨体 body of pubis
6. 耻骨肌 pectineus
7. 腹股沟浅淋巴结 superficial inguinal lymph nodes
8. 股神经 femoral nerve
9. 缝匠肌 sartorius
10. 阔筋膜张肌 tensor fasciae latae
11. 髂股韧带 iliofemoral ligament
12. 股骨头 femoral head
13. 髋臼唇 acetabular labrum
14. 坐骨体 body of ischium
15. 臀大肌 gluteus maximus
16. 肛提肌 levator ani
17. 精囊 seminal vesicle
18. 直肠膀胱陷凹 rectovesical pouch
19. 输精管 ductus deferens
20. 直肠 rectum
21. 尾骨 coccyx
22. 输尿管 ureter
23. 尾骨肌 coccygeus
24. 膀胱静脉丛 vesical venous plexus
25. 闭孔内肌 obturator internus
26. 股骨头韧带 ligament of head of femur
27. 髋关节 hip joint
28. 坐骨棘 ischial spine
29. 坐骨神经 sciatic nerve
30. 坐股韧带 ischiofemoral ligament
31. 大转子 greater trochanter
32. 臀中肌 gluteus medius
33. 阔筋膜 fasciae lata
34. 股直肌 rectus femoris
35. 髂腰肌 iliopsoas
36. 股动、静脉 femoral artery and vein
37. 精索 spermatic cord
38. 闭孔淋巴结 glandulae foraminis obturatorii
39. 骶前间隙 presacral space

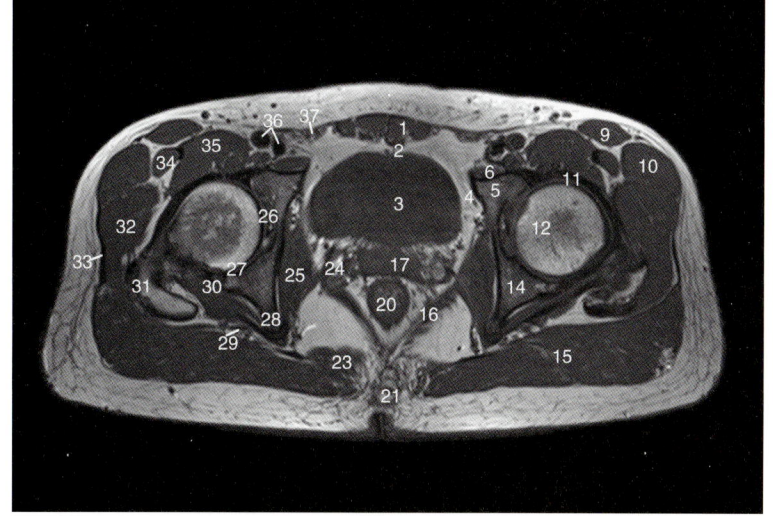

B. T1W1

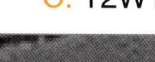

C. T2W1

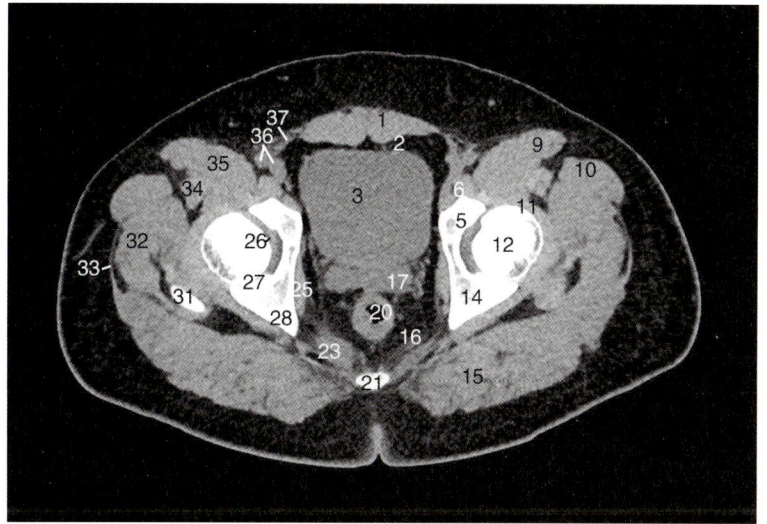

D. CT 平扫

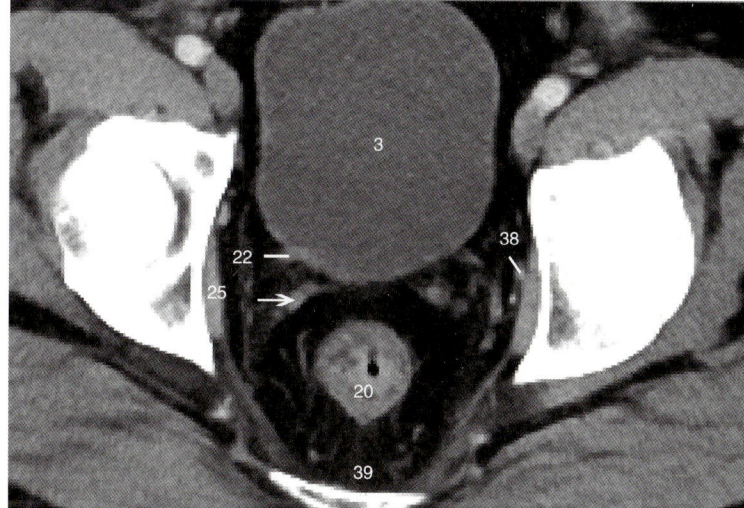

E. CT 增强

关键结构：膀胱，直肠，坐骨。

此断面为男性经股骨头中份横断面。断面内髋骨相对内移，盆腔横径缩小。盆腔侧壁主要为髋骨及其内面的闭孔内肌，髋骨恰经髋臼窝，显示髋臼底的骨质较薄，髋骨的后端为锥状的坐骨棘。在髋关节前方，髂腰肌与耻骨肌之间可见股神经与股动、静脉及腹股沟深淋巴结。髋臼内侧为闭孔内肌，在该肌前外缘与耻骨上支之间可见位于闭膜管内的闭孔动、静脉，闭孔神经及少量脂肪组织，闭膜管的脂肪组织在 CT 上呈明显低密度，血管和神经呈等密度，T1WI 及 T2WI 上脂肪均呈明显高信号，能把呈低信号的血管与神经衬托出来。盆腔后壁为尾骨和盆膈，后者位于尾骨与坐骨棘之间，主要由尾骨肌和肛提肌构成。盆后壁为尾骨，两侧可见起自尾骨至坐骨的尾骨肌及其前方髂尾肌，髂尾肌、耻尾肌和耻骨直肠肌构成肛提肌。盆腔前壁为腹直肌。盆腔自此平面向下逐层变窄，而会阴结构逐渐显现。盆腔前部主要为膀胱，后部为直肠，二者间有精囊、输精管壶腹和膀胱静脉丛。膀胱后壁明显增厚，已达膀胱三角区，在膀胱后壁两侧的壁内见由外侧向内侧斜行的输尿管。直肠两侧和后方与盆壁之间分别为直肠旁间隙和骶前间隙。直肠旁间隙位于盆底腹膜与盆膈之间、直肠筋膜的周围，被直肠侧韧带（由直肠下动、静脉及周围结缔组织构成）分为前、后两部。前部称直肠前隙或骨盆直肠间隙，其前方为直肠膀胱隔（男）或直肠阴道隔（女），后方为直肠和直肠侧韧带；后部为直肠后隙，又称为骶前间隙，位于直肠侧韧带与骶骨之间，向上与腹膜后间隙相通，下至盆膈[31]。

男性盆部连续横断层 7（MH.6520）

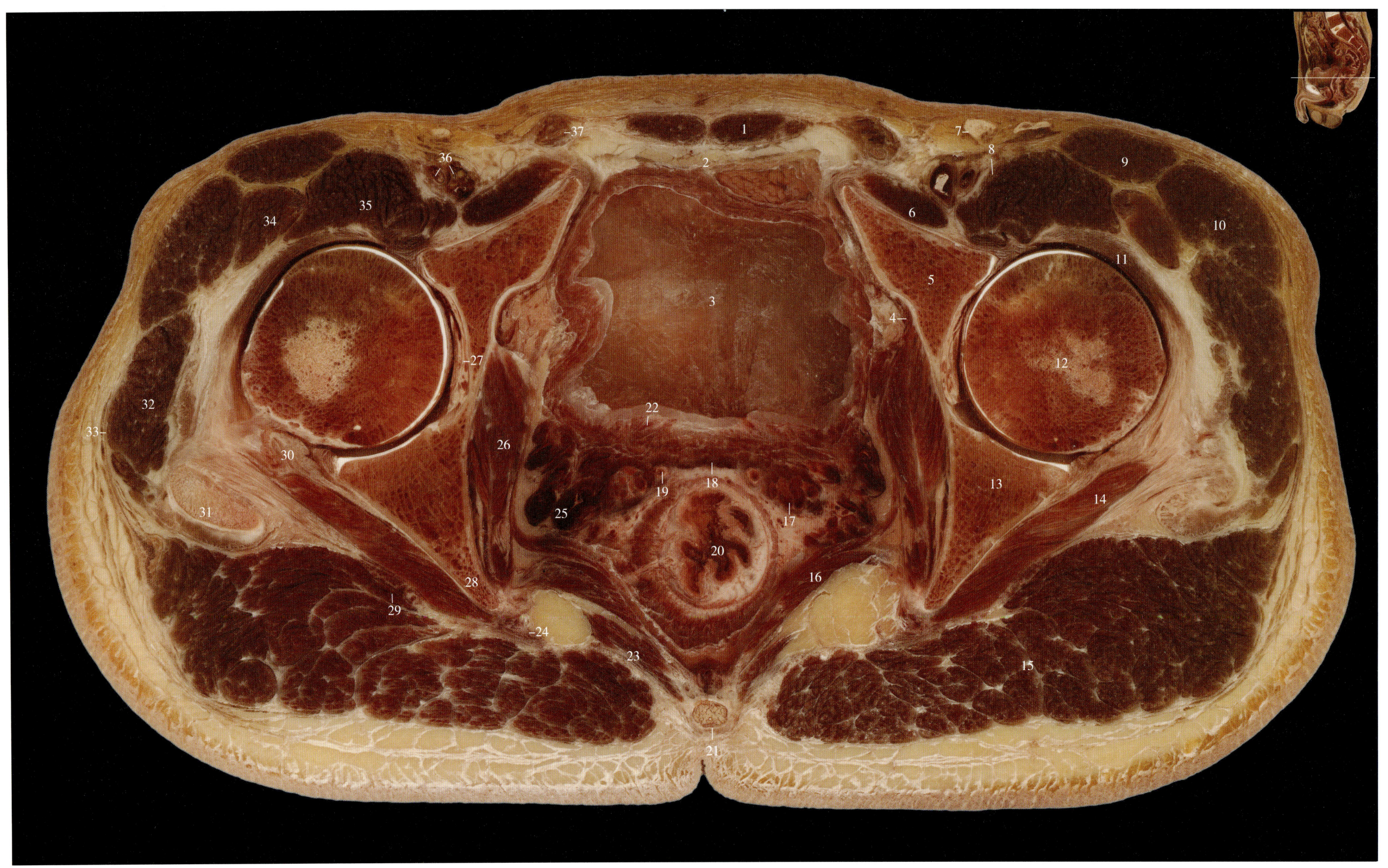

A. 断层标本图像

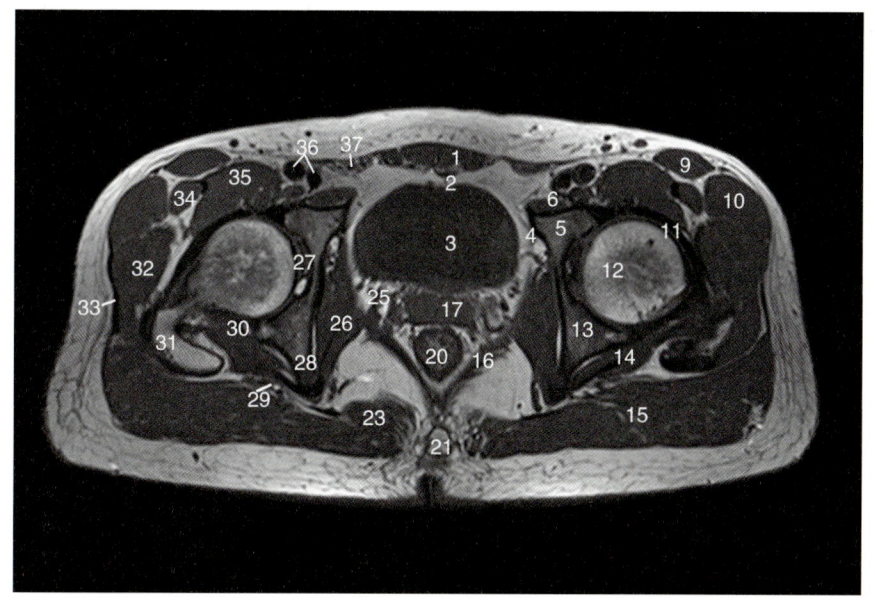
B. MR T1WI

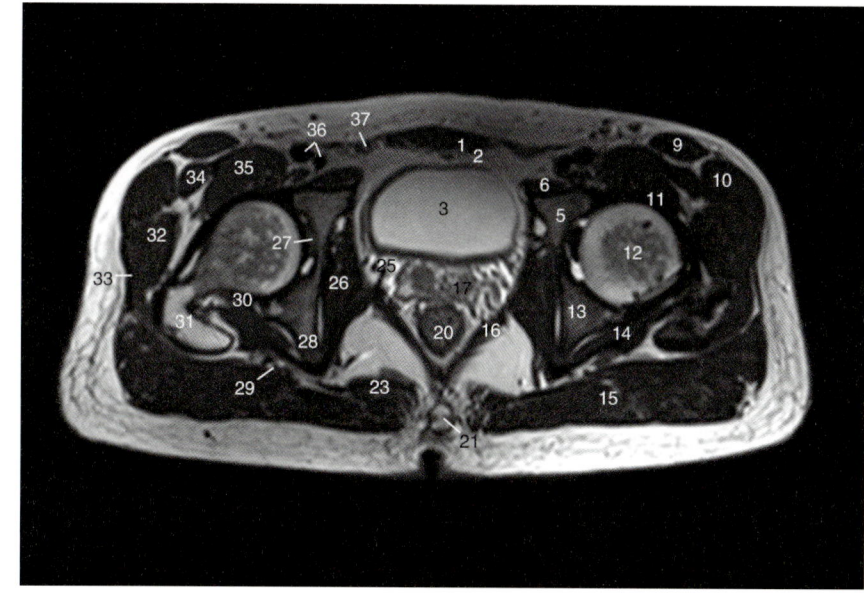
C. MR T2WI

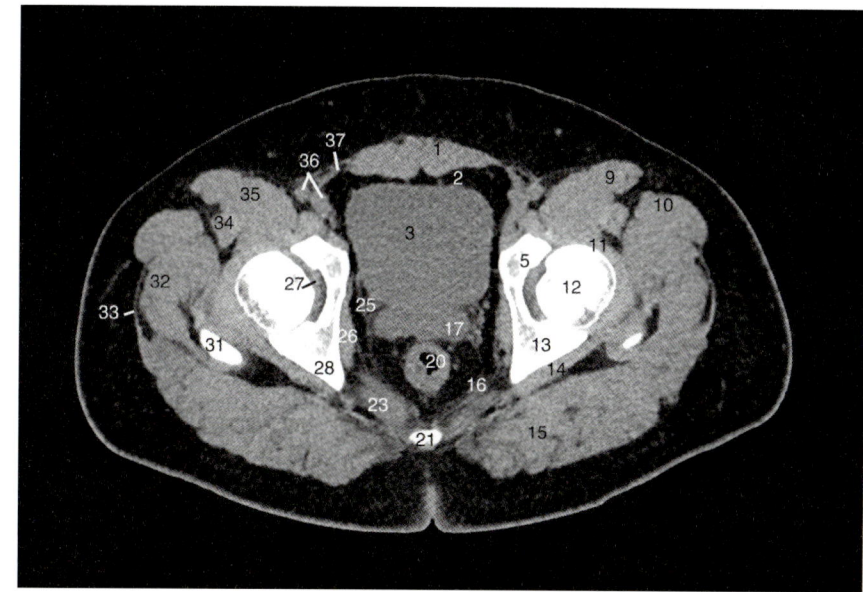
D. CT 平扫图像

1. 腹直肌 rectus abdominis
2. 膀胱前间隙 prevesical space
3. 膀胱 urinary bladder
4. 闭孔血管和神经 obturator blood vessels and nerve
5. 耻骨体 body of pubis
6. 耻骨肌 pectineus
7. 腹股沟浅淋巴结 superficial inguinal lymph nodes
8. 股神经 femoral nerve
9. 缝匠肌 sartorius
10. 阔筋膜张肌 tensor fasciae latae
11. 髂股韧带 iliofemoral ligament
12. 股骨头 femoral head
13. 坐骨体 body of ischium
14. 上孖肌 gemellus superior
15. 臀大肌 gluteus maximus
16. 肛提肌 levator ani
17. 精囊 seminal vesicle
18. 直肠膀胱陷凹 rectovesical pouch
19. 输精管 ductus deferens
20. 直肠 rectum
21. 尾骨 coccyx
22. 输尿管 ureter
23. 尾骨肌 coccygeus
24. 阴部内血管和阴部神经 internal pudendal blood vessels and pudendal nerve
25. 膀胱静脉丛 vesical venous plexus
26. 闭孔内肌 obturator internus
27. 股骨头韧带 ligament of head of femur
28. 坐骨棘 ischial spine
29. 坐骨神经 sciatic nerve
30. 坐股韧带 ischiofemoral ligament
31. 大转子 greater trochanter
32. 臀中肌 gluteus medius
33. 阔筋膜 fasciae lata
34. 股直肌 rectus femoris
35. 髂腰肌 iliopsoas
36. 股动、静脉 femoral artery and vein
37. 精索 spermatic cord
38. 前列腺 prostate

关键结构：直肠，精囊，输精管。

此断面经过股骨头中份。盆腔内前为膀胱，三角区膀胱壁增厚，输尿管壁内段明显变短。膀胱后方可见精囊，精囊内前方为输精管，周围脂肪间隙内可见膀胱静脉丛，后为直肠。直肠在第3骶椎平面续于乙状结肠，向下穿盆膈移行为肛管，全长约为11 cm。直肠在矢状面上有两个弯曲，即上部的骶曲和下部的会阴区，骶曲与骶骨盆面弯曲度一致，凸向后方。会阴区在尾骨尖处，凸向前方。直肠下部较为膨大称为直肠壶腹。直肠腔内黏膜常有3条横行的半月状皱襞称直肠皱襞。其中第二横襞较为恒定，位于直肠右侧壁，离肛门约11 cm，常作为直肠镜检的定位标志之一。直肠的上1/3腹膜覆盖其前面和两侧面，中1/3仅前方有腹膜覆盖，下1/3无腹膜覆盖。男性直肠在腹膜反折线以上隔直肠膀胱陷凹与膀胱底上部和精囊相邻，腹膜反折线以下则借直肠膀胱隔与膀胱底下部、精囊、输尿管壶腹、前列腺及输精管盆部相邻。直肠的动脉主要有直肠上、下动脉及骶正中动脉，彼此间有吻合。直肠上动脉是肠系膜下动脉的延续。该动脉经乙状结肠系膜根入盆腔，在第3骶椎平面分为左、右两支，沿着直肠两侧下降，分支供给直肠。由于第3骶椎平面在外科手术中较难确定，可用骶骨岬作为标志。从骶骨岬至直肠上动脉分为两终支处，其长度成年男性约为5.5 cm，女性约为5.1 cm[41]。直肠下动脉起自髂内动脉前干，行向前下，营养直肠下段。

203

男性盆部连续横断层 8（MH.6510）

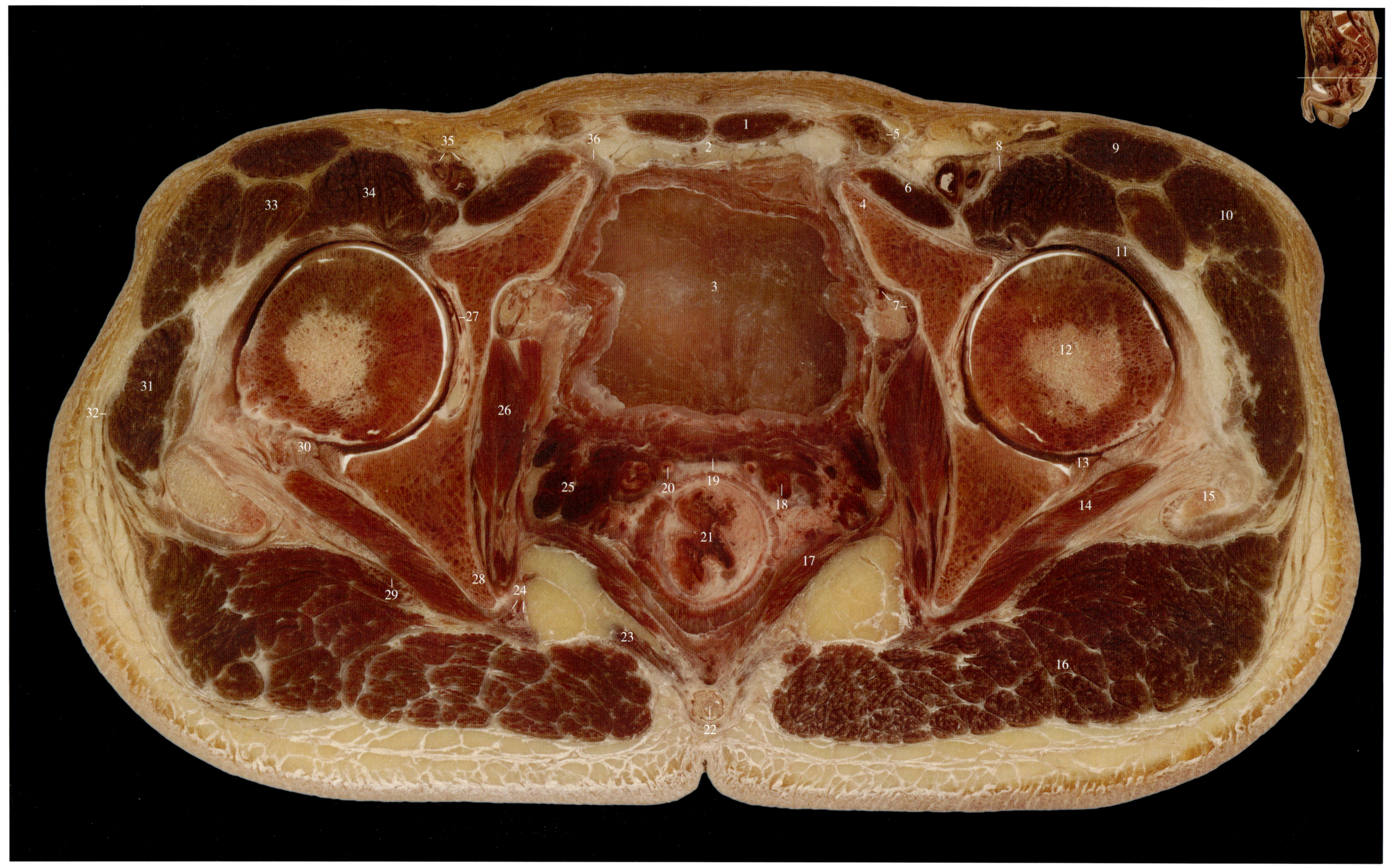

A. 断层标本图像

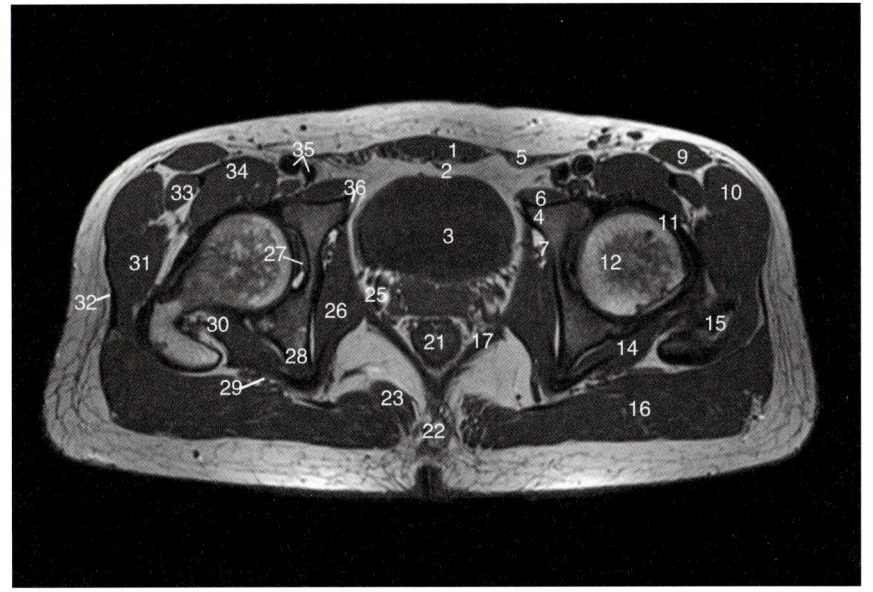
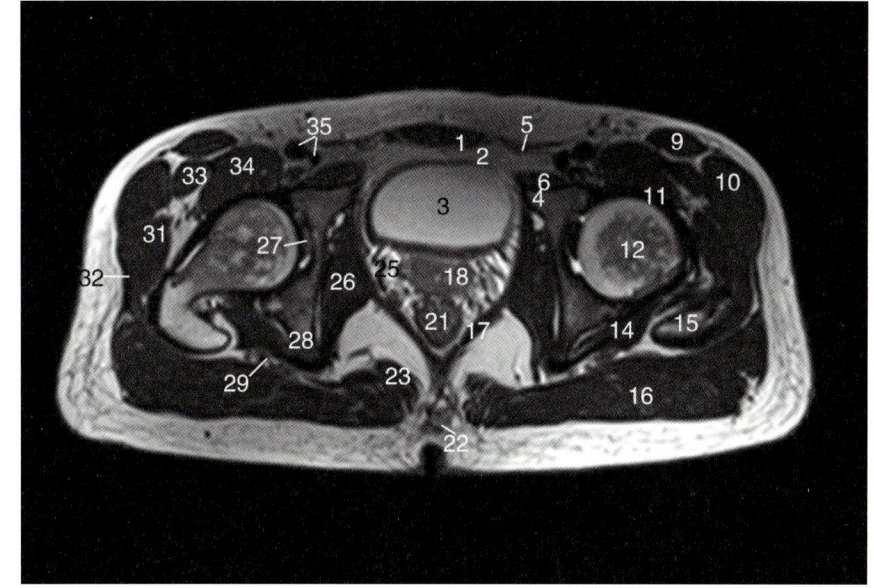
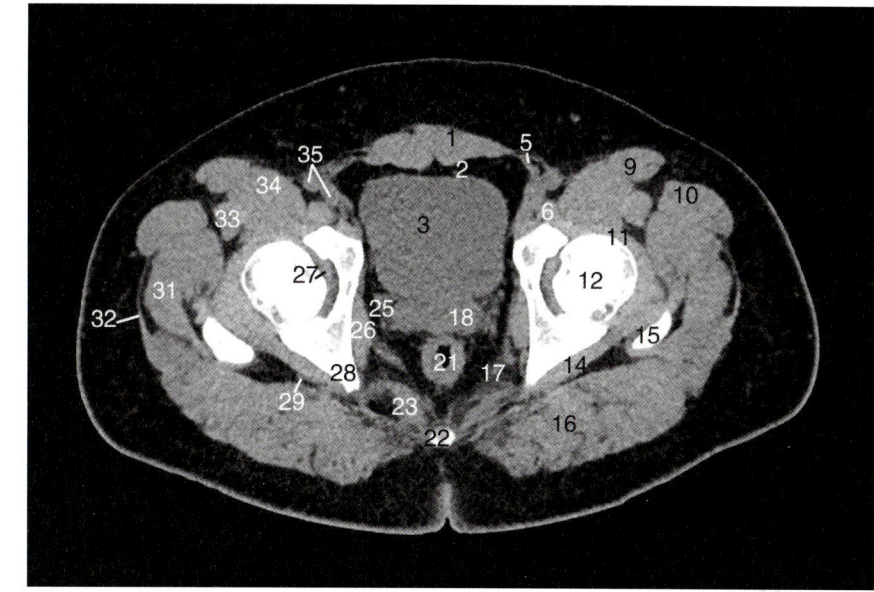

B. MR T1WI　　　　　　　　　　　　C. MR T2WI　　　　　　　　　　　　D. CT 平扫图像

关键结构：膀胱，精囊，直肠。

　　此断面经过股骨头中份。盆腔内，前部回肠袢即将消失，其所在部位为膀胱底所替代，后部为直肠，二者之间可见直肠膀胱陷凹。膀胱后壁输尿管壁内段走进膀胱。紧贴膀胱底后壁可见精囊，表面凹凸不平，左右各一，其排泄管与输精管壶腹的末端汇合成射精管。精囊主要位于股骨头中部至耻骨联合上部断面内，两侧长度之和约为 6 cm，在断面上呈对称性的囊泡状结构，其形态可分为卵圆形（70%）、管状（20%）和圆形（10%）3 种[1]，在 MRI 上呈等 T1 长 T2 信号。精囊向内侧与输精管汇合处有脂肪组织将其与膀胱后壁分隔开，使之与膀胱后壁之间形成夹角，即膀胱精囊角。于仰卧位扫描时呈锐角，平均为 28.75°cm±4.55°，该角在冠状位上也可观察到，患膀胱、精囊和前列腺肿瘤时该角减小或消失，在影像诊断中有重要价值。另外，在矢状位上，前列腺与直肠间存在直肠前列腺角，该角由精囊后界及直肠壁的前界构成，其内为前列腺与直肠间的软组织构成，用以外科评估前列腺及直肠肿瘤[45]。

1. 腹直肌 rectus abdominis
2. 膀胱前间隙 prevesical space
3. 膀胱 urinary bladder
4. 耻骨上支 superior ramus of pubis
5. 精索 spermatic cord
6. 耻骨肌 pectineus
7. 闭孔血管和神经 obturator blood vessels and nerve
8. 股神经 femoral nerve
9. 缝匠肌 sartorius
10. 阔筋膜张肌 tensor fasciae latae
11. 髂股韧带 iliofemoral ligament
12. 股骨头 femoral head
13. 髋臼唇 acetabular labrum
14. 上孖肌 gemellus superior
15. 大转子 greater trochanter
16. 臀大肌 gluteus maximus
17. 肛提肌 levator ani
18. 精囊 seminal vesicle
19. 直肠膀胱陷凹 rectovesical pouch
20. 输精管 ductus deferens
21. 直肠 rectum
22. 尾骨 coccyx
23. 尾骨肌 coccygeus
24. 阴部内血管和阴部神经 internal pudendal blood vessels and pudendal nerve
25. 膀胱静脉丛 vesical venous plexus
26. 闭孔内肌 obturator internus
27. 股骨头韧带 ligament of head of femur
28. 坐骨棘 ischial spine
29. 坐骨神经 sciatic nerve
30. 坐股韧带 ischiofemoral ligament
31. 臀中肌 gluteus medius
32. 阔筋膜 fasciae lata
33. 股直肌 rectus femoris
34. 髂腰肌 iliopsoas
35. 股动、静脉 femoral artery and vein
36. 耻骨上韧带 superior public ligament

男性盆部连续横断层 9（MH.6500）

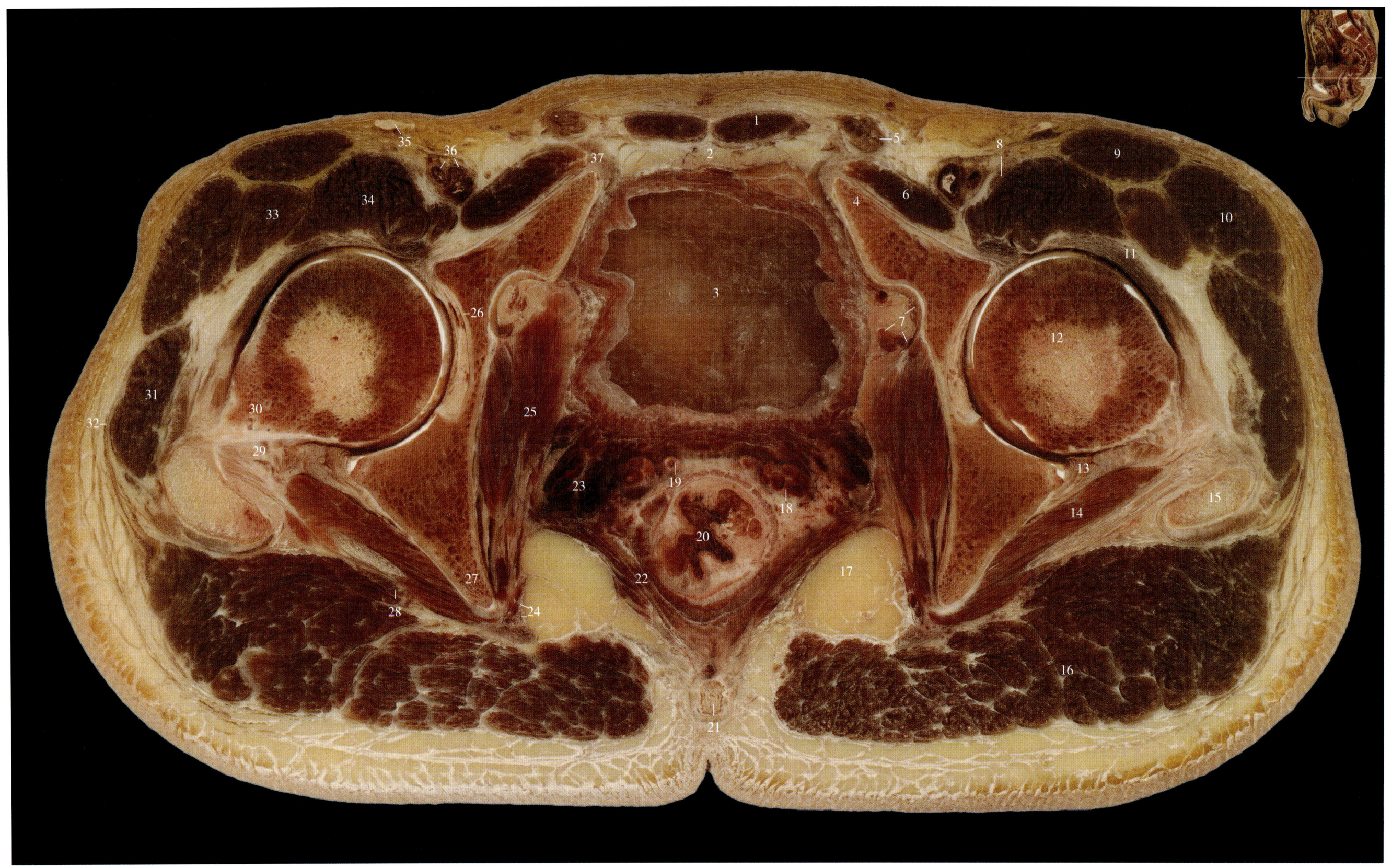

A. 断层标本图像

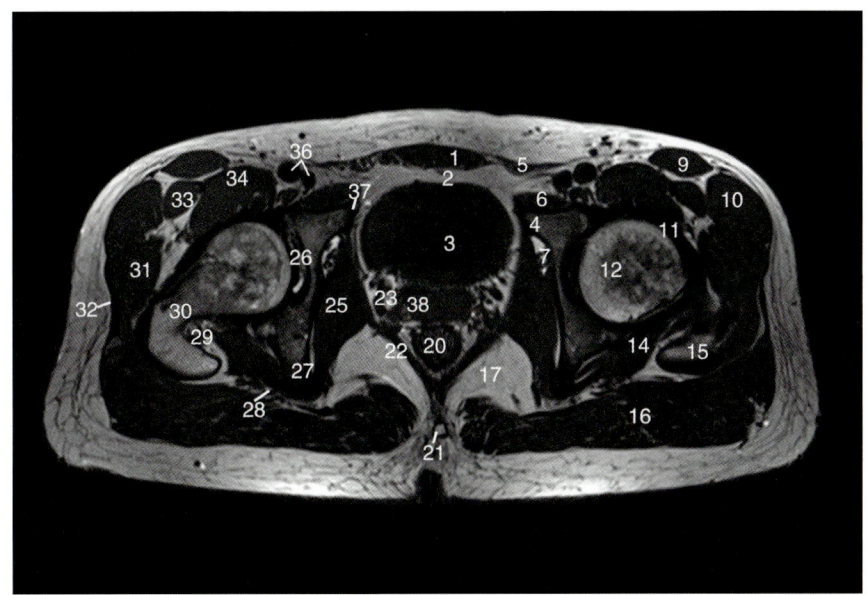
B. MR T1WI

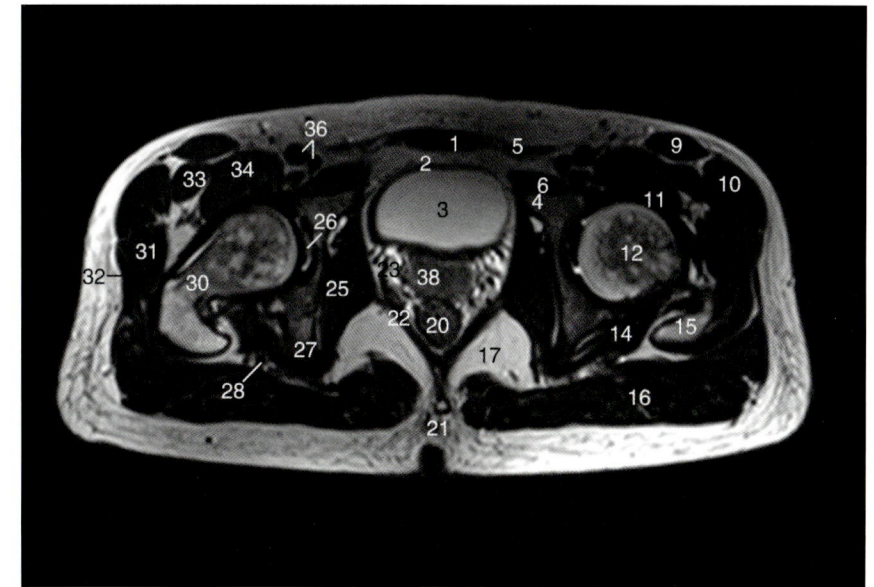
C. MR T2WI

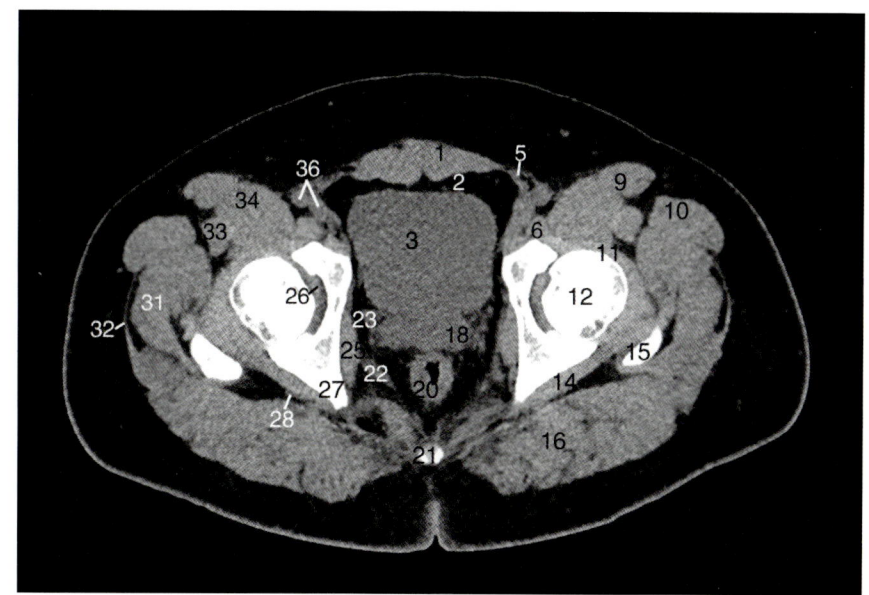
D. CT 平扫图像

1. 腹直肌 rectus abdominis
2. 膀胱前间隙 prevesical space
3. 膀胱 urinary bladder
4. 耻骨上支 superior ramus of pubis
5. 精索 spermatic cord
6. 耻骨肌 pectineus
7. 闭孔血管和神经 obturator blood vessels and nerve
8. 股神经 femoral nerve
9. 缝匠肌 sartorius
10. 阔筋膜张肌 tensor fasciae latae
11. 髂股韧带 iliofemoral ligament
12. 股骨头 femoral head
13. 髋臼唇 acetabular labrum
14. 上孖肌 gemellus superior
15. 大转子 greater trochanter
16. 臀大肌 gluteus maximus
17. 坐骨肛门窝 ischioanal fossa
18. 精囊 seminal vesicle
19. 输精管 ductus deferens
20. 直肠 rectum
21. 尾骨 coccyx
22. 肛提肌 levator ani
23. 膀胱静脉丛 vesical venous plexus
24. 阴部内血管和阴部神经 internal pudendal blood vessels and pudendal nerve
25. 闭孔内肌 obturator internus
26. 股骨头韧带 ligament of head of femur
27. 坐骨棘 ischial spine
28. 坐骨神经 sciatic nerve
29. 坐股韧带 ischiofemoral ligament
30. 股骨颈 neck of femur
31. 臀中肌 gluteus medius
32. 阔筋膜 fasciae lata
33. 股直肌 rectus femoris
34. 髂腰肌 iliopsoas
35. 腹股沟浅淋巴结 superficial inguinal lymph nodes
36. 股动、静脉 femoral artery and vein
37. 耻骨上韧带 superior public ligament
38. 前列腺 prostate

关键结构：精索，闭孔内肌，坐骨神经。

此断面经过股骨头中下份。

在髋关节前方，髂腰肌与耻骨肌之间可见股神经与股动、静脉及腹股沟深淋巴结。精索为一对圆索状结构，位于腹股沟管腹环至睾丸后上缘之间。精索是由输精管、睾丸动脉、输精管动脉、蔓状静脉丛、神经、淋巴管、鞘突剩件及包绕它们的鞘突被膜组成。精索的被膜共有3层，由外侧向内侧为：精索外筋膜，是腹外斜肌腱膜的延续；提睾肌，呈分散状，来自腹内斜肌和腹横肌的肌纤维；精索内筋膜，是腹横筋膜的延续[12, 46]。本断面可见腹直肌外侧的精索已出腹股沟管皮下环，在此断面中可分辨精索内的输精管及血管，在MR图像上根据信号强度亦可区分二者，前者呈中等强度信号，血管在T2WI上呈现流空低信号。髋臼内侧为闭孔内肌，在该肌前外缘与耻骨上支之间可见位于闭膜管内的闭膜动、静脉与闭孔神经及少量脂肪组织。闭孔内肌向后集中成腱，绕过坐骨小切迹至臀区，附于股骨大转子内侧。在臀区闭孔内肌肌腱后方，臀大肌深面可见坐骨神经下行。盆后壁为尾骨，两侧的尾骨肌在此断面消失，可见尾骨前方的肛提肌。盆腔内前为膀胱，后为直肠，二者之间的直肠膀胱陷凹即将消失，膀胱后方可见精囊。在髋臼与股骨头各断面中，髋臼与其邻近血管、神经的位置关系较密切，其中髋臼上份的前内侧与髂外动、静脉紧邻，髋臼下份的前内侧与闭孔动、静脉紧邻，且该处髋臼骨质较薄，故在行全髋关节置换术于臼内安放螺丝钉时，应予注意。

男性盆部连续横断层 10（MH.6490）

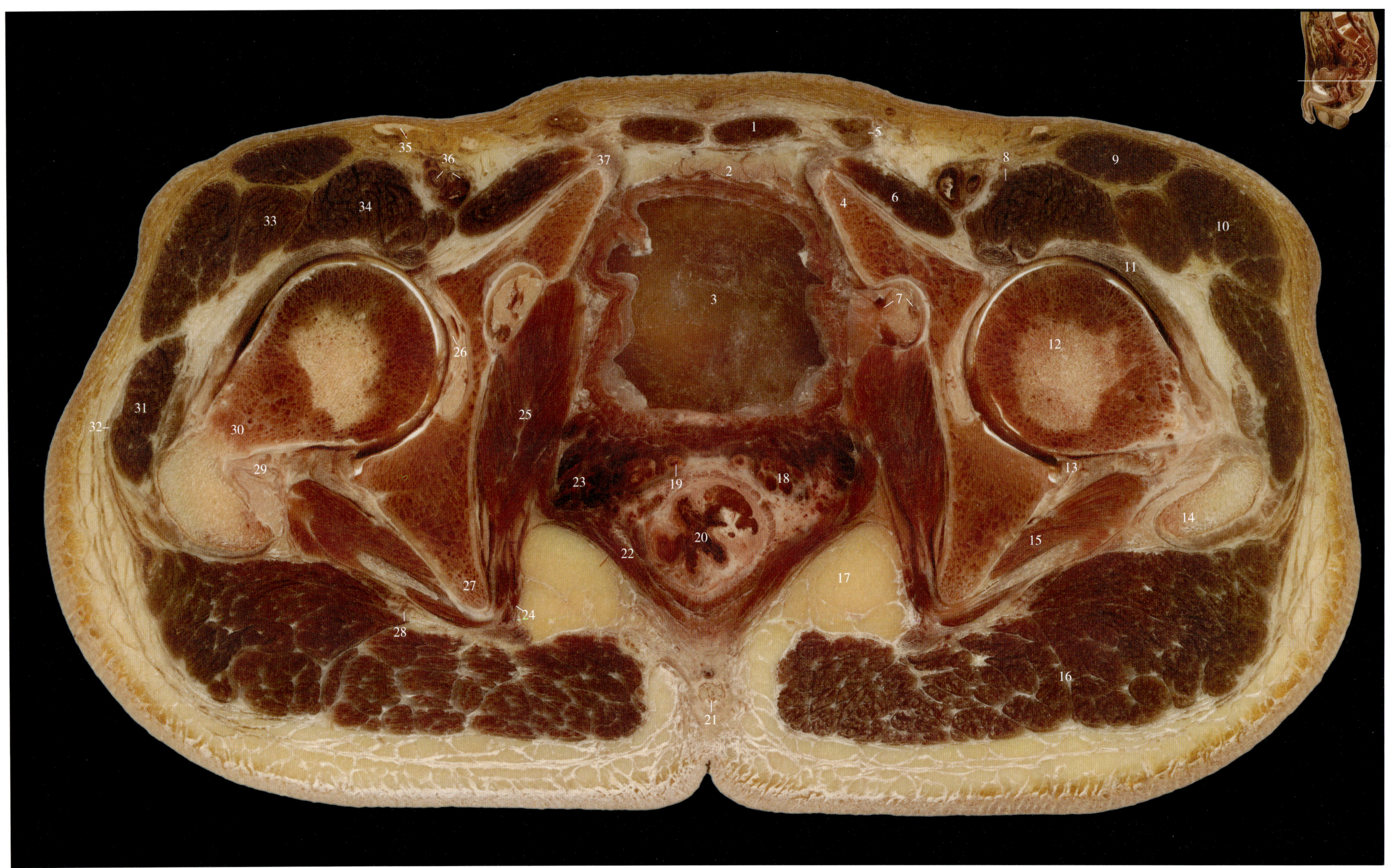

A. 断层标本图像

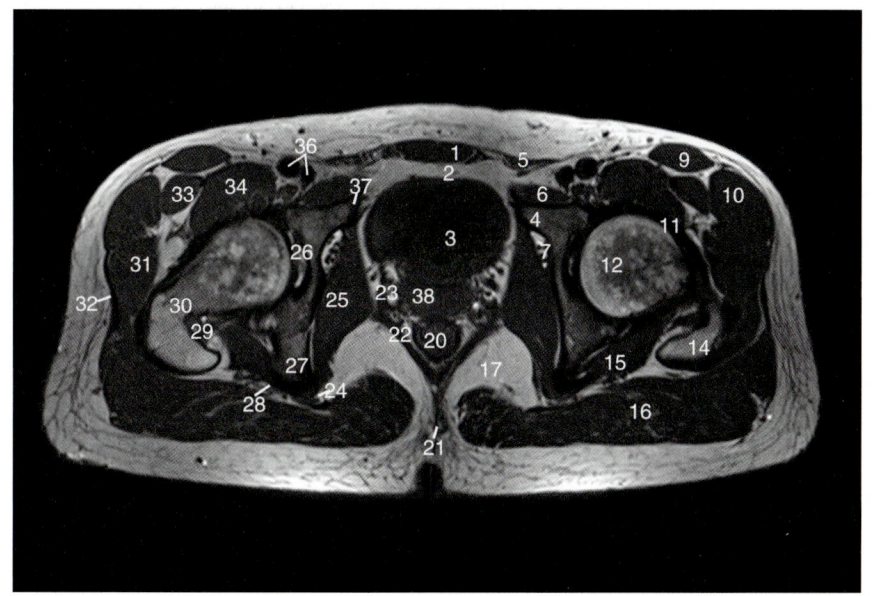

B. MR T1WI

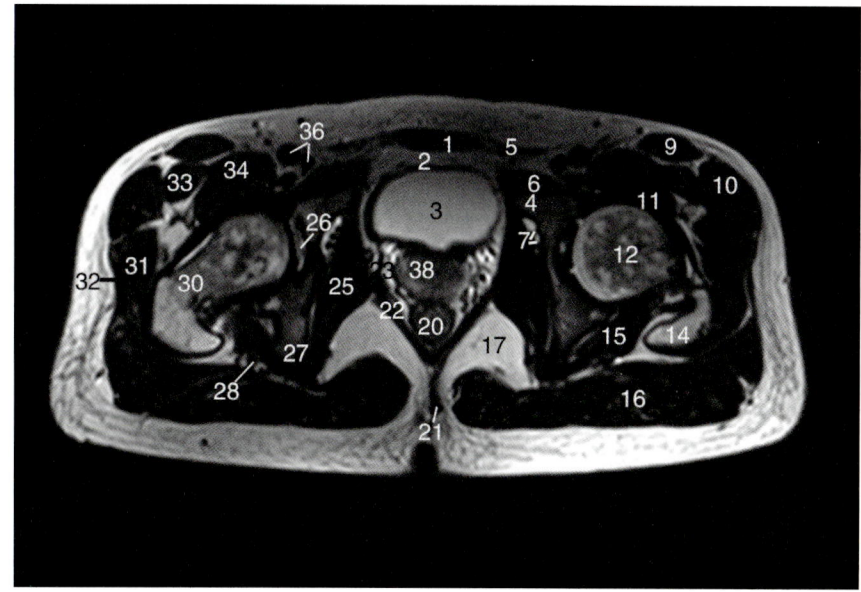

C. MR T2WI

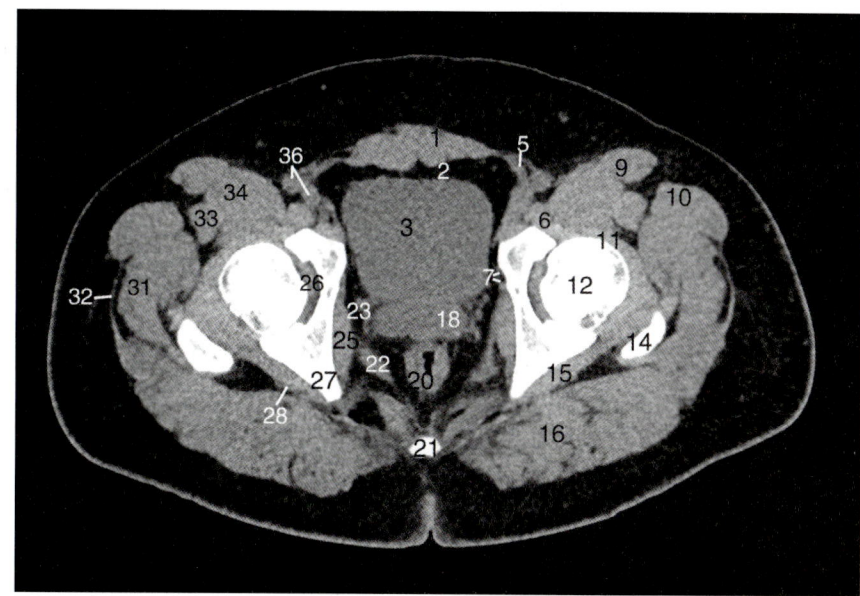

D. CT 平扫图像

关键结构：直肠，坐骨直肠窝，阴部管。

此断面经过股骨头中下份。精索逐渐向中线移行，接近腹直肌。盆腔内回肠襻消失，膀胱底前壁与腹壁间为充满脂肪的膀胱前间隙。膀胱后壁输尿管消失，为膀胱三角区。膀胱后方为直肠。直肠有丰富的静脉丛，直肠内静脉丛位于直肠黏膜下层，直肠外静脉丛位于肌层外，二者有丰富的吻合，形成直肠上静脉回流到肠系膜下静脉。直肠上部的淋巴结注入直肠壁外的直肠旁淋巴结，其输出管注入直肠上淋巴结和肠系膜下淋巴结。直肠下部的淋巴结注入髂内淋巴结和骶淋巴结[41]。MRI 在直肠及肛周病变诊断中的应用较 CT 具有明显优势。在直肠两侧，肛提肌、闭孔内肌和臀大肌之间为坐骨肛门窝（也称坐骨直肠窝），窝的外侧壁上可见行于阴部管内的阴部内血管和阴部神经。在坐骨肛门窝内，有大量的脂肪组织和纤维隔，称坐骨肛门窝脂体，具有弹性缓冲作用。窝内脂肪的血供较差，感染时易形成脓肿或瘘管。在 CT 图像上，坐骨肛门窝为坐骨结节、肛管和臀大肌所围成的三角形低密度区域；在 MRI 上为短 T1 长 T2 信号。

1. 腹直肌 rectus abdominis
2. 膀胱前间隙 prevesical space
3. 膀胱 urinary bladder
4. 耻骨上支 superior ramus of pubis
5. 精索 spermatic cord
6. 耻骨肌 pectineus
7. 闭孔血管和神经 obturator blood vessels and nerve
8. 股神经 femoral nerve
9. 缝匠肌 sartorius
10. 阔筋膜张肌 tensor fasciae latae
11. 髂股韧带 iliofemoral ligament
12. 股骨头 femoral head
13. 髋臼唇 acetabular labrum
14. 大转子 greater trochanter
15. 上孖肌 gemellus superior
16. 臀大肌 gluteus maximus
17. 坐骨肛门窝 ischioanal fossa
18. 精囊 seminal vesicle
19. 输精管 ductus deferens
20. 直肠 rectum
21. 尾骨 coccyx
22. 肛提肌 levator ani
23. 膀胱静脉丛 vesical venous plexus
24. 阴部内血管和阴部神经 internal pudendal blood vessels and pudendal nerve
25. 闭孔内肌 obturator internus
26. 股骨头韧带 ligament of head of femur
27. 坐骨棘 ischial spine
28. 坐骨神经 sciatic nerve
29. 坐股韧带 ischiofemoral ligament
30. 股骨颈 neck of femur
31. 臀中肌 gluteus medius
32. 阔筋膜 fasciae lata
33. 股直肌 rectus femoris
34. 髂腰肌 iliopsoas
35. 腹股沟浅淋巴结 superficial inguinal lymph nodes
36. 股动、静脉 femoral artery and vein
37. 耻骨上韧带 superior public ligament
38. 前列腺 prostate

男性盆部连续横断层 11（MH.6480）

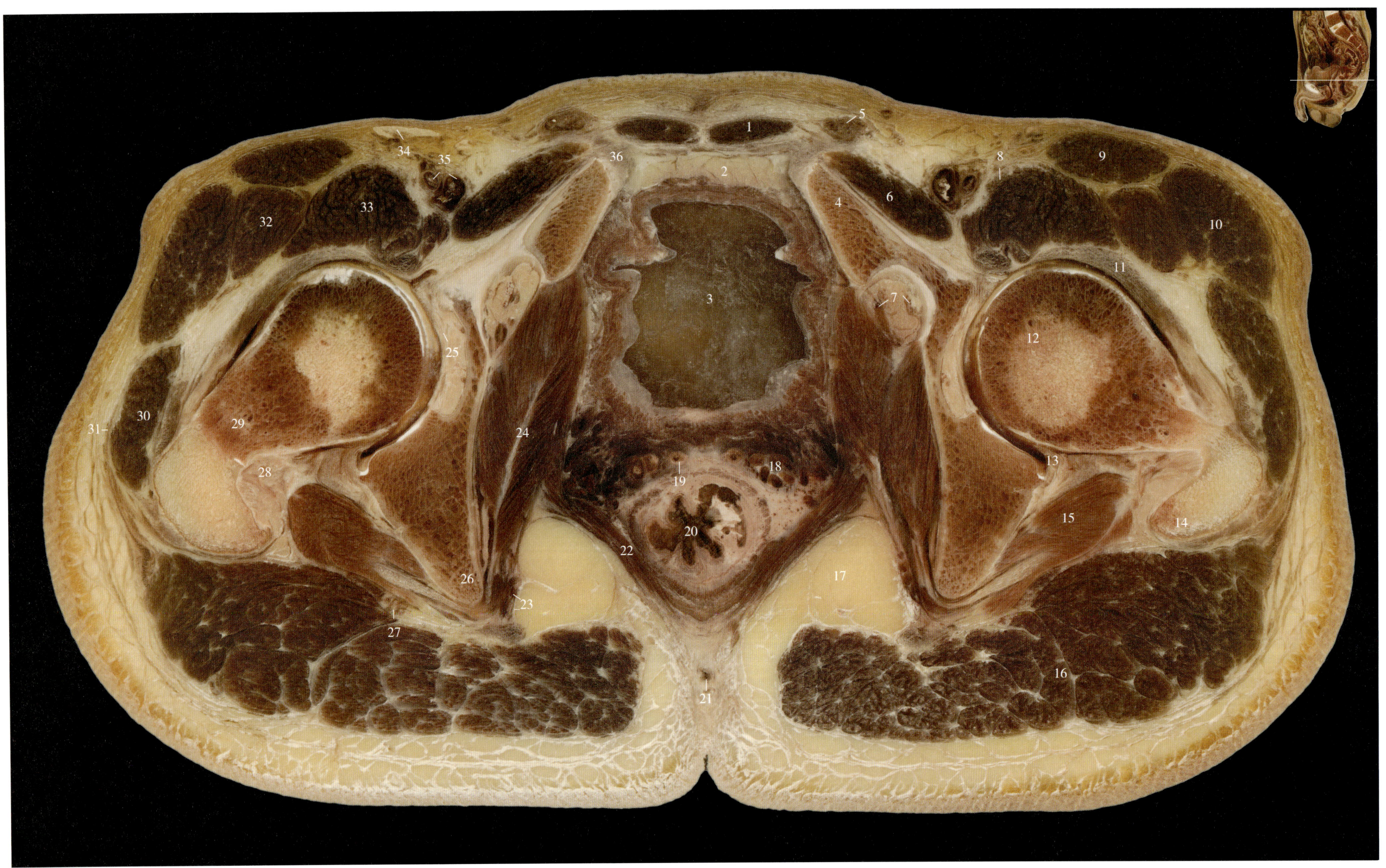

A. 断层标本图像

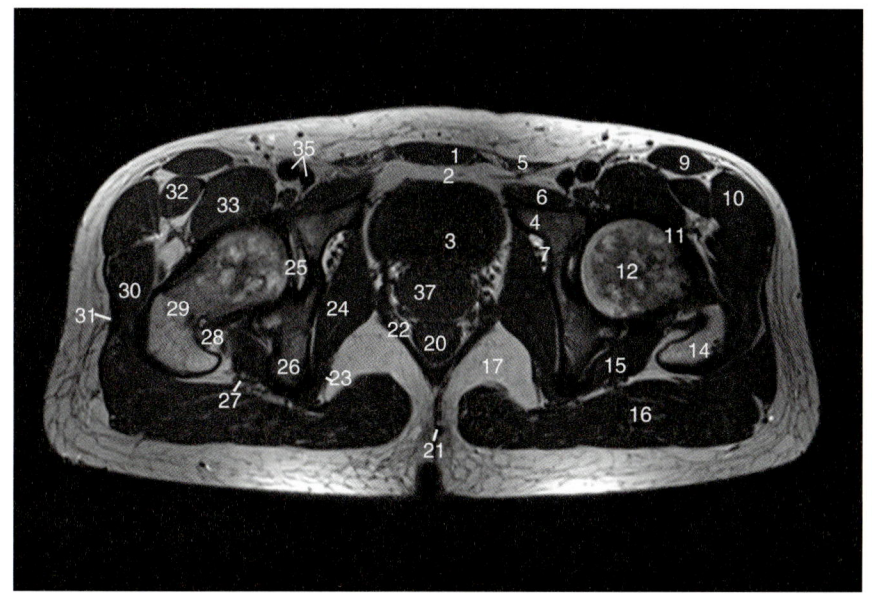

B. MR T1WI

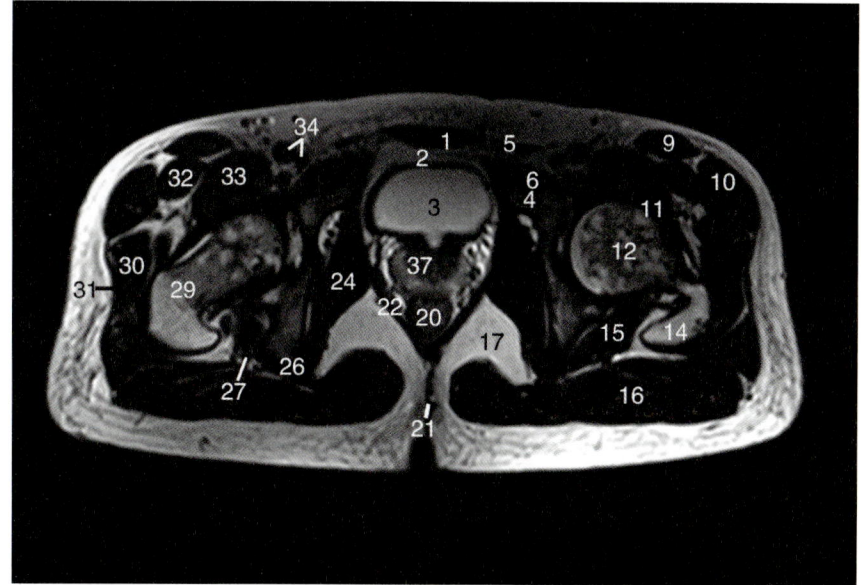

C. MR T2WI

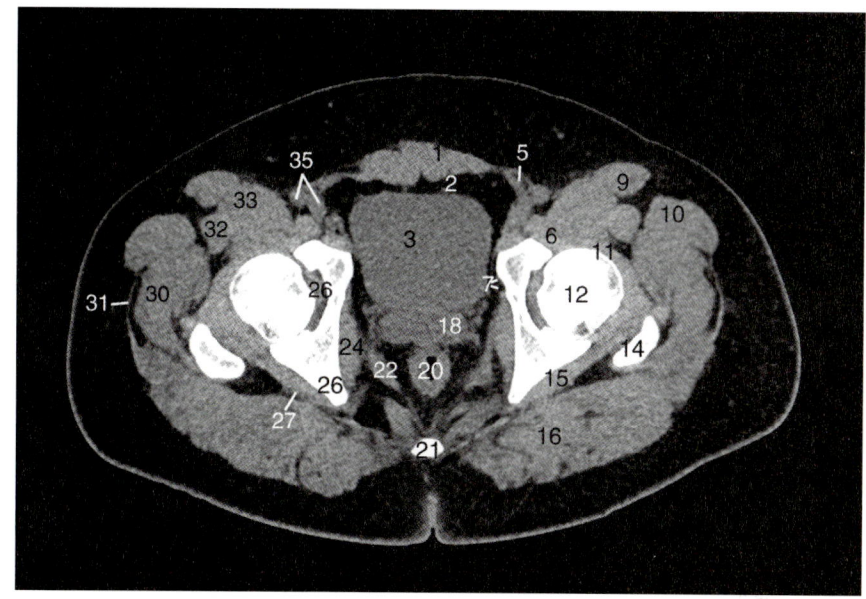

D. CT 平扫图像

1. 腹直肌 rectus abdominis
2. 膀胱前间隙 prevesical space
3. 膀胱 urinary bladder
4. 耻骨上支 superior ramus of pubis
5. 精索 spermatic cord
6. 耻骨肌 pectineus
7. 闭孔血管和神经 obturator blood vessels and nerve
8. 股神经 femoral nerve
9. 缝匠肌 sartorius
10. 阔筋膜张肌 tensor fasciae latae
11. 髂股韧带 iliofemoral ligament
12. 股骨头 femoral head
13. 髋臼唇 acetabular labrum
14. 大转子 greater trochanter
15. 下孖肌 gemellus inferior
16. 臀大肌 gluteus maximus
17. 坐骨肛门窝 ischioanal fossa
18. 精囊 seminal vesicle
19. 输精管壶腹 ampulla of ductus deferens
20. 直肠 rectum
21. 尾骨 coccyx
22. 肛提肌 levator ani
23. 阴部内血管和阴部神经 internal pudental blood vessels and pudendal nerve
24. 闭孔内肌 obturator internus
25. 股骨头韧带 ligament of head of femur
26. 坐骨棘 ischial spine
27. 坐骨神经 sciatic nerve
28. 坐股韧带 ischiofemoral ligament
29. 股骨颈 neck of femur
30. 臀中肌 gluteus medius
31. 阔筋膜 fasciae lata
32. 股直肌 rectus femoris
33. 髂腰肌 iliopsoas
34. 腹股沟浅淋巴结 superficial inguinal lymph nodes
35. 股动、静脉 femoral artery and vein
36. 耻骨上韧带 superior public ligament
37. 前列腺 prostate

关键结构：精索，膀胱，精囊。

此断面经过股骨头中下份。骨盆侧壁见股骨头向外走行、变细，移行为股骨颈，股骨颈与股骨体连接处上外侧的方形隆起为大转子，是判断股骨颈骨折或髋关节脱位的重要标志。股骨颈前后方可见关节囊，囊壁厚为 2~3 mm[1]，大转子位居关节囊外。盆腔内前为膀胱，后为直肠，膀胱后方可见精囊及输精管壶腹。膀胱的主要供血动脉是膀胱上动脉，1~2 支，约在耻骨上缘平面起自髂内动脉的分支脐动脉的根部，斜行至膀胱，分布于膀胱上壁和两侧。膀胱下动脉多起自髂内动脉前干或阴部内动脉，位于闭孔动脉后下方，沿盆侧壁向后下行，营养膀胱下部、精囊腺、前列腺等。膀胱淋巴结多注入髂外淋巴结，少数注入髂内淋巴结和髂总淋巴结。分布于膀胱的神经来自盆丛的膀胱丛，其中交感神经来自 T11、T12 和 L1、L2 脊髓节，使逼尿肌松弛、尿道内括约肌收缩，有利于尿的贮存；副交感神经来自盆内脏神经，使逼尿肌收缩、尿道内括约肌松弛排尿[41]。盆前壁为腹直肌，膀胱与腹直肌之间称膀胱前间隙，此间隙内男性有耻骨前列腺韧带，此间隙中还有丰富的结缔组织和静脉丛。膀胱静脉在膀胱外下部形成膀胱静脉丛，围绕膀胱颈，然后汇集成与伴行动脉同名的静脉注入髂内静脉。

211

男性盆部连续横断层 12（MH.6470）

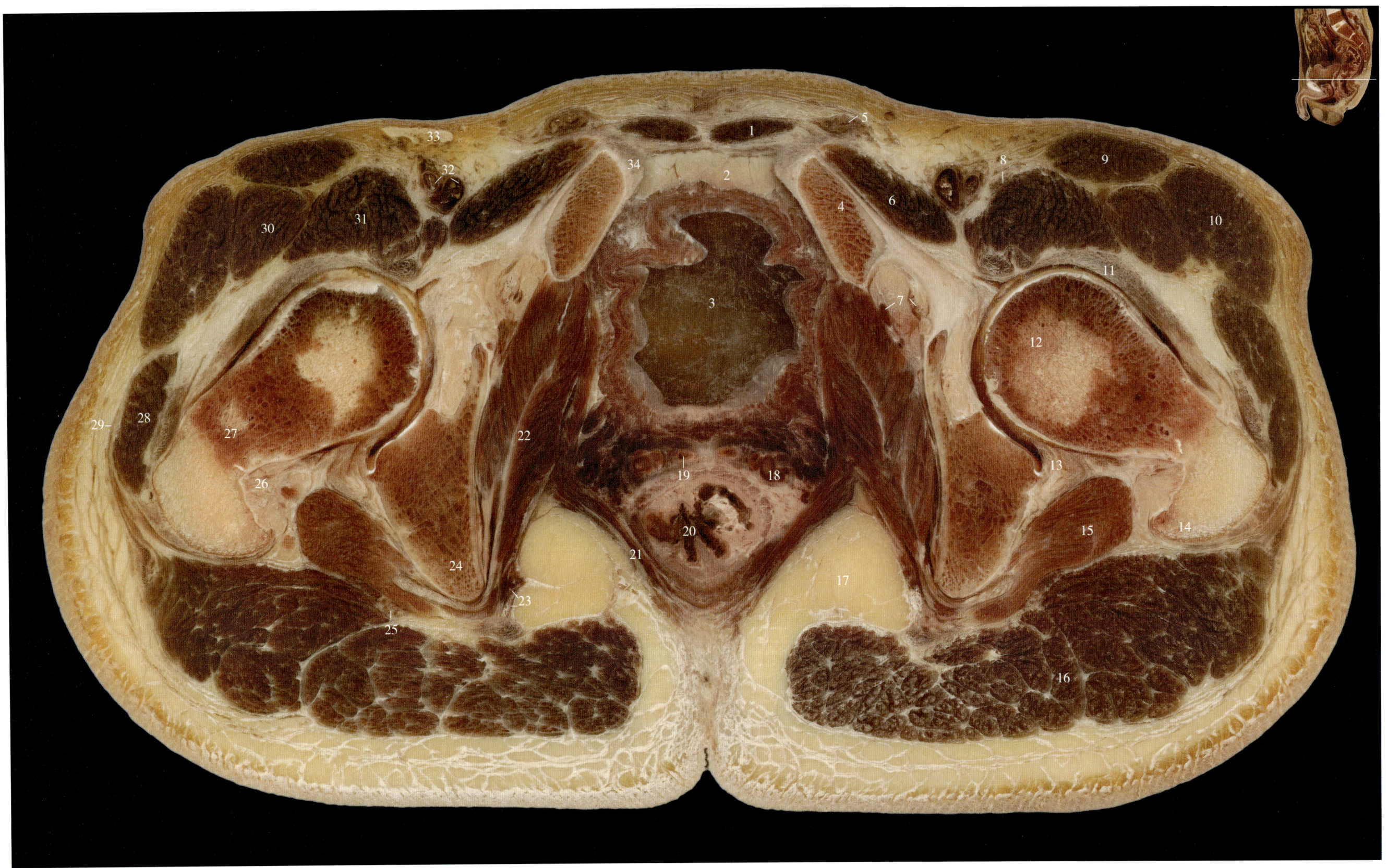

A. 断层标本图像

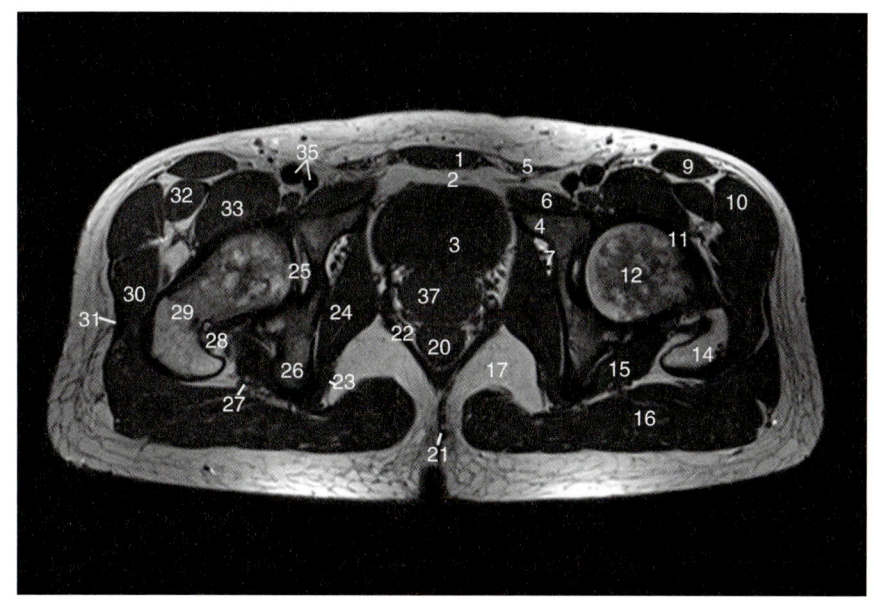

B. MR T1WI

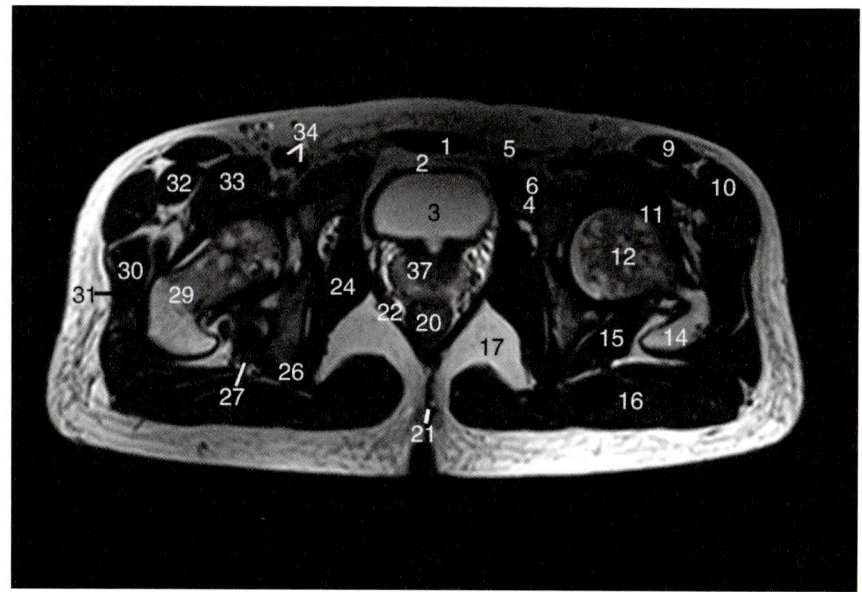

C. MR T2WI

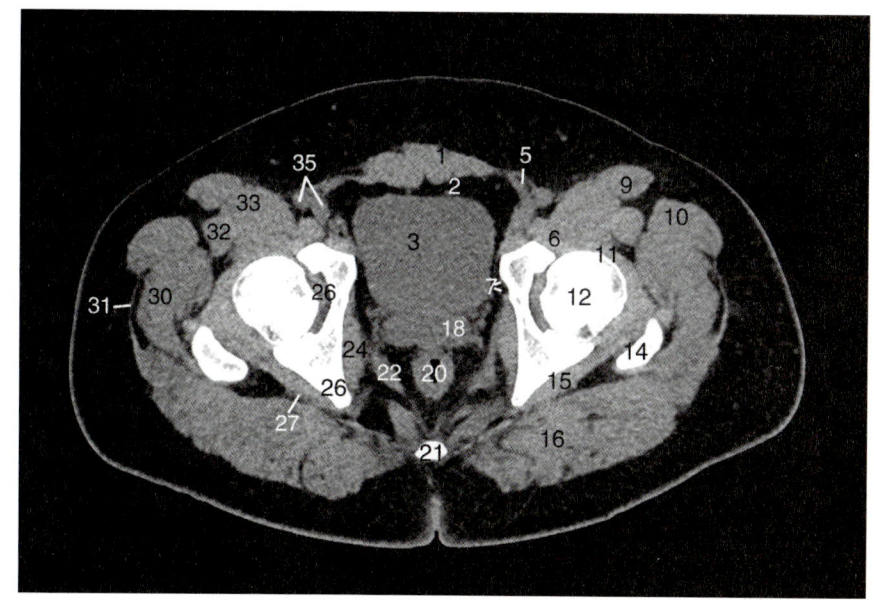

D. CT 平扫图像

1. 腹直肌 rectus abdominis
2. 膀胱前间隙 prevesical space
3. 膀胱 urinary bladder
4. 耻骨上支 superior ramus of pubis
5. 精索 spermatic cord
6. 耻骨肌 pectineus
7. 闭孔血管和神经 obturator blood vessels and nerve
8. 股神经 femoral nerve
9. 缝匠肌 sartorius
10. 阔筋膜张肌 tensor fasciae latae
11. 髂股韧带 iliofemoral ligament
12. 股骨头 femoral head
13. 髋臼唇 acetabular labrum
14. 大转子 greater trochanter
15. 下孖肌 gemellus inferior
16. 臀大肌 gluteus maximus
17. 坐骨肛门窝 ischioanal fossa
18. 精囊 seminal vesicle
19. 输精管壶腹 ampulla of ductus deferens
20. 直肠 rectum
21. 尾骨 coccyx
22. 肛提肌 levator ani
23. 阴部内血管和阴部神经 internal pudendal blood vessels and pudendal nerve
24. 闭孔内肌 obturator internus
25. 股骨头韧带 ligament of head of femur
26. 坐骨棘 ischial spine
27. 坐骨神经 sciatic nerve
28. 坐股韧带 ischiofemoral ligament
29. 股骨颈 neck of femur
30. 臀中肌 gluteus medius
31. 阔筋膜 fasciae lata
32. 股直肌 rectus femoris
33. 髂腰肌 iliopsoas
34. 腹股沟浅淋巴结 superficial inguinal lymph nodes
35. 股动、静脉 femoral artery and vein
36. 耻骨上韧带 superior public ligament
37. 前列腺 prostate

关键结构：精索，膀胱，精囊。

此断面经过股骨头中下份。骨盆侧壁见股骨头向外走行、变细，移行为股骨颈，股骨颈与股骨体连接处上外侧的方形隆起为大转子，是判断股骨颈骨折或髋关节脱位的重要标志。股骨颈前后方可见关节囊，囊壁厚为 2~3 mm[1]，大转子位居关节囊外。盆腔内前为膀胱，后为直肠，膀胱后方可见精囊及输精管壶腹。膀胱的主要供血动脉是膀胱上动脉，1~2 支，约在耻骨上缘平面起自髂内动脉的分支脐动脉的根部，斜行至膀胱，分布于膀胱上壁和两侧。膀胱下动脉多起自髂内动脉前干或阴部内动脉，位于闭孔动脉后下方，沿盆侧壁向后下行，营养膀胱下部、精囊腺、前列腺等。膀胱淋巴结多注入髂外淋巴结，少数注入髂内淋巴结和髂总淋巴结。分布于膀胱的神经来自盆丛的膀胱丛，其中交感神经来自T11、T12和L1、L2脊髓节，使逼尿肌松弛、尿道内括约肌收缩，有利于尿的贮存；副交感神经来自盆内脏神经，使逼尿肌收缩、尿道内括约肌松弛排尿[41]。盆前壁为腹直肌，膀胱与腹直肌之间称膀胱前间隙，此间隙内男性有耻骨前列腺韧带，此间隙中还有丰富的结缔组织和静脉丛。膀胱静脉在膀胱外下部形成膀胱静脉丛，围绕膀胱颈，然后汇集成与伴行动脉同名的静脉注入髂内静脉。

男性盆部连续横断层 12（MH.6470）

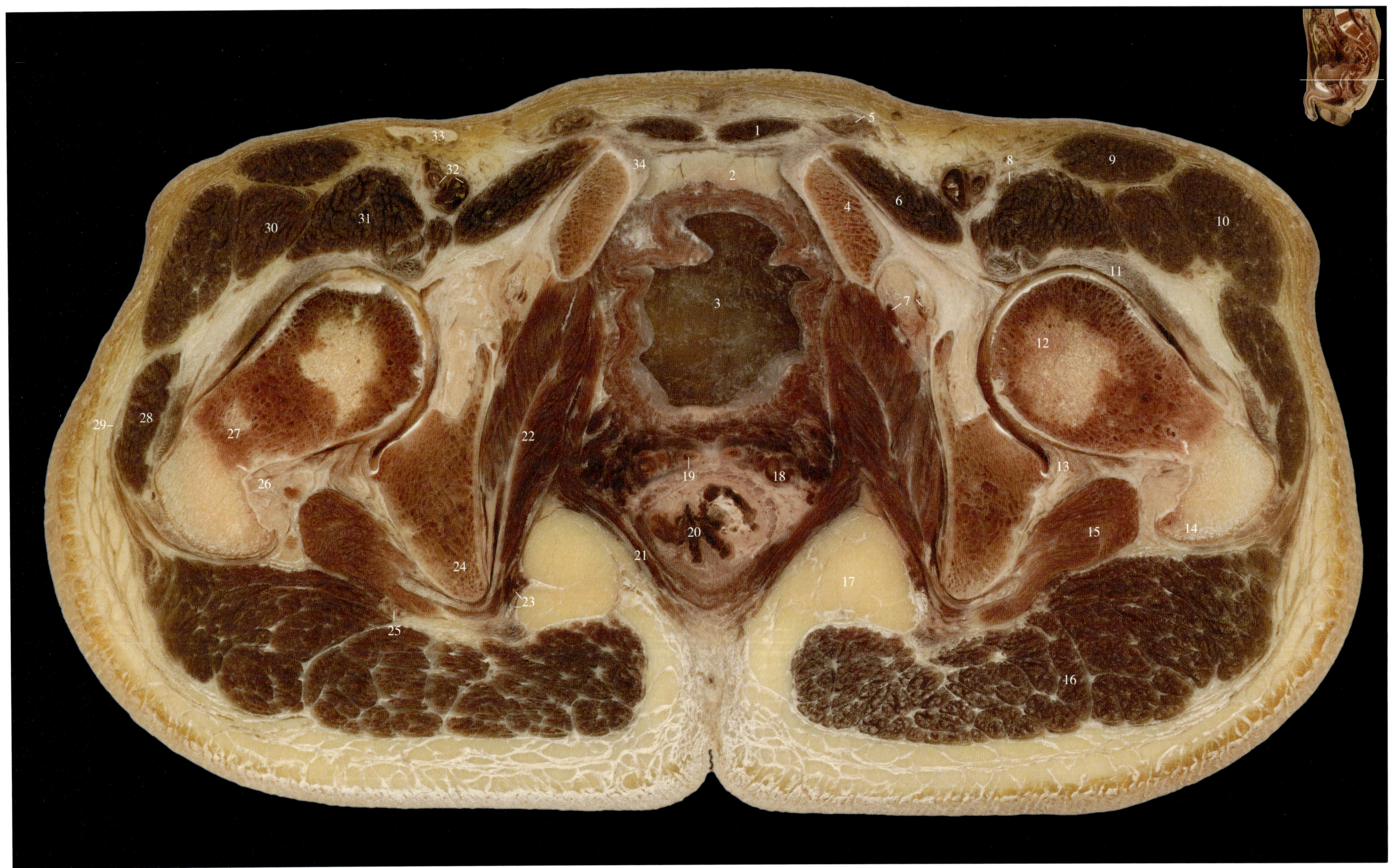

A. 断层标本图像

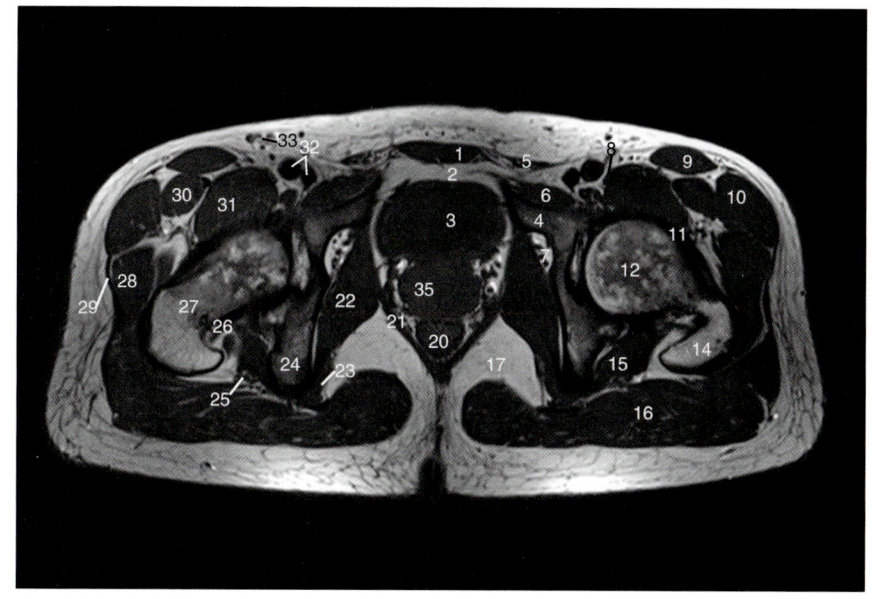

B. MR T1WI

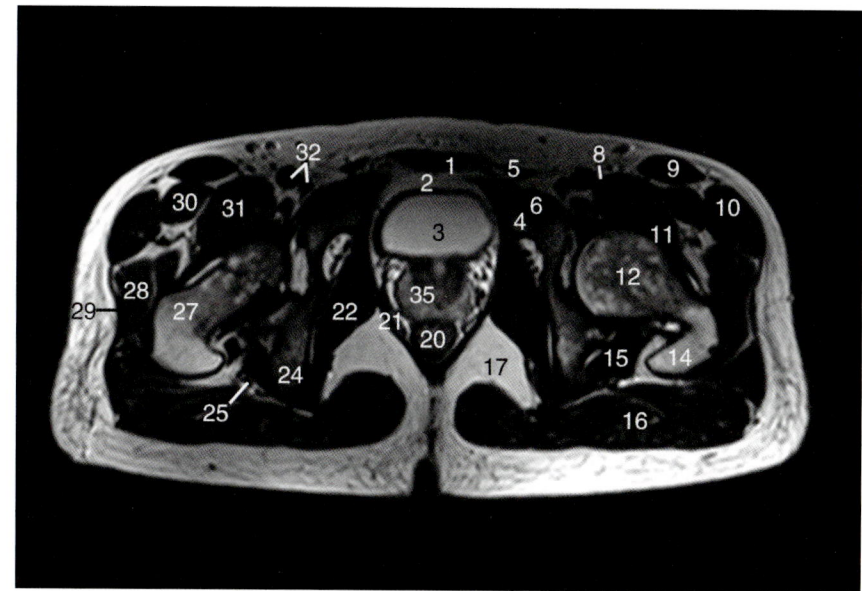

C. MR T2WI

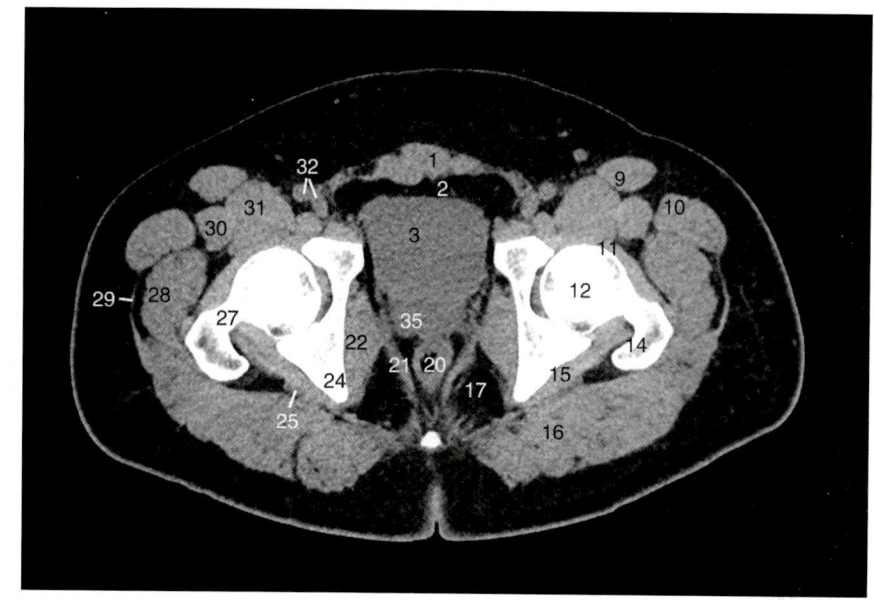

D. CT 平扫图像

1. 腹直肌 rectus abdominis
2. 膀胱前间隙 prevesical space
3. 膀胱 urinary bladder
4. 耻骨上支 superior ramus of pubis
5. 精索 spermatic cord
6. 耻骨肌 pectineus
7. 闭孔血管和神经 obturator blood vessels and nerve
8. 股神经 femoral nerve
9. 缝匠肌 sartorius
10. 阔筋膜张肌 tensor fasciae latae
11. 髂股韧带 iliofemoral ligament
12. 股骨头 femoral head
13. 髋臼唇 acetabular labrum
14. 大转子 greater trochanter
15. 下孖肌 gemellus inferior
16. 臀大肌 gluteus maximus
17. 坐骨肛门窝 ischioanal fossa
18. 精囊 seminal vesicle
19. 输精管壶腹 ampulla of ductus deferens
20. 直肠 rectum
21. 肛提肌 levator ani
22. 闭孔内肌 obturator internus
23. 阴部内血管和阴部神经 internal pudendal blood vessels and pudendal nerve
24. 坐骨结节 ischial tuberosity
25. 坐骨神经 sciatic nerve
26. 坐股韧带 ischiofemoral ligament
27. 股骨颈 neck of femur
28. 臀中肌 gluteus medius
29. 阔筋膜 fasciae lata
30. 股直肌 rectus femoris
31. 髂腰肌 iliopsoas
32. 股动、静脉 femoral artery and vein
33. 腹股沟浅淋巴结 superficial inguinal lymph nodes
34. 耻骨上韧带 superior public ligament
35. 前列腺 prostate

关键结构：输精管，膀胱，精索。

此断面经过耻骨上支。盆壁骨性部分由两侧的髋关节构成，股骨头下份断面缩小，耻骨体消失，耻骨上支间见膀胱前间隙（亦称耻骨后间隙）[1]，髋关节的中部主要由两侧的坐骨支构成，断面后部的尾骨消失。在髋关节前方，髂腰肌与耻骨肌之间可见股神经与股动、静脉及腹股沟浅淋巴结，耻骨肌前方皮下见精索。盆腔内结构从前往后是膀胱、直肠，二者之间见精囊及输精管壶腹部。输精管是附睾管的直接延续，成人输精管左侧长度为 31.24 cm ± 3.50 cm，右侧为 32.12 cm ± 3.69 cm[16]；输精管盆部自腹股沟深环处接腹股沟管部，从外侧绕腹壁下动脉的起始部，急转向内下方，越过髂外动、静脉前方进入盆腔。沿盆侧壁行向后下，跨过膀胱上血管和闭孔血管，从前内侧与输尿管交叉，继而转至膀胱底。膀胱黏膜层和肌层有丰富的淋巴网络，经集合淋巴管，汇聚到膀胱前间隙，流入髂外淋巴结的中间和内侧组。具体途径是：膀胱的前壁通过集合位于外侧膀胱边界中部 3/1 处的淋巴管引流，朝着脐动脉和膀胱上动脉的起源下降，与后壁的集合淋巴管汇合，并汇入髂外淋巴结。后壁的集合淋巴管要么延伸到膀胱的后外侧角，越过脐动脉并流入内侧和中间髂外淋巴结，要么流到膀胱三角区的集合淋巴管中，伴行于子宫或输精管动脉，最终汇入髂外淋巴结的内侧和中间组[47]。

男性盆部连续横断层 13（MH.6460）

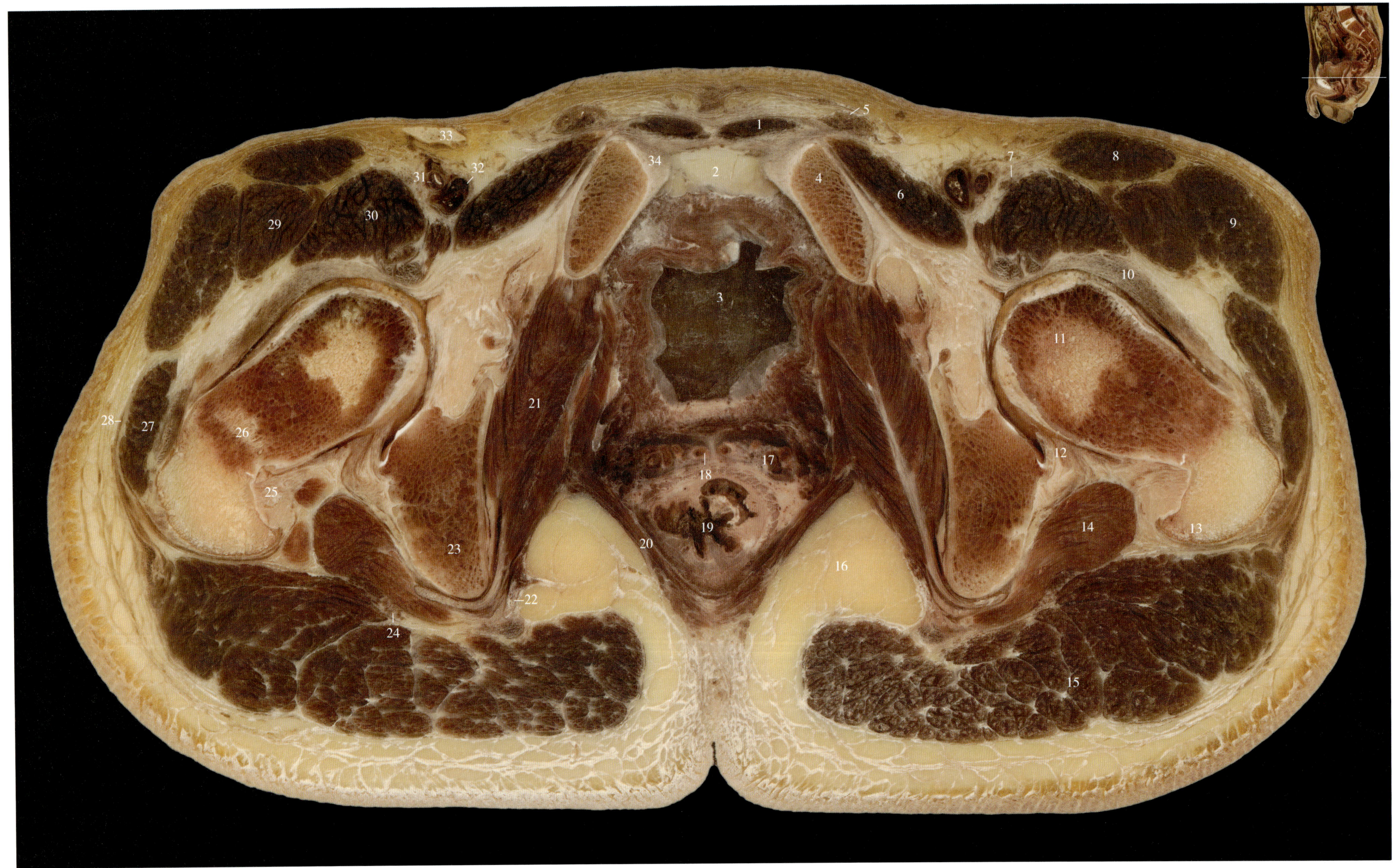

A. 断层标本图像

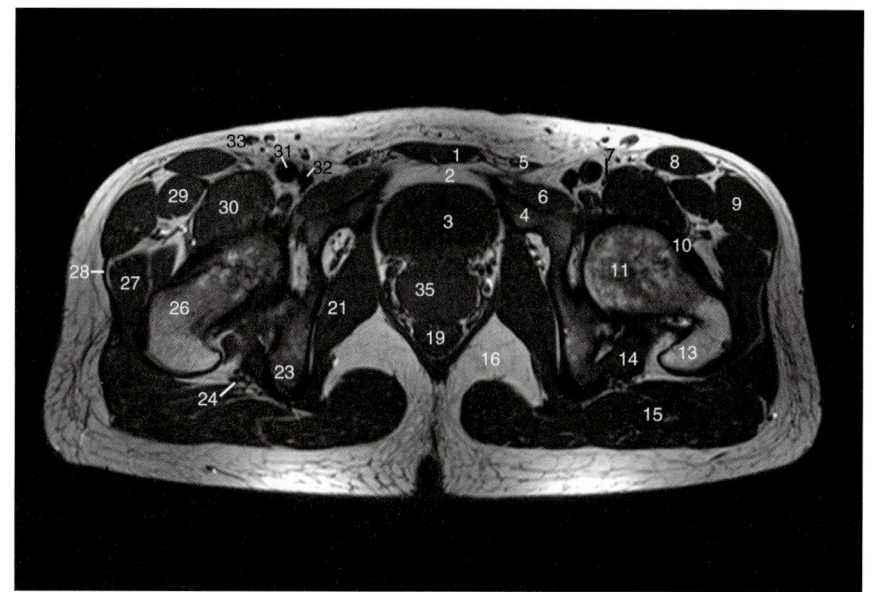

B. MR T1WI

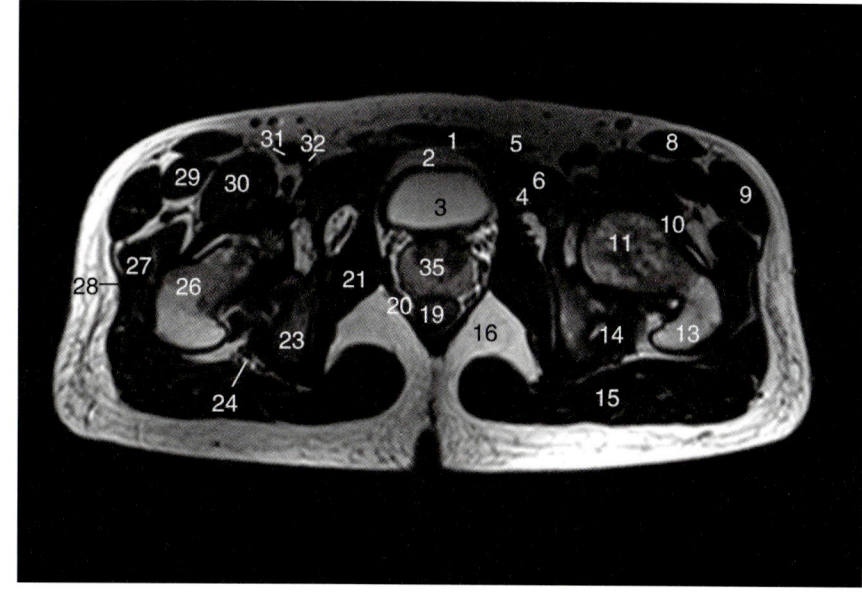

C. MR T2WI

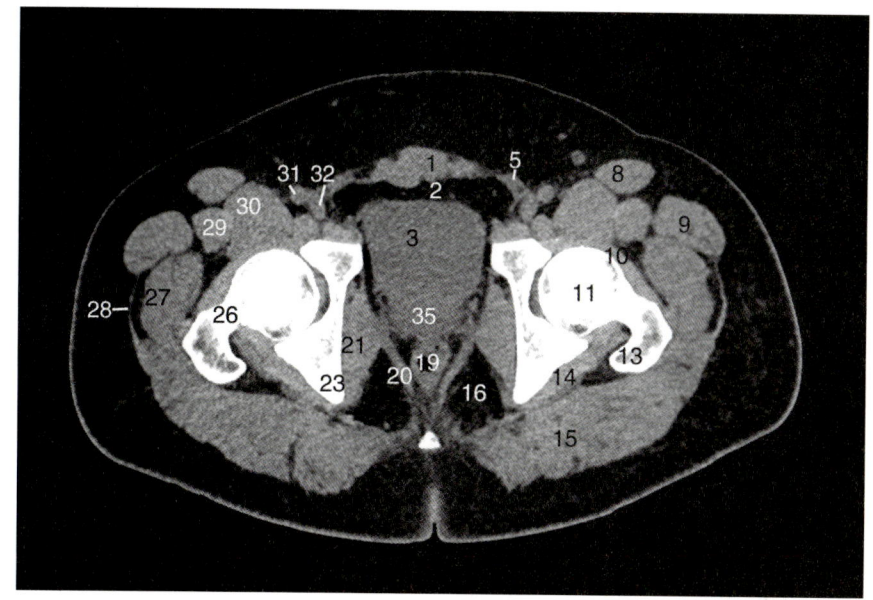

D. CT 平扫图像

1. 腹直肌 rectus abdominis
2. 膀胱前间隙 prevesical space
3. 膀胱 urinary bladder
4. 耻骨上支 superior ramus of pubis
5. 精索 spermatic cord
6. 耻骨肌 pectineus
7. 股神经 femoral nerve
8. 缝匠肌 sartorius
9. 阔筋膜张肌 tensor fasciae latae
10. 髂股韧带 iliofemoral ligament
11. 股骨头 femoral head
12. 髋臼唇 acetabular labrum
13. 大转子 greater trochanter
14. 下孖肌 gemellus inferior
15. 臀大肌 gluteus maximus
16. 坐骨肛门窝 ischioanal fossa
17. 精囊 seminal vesicle
18. 输精管壶腹 ampulla of ductus deferens
19. 直肠 rectum
20. 肛提肌 levator ani
21. 闭孔内肌 obturator internus
22. 阴部神经 pudendal nerve
23. 坐骨结节 ischial tuberosity
24. 坐骨神经 sciatic nerve
25. 坐股韧带 ischiofemoral ligament
26. 股骨颈 neck of femur
27. 臀中肌 gluteus medius
28. 阔筋膜 fasciae lata
29. 股直肌 rectus femoris
30. 髂腰肌 iliopsoas
31. 股动脉 femoral artery
32. 股静脉 femoral vein
33. 腹股沟浅淋巴结 superficial inguinal lymph nodes
34. 耻骨上韧带 superior public ligament
35. 前列腺 prostate

关键结构：股骨颈，精囊，输精管壶腹。

此断面经过耻骨上支。两侧中部主要由坐骨支构成，股骨头基本消失，髋关节内主要为股骨头基底部与股骨颈近端。此处常见良性囊样病变：股骨颈疝窝，CT 表现为有硬化边的小囊样低密度，MRI 表现为含有液体的囊状信号。国内有学者认为，此窝的形成与股骨颈外侧的髂股韧带机械压力有关。盆腔内前部为膀胱，膀胱后方为精囊，精囊的前内侧为输精管壶腹。直肠居于盆腔的后部，直肠后及外缘由肛提肌环绕。两侧输精管壶腹部已经接近中线，输精管依其行程可分为：①睾丸部，始于附睾尾，最短，较迂曲，沿睾丸后缘、附睾内侧行至睾丸上端，输精管睾丸部左侧长度为 $4.38\ cm \pm 0.55\ cm$，右侧为 $4.42\ cm \pm 0.49\ cm$；②精索部，介于睾丸上端与腹股沟管皮下环之间，此段位置表浅，易于触及，输精管精索部左侧长度为 $7.22\ cm \pm 2.60\ cm$，右侧长度为 $6.75\ cm + 2.06\ cm$；③腹股沟管部，全程位于腹股沟管的精索内，左侧长度为 $4.62\ cm \pm 0.98\ cm$，右侧长度为 $4.53\ cm \pm 0.80\ cm$；④盆部，为输精管最长一段，左侧为 $15.02\ cm \pm 2.21\ cm$，右侧 $16.42\ cm \pm 2.85\ cm$[16]，经腹环出腹股沟管后，弯向内下，越过髂外血管，沿盆侧壁腹膜外行向后下，跨过输尿管末端前内方至膀胱底的后面和直肠前面；两侧输精管在此逐渐接近，膨大形成输精管壶腹。输精管壶腹末端变细，穿过前列腺，与精囊的输出管汇合成射精管，射精时精子经输精管、射精管和尿道排出体外[25, 48]。

男性盆部连续横断层 14（MH.6450）

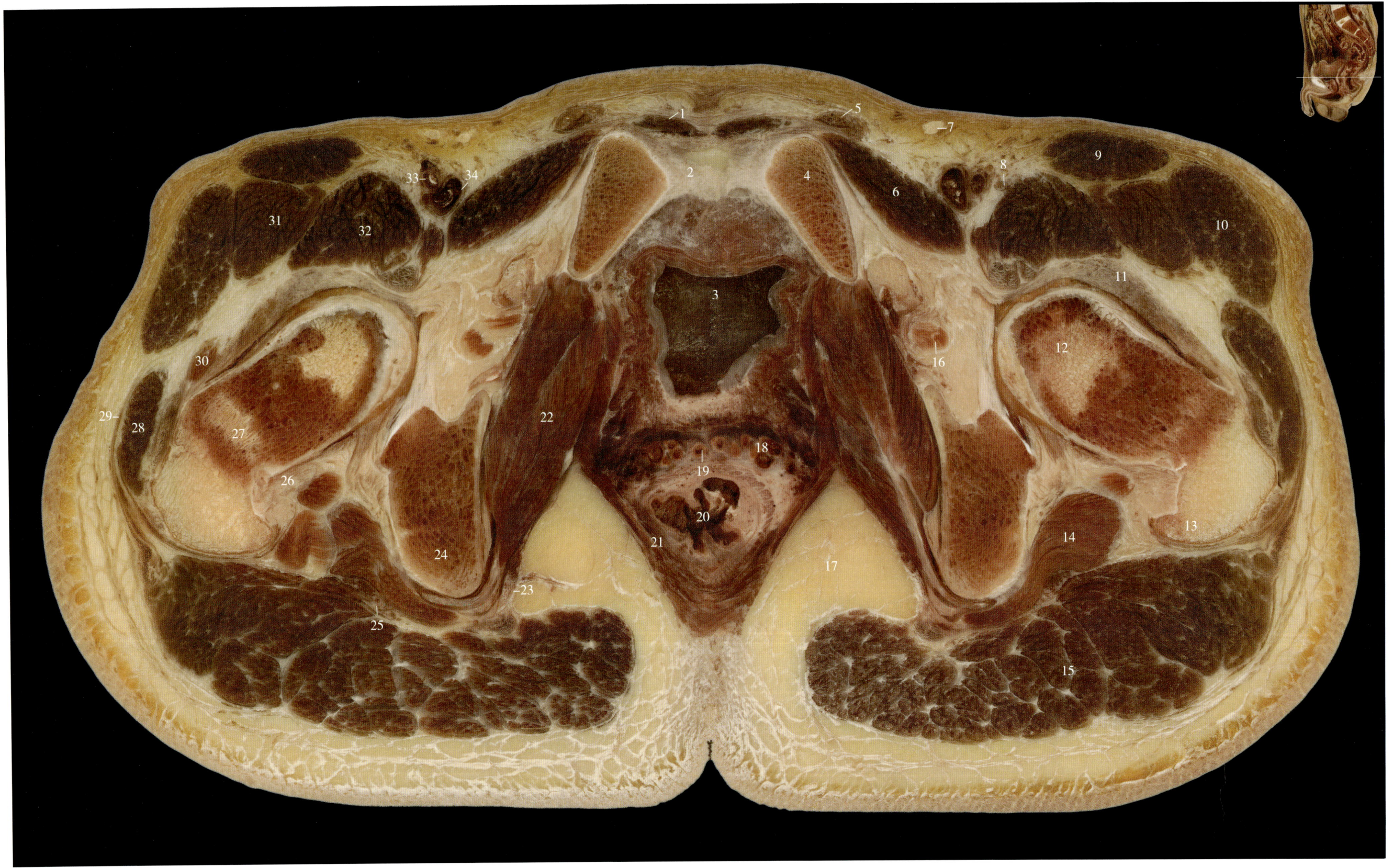

A. 断层标本图像

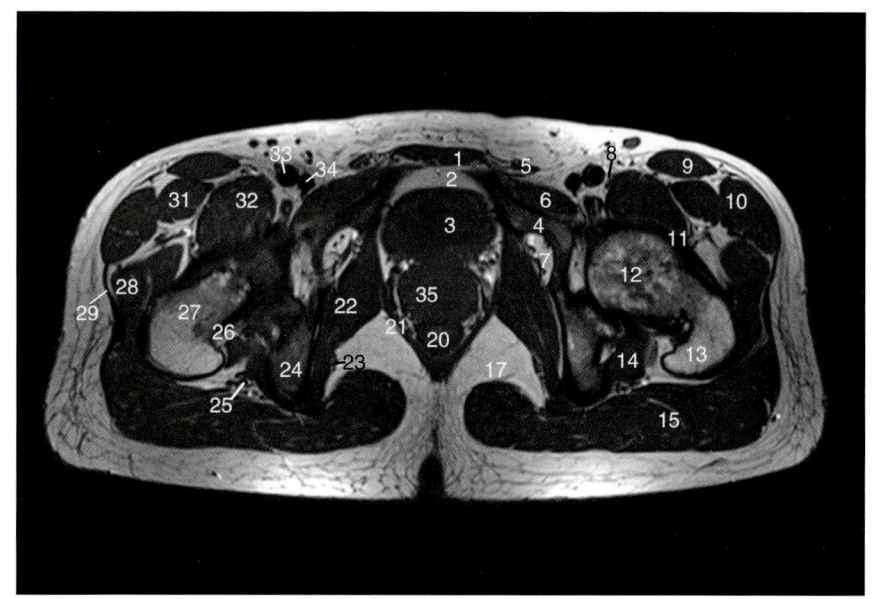
B. MR T1WI

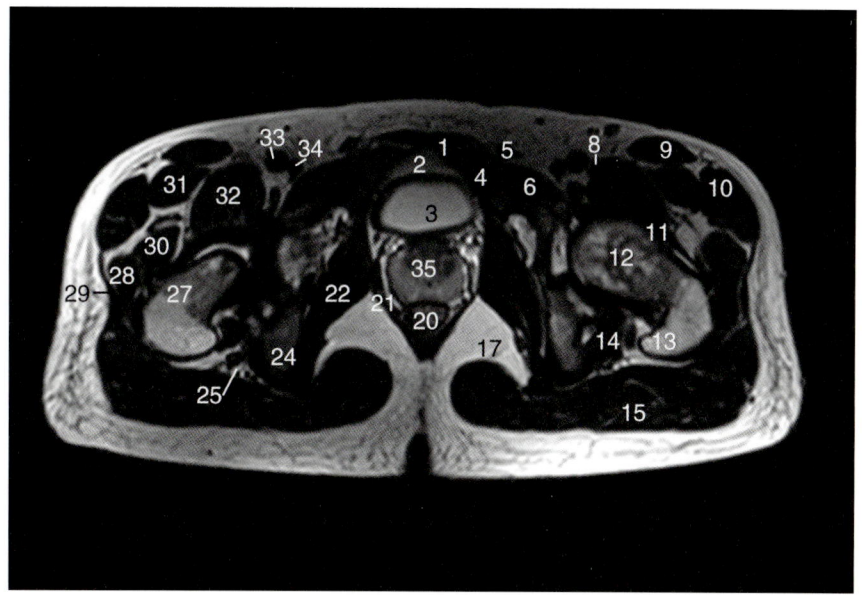
C. MR T2WI

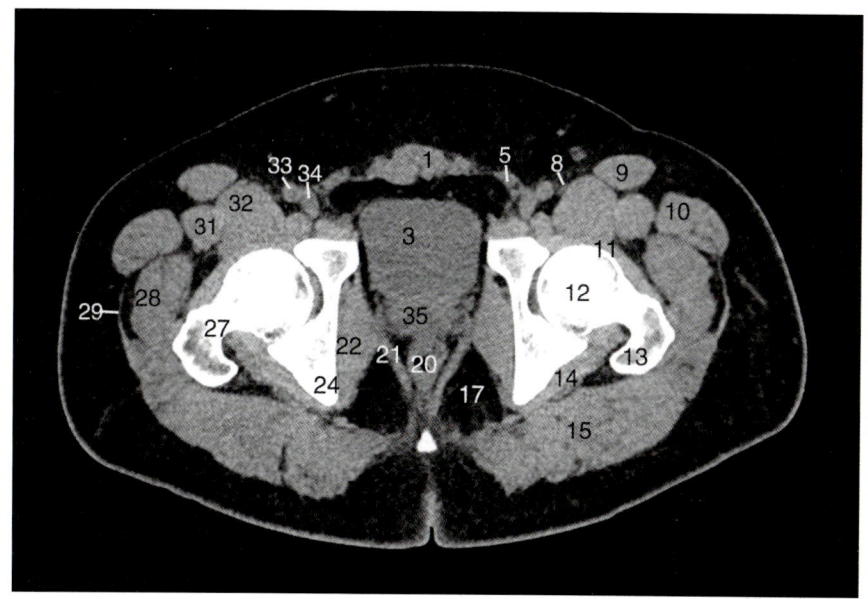
D. CT 平扫图像

1. 腹直肌 rectus abdominis
2. 耻骨上韧带 superior public ligament
3. 膀胱 urinary bladder
4. 耻骨上支 superior ramus of pubis
5. 精索 spermatic cord
6. 耻骨肌 pectineus
7. 腹股沟浅淋巴结 superficial inguinal lymph nodes
8. 股神经 femoral nerve
9. 缝匠肌 sartorius
10. 阔筋膜张肌 tensor fasciae latae
11. 髂股韧带 iliofemoral ligament
12. 股骨头 femoral head
13. 大转子 greater trochanter
14. 下孖肌 gemellus inferior
15. 臀大肌 gluteus maximus
16. 闭孔外肌 obturator externus
17. 坐骨肛门窝 ischioanal fossa
18. 精囊 seminal vesicle
19. 输精管 ductus deferens
20. 直肠 rectum
21. 肛提肌 levator ani
22. 闭孔内肌 obturator internus
23. 阴部神经 pudendal nerve
24. 坐骨结节 ischial tuberosity
25. 坐骨神经 sciatic nerve
26. 坐股韧带 ischiofemoral ligament
27. 股骨颈 neck of femur
28. 臀中肌 gluteus medius
29. 阔筋膜 fasciae lata
30. 股外侧肌 vastus lateralis
31. 股直肌 rectus femoris
32. 髂腰肌 iliopsoas
33. 股动脉 femoral artery
34. 股静脉 femoral vein
35. 前列腺 prostate

关键结构：膀胱，精索，输精管。

此断面经过耻骨上支。骨盆侧壁的前部和后部分别是耻骨上支与坐骨结节，中部见股骨颈及将消失的股骨头，髋关节内侧是闭孔，闭孔前部见闭膜管及其内通过的血管与神经。髋关节前内方，髂腰肌与耻骨肌之间可见股神经与股动、静脉及腹股沟淋巴结。臀大肌深面可见坐骨神经下行。盆腔内前为膀胱，膀胱后方可见精囊及输精管，后部为直肠，其后外侧有肛提肌，两侧为坐骨肛门窝。此断面膀胱已达膀胱颈部，后壁为膀胱三角区，此处是膀胱肿瘤好发部位。膀胱癌主要为移行细胞癌，少数为鳞癌和腺癌，膀胱癌呈浸润性生长，造成膀胱壁增厚、僵硬、凹凸不平。膀胱癌可向外侵犯肌层，进而延伸至周围组织和器官。若肿瘤侵犯输尿管口，可导致输尿管和肾积水；累及膀胱周围组织时，膀胱周围脂肪层分界模糊。MRI在膀胱癌的TNM分期中起到重要作用[49]。来自膀胱、前列腺和子宫颈的淋巴液主要流入髂外淋巴结，部分流入髂总淋巴结。直肠的淋巴结流入髂内和髂总淋巴结。睾丸的区域淋巴结流入腰丛淋巴结，此淋巴通道是胎儿性腺下降的残余。腹股沟的淋巴结聚集在大隐静脉末端的周围沿着腹股沟韧带。除此之外，它们还有引流下肢淋巴的功能，接受来自盆腔器官的淋巴比如外生殖器和阴道的下3/1的淋巴结[47]。

男性盆部连续横断层 15（MH.6440）

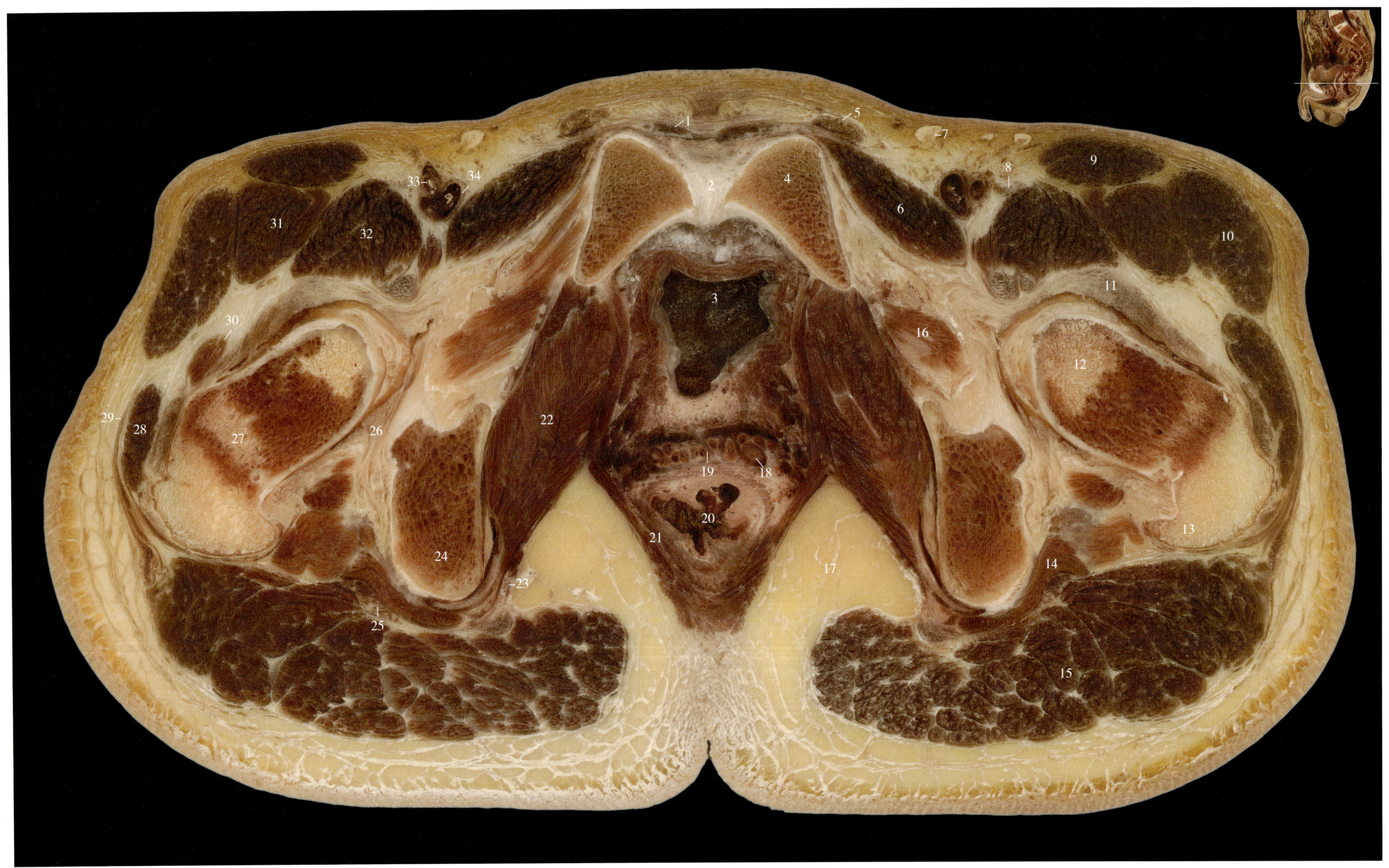

A. 断层标本图像

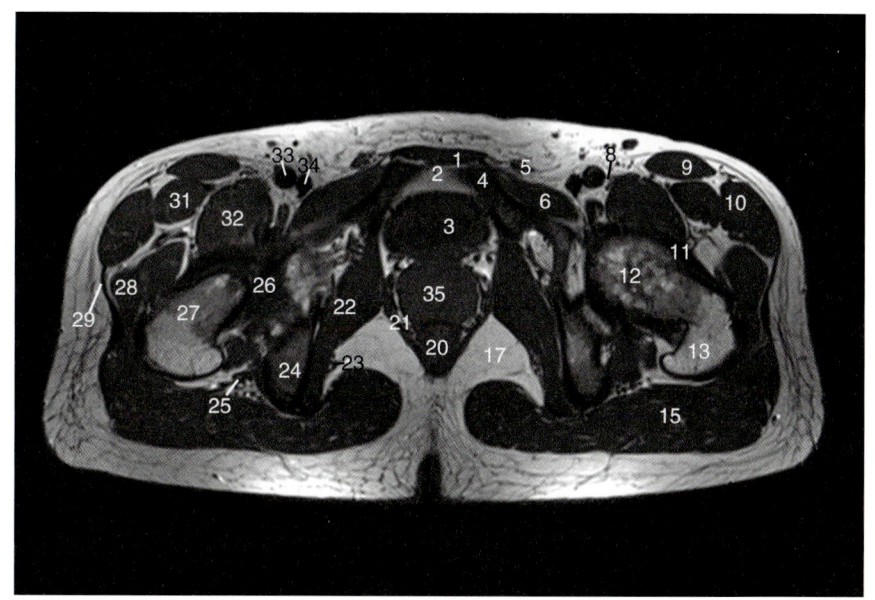
B. MR T1WI

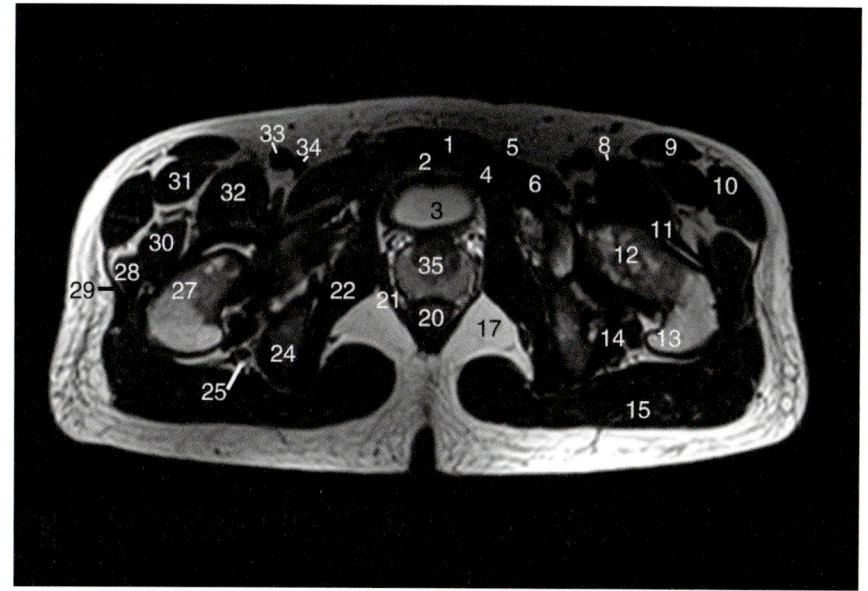
C. MR T2WI

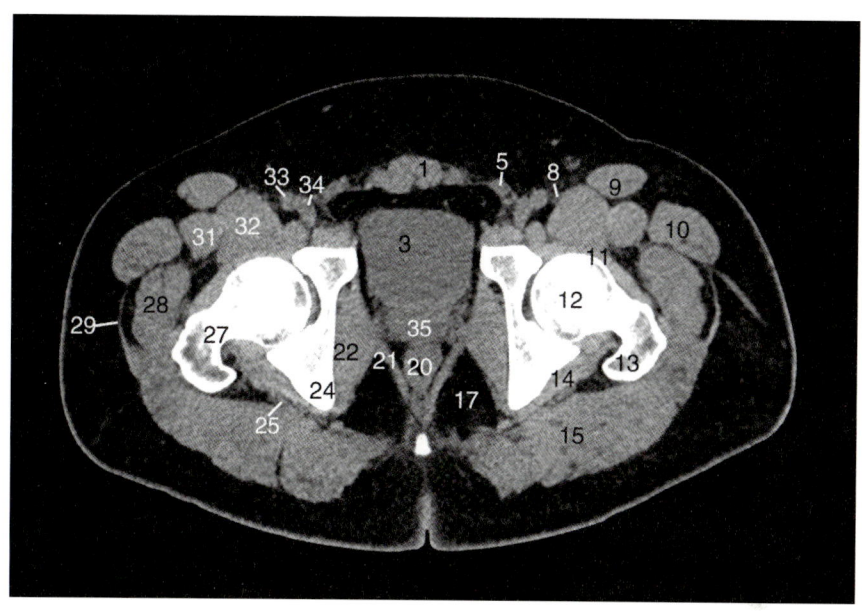
D. CT 平扫图像

1. 腹直肌 rectus abdominis
2. 耻骨联合 pubic symphysis
3. 膀胱 urinary bladder
4. 耻骨上支 superior ramus of pubis
5. 精索 spermatic cord
6. 耻骨肌 pectineus
7. 腹股沟浅淋巴结 superficial inguinal lymph nodes
8. 股神经 femoral nerve
9. 缝匠肌 sartorius
10. 阔筋膜张肌 tensor fasciae latae
11. 髂股韧带 iliofemoral ligament
12. 股骨头 femoral head
13. 大转子 greater trochanter
14. 下孖肌 gemellus inferior
15. 臀大肌 gluteus maximus
16. 闭孔外肌 obturator externus
17. 坐骨肛门窝 ischioanal fossa
18. 精囊 seminal vesicle
19. 输精管 ductus deferens
20. 直肠 rectum
21. 肛提肌 levator ani
22. 闭孔内肌 obturator internus
23. 阴部神经 pudendal nerve
24. 坐骨结节 ischial tuberosity
25. 坐骨神经 sciatic nerve
26. 坐股韧带 ischiofemoral ligament
27. 股骨颈 neck of femur
28. 臀中肌 gluteus medius
29. 阔筋膜 fasciae lata
30. 股外侧肌 vastus lateralis
31. 股直肌 rectus femoris
32. 髂腰肌 iliopsoas
33. 股动脉 femoral artery
34. 股静脉 femoral vein
35. 前列腺 prostate

关键结构：直肠，膀胱，输精管。

此断面经过耻骨联合上份。盆前壁见由左、右两侧耻骨联合面及其间的耻骨间盘构成耻骨联合上份，其前外侧皮下组织内可见精索；盆侧壁主要由衬贴于髋臼内侧的闭孔内肌所构成，该肌起自耻骨后方及闭孔膜的内面，其前外缘与耻骨上支之间为闭膜管，闭孔血管及神经经此管离开盆腔进入股内侧区；该侧面于闭孔内肌的外侧出现闭孔外肌。盆腔内脏器自前往后分别是膀胱、输精管末端和精囊及其后方的直肠。上述脏器周围有丰富的静脉丛。直肠癌直接向前可浸润前列腺、精囊腺及膀胱。MRI 可明确判断肠壁肿瘤的范围及是否突破肠壁；如肠壁外系膜模糊不清或伴有系膜内条索或结节影，表明肿瘤突破肠壁侵犯系膜。直肠供血动脉有直肠上动脉、直肠下动脉及骶正中动脉。直肠上动脉为肠系膜下动脉的终支，在乙状结肠系膜内下行至第 3 骶椎高度，分为左、右支，自直肠侧壁进入直肠。直肠下动脉来自髂内动脉，较为细小，其分支至直肠下部和肛管上部。骶正中动脉发出分支经直肠背面分布于直肠后壁。直肠静脉来自直肠肛管静脉丛，此丛可分为黏膜下及肛管皮下的直肠肛管内丛和位于腹膜反折线以下、肌层表面的直肠肛管外丛。以齿状线为界，直肠肛管内丛分为上丛和下丛；直肠肛管内丛静脉曲张形成痔，齿状线以下为外痔，齿状线以上为内痔[50]。

男性盆部连续横断层 16（MH.6430）

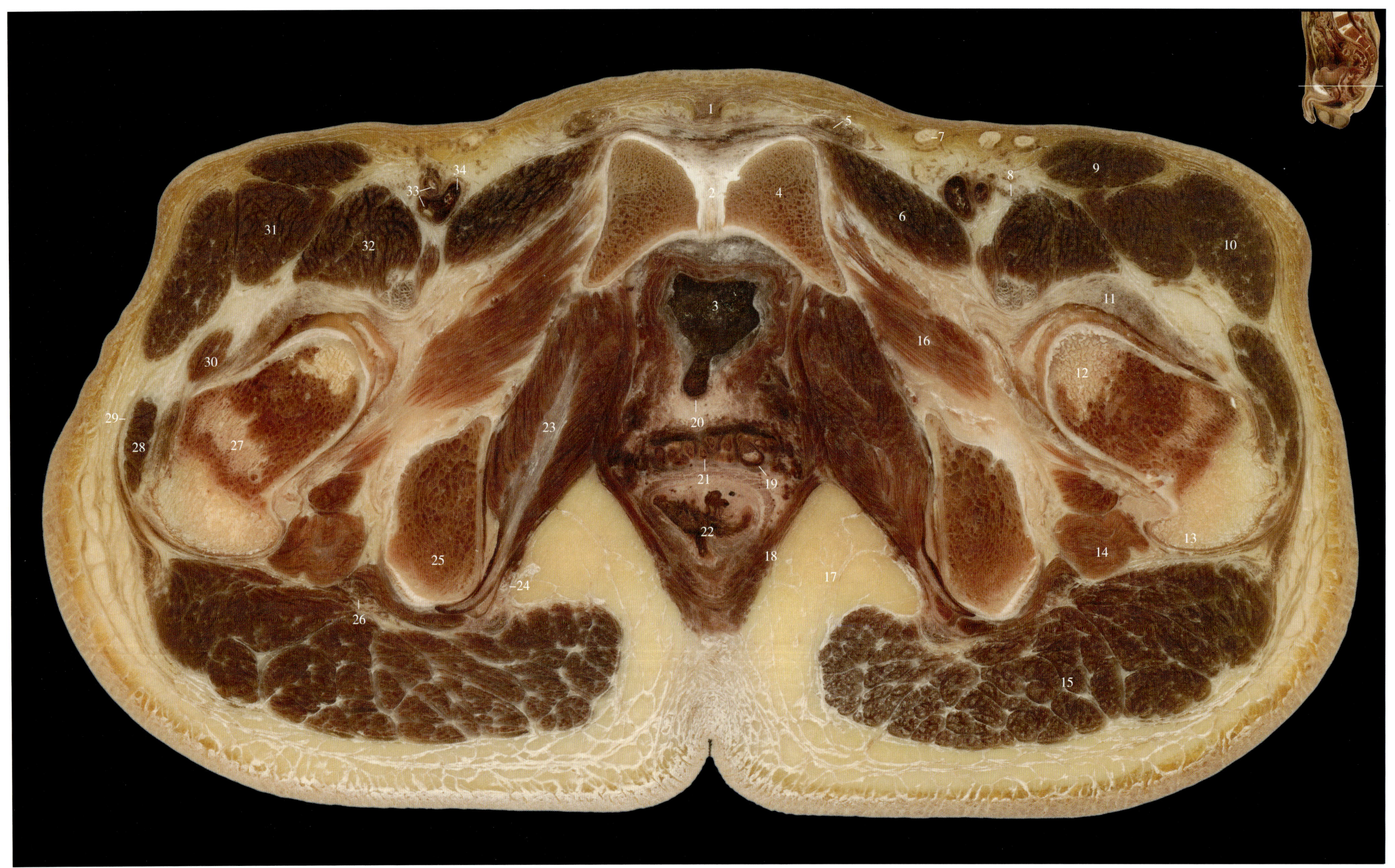

A. 断层标本图像

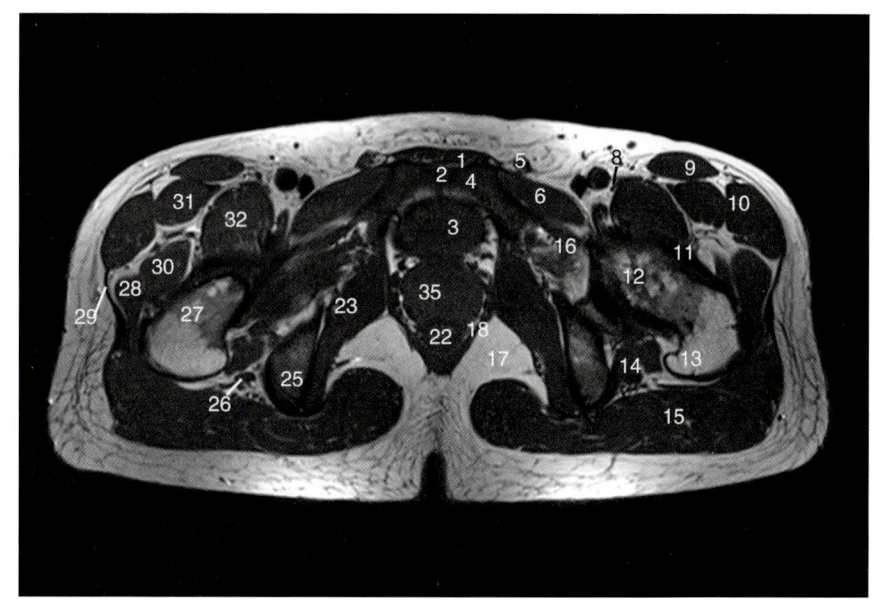
B. MR T1WI

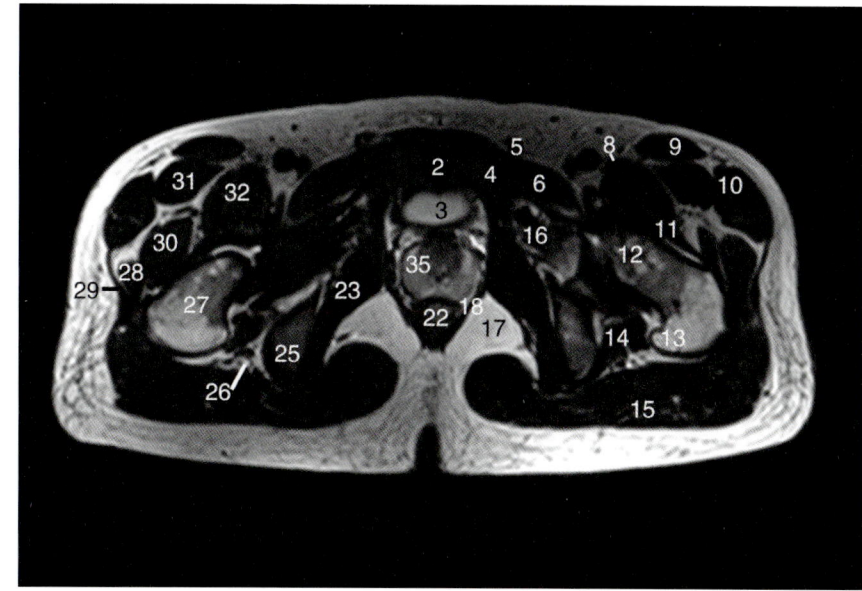
C. MR T2WI

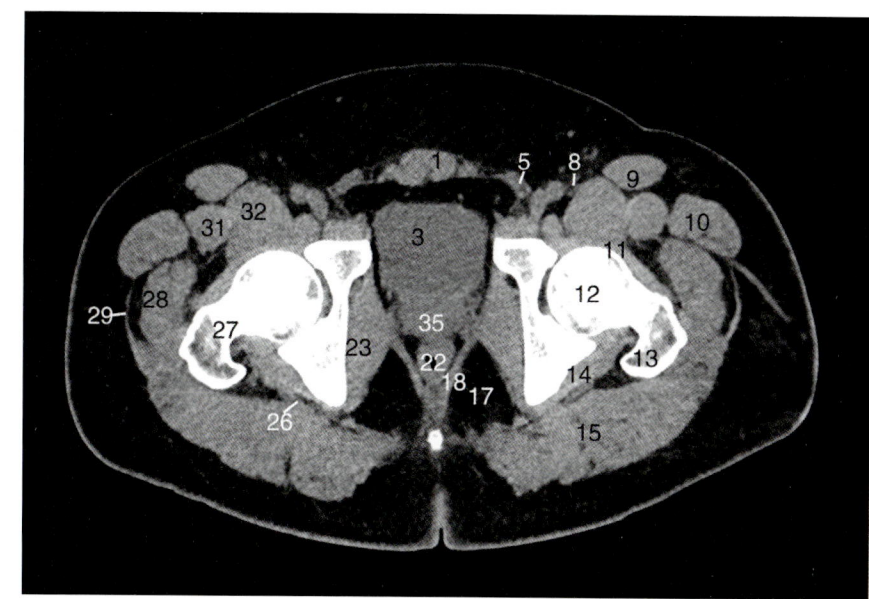
D. CT 平扫图像

关键结构：阴部管，精索，输精管壶腹。

此断面经过耻骨联合上份。盆腔断面明显缩小。盆腔前壁耻骨联合代替了腹直肌，耻骨联合正前方出现阴茎悬韧带，侧方皮下为精索。盆腔侧壁股骨头消失，可见股骨颈及大转子，股骨与坐骨间下孖肌消失，出现股方肌。盆腔内，前方的膀胱近消失，出现尿道内口。盆腔内后方为直肠，二者间有精囊和输精管壶腹。直肠两侧坐骨肛门窝的外侧壁上可见行于阴部管（Alcock 管）内的阴部内血管和阴部神经。阴部内动脉起自髂内动脉干，亦可与臀下动脉共干，经梨状肌下孔出盆腔，再经坐骨小孔入坐骨肛门窝。主干沿外侧壁上的阴部管前行，在阴部管内阴部内动脉发出肛动脉，横行分布于肛门周围的结构。在阴部管前端阴部内动脉分为会阴动脉和阴茎动脉进入尿生殖区。阴部内静脉与同名动脉伴行，汇入髂内静脉。阴部神经由骶丛发出，与阴部内血管伴行，在坐骨肛门窝的阴部管内分出肛神经、会阴神经及阴茎背神经，与同名动脉伴行[16]。由于阴部神经在行程中绕过坐骨棘，故在行会阴手术时，在坐骨结节与肛门连线的中点刺向坐骨棘的下方，进行阴部神经阻滞麻醉。

1. 悬韧带 suspensory ligament
2. 耻骨联合 pubic symphysis
3. 膀胱 urinary bladder
4. 耻骨上支 superior ramus of pubis
5. 精索 spermatic cord
6. 耻骨肌 pectineus
7. 腹股沟浅淋巴结 superficial inguinal lymph nodes
8. 股神经 femoral nerve
9. 缝匠肌 sartorius
10. 阔筋膜张肌 tensor fasciae latae
11. 髂股韧带 iliofemoral ligament
12. 股骨头 femoral head
13. 大转子 greater trochanter
14. 股方肌 quadratus femoris
15. 臀大肌 gluteus maximus
16. 闭孔外肌 obturator externus
17. 坐骨肛门窝 ischioanal fossa
18. 肛提肌 levator ani
19. 精囊 seminal vesicle
20. 尿道内口 internal urethra orifice
21. 输精管 ductus deferens
22. 直肠 rectum
23. 闭孔内肌 obturator internus
24. 阴部神经 pudendal nerve
25. 坐骨结节 ischial tuberosity
26. 坐骨神经 sciatic nerve
27. 股骨颈 neck of femur
28. 臀中肌 gluteus medius
29. 阔筋膜 fasciae lata
30. 股外侧肌 vastus lateralis
31. 股直肌 rectus femoris
32. 髂腰肌 iliopsoas
33. 股动、静脉 femoral artery and vein
34. 大隐静脉 great saphenous vein
35. 前列腺 prostate

男性盆部连续横断层 17（MH.6420）

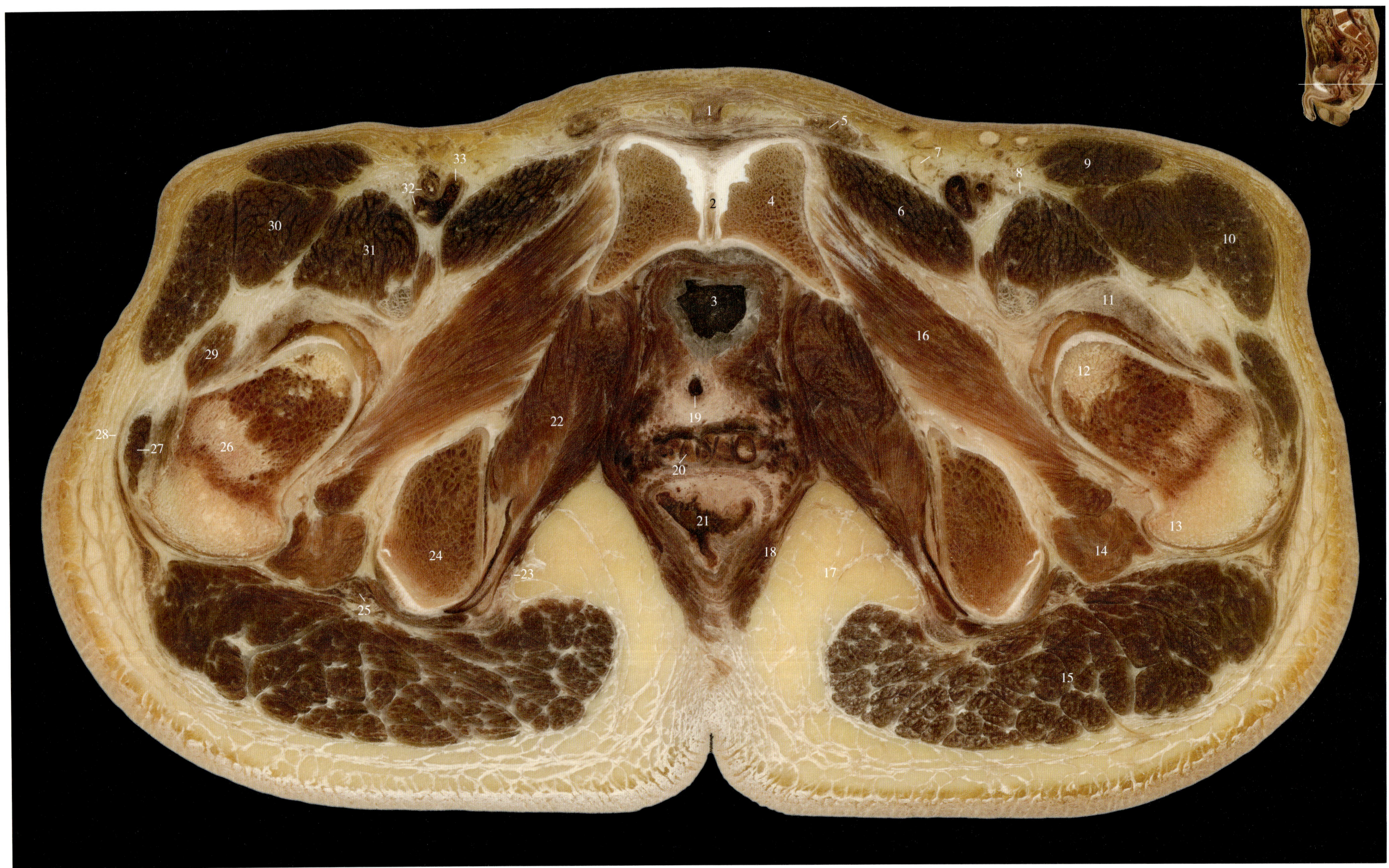

A. 断层标本图像

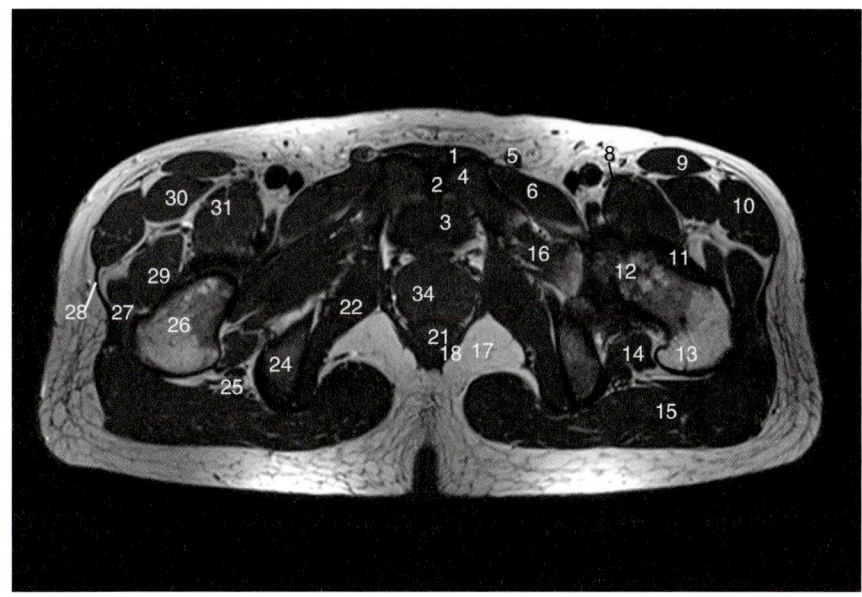

B. MR T1WI

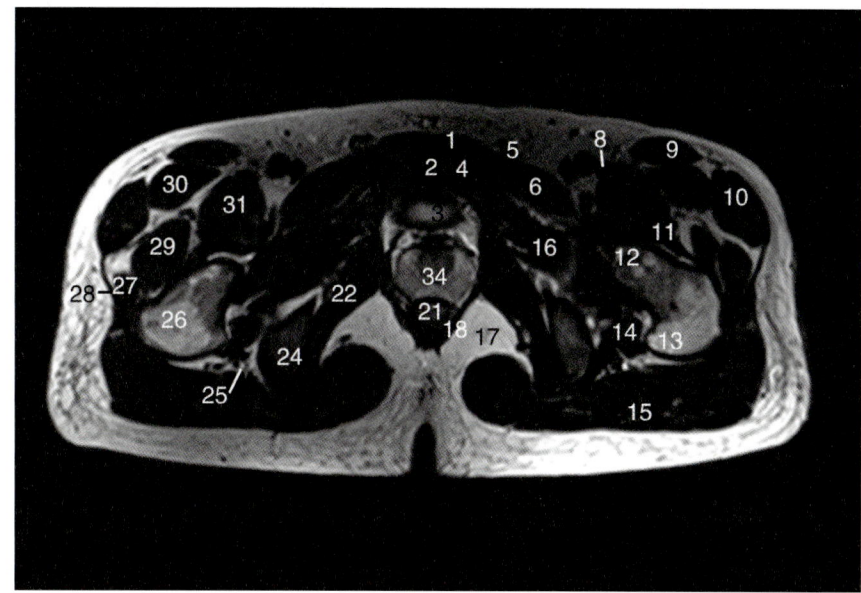

C. MR T2WI

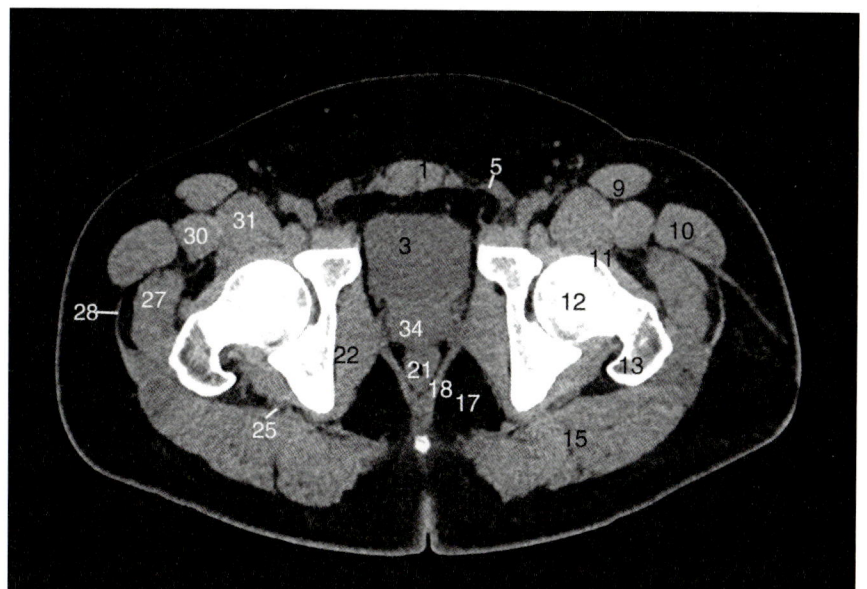

D. CT 平扫图像

关键结构：耻骨联合，尿道，直肠。

　　此断面经过耻骨联合中份。耻骨上、下支相互移行处内侧是耻骨联合面，两侧联合面借纤维软骨相接，构成耻骨联合，耻骨间盘内常有一矢状裂隙，称耻骨联合腔。耻骨联合位于腹前壁前正中线的下端，是骨盆入口的标志之一，是重要的体表标志。女性耻骨间盘较厚，且耻骨联合腔较男性大。在耻骨联合上、下方分别有耻骨上韧带和耻骨弓状韧带加强。此断面耻骨联合前方可见阴茎悬韧带及两侧的精索，侧壁的髋关节消失。盆腔前部膀胱即将消失，出现尿道，尿道后方可见精囊，盆腔后部为直肠。直肠淋巴引流主要朝上，黏膜层的淋巴滤泡引流至紧贴直肠外表面的直肠上淋巴结和直肠旁的直肠旁淋巴结，然后沿直肠上血管到达肠系膜下动脉起始处的主动脉前淋巴结。直肠下份的淋巴管可沿直肠下动脉和肛动脉到达髂内淋巴结。直肠的神经支配：直肠和肛管齿状线以上由交感神经和副交感神经支配。交感神经来自上腹下丛和盆丛，副交感神经是直肠功能的主要调节神经，纤维来自盆内脏神经，通过直肠侧韧带分布于直肠和肛管。与排便反射相关的传入纤维也经盆内脏神经传入[22]。

1. 悬韧带 suspensory ligament
2. 耻骨联合 pubic symphysis
3. 膀胱 urinary bladder
4. 耻骨上支 superior ramus of pubis
5. 精索 spermatic cord
6. 耻骨肌 pectineus
7. 腹股沟浅淋巴结 superficial inguinal lymph nodes
8. 股神经 femoral nerve
9. 缝匠肌 sartorius
10. 阔筋膜张肌 tensor fasciae latae
11. 髂股韧带 iliofemoral ligament
12. 股骨头 femoral head
13. 大转子 greater trochanter
14. 股方肌 quadratus femoris
15. 臀大肌 gluteus maximus
16. 闭孔外肌 obturator externus
17. 坐骨肛门窝 ischioanal fossa
18. 肛提肌 levator ani
19. 尿道 urethra
20. 精囊 seminal vesicle
21. 直肠 rectum
22. 闭孔内肌 obturator internus
23. 阴部神经 pudendal nerve
24. 坐骨结节 ischial tuberosity
25. 坐骨神经 sciatic nerve
26. 股骨颈 neck of femur
27. 臀中肌 gluteus medius
28. 阔筋膜 fasciae lata
29. 股外侧肌 vastus lateralis
30. 股直肌 rectus femoris
31. 髂腰肌 iliopsoas
32. 股动、静脉 femoral artery and vein
33. 大隐静脉 great saphenous vein
34. 前列腺 prostate

男性盆部连续横断层 18（MH.6410）

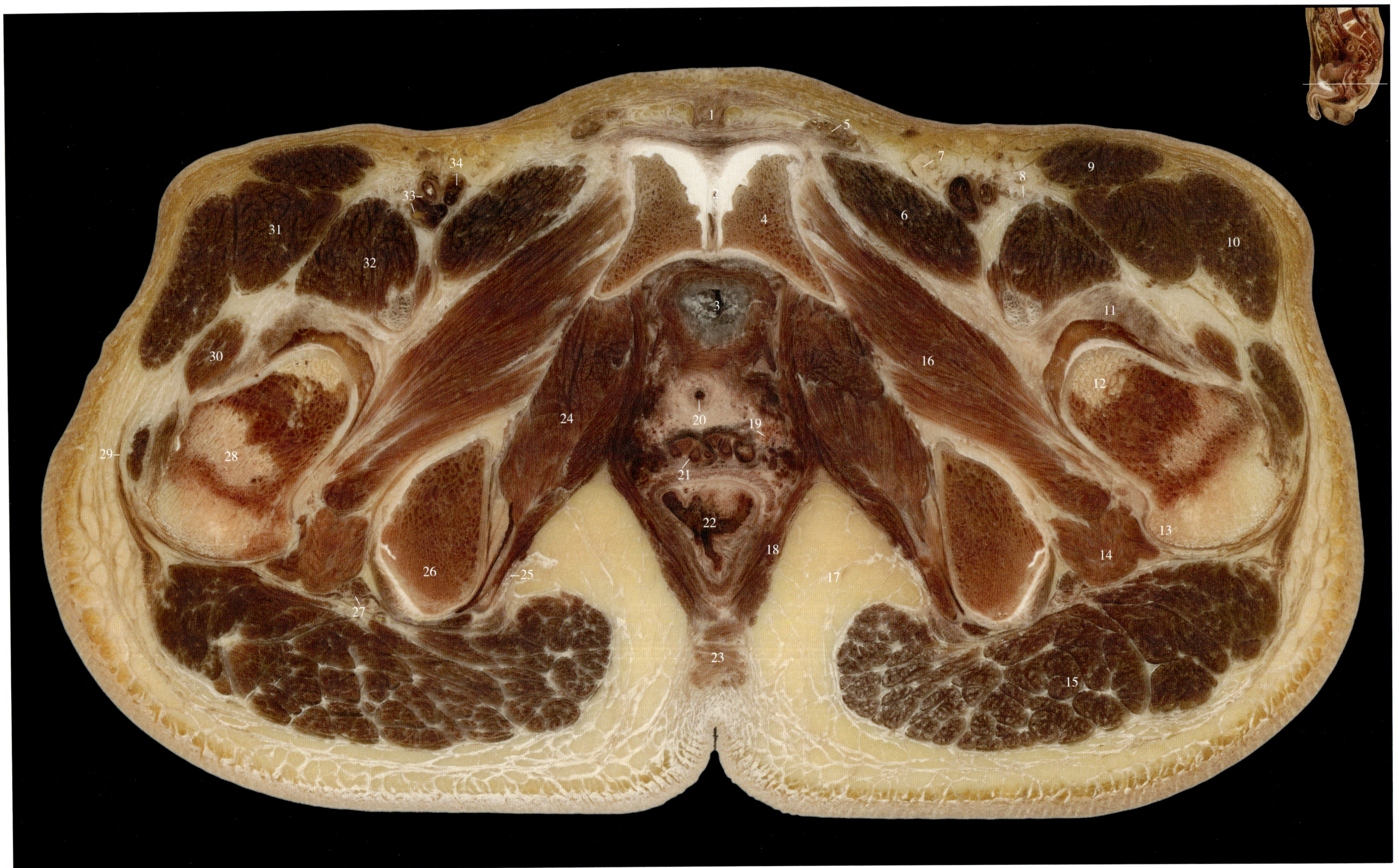

A. 断层标本图像

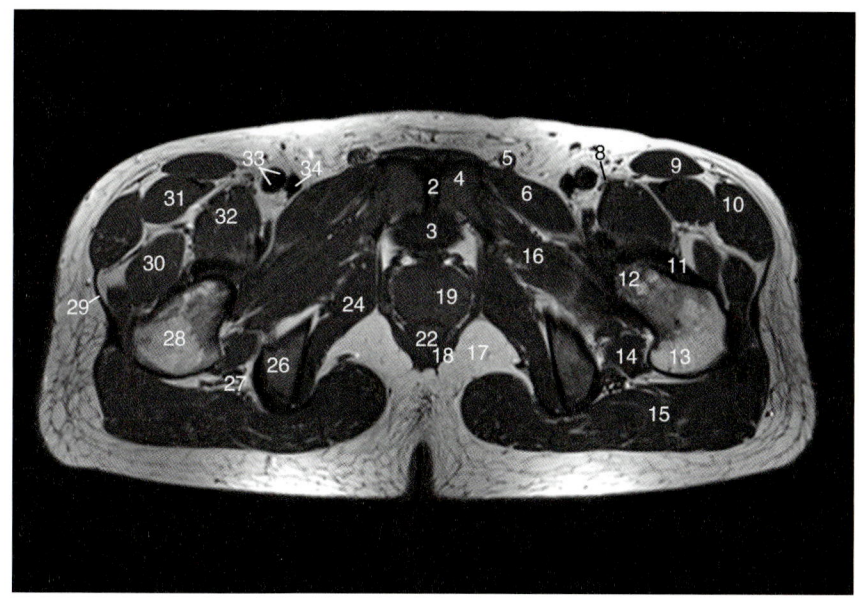

B. MR T1WI

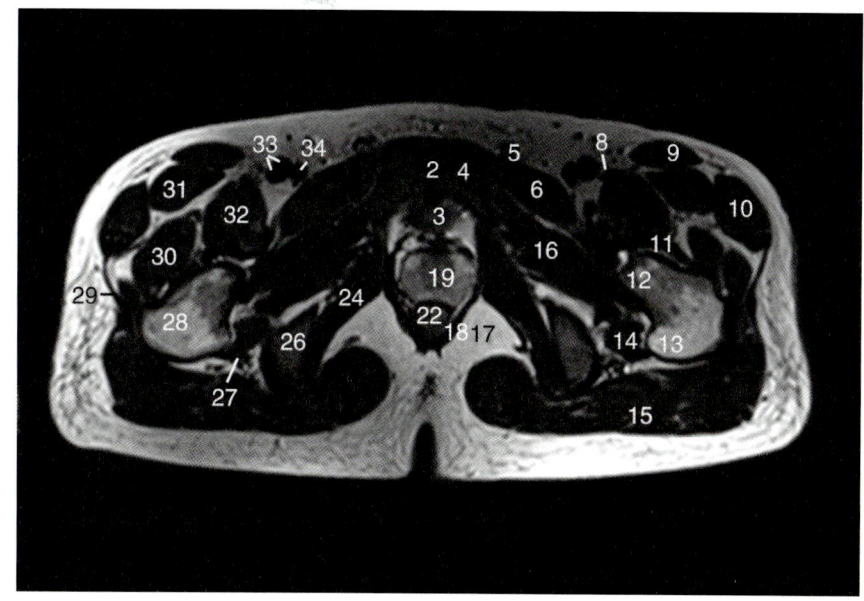

C. MR T2WI

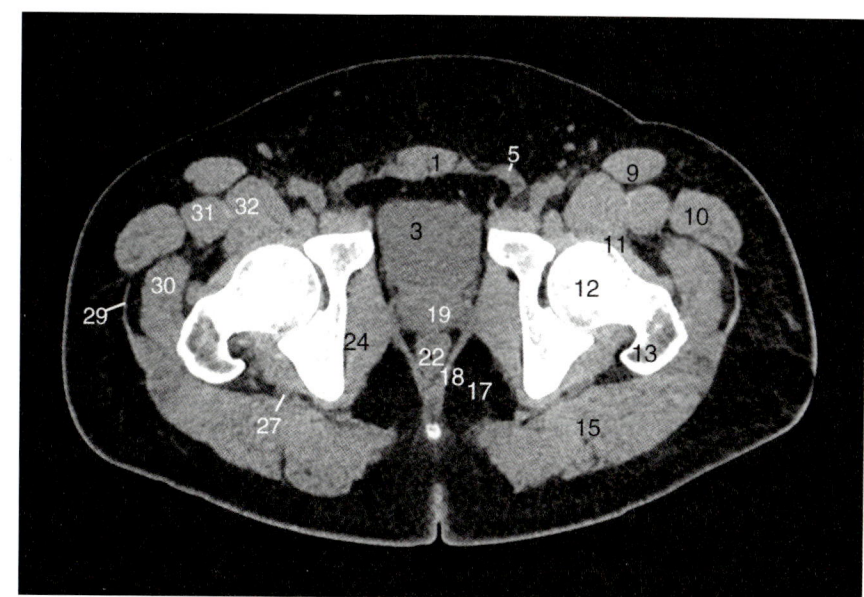

D. CT 平扫图像

1. 悬韧带 suspensory ligament
2. 耻骨联合 pubic symphysis
3. 膀胱 urinary bladder
4. 耻骨上支 superior ramus of pubis
5. 精索 spermatic cord
6. 耻骨肌 pectineus
7. 腹股沟浅淋巴结 superficial inguinal lymph nodes
8. 股神经 femoral nerve
9. 缝匠肌 sartorius
10. 阔筋膜张肌 tensor fasciae latae
11. 髂股韧带 iliofemoral ligament
12. 股骨头 femoral head
13. 大转子 greater trochanter
14. 股方肌 quadratus femoris
15. 臀大肌 gluteus maximus
16. 闭孔外肌 obturator externus
17. 坐骨肛门窝 ischioanal fossa
18. 肛提肌 levator ani
19. 前列腺 prostate
20. 尿道 urethra
21. 精囊 seminal vesicle
22. 直肠 rectum
23. 肛门外括约肌 sphincter ani externus
24. 闭孔内肌 obturator internus
25. 阴部神经 pudendal nerve
26. 坐骨结节 ischial tuberosity
27. 坐骨神经 sciatic nerve
28. 股骨颈 neck of femur
29. 阔筋膜 fasciae lata
30. 股外侧肌 vastus lateralis
31. 股直肌 rectus femoris
32. 髂腰肌 iliopsoas
33. 股动、静脉 femoral artery and vein
34. 大隐静脉 great saphenous vein

关键结构：耻骨后间隙，精囊腺，前列腺。

此断面经过耻骨联合中份。耻骨联合位居盆腔前壁，前方可见两侧的精索。盆腔内前部为即将消失的膀胱，膀胱与耻骨联合之间为耻骨后间隙，膀胱后出现尿道及前列腺基底部，前列腺后方为直肠，二者之间见精囊、膀胱、前列腺及直肠被两侧的肛提肌呈"U"形包绕。耻骨后间隙也称膀胱前隙，前界为耻骨联合、耻骨上支及闭孔内肌筋膜；后界在男性为膀胱和前列腺，女性为膀胱；两侧界为脐内侧韧带；上界为壁腹膜至膀胱上面的反折处；下界在男性为盆膈和耻骨前列腺韧带（连前列腺至耻骨联合下缘），在女性为盆膈和耻骨膀胱韧带。间隙内为疏松结缔组织和静脉丛等。耻骨折引起的血肿和膀胱前壁损伤的尿外渗常潴留在此间隙内。耻骨上腹膜外引流、膀胱及子宫下部等手术，均通过此间隙进行，此时应避免伤及腹膜。此断面显示精囊腺呈多囊样改变，双侧对称分布，体积较大。精囊的体积及最大水平面积从60岁开始随年龄的增长有下降趋势，精囊的输出管与输精管壶腹部的末端汇合成射精管。精囊分泌的液体参与精液的组成。CT上精囊腺呈"八"形均匀软组织密度影，CT值37~75HU不等，双侧共长60 mm左右[16]，边缘常呈小分叶状。MRI上精囊腺由卷曲的细管构成，其内充盈液体。在T1WI上呈均一低信号，T2WI呈"铺路石"样高信号，壁为低信号。精囊超声表现为纤细、蜿蜒条状低回声。

男性盆部连续横断层 19（MH.6400）

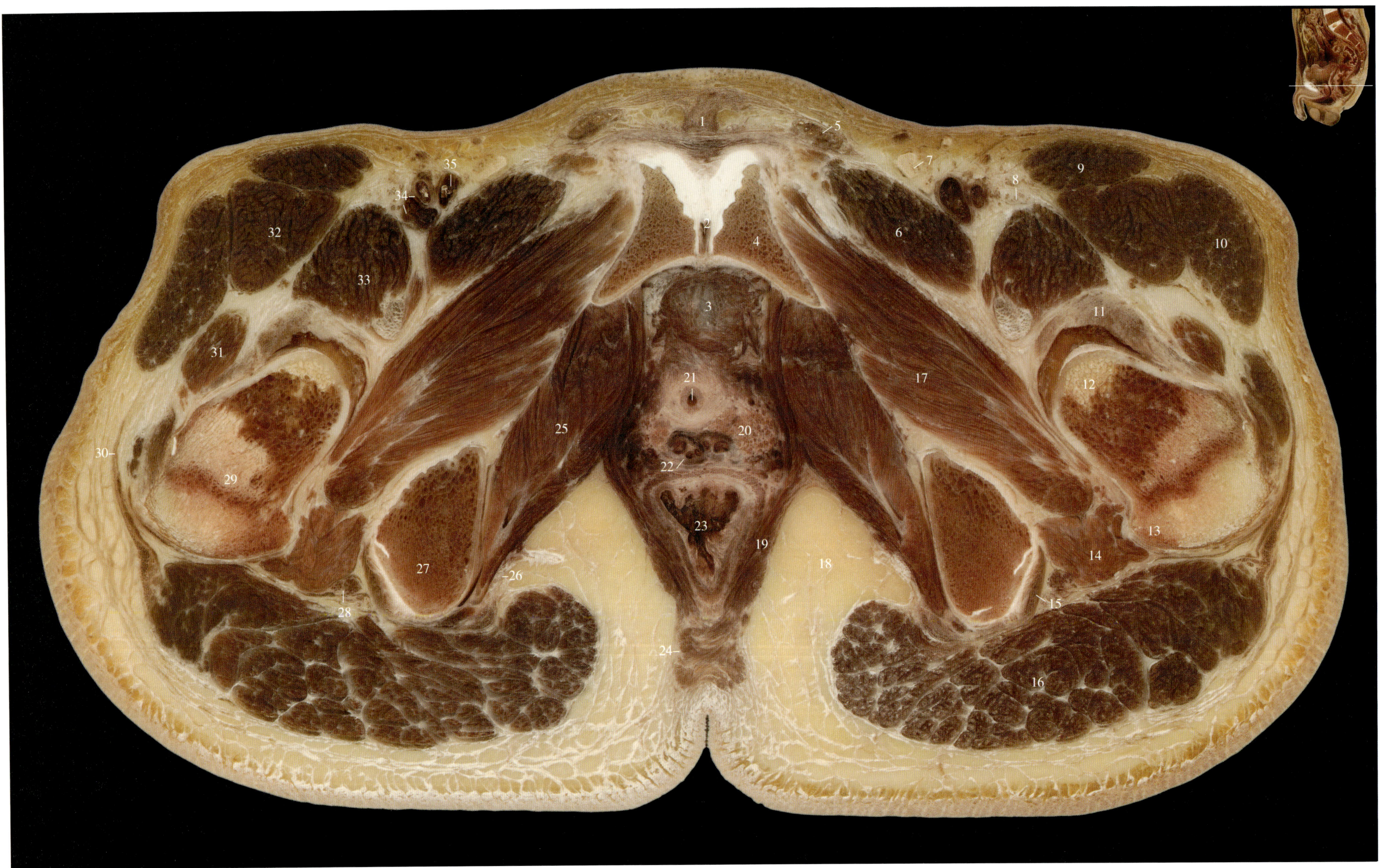

A. 断层标本图像

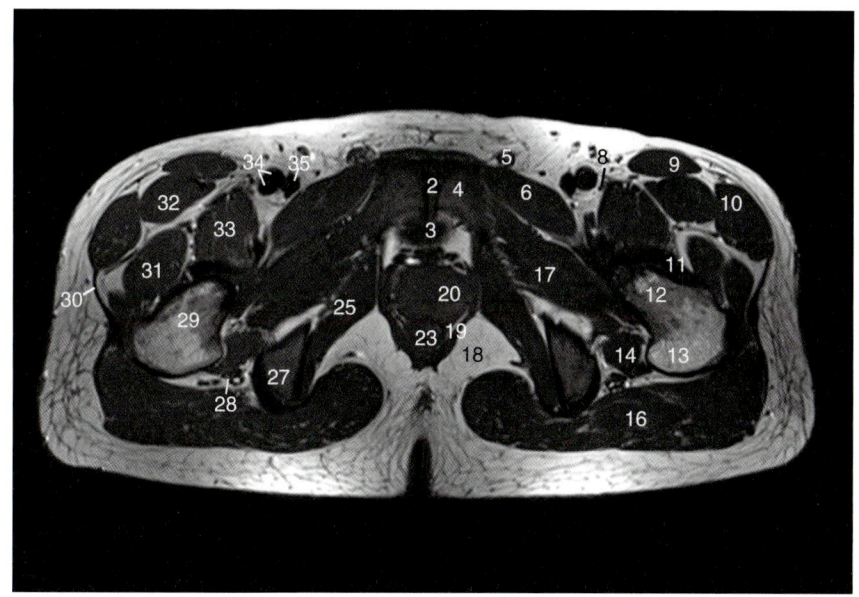

B. MR T1WI

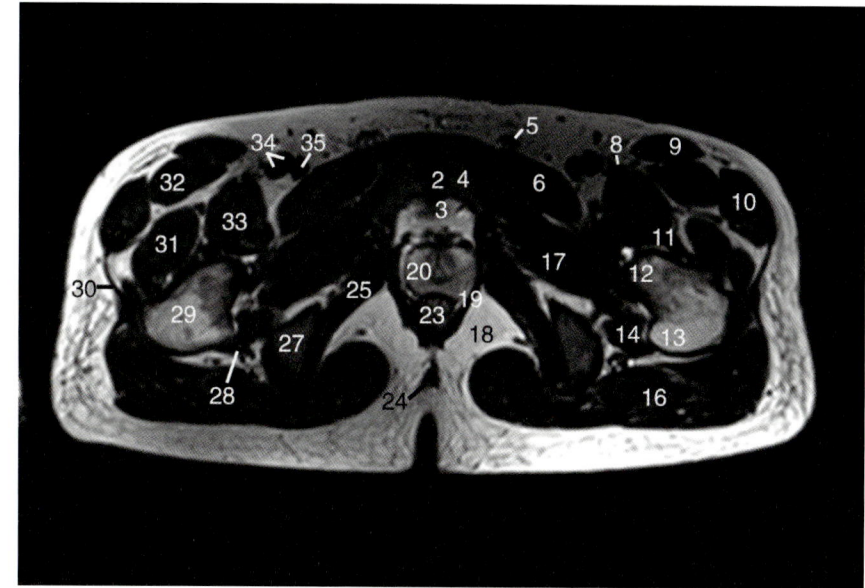

C. MR T2WI

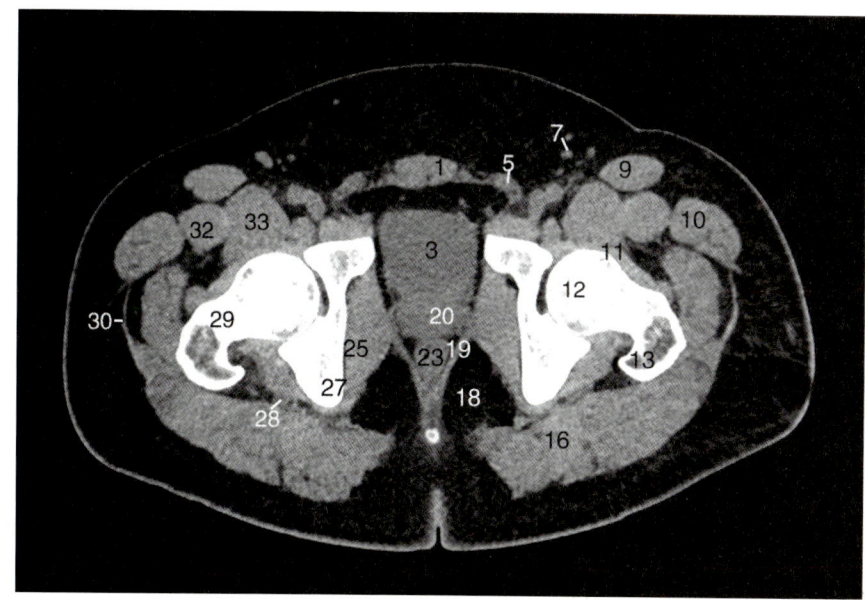

D. CT 平扫图像

1. 悬韧带 suspensory ligament
2. 耻骨联合 pubic symphysis
3. 膀胱 urinary bladder
4. 耻骨上支 superior ramus of pubis
5. 精索 spermatic cord
6. 耻骨肌 pectineus
7. 腹股沟浅淋巴结 superficial inguinal lymph nodes
8. 股神经 femoral nerve
9. 缝匠肌 sartorius
10. 阔筋膜张肌 tensor fasciae latae
11. 髂股韧带 iliofemoral ligament
12. 股骨头 femoral head
13. 大转子 greater trochanter
14. 股方肌 quadratus femoris
15. 半膜肌肌腱 tendon of semimembranosus
16. 臀大肌 gluteus maximus
17. 闭孔外肌 obturator externus
18. 坐骨肛门窝 ischioanal fossa
19. 肛提肌 levator ani
20. 前列腺 prostate
21. 尿道前列腺部 prostatic portion of urethra
22. 精囊 seminal vesicle
23. 直肠 rectum
24. 肛门外括约肌 sphincter ani externus
25. 闭孔内肌 obturator internus
26. 阴部神经 pudendal nerve
27. 坐骨结节 ischial tuberosity
28. 坐骨神经 sciatic nerve
29. 股骨颈 neck of femur
30. 阔筋膜 fasciae lata
31. 股外侧肌 vastus lateralis
32. 股直肌 rectus femoris
33. 髂腰肌 iliopsoas
34. 股动、静脉 femoral artery and vein
35. 大隐静脉 great saphenous vein

关键结构：前列腺，耻骨后间隙，直肠。

此断面经过耻骨联合中份。耻骨联合位居盆腔前壁，前方可见阴茎悬韧带及两侧的精索。耻骨联合之间为耻骨后间隙。盆腔壁层筋膜在前列腺前方增厚形成耻骨前列腺韧带，连接前列腺和耻骨；背深静脉复合体位于两侧耻骨前列腺韧带之间、耻骨尿道韧带之上，前缘与前列腺筋膜、后缘与前列腺连接紧密；前列腺筋膜前方为填充脂肪组织的耻骨后间隙；在背深静脉复合体底部，耻骨尿道韧带连接耻骨与尿道。前列腺两侧筋膜由内向外依次为前列腺包囊、前列腺筋膜和盆腔壁层筋膜，前列腺包囊和前列腺筋膜间存在丰富的前列腺静脉丛；前列腺包囊、前列腺静脉丛和前列腺筋膜三者在前列腺两侧相互融合形成前列腺纤维鞘，纤维鞘内侧缘与前列腺连接紧密，外侧缘与盆腔壁层筋膜之间为一疏松的、无血管神经的筋膜间隙。Denonvilliers 筋膜和直肠固有筋膜在前列腺后方构成直肠膀胱隔，两层筋膜之间为一无血管神经的间隙；在前列腺后外侧，两层筋膜分离走行，与外侧的盆腔壁层筋膜构成神经血管束三角。前列腺根治术手术中紧贴前列腺筋膜和 Denonvilliers 筋膜的外侧面分离，有利于减少手术中神经、血管的损伤[51]。盆腔内前部为即将消失的膀胱，中部是前列腺及尿道前列腺部，后部为直肠。精囊即将消失。

男性盆部连续横断层 20（MH.6390）

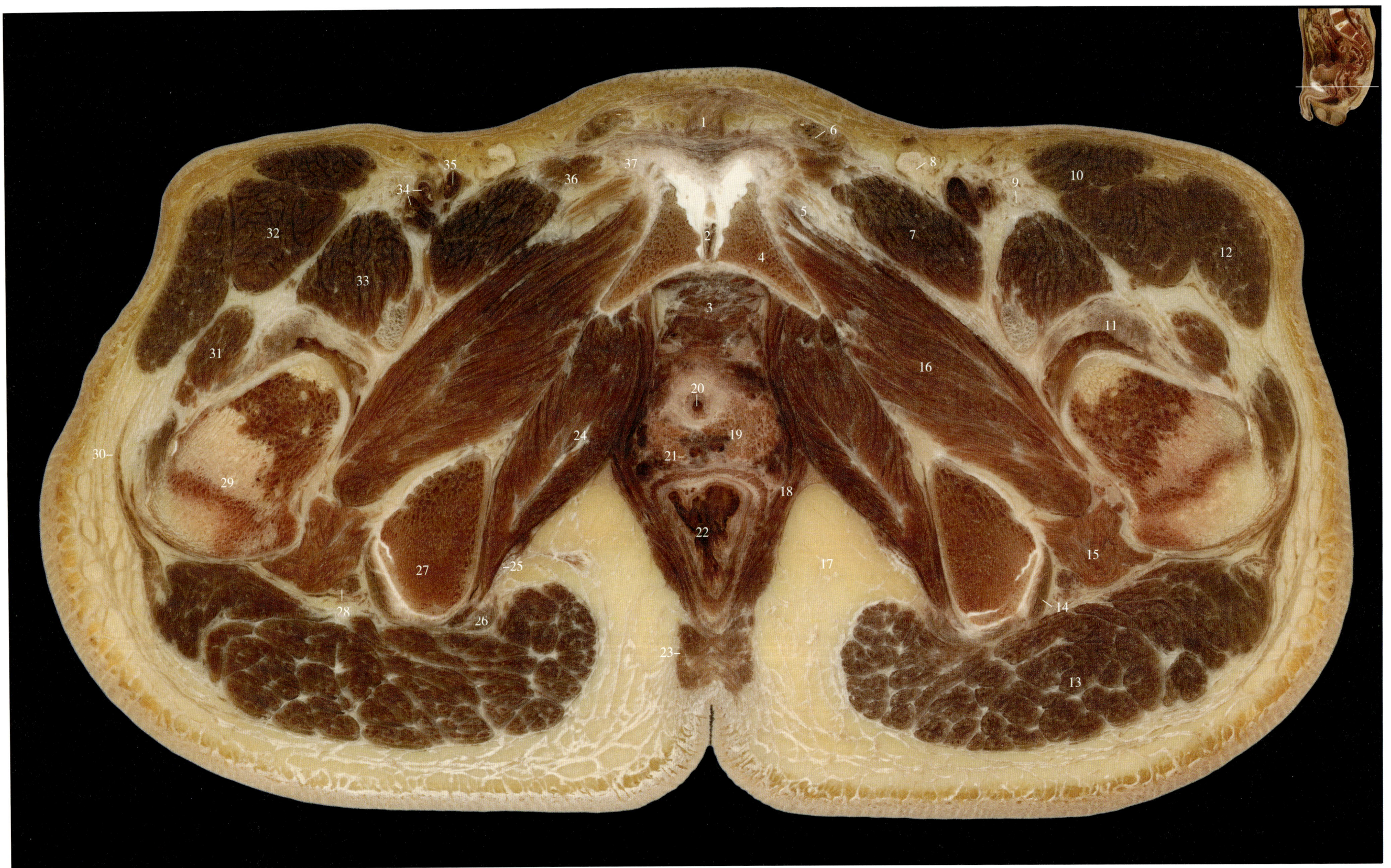

A. 断层标本图像

1. 悬韧带 suspensory ligament
2. 耻骨联合 pubic symphysis
3. 膀胱 urinary bladder
4. 耻骨下支 inferior ramus of pubis
5. 短收肌 adductor brevis
6. 精索 spermatic cord
7. 耻骨肌 pectineus
8. 腹股沟浅淋巴结 superficial inguinal lymph nodes
9. 股神经 femoral nerve
10. 缝匠肌 sartorius
11. 髂股韧带 iliofemoral ligament
12. 阔筋膜张肌 tensor fasciae latae
13. 臀大肌 gluteus maximus
14. 半膜肌肌腱 tendon of semimembranosus
15. 股方肌 quadratus femoris
16. 闭孔外肌 obturator externus
17. 坐骨肛门窝 ischioanal fossa
18. 肛提肌 levator ani
19. 前列腺 prostate
20. 尿道前列腺部 prostatic portion of urethra
21. 射精管 ejaculatory
22. 直肠 rectum
23. 肛门外括约肌 sphincter ani externus
24. 闭孔内肌 obturator internus
25. 阴部神经 pudendal nerve
26. 股二头肌长头和半腱肌 long head of biceps femoris and semitendinosus
27. 坐骨结节 ischial tuberosity
28. 坐骨神经 sciatic nerve
29. 股骨颈 neck of femur
30. 阔筋膜 fasciae lata
31. 股外侧肌 vastus lateralis
32. 股直肌 rectus femoris
33. 髂腰肌 iliopsoas
34. 股动、静脉 femoral artery and vein
35. 大隐静脉 great saphenous vein
36. 长收肌 adductor longus
37. 耻骨弓状韧带 arcuate pubic ligament

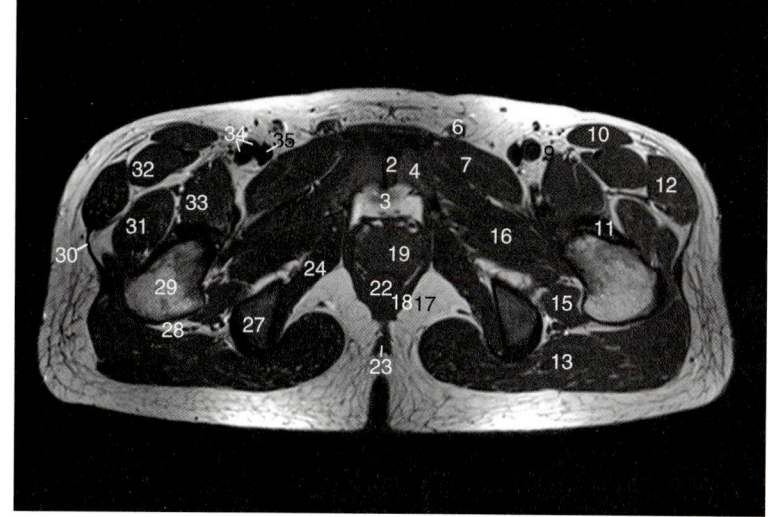

B. T1W1   C. T2W1

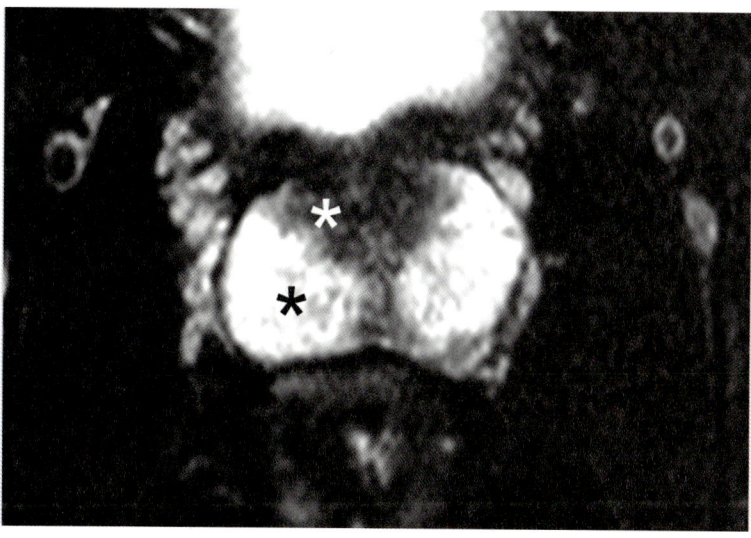   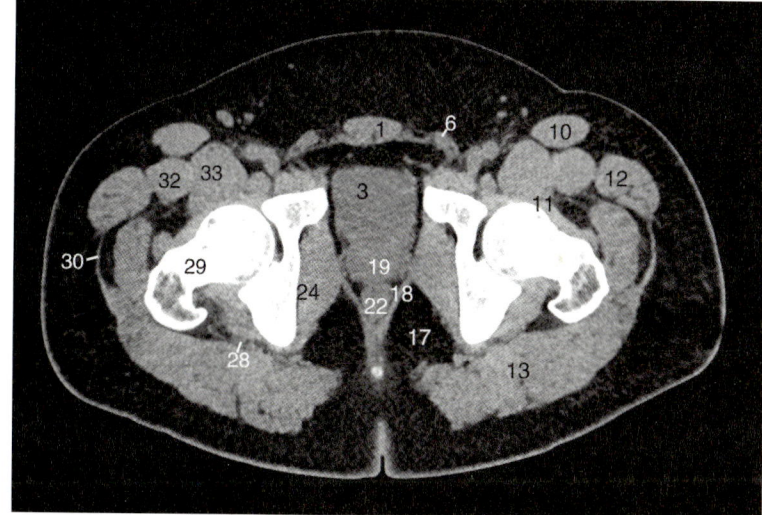

D. FS-T2WI   E. CT 平扫图像

关键结构：前列腺，射精管，肛管。

此断面经过耻骨联合中份。耻骨联合位于盆前壁中央，其前方可见耻骨弓状韧带、阴茎悬韧带及其两侧的精索。盆侧壁为闭孔。盆腔内，前方的膀胱近消失，前列腺居中，在前列腺断面中，前部有尿道前列腺部通过，其后偏外部可见成对的射精管穿行。盆腔内后方为肛管，其两侧为肛提肌（男性肛提肌包括前列腺提肌、耻骨直肠肌、耻尾肌、髂尾肌）。在 CT 及 MRI T1WI 上，不能区分前列腺其内的管道结构及带区；在 T2WI（尤其在高分辨脂肪抑制 T2WI）上，各解剖带区因成分不同（特别是含水量差别）呈不同信号强度，移行区呈等低信号（见 FS-T2WI 白 *），外周区呈明显高信号（见 FS-T2WI 黑 *），在前列腺病变的诊断与鉴别诊断中，还需要结合扩散加权成像（DWI）。前列腺基底部的后份见一对射精管，射精管长约 2 cm[16]，由输精管壶腹末端与精囊管以锐角的形式汇合成，它向前内下方贯穿于前列腺后叶、中叶和侧叶之间，管径越向终端越细，其下段行于前列腺小囊的两侧，末端呈裂隙状开口于尿道前列腺部的精阜上、前列腺小囊的两侧。射精管的走行与前列腺小囊开口的形态有关。射精管管壁有平滑肌纤维，能够产生有力的收缩，帮助精液的排出[25]。

男性盆部连续横断层 21（MH.6380）

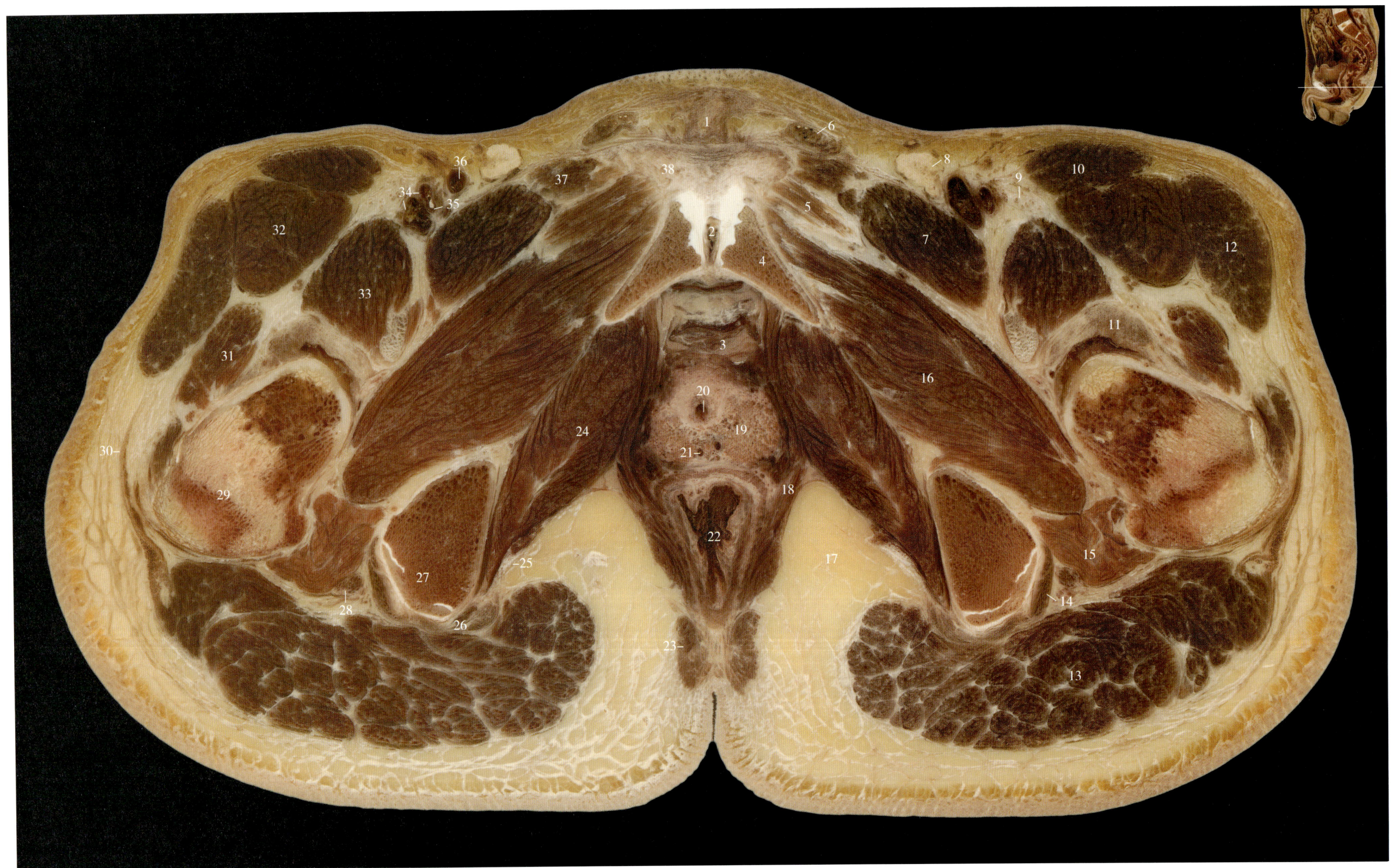

A. 断层标本图像

1. 悬韧带 suspensory ligament
2. 耻骨联合 pubic symphysis
3. 膀胱 urinary bladder
4. 耻骨下支 inferior ramus of pubis
5. 短收肌 adductor brevis
6. 精索 spermatic cord
7. 耻骨肌 pectineus
8. 腹股沟浅淋巴结 superficial inguinal lymph nodes
9. 股神经 femoral nerve
10. 缝匠肌 sartorius
11. 髂股韧带 iliofemoral ligament
12. 阔筋膜张肌 tensor fasciae latae
13. 臀大肌 gluteus maximus
14. 半膜肌肌腱 tendon of semimembranosus
15. 股方肌 quadratus femoris
16. 闭孔外肌 obturator externus
17. 坐骨肛门窝 ischioanal fossa
18. 肛提肌 levator ani
19. 前列腺 prostate
20. 尿道前列腺部 prostatic portion of urethra
21. 射精管 ejaculatory
22. 肛管 anal canal
23. 肛门外括约肌 sphincter ani externus
24. 闭孔内肌 obturator internus
25. 阴部神经 pudendal nerve
26. 股二头肌长头和半腱肌 long head of biceps femoris and semitendinosus
27. 坐骨结节 ischial tuberosity
28. 坐骨神经 sciatic nerve
29. 股骨颈 neck of femur
30. 阔筋膜 fasciae lata
31. 股外侧肌 vastus lateralis
32. 股直肌 rectus femoris
33. 髂腰肌 iliopsoas
34. 股动、静脉 femoral artery and vein
35. 股深动脉 deep femoral artery
36. 大隐静脉 great saphenous vein
37. 长收肌 adductor longus
38. 耻骨弓状韧带 arcuate pubic ligament

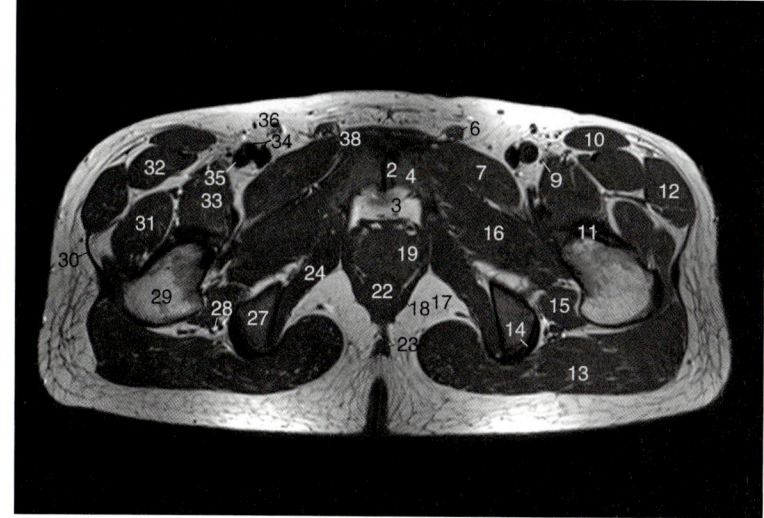

B. T1WI

C. T2WI

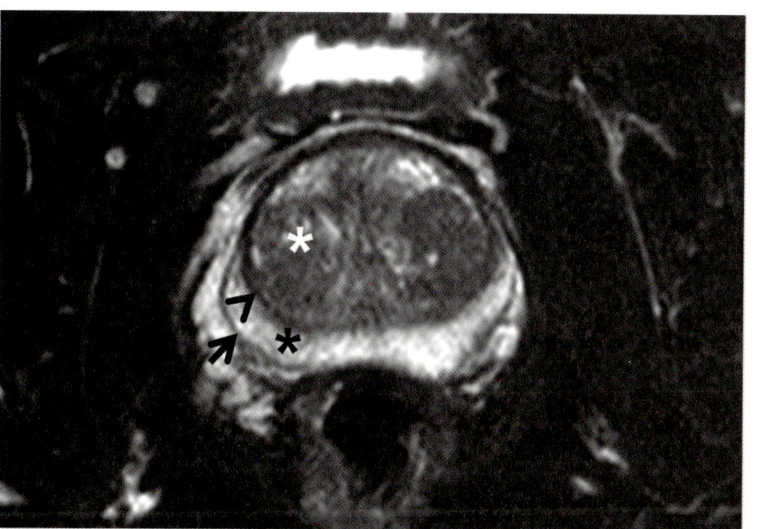

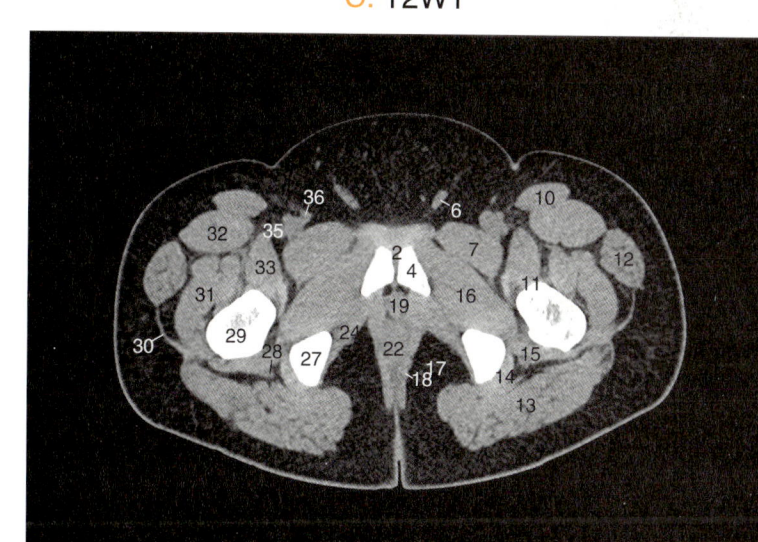

D. FS-T2WI

E. CT 平扫图像

关键结构：前列腺，耻骨联合，精索。

此断面经过耻骨联合中份。

盆腔内前部为部分膀胱壁，尿道前列腺部及前列腺居于盆腔中部，后部为直肠。前列腺主要由腺体、肌肉和纤维组成，外形似一个锥形，位于小骨盆的下部，耻骨联合下缘和耻骨弓的后方，直肠壶腹的前方。前列腺大小随年龄变化而变化，47~50 岁之后，大部分男性前列腺可能出现良性肥大（BPH）。FS-T2WI 图中显示前列腺移行区明显增大（白 * 所示），呈结节状混杂信号；外周带（黑 * 所示）受压变薄，呈明显高信号。移行区与外周带间见线状低信号为外科包膜（↗所示）。外周带周围低信号为前列腺被膜（↗所示），被膜之外高信号为静脉丛。前列腺的血液供应主要来自膀胱下动脉、输精管动脉、直肠下动脉、髂内动脉的前支及脐动脉等。这些血管沿腺体后外侧膀胱前列腺沟进入。前列腺筋膜鞘的前份和外侧份有前列腺静脉丛。前列腺血供十分丰富，在行前列腺摘除时，彻底止血尤为重要[52]。在成年男性，在耻骨联合上部至其下缘这段范围内行 CT 和 MRI 扫描，均可观察到前列腺影像。CT 对前列腺病变的显示不敏感，MRI 的 T2WI 及 DWI 序列是前列腺分区及疾病诊断的首选影像学手段。多参数磁共振成像（mpMRI），可提高前列腺病变检测、分类和体积定量准确性，减少过度诊疗[53]；而机器学习是人工智能的一个分支，它可以快速准确地分析 mpMR 图像，在识别前列腺病变和增强前列腺癌管理方面具有更好的标准化和一致性，有着良好的前景[54]。

男性盆部连续横断层 22（MH.6370）

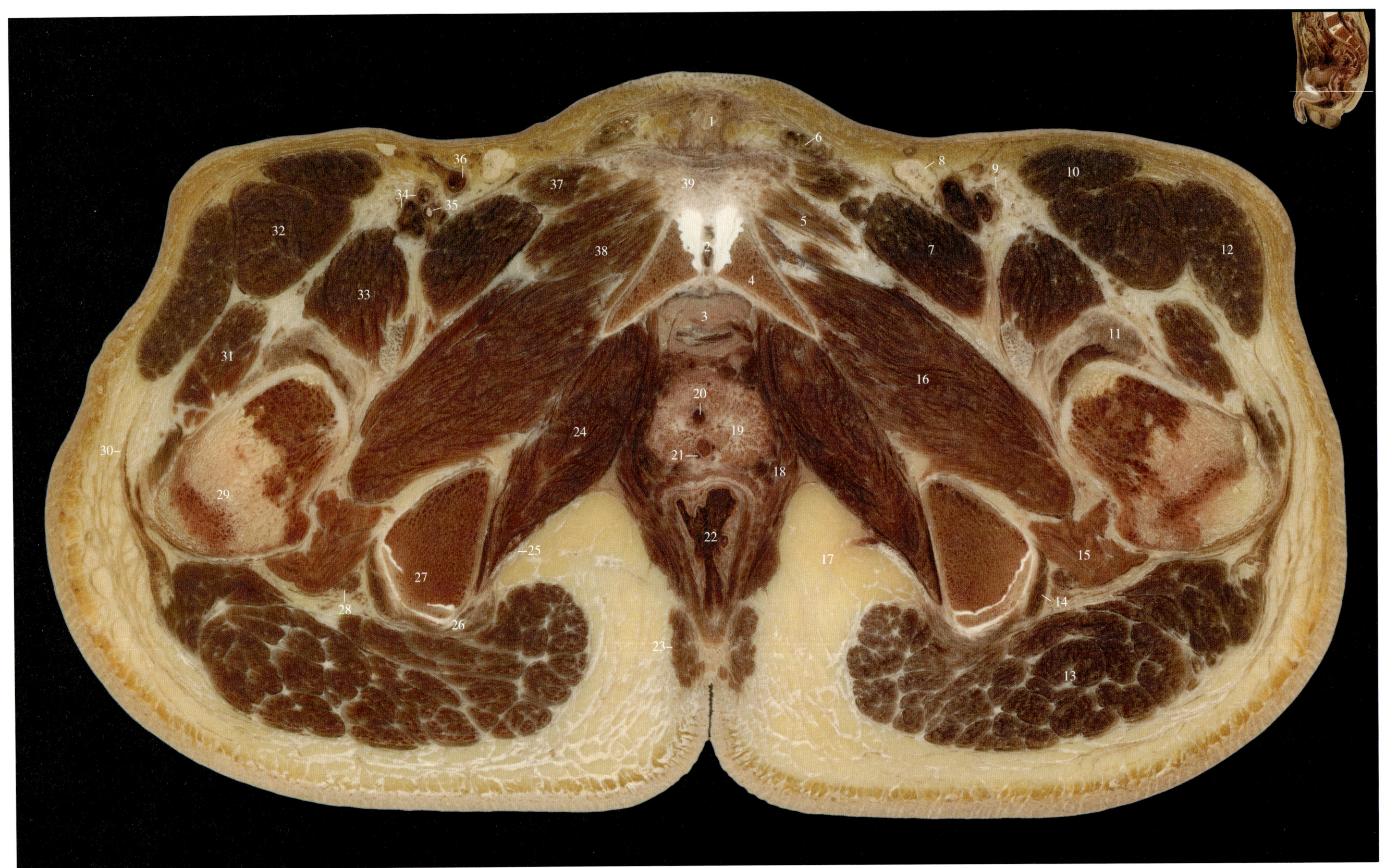

A. 断层标本图像

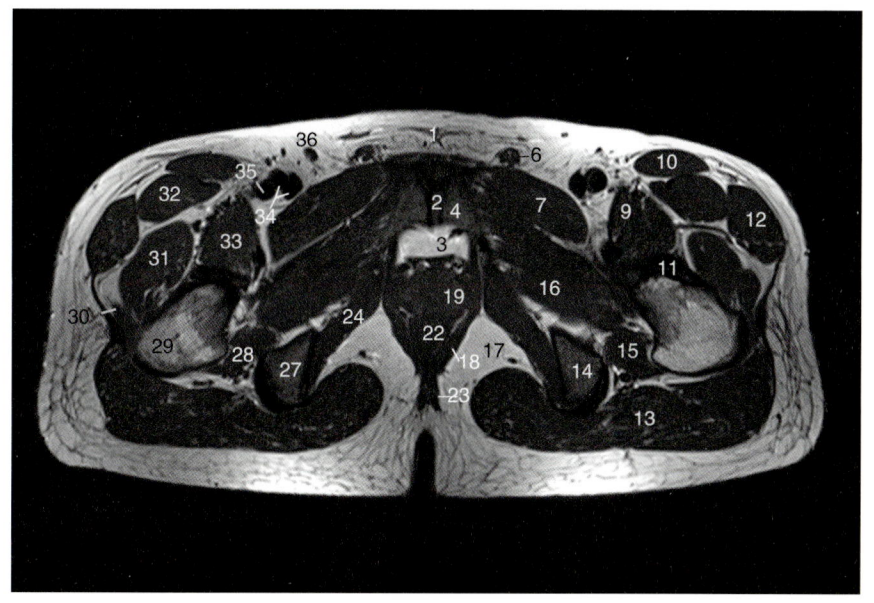
B. MR T1WI

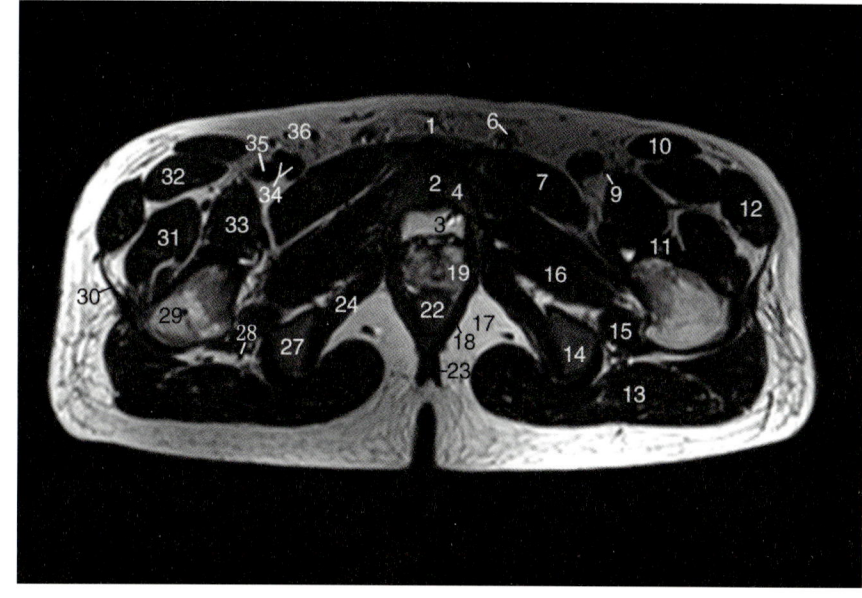
C. MR T2WI

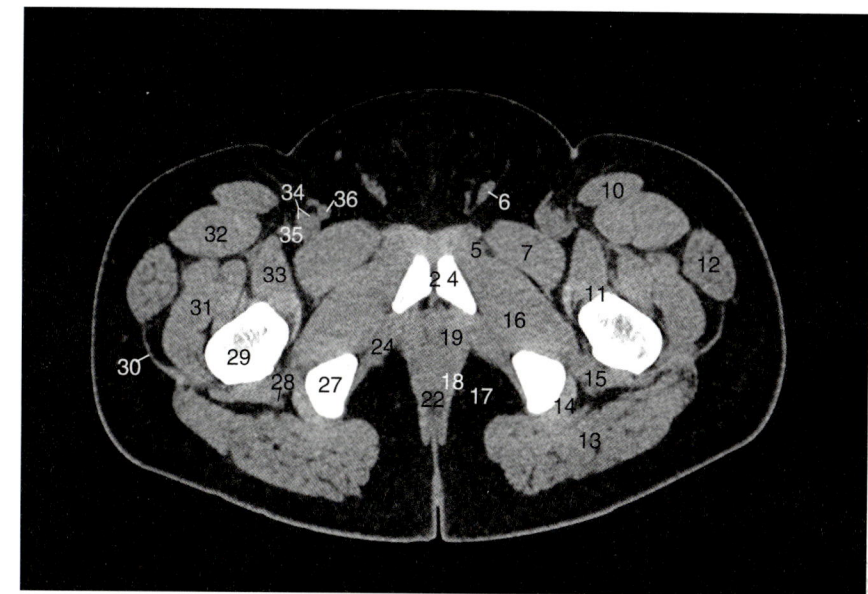
D. CT 平扫图像

1. 悬韧带 suspensory ligament
2. 耻骨联合 pubic symphysis
3. 耻骨后间隙 retropubic space
4. 耻骨下支 inferior ramus of pubis
5. 短收肌 adductor brevis
6. 精索 spermatic cord
7. 耻骨肌 pectineus
8. 腹股沟浅淋巴结 superficial inguinal lymph nodes
9. 股神经 femoral nerve
10. 缝匠肌 sartorius
11. 髂股韧带 iliofemoral ligament
12. 阔筋膜张肌 tensor fasciae latae
13. 臀大肌 gluteus maximus
14. 半膜肌肌腱 tendon of semimembranosus
15. 股方肌 quadratus femoris
16. 闭孔外肌 obturator externus
17. 坐骨肛门窝 ischioanal fossa
18. 肛提肌 levator ani
19. 前列腺 prostate
20. 尿道前列腺部 prostatic portion of urethra
21. 射精管 ejaculatory
22. 肛管 anal canal
23. 肛门外括约肌 sphincter ani externus
24. 闭孔内肌 obturator internus
25. 阴部神经 pudendal nerve
26. 股二头肌长头和半腱肌 long head of biceps femoris and semitendinosus
27. 坐骨结节 ischial tuberosity
28. 坐骨神经 sciatic nerve
29. 股骨颈 neck of femur
30. 阔筋膜 fasciae lata
31. 股外侧肌 vastus lateralis
32. 股直肌 rectus femoris
33. 髂腰肌 iliopsoas
34. 股动、静脉 femoral artery and vein
35. 股深动脉 deep femoral artery
36. 大隐静脉 great saphenous vein
37. 长收肌 adductor longus
38. 大收肌 adductor magnus
39. 耻骨弓状韧带 arcuate pubic ligament

关键结构：耻骨后间隙，尿道前列腺部，前列腺。

此断面经过耻骨联合中份。盆前壁中央为耻骨联合，其前方可见耻骨弓状韧带、阴茎悬韧带及其两侧的精索，其后方与膀胱之间为耻骨后间隙，耻骨后间隙上界为腹膜返折线，下界是尿生殖膈，两侧为盆筋膜形成的韧带，内为疏松结缔组织和静脉丛等，其内的脂肪在 CT 图像上呈低密度影，在 T1WI 和 T2WI 上呈高信号。盆侧壁为闭孔内肌。盆腔内前列腺居前，肛管居后，前列腺内有尿道和射精管穿行。男性尿道分为前列腺部、膜部和海绵体部。临床上将海绵体部称为前尿道，长为 138.81 mm ± 32.03 mm；膜部和前列腺部称为后尿道，长为 33.05 mm ± 4.96 mm[16]。尿道前列腺部为尿道穿过前列腺的部分，长约 3 cm；后壁有一纵行隆起称为尿道嵴，嵴中部隆起称为精阜。精阜中央小凹称为前列腺小囊，两侧各有一个细小的射精管口及许多细小的前列腺输出管的开口。前列腺的神经来自自主神经下腹下丛下部分出的前列腺丛，随前列腺的动脉由前列腺底部和两侧进入前列腺。前列腺丛还分布于精囊、尿道前列腺部、射精管、尿道膜部和尿道海绵体部、阴茎的海绵体，及尿道球腺。

男性盆部连续横断层 23（MH.6360）

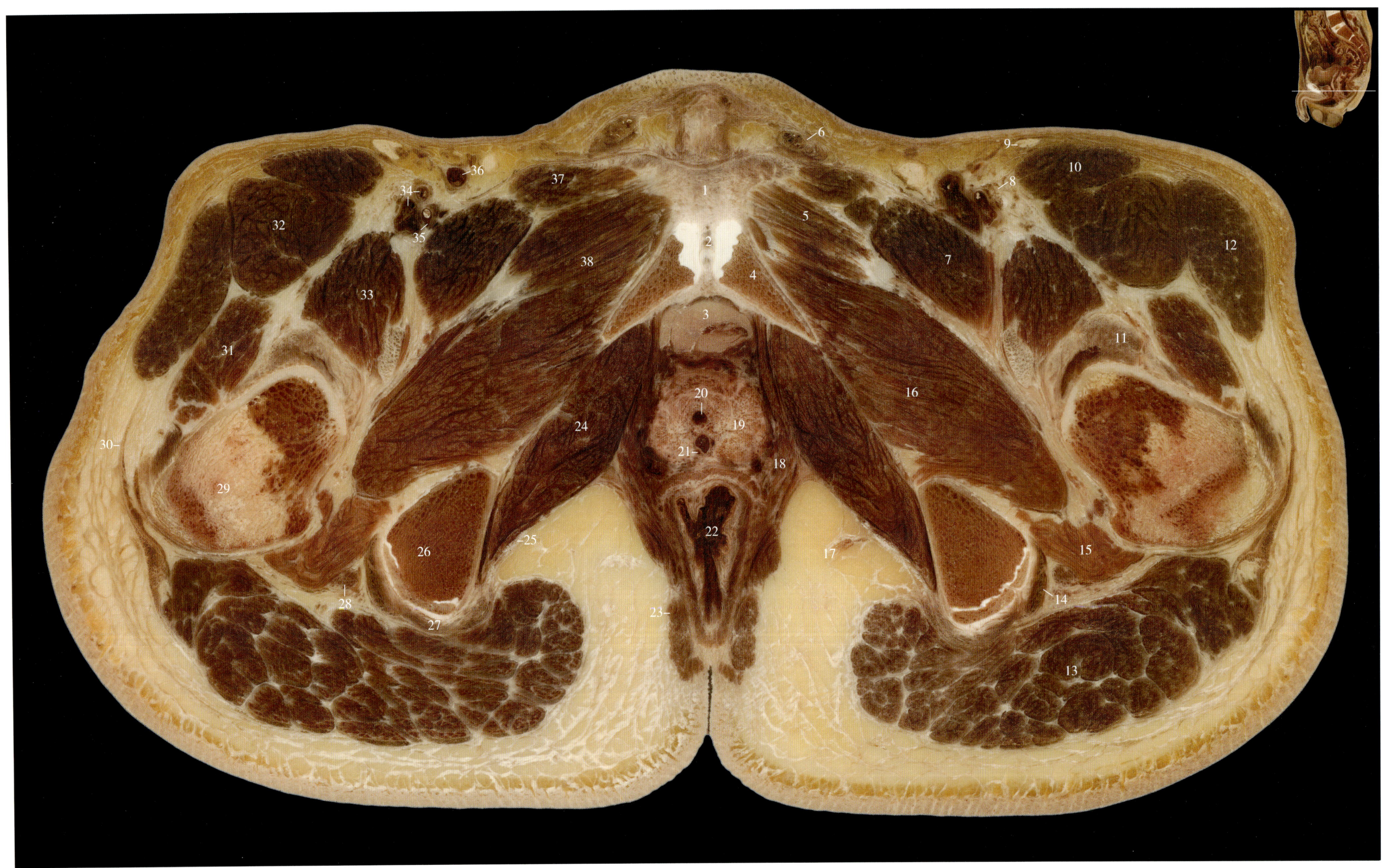

A. 断层标本图像

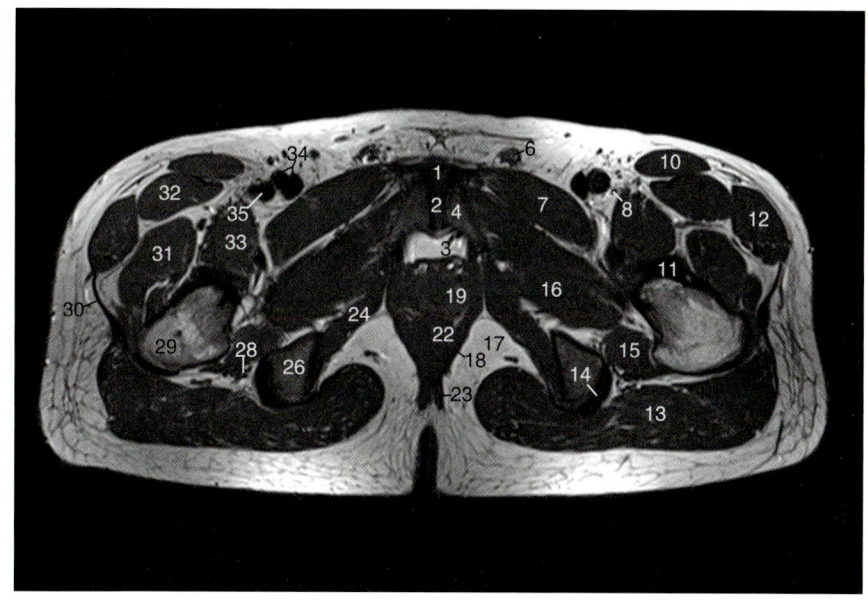
B. MR T1WI

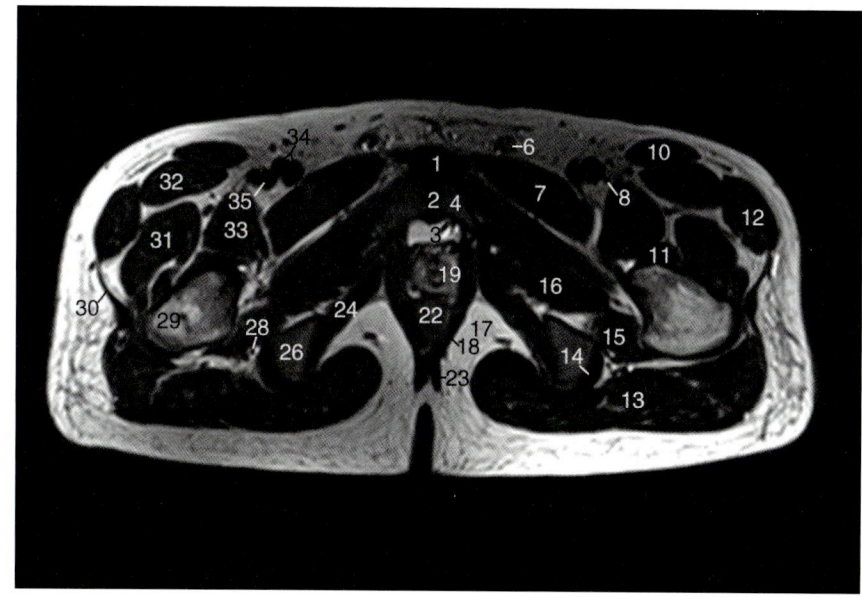
C. MR T2WI

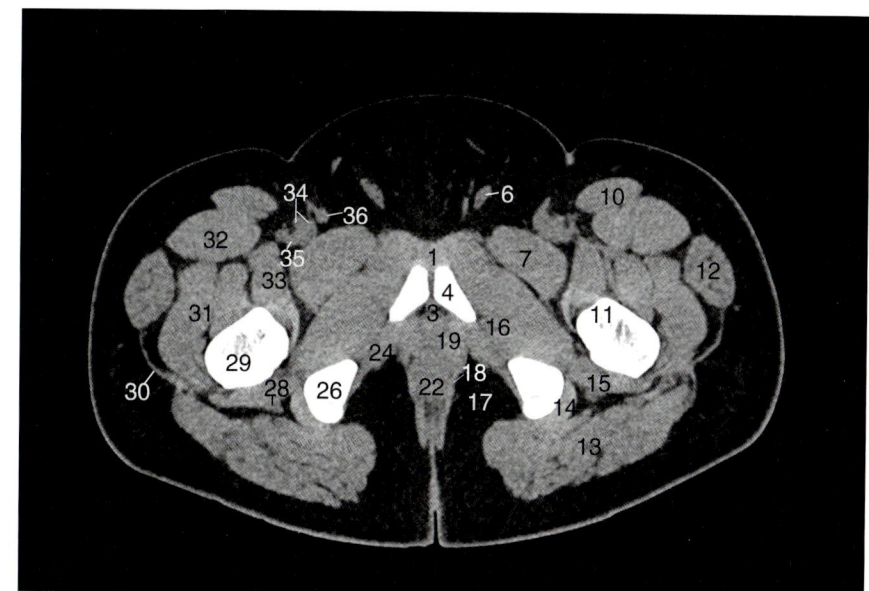
D. CT 平扫图像

1. 耻骨弓状韧带 arcuate pubic ligament
2. 耻骨联合 pubic symphysis
3. 耻骨后间隙 retropubic space
4. 耻骨下支 inferior ramus of pubis
5. 短收肌 adductor brevis
6. 精索 spermatic cord
7. 耻骨肌 pectineus
8. 股神经 femoral nerve
9. 腹股沟浅淋巴结 superficial inguinal lymph nodes
10. 缝匠肌 sartorius
11. 髂股韧带 iliofemoral ligament
12. 阔筋膜张肌 tensor fasciae latae
13. 臀大肌 gluteus maximus
14. 半膜肌肌腱 tendon of semimembranosus
15. 股方肌 quadratus femoris
16. 闭孔外肌 obturator externus
17. 坐骨肛门窝 ischioanal fossa
18. 肛提肌 levator ani
19. 前列腺 prostate
20. 尿道前列腺部 prostatic portion of urethra
21. 射精管 ejaculatory
22. 肛管 anal canal
23. 肛门外括约肌 sphincter ani externus
24. 闭孔内肌 obturator internus
25. 阴部神经 pudendal nerve
26. 坐骨结节 ischial tuberosity
27. 股二头肌长头和半腱肌 long head of biceps femoris and semitendinosus
28. 坐骨神经 sciatic nerve
29. 股骨颈 neck of femur
30. 阔筋膜 fasciae lata
31. 股外侧肌 vastus lateralis
32. 股直肌 rectus femoris
33. 髂腰肌 iliopsoas
34. 股动、静脉 femoral artery and vein
35. 股深动脉 deep femoral artery
36. 大隐静脉 great saphenous vein
37. 长收肌 adductor longus
38. 大收肌 adductor magnus

关键结构：前列腺，肛管，肛门括约肌。

此断面经过耻骨联合下缘。

盆前壁中央为耻骨联合，其前方可见耻骨弓状韧带、阴茎悬韧带及其两侧的精索，其后方为耻骨后间隙。盆侧壁为闭孔内肌，张于坐骨结节与耻骨下支之间。闭孔内肌内侧为肛提肌。盆腔内，居前的前列腺内有尿道和射精管穿行，肛管居后。直肠在第3骶椎平面与乙状结肠相接，在尾骨尖前2~3 cm穿过盆膈后延续为肛管，止于肛门。以齿状线为界肛管分为上下两部分，成人长为 4.41 cm ± 0.67 cm，儿童为 3.12 cm ± 0.32 cm，新生儿为 1.48 cm ± 0.22 cm（男婴为 1.40 cm ± 0.4 cm，女婴为 1.70 cm ± 0.30 cm）。断面上可见环绕肛管的肛门内、外括约肌。内括约肌为肛管壁内环行肌层增厚形成，各径：宽度为 3.06 cm ± 0.27 cm，儿童为 2.02 cm ± 0.21 cm；成人厚度为 0.20 cm+0.01 cm，儿童为 0.15 cm ± 0.01 cm。肛门外括约肌环绕肛门内括约肌周围，为横纹肌，各径为：浅部和深部的宽度均为 0.40 cm ± 0.10 cm；厚度均为 0.10 cm ± 0.10 cm，高度均为 2.30 cm ± 0.65 cm；小儿为 1.21 cm ± 0.20 cm[16]。肛门外括约肌按其纤维的位置分为三部分：①皮下部，位肛管下端皮下；②浅部，在皮下部之上，围绕肛门内括约肌下部；③深部，肌束厚，环绕内括约肌上部。直肠血供来自直肠上动脉（肠系膜下动脉分支）、直肠下动脉（髂内或阴部内动脉分支）及肛门动脉（阴部内动脉分支）、骶正中动脉（腹主动脉分支，部分阙如）[41]。齿状线以下的肛管及其周围结构主要由阴部神经的分支支配。肛管、肛门外括约肌、肛门周围皮下的淋巴汇入腹股沟浅淋巴结，然后至髂外淋巴结。也有部分坐骨直肠窝的淋巴沿肛血管和阴部内血管汇入髂内淋巴结[55]。

男性盆部连续横断层 24（MH.6350）

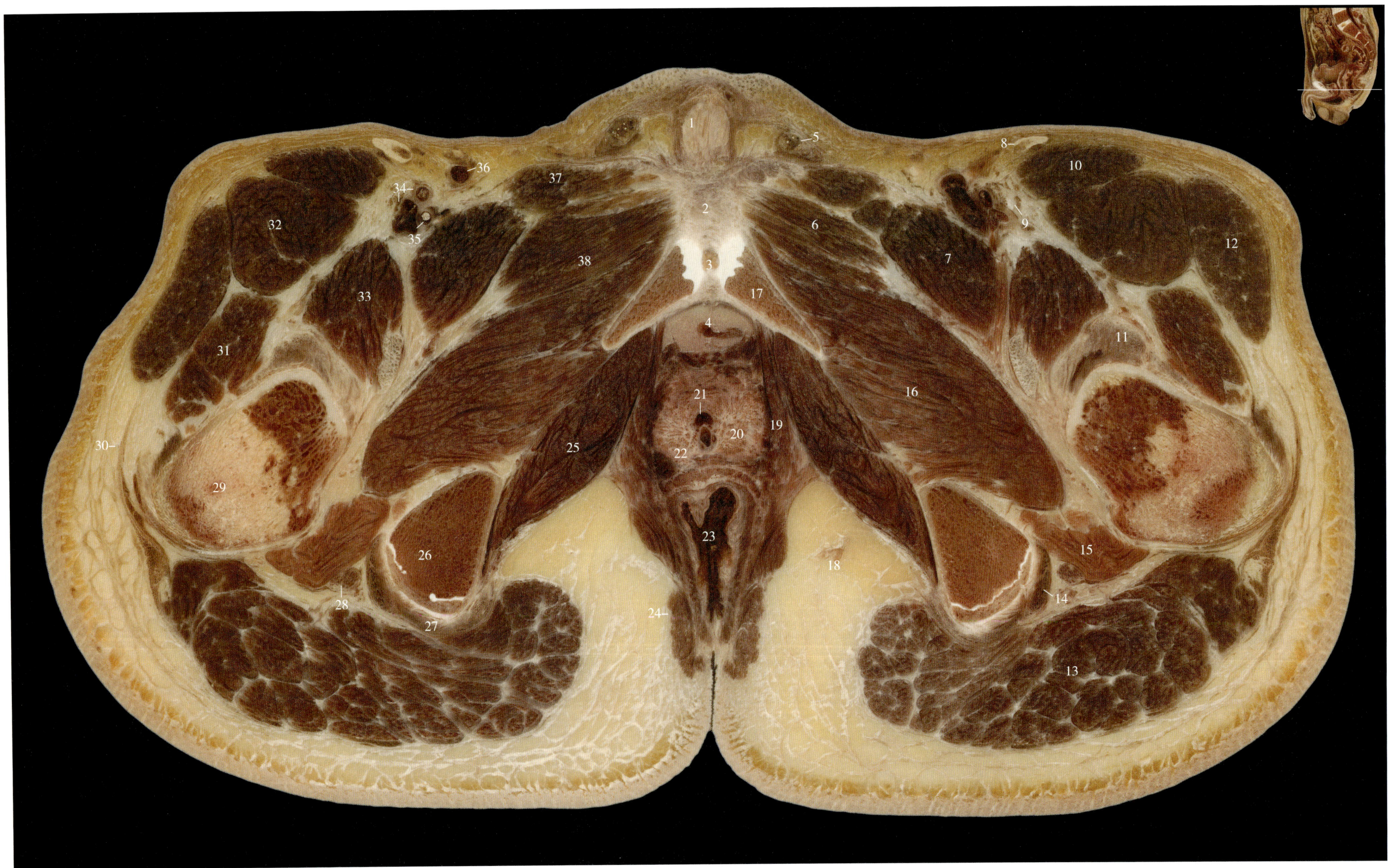

A. 断层标本图像

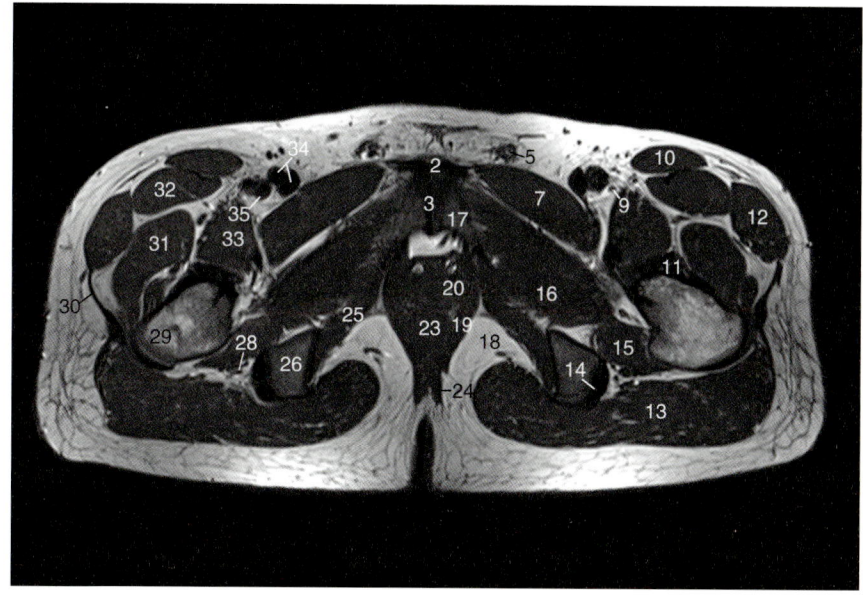
B. MR T1WI

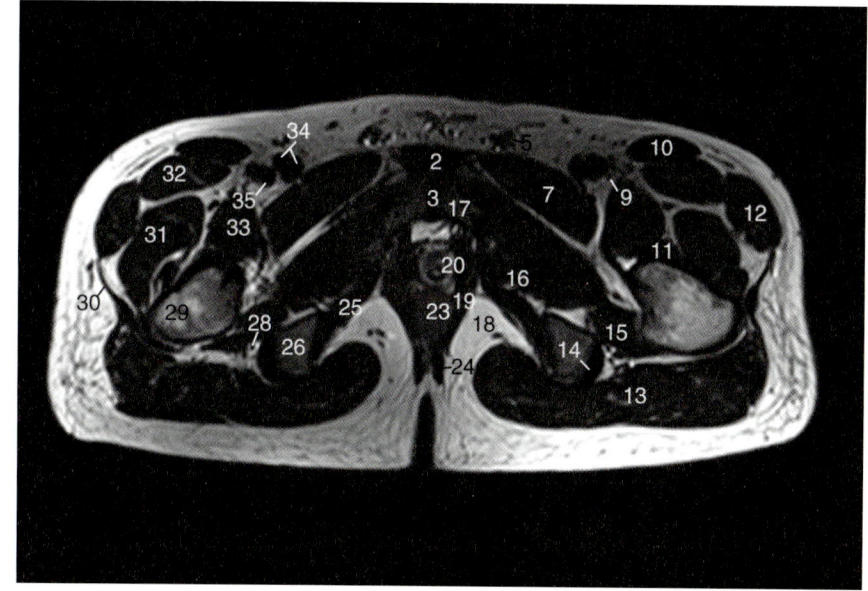
C. MR T2WI

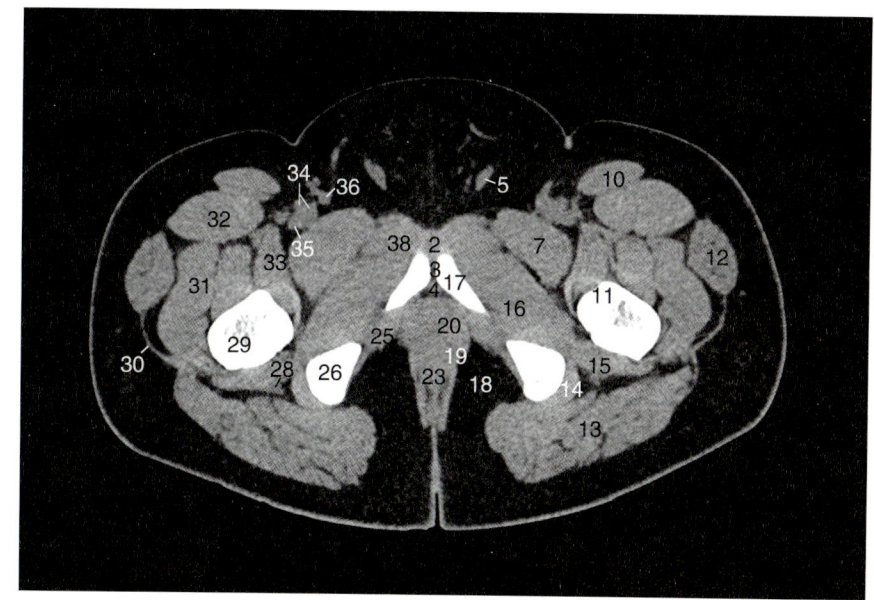
D. CT 平扫图像

关键结构：耻骨弓状韧带，前列腺沟，坐骨肛门窝。

此断面经过耻骨联合下缘层面。耻骨联合位居盆腔前壁，前方为耻骨弓状韧带及初现的阴茎海绵体，其两侧为精索；耻骨弓状韧带在耻骨联合下方附于两侧耻骨下支，加固耻骨联合，维持骨盆两侧的约束。盆腔侧壁为闭孔内肌，闭孔内肌与内侧的肛提肌及其后方的臀大肌之间为锥体形坐骨肛门窝，窝尖朝上，为盆膈下筋膜与闭孔内肌筋膜之交接处；窝底向下，为肛门三角区的皮肤及浅筋膜，窝内充满大量脂肪，缺少血供，是肛区皮肤与肛提肌之间的潜在间隙，允许肛管扩张，易感染并向上或经肛管后方向对侧蔓延；坐骨肛门窝向前延伸至肛提肌与尿生殖膈之间，形成前隐窝；向后延伸至臀大肌、骶结节韧带与尾骨肌之间形成的后隐窝。盆腔内部为前列腺，断面形似板栗状，前面与耻骨联合之间为耻骨后间隙，其间有静脉丛通过；两侧隆凸与肛提肌及其筋膜相贴；后面平坦，正中有一浅沟，此即前列腺沟，肛门指检时可能触及，前列腺增生时，此沟消失[1]。前列腺内前有尿道通过，后有射精管穿行。

1. 阴茎海绵体 cavernous body of penis
2. 耻骨弓状韧带 arcuate pubic ligament
3. 耻骨联合 pubic symphysis
4. 耻骨后间隙 retropubic space
5. 精索 spermatic cord
6. 短收肌 adductor brevis
7. 耻骨肌 pectineus
8. 腹股沟浅淋巴结 superficial inguinal lymph nodes
9. 股神经 femoral nerve
10. 缝匠肌 sartorius
11. 髂股韧带 iliofemoral ligament
12. 阔筋膜张肌 tensor fasciae latae
13. 臀大肌 gluteus maximus
14. 半膜肌肌腱 tendon of semimembranosus
15. 股方肌 quadratus femoris
16. 闭孔外肌 obturator externus
17. 耻骨下支 inferior ramus of pubis
18. 坐骨肛门窝 ischioanal fossa
19. 肛提肌 levator ani
20. 前列腺 prostate
21. 尿道前列腺部 prostatic portion of urethra
22. 射精管 ejaculatory
23. 肛管 anal canal
24. 肛门外括约肌 sphincter ani externus
25. 闭孔内肌 obturator internus
26. 坐骨结节 ischial tuberosity
27. 股二头肌长头和半腱肌 long head of biceps femoris and semitendinosus
28. 坐骨神经 sciatic nerve
29. 股骨颈 neck of femur
30. 阔筋膜 fasciae lata
31. 股外侧肌 vastus lateralis
32. 股直肌 rectus femoris
33. 髂腰肌 iliopsoas
34. 股动、静脉 femoral artery and vein
35. 股深动脉 deep femoral artery
36. 大隐静脉 great saphenous vein
37. 长收肌 adductor longus
38. 大收肌 adductor magnus

男性盆部连续横断层 25（MH.6340）

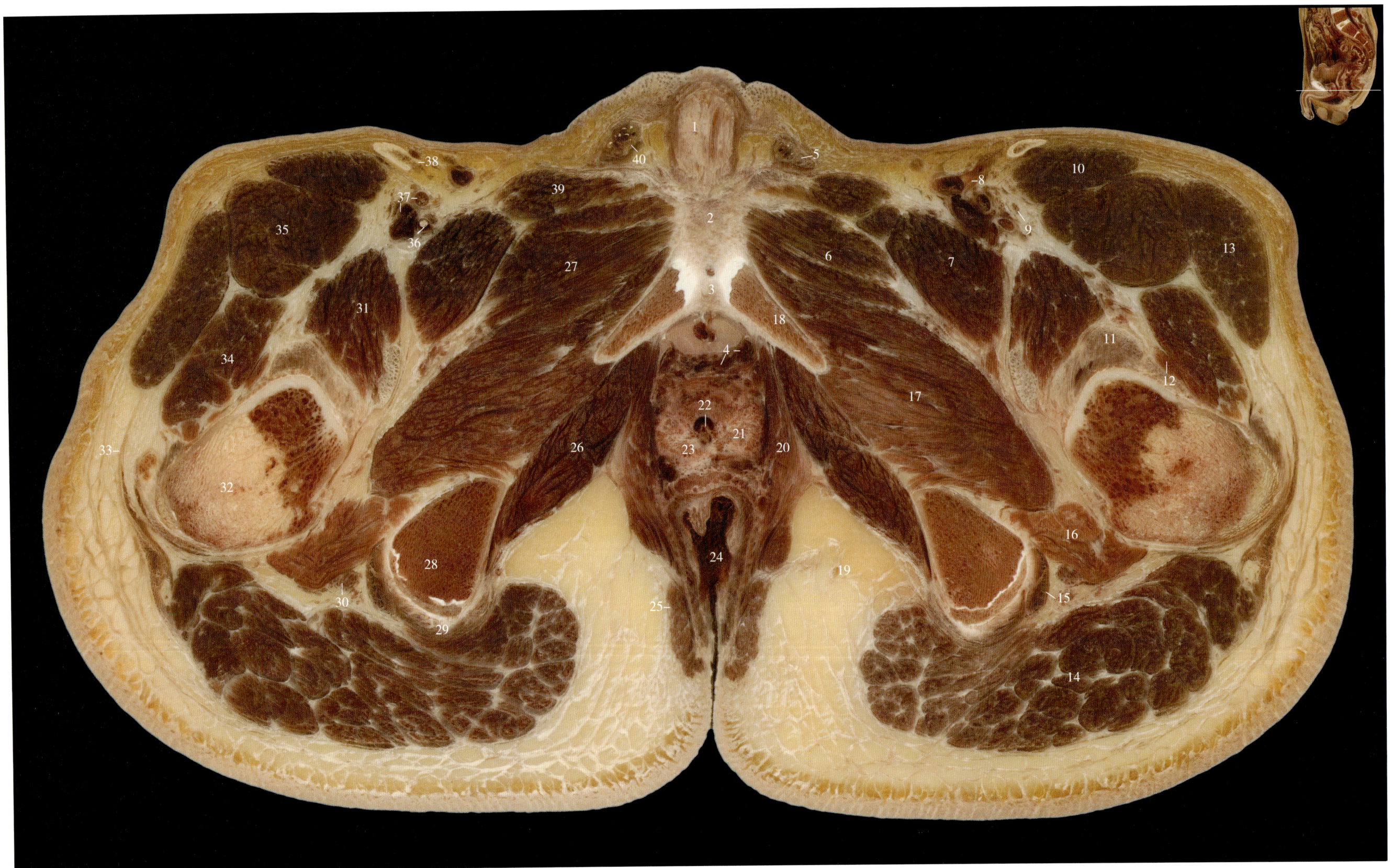

A. 断层标本图像

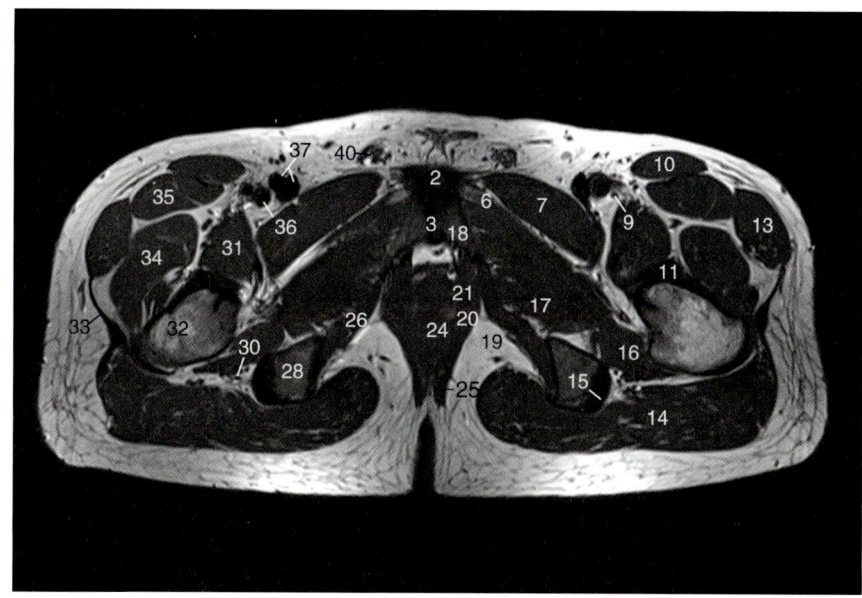
B. MR T1WI

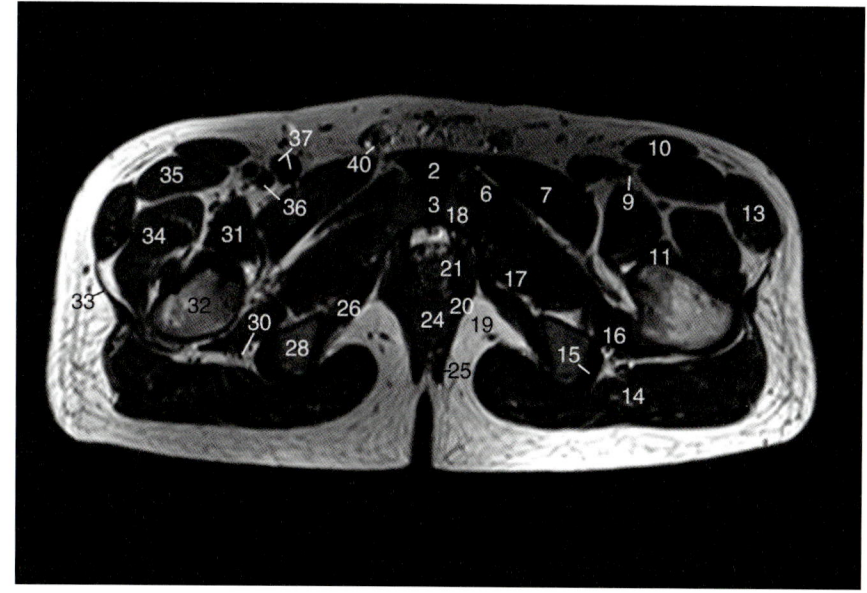
C. MR T2WI

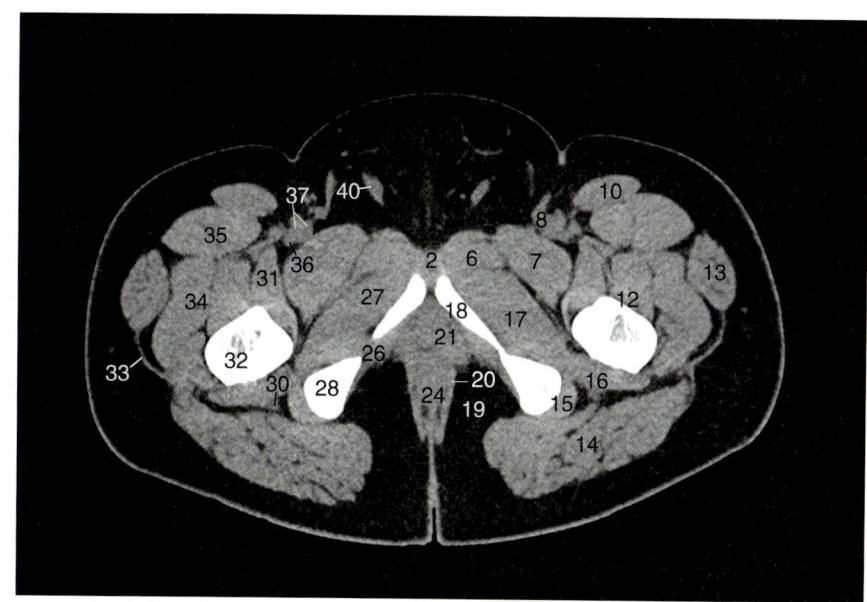
D. CT 平扫图像

1. 阴茎海绵体 cavernous body of penis
2. 耻骨弓状韧带 arcuate pubic ligament
3. 耻骨联合 pubic symphysis
4. 前列腺静脉丛 prostatic venous plexus
5. 输精管 ductus deferens
6. 短收肌 adductor brevis
7. 缝匠肌 sartorius
8. 大隐静脉 great saphenous vein
9. 股神经 femoral nerve
10. 耻骨肌 pectineus
11. 髂股韧带 iliofemoral ligament
12. 股中间肌 vastus intermedius
13. 阔筋膜张肌 tensor fasciae latae
14. 臀大肌 gluteus maximus
15. 半膜肌肌腱 tendon of semimembranosus
16. 股方肌 quadratus femoris
17. 闭孔外肌 obturator externus
18. 耻骨下支 inferior ramus of pubis
19. 坐骨肛门窝 ischioanal fossa
20. 肛提肌 levator ani
21. 前列腺 prostate
22. 尿道嵴 urethral ridge
23. 射精管 ejaculatory
24. 肛管 anal canal
25. 肛门外括约肌 sphincter ani externus
26. 闭孔内肌 obturator internus
27. 大收肌 adductor magnus
28. 坐骨结节 ischial tuberosity
29. 股二头肌长头和半腱肌 long head of biceps femoris and semitendinosus
30. 坐骨神经 sciatic nerve
31. 髂腰肌 iliopsoas
32. 股骨颈 neck of femur
33. 阔筋膜 fasciae lata
34. 股外侧肌 vastus lateralis
35. 股直肌 rectus femoris
36. 股深动脉 deep femoral artery
37. 股动、静脉 femoral artery and vein
38. 腹股沟浅淋巴结 superficial inguinal lymph nodes
39. 长收肌 adductor longus
40. 精索 spermatic cord

关键结构：前列腺，精阜，阴茎海绵体。

此断面经过耻骨联合下缘层面。盆腔前壁正中为耻骨联合下份，其前方为耻骨弓状韧带及阴茎海绵体，其两侧为精索。盆腔内前部为前列腺，前列腺前与耻骨联合之间为耻骨后间隙，内见颜色较深的静脉丛。前列腺断面中央偏前处有尿道前列腺部通过，在尿道后壁正中有突向腔内的隆起，此系尿道嵴，嵴的中部突起膨大称为精阜，精阜中央有一小凹，称前列腺小囊[41]，其两侧有射精管的开口。在成年男性，耻骨联合上部至其下缘这段范围内扫描，绝大多数均可观察到前列腺影像。前列腺的大小随年龄变化，在 CT 和 MRI 上，30 岁以下，前后径为 2.0~2.3 cm，横径为 3.1~4.1 cm；60~70 岁，前列腺平均值增大，前后径为 4.3 cm，横径为 4.8 cm。断层解剖测值：前后径为 2.54 cm ± 0.57 cm，横径为 3.38 cm ± 0.72 cm [1]。成人前列腺各径的超声数值（cm）：左右径为 4.40 cm ± 0.21 cm；前后径为 2.44 cm ± 0.16 cm；前后径/左右径为 1:1.80 [16]。所有测值均为横径明显大于前后径，而在前列腺病变时，前后径明显增大，等于或超过横径。

男性盆部连续横断层 26（MH.6330）

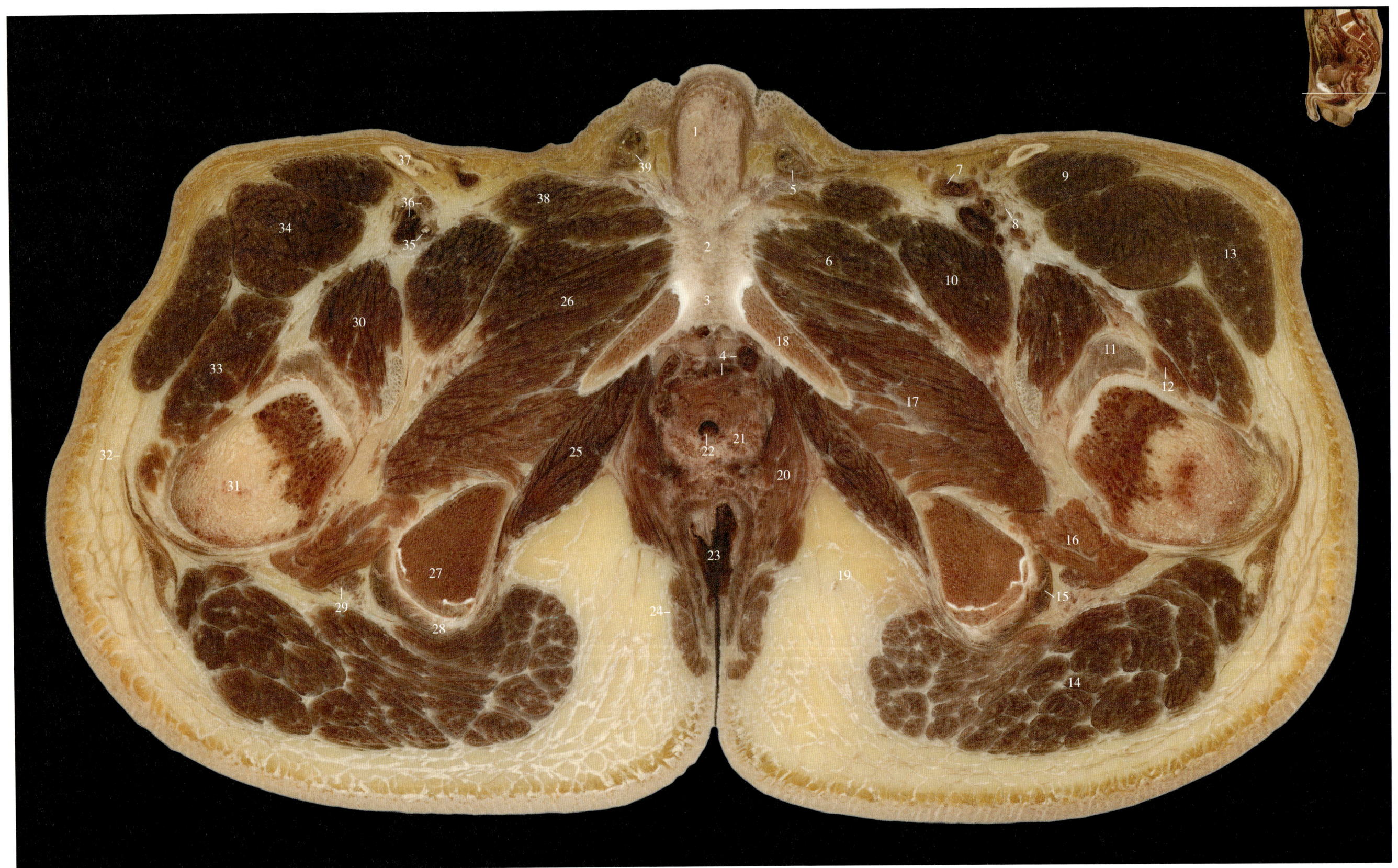

A. 断层标本图像

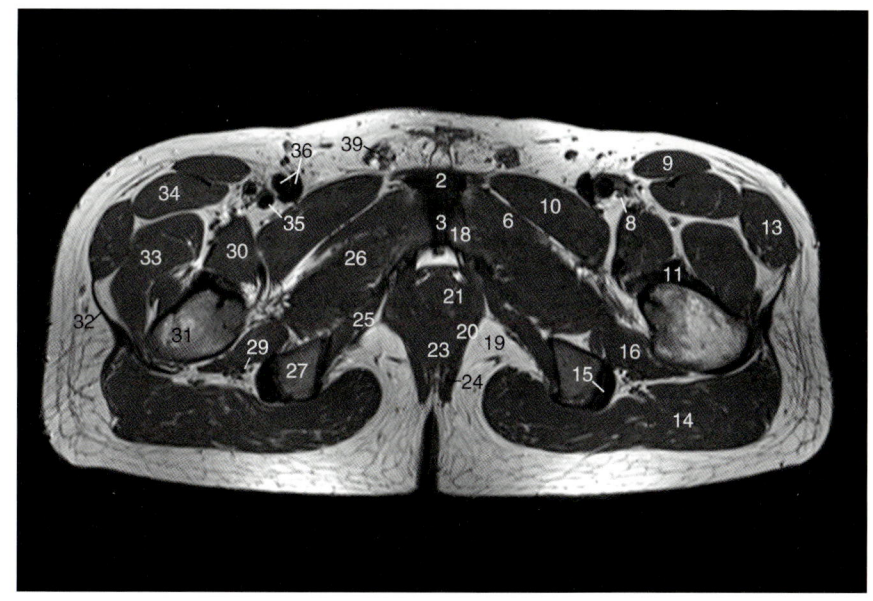
B. MR T1WI

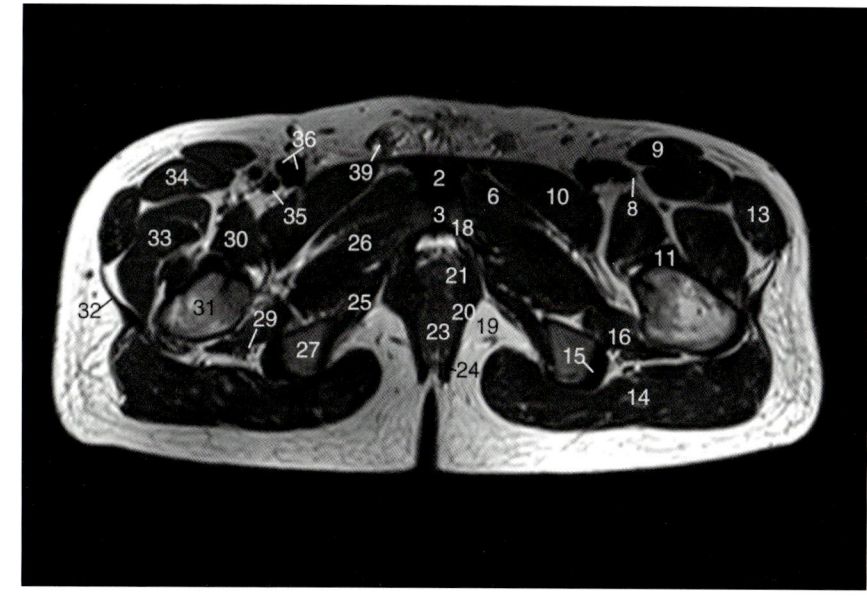
C. MR T2WI

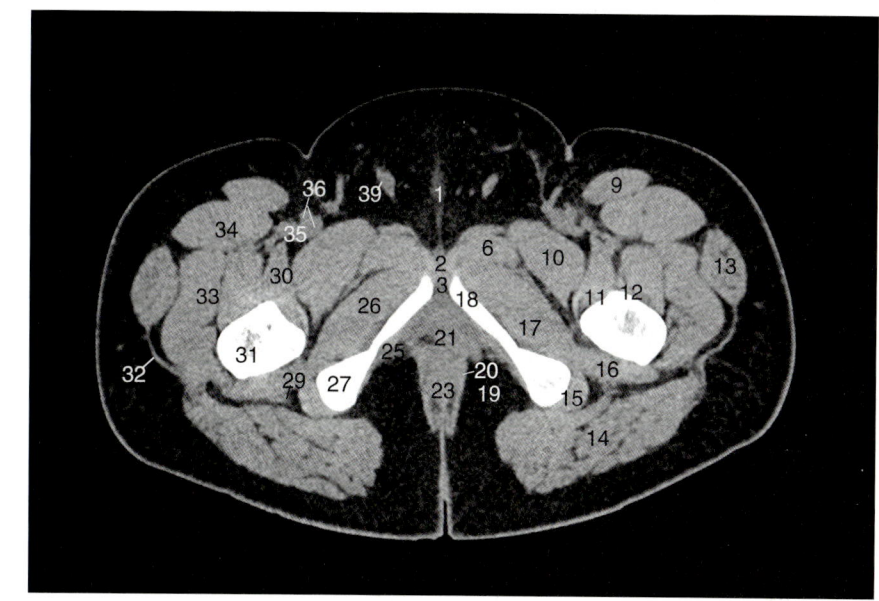
D. CT 平扫图像

1. 阴茎海绵体 cavernous body of penis
2. 耻骨弓状韧带 arcuate pubic ligament
3. 耻骨联合 pubic symphysis
4. 前列腺静脉丛 prostatic venous plexus
5. 输精管 ductus deferens
6. 短收肌 adductor brevis
7. 大隐静脉 great saphenous vein
8. 股神经 femoral nerve
9. 缝匠肌 sartorius
10. 耻骨肌 pectineus
11. 髂股韧带 iliofemoral ligament
12. 股中间肌 vastus intermedius
13. 阔筋膜张肌 tensor fasciae latae
14. 臀大肌 gluteus maximus
15. 半膜肌肌腱 tendon of semimembranosus
16. 股方肌 quadratus femoris
17. 闭孔外肌 obturator externus
18. 耻骨下支 inferior ramus of pubis
19. 坐骨肛门窝 ischioanal fossa
20. 肛提肌 levator ani

21. 前列腺 prostate
22. 尿道嵴 urethral ridge
23. 肛管 anal canal
24. 肛门外括约肌 sphincter ani externus
25. 闭孔内肌 obturator internus
26. 大收肌 adductor magnus
27. 坐骨结节 ischial tuberosity
28. 股二头肌长头和半腱肌 long head of biceps femoris and semitendinosus
29. 坐骨神经 sciatic nerve
30. 髂腰肌 iliopsoas
31. 股骨颈 neck of femur
32. 阔筋膜 fasciae lata
33. 股外侧肌 vastus lateralis
34. 股直肌 rectus femoris
35. 股深动脉 deep femoral artery
36. 股动、静脉 femoral artery and vein
37. 腹股沟浅淋巴结 superficial inguinal lymph nodes
38. 长收肌 adductor longus
39. 精索 spermatic cord

关键结构：前列腺，前列腺静脉丛，阴茎海绵体。

此断面经过耻骨下支层面。前列腺位于盆腔前部，内有尿道前列腺部通过，前列腺内射精管消失。其与耻骨联合之间的耻骨后间隙有静脉丛通过；前列腺两侧隆凸与肛提肌及其筋膜相贴；后与肛管相邻。在前列腺的前面和两侧的固有囊与筋膜鞘之间可见由前列腺静脉形成的前列腺静脉丛，其接受阴茎背深静脉的汇合[1]。前列腺静脉丛与阴部静脉丛和膀胱静脉丛有交通支，经膀胱下静脉汇入髂内静脉或髂内静脉的其他属支；前列腺静脉和痔静脉丛有吻合，通过直肠上静脉引流到肝门静脉系，这是前列腺癌引起肝转移的主要原因。前列腺静脉与椎内静脉及髂骨的静脉有许多交通，这是前列腺癌在骨转移时首先表现为骶骨、腰椎和髂骨转移的原因。前列腺的淋巴流向有3个途经：①前列腺前部集合淋巴管沿膀胱上动脉的分支走行，注入膀胱前淋巴结，最后注入髂内淋巴结和髂外淋巴结；②前列腺后部发出的集合淋巴管大部分与精囊的淋巴管汇合，主要注入髂内淋巴结；③前列腺外侧部的集合淋巴管注入骶淋巴结或主动脉下淋巴结[56]。T2WI可分辨前列腺各带区：尿道表现为前列腺前1/3内的高信号区；尿道两侧的移行区与射精管旁的中央区呈等信号；外周区表现为前列腺后外两侧对称的新月形明显高信号；前纤维肌肉肌质区信号很低，居前列腺最前份。

男性盆部连续横断层 27（MH.6320）

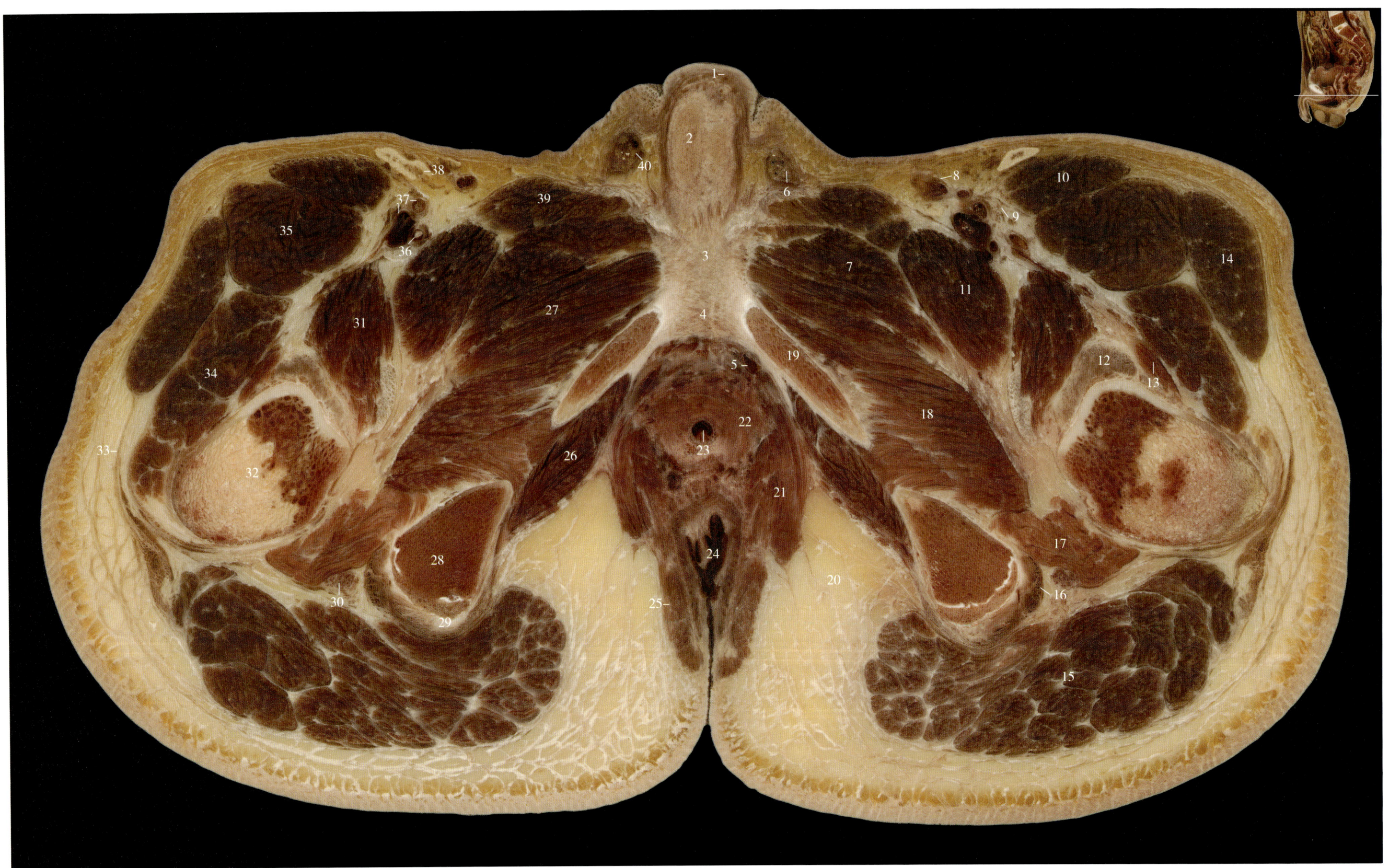

A. 断层标本图像

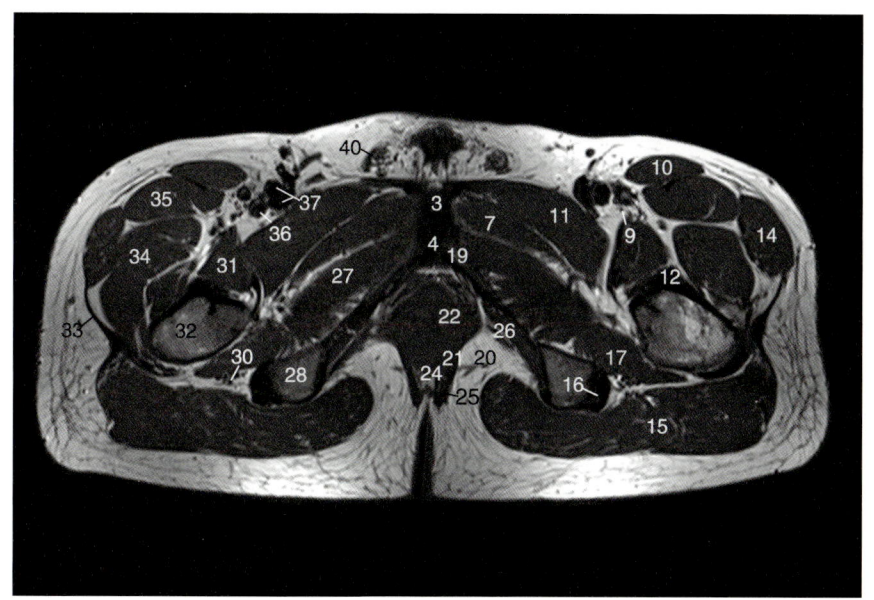

B. MR T1WI

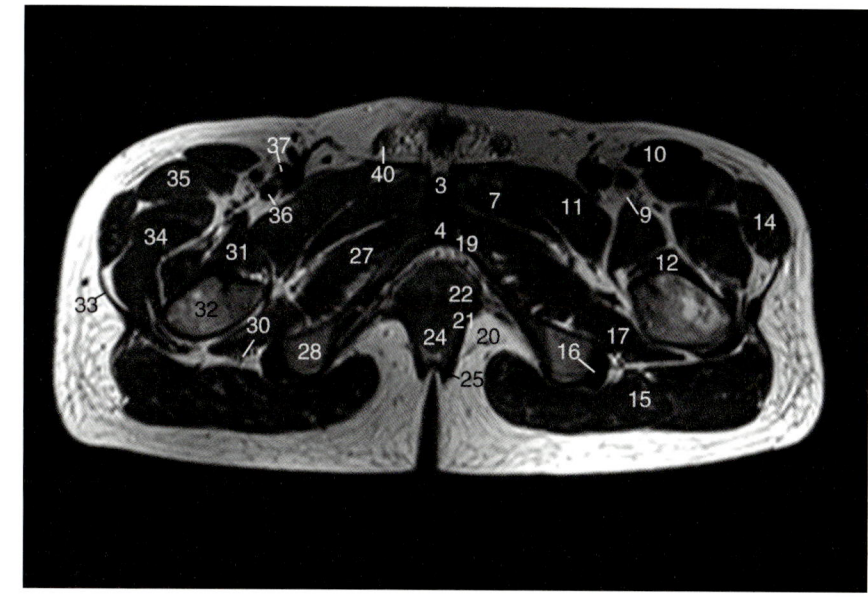

C. MR T2WI

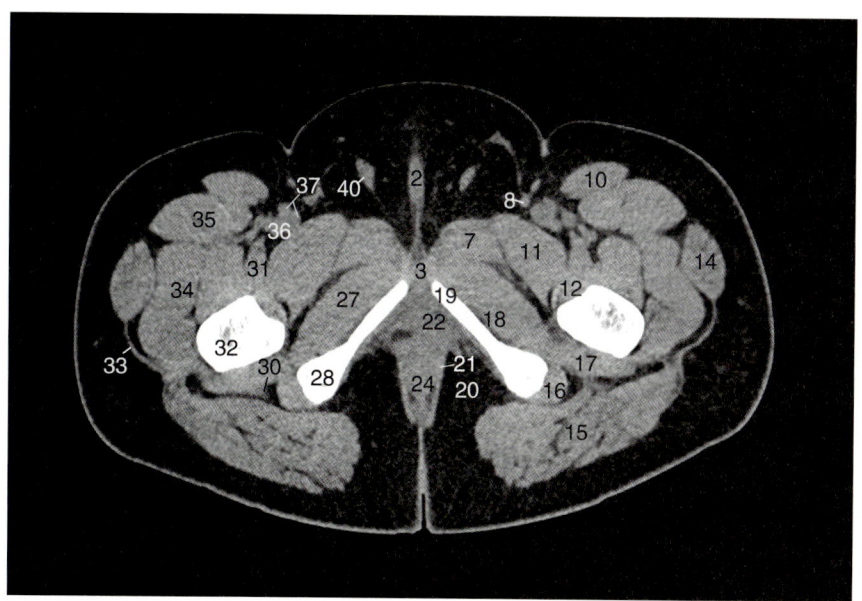

D. CT 平扫图像

1. 阴茎背浅静脉 superficial dorsal vein of penis
2. 阴茎海绵体 cavernous body of penis
3. 耻骨弓状韧带 arcuate pubic ligament
4. 耻骨联合 pubic symphysis
5. 前列腺静脉丛 prostatic venous plexus
6. 输精管 ductus deferens
7. 短收肌 adductor brevis
8. 大隐静脉 great saphenous vein
9. 股神经 femoral nerve
10. 缝匠肌 sartorius
11. 耻骨肌 pectineus
12. 髂股韧带 iliofemoral ligament
13. 股中间肌 vastus intermedius
14. 阔筋膜张肌 tensor fasciae latae
15. 臀大肌 gluteus maximus
16. 半膜肌肌腱 tendon of semimembranosus
17. 股方肌 quadratus femoris
18. 闭孔外肌 obturator externus
19. 耻骨下支 inferior ramus of pubis
20. 坐骨肛门窝 ischioanal fossa

21. 肛提肌 levator ani
22. 会阴深横肌 deep transverse muscles of perineum
23. 尿道膜部 membranous portion of urethra
24. 肛管 anal canal
25. 肛门外括约肌 sphincter ani externus
26. 闭孔内肌 obturator internus
27. 大收肌 adductor magnus
28. 坐骨结节 ischial tuberosity
29. 股二头肌长头和半腱肌 long head of biceps femoris and semitendinosus
30. 坐骨神经 sciatic nerve
31. 髂腰肌 iliopsoas
32. 股骨颈 neck of femur
33. 阔筋膜 fasciae lata
34. 股外侧肌 vastus lateralis
35. 股直肌 rectus femoris
36. 股深动脉 deep femoral artery
37. 股动、静脉 femoral artery and vein
38. 腹股沟浅淋巴结 superficial inguinal lymph nodes
39. 长收肌 adductor longus
40. 精索 spermatic cord

关键结构：阴囊，阴茎背浅静脉，肛提肌。

此断面经过耻骨联合下缘。本断面两侧出现耻骨下支，耻骨弓状韧带前方阴茎的断面中可见阴茎背浅静脉及成对的阴茎海绵体，两侧为圆索状的精索，精索已进入阴囊。盆腔内，前部为前列腺尖部，其周围可见大量静脉丛；后部为肛管。从前列腺所在各断面中可以看出，前列腺基底部和中部与耻骨联合和肛提肌之间相对有较多的脂肪组织间隔，故在 CT、MRI 上较易区别各相邻结构，但在腺体尖部，由于与两侧的肛提肌及后方的直肠紧贴，CT 有时难以辨别前列腺、肛提肌和直肠。阴茎的血供主要来自阴茎背动脉和阴茎深动脉[41]。阴茎背动脉穿行于阴茎深筋膜与白膜之间，阴茎深动脉则经阴茎脚进入阴茎海绵体。阴茎有阴茎背浅静脉和阴茎背深静脉，前者收集阴茎包皮及皮下的小静脉，经阴部外浅静脉汇入大隐静脉；后者收集阴茎海绵体和阴茎头的静脉血，向后穿过耻骨弓状韧带与会阴横韧带之间进入盆腔，分左、右支汇入前列腺静脉丛。

男性盆部连续横断层 28（MH.6310）

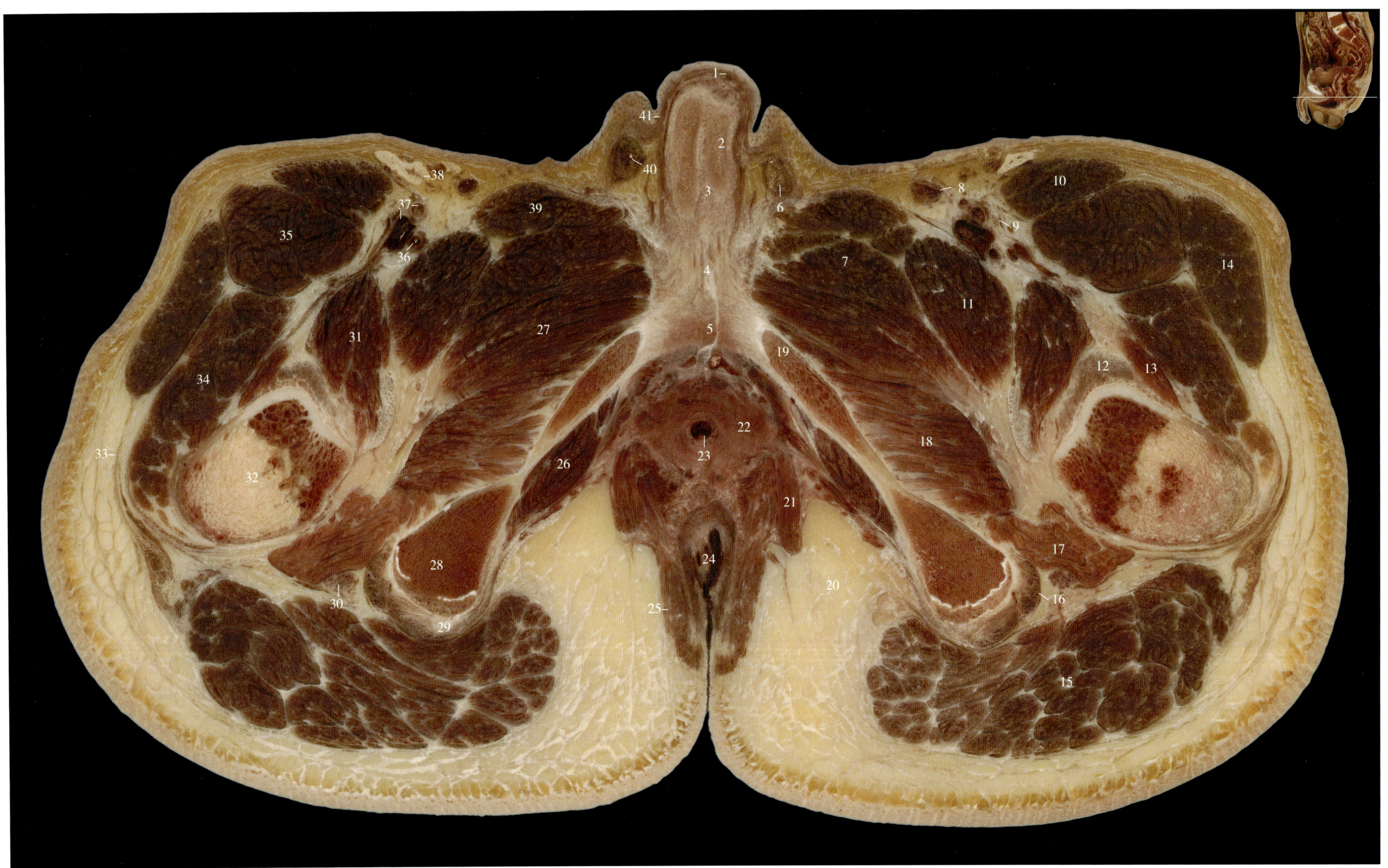

A. 断层标本图像

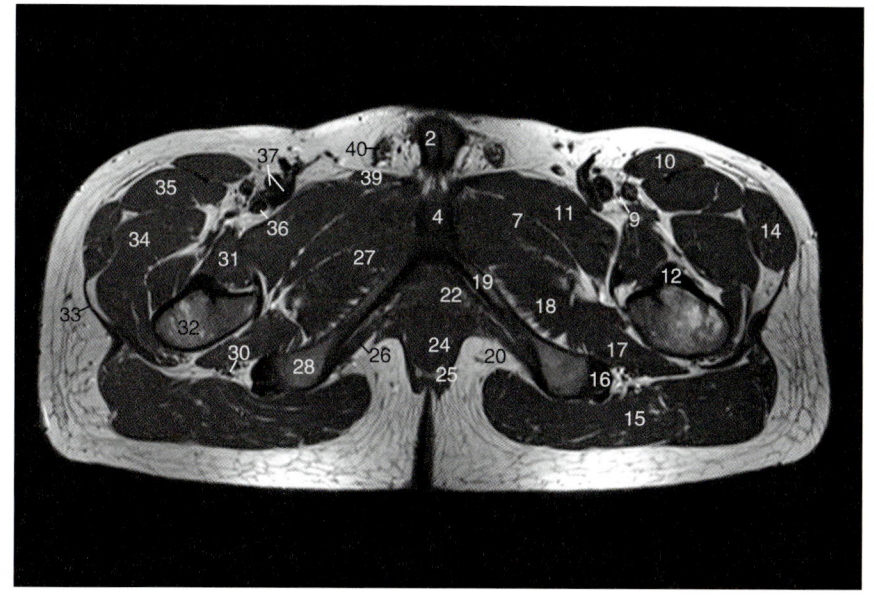
B. MR T1WI

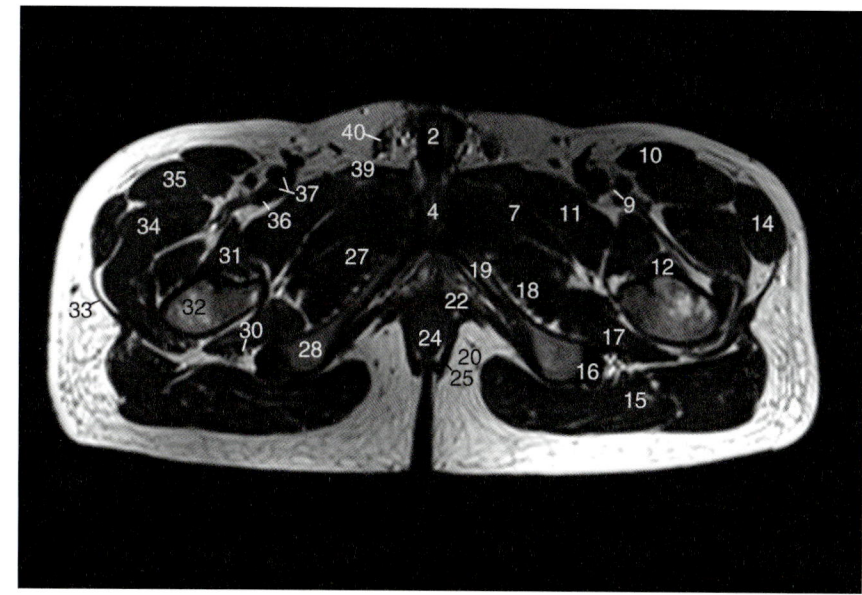
C. MR T2WI

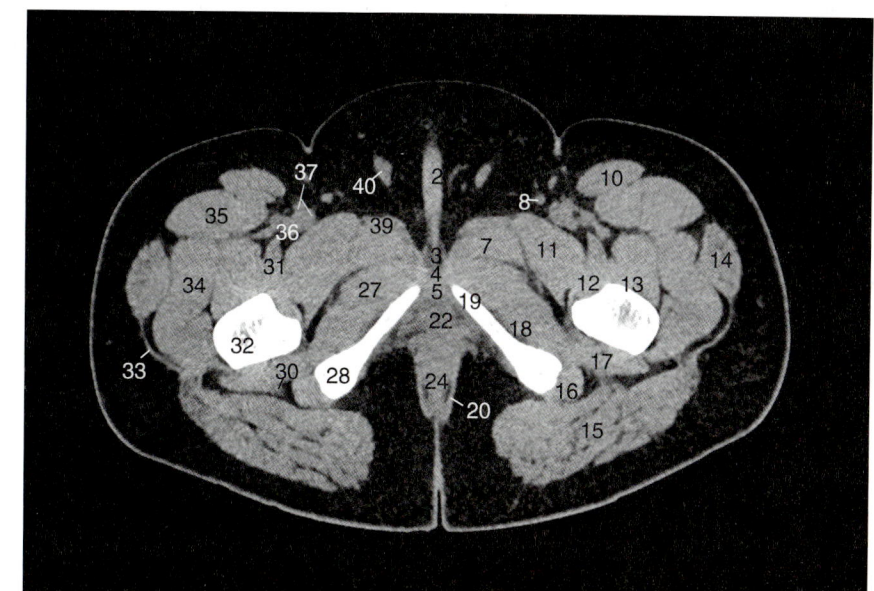
D. CT 平扫图像

1. 阴茎背浅静脉 superficial dorsal vein of penis
2. 阴茎海绵体 cavernous body of penis
3. 阴茎中隔 septum of penis
4. 耻骨弓状韧带 arcuate pubic ligament
5. 耻骨联合 pubic symphysis
6. 输精管 ductus deferens
7. 短收肌 adductor brevis
8. 大隐静脉 great saphenous vein
9. 股神经 femoral nerve
10. 缝匠肌 sartorius
11. 耻骨肌 pectineus
12. 髂股韧带 iliofemoral ligament
13. 股中间肌 vastus intermedius
14. 阔筋膜张肌 tensor fasciae latae
15. 臀大肌 gluteus maximus
16. 半膜肌肌腱 tendon of semimembranosus
17. 股方肌 quadratus femoris
18. 闭孔外肌 obturator externus
19. 耻骨下支 inferior ramus of pubis
20. 坐骨肛门窝 ischioanal fossa
21. 肛提肌 levator ani
22. 会阴深横肌 deep transverse muscles of perineum
23. 尿道膜部 membranous portion of urethra
24. 肛管 anal canal
25. 肛门外括约肌 sphincter ani externus
26. 闭孔内肌 obturator internus
27. 大收肌 adductor magnus
28. 坐骨结节 ischial tuberosity
29. 股二头肌长头和半腱肌 long head of biceps femoris and semitendinosus
30. 坐骨神经 sciatic nerve
31. 髂腰肌 iliopsoas
32. 股骨颈 neck of femur
33. 阔筋膜 fasciae lata
34. 股外侧肌 vastus lateralis
35. 股直肌 rectus femoris
36. 股深动脉 deep femoral artery
37. 股动、静脉 femoral artery and vein
38. 腹股沟浅淋巴结 superficial inguinal lymph nodes
39. 长收肌 adductor longus
40. 精索 spermatic cord
41. 肉膜 dartos coat

关键结构：精索，前列腺，肛管。

此断面经过耻骨联合下缘。自该断面至阴囊消失断面，为男性盆部与会阴部的第 3 段，主要结构包括会阴肌、男性外生殖器（阴茎、阴囊）、睾丸、附睾、精索、男性尿道、肛管、肛门外括约肌等。该断面前份正中为耻骨联合下缘，其前方为耻骨弓状韧带，弓状韧带前正中为阴茎，两侧为阴囊及阴囊内的精索。阴茎内可见阴茎背浅静脉、阴茎海绵体、尿道海绵体。盆腔内前部为会阴深横肌，其中心为尿道膜部，前列腺尖部消失；盆腔内后部为肛管，在肛管两侧前部可见肛提肌，后部有肛门外括约肌环绕。阴囊容纳睾丸、附睾和精索下部，悬于耻骨联合下方。阴囊神经有髂腹股沟神经、生殖股神经的生殖支、会阴神经的阴囊后神经和股后皮神经的会阴支[56]。前 2 支神经主要来自第 1 腰脊髓节段，支配阴囊的前 2/3；而后 2 支主要来自第 3 骶脊髓节段，支配阴囊的后 1/3。

男性盆部连续横断层 29（MH.6300）

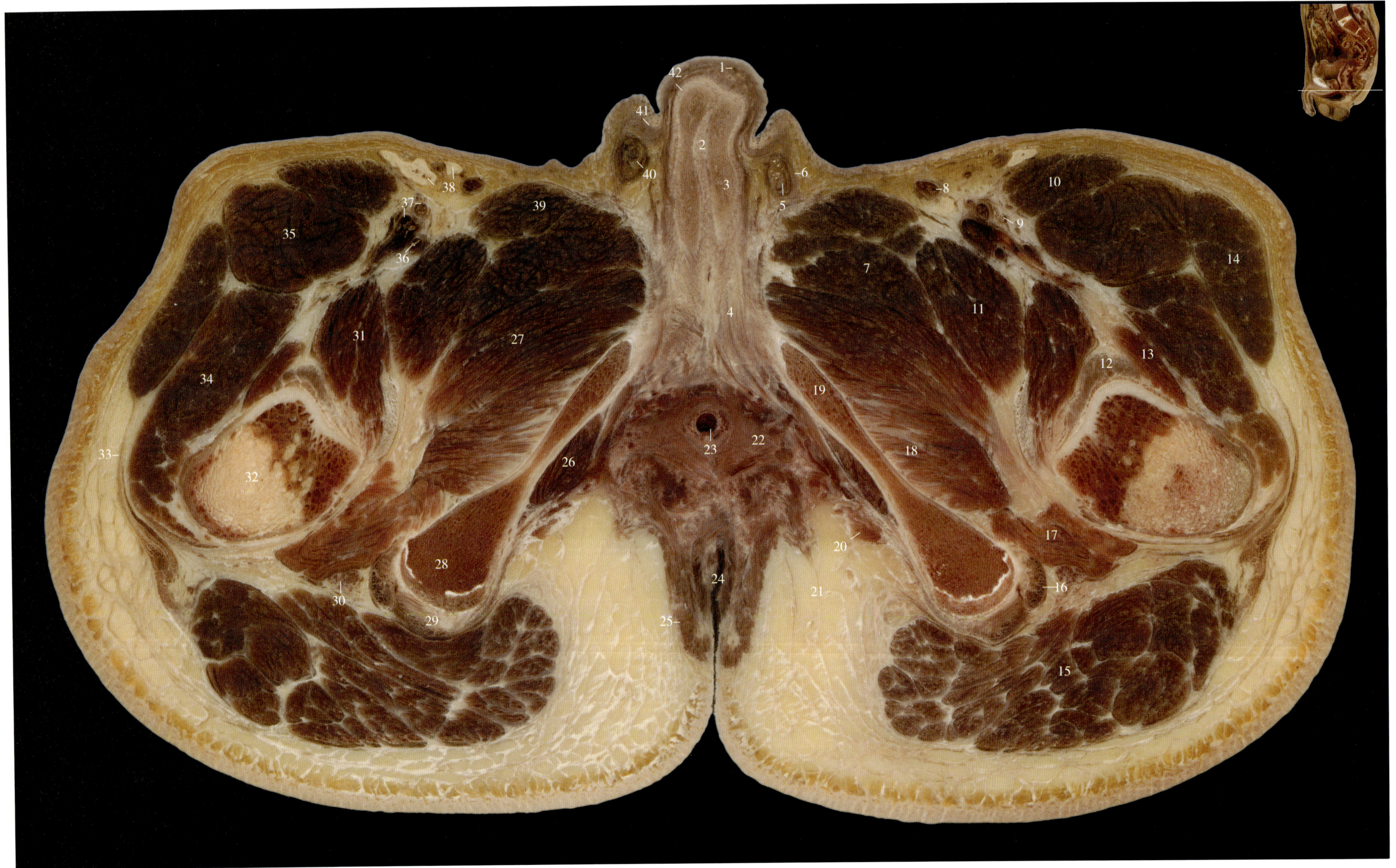

A. 断层标本图像

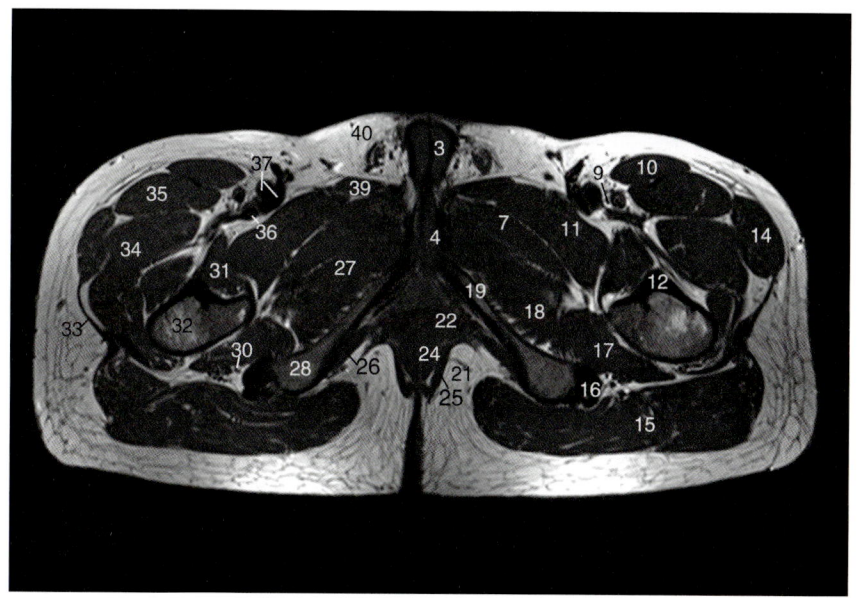
B. MR T1WI

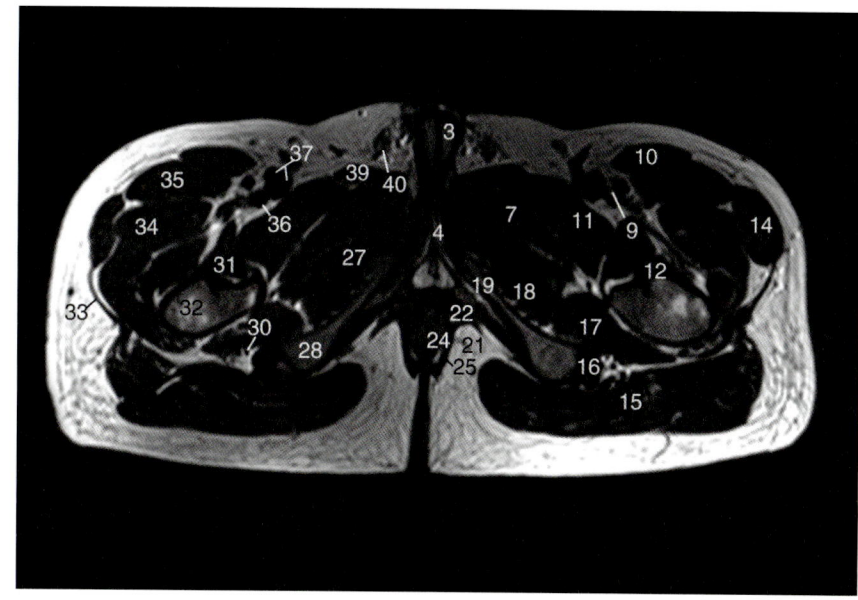
C. MR T2WI

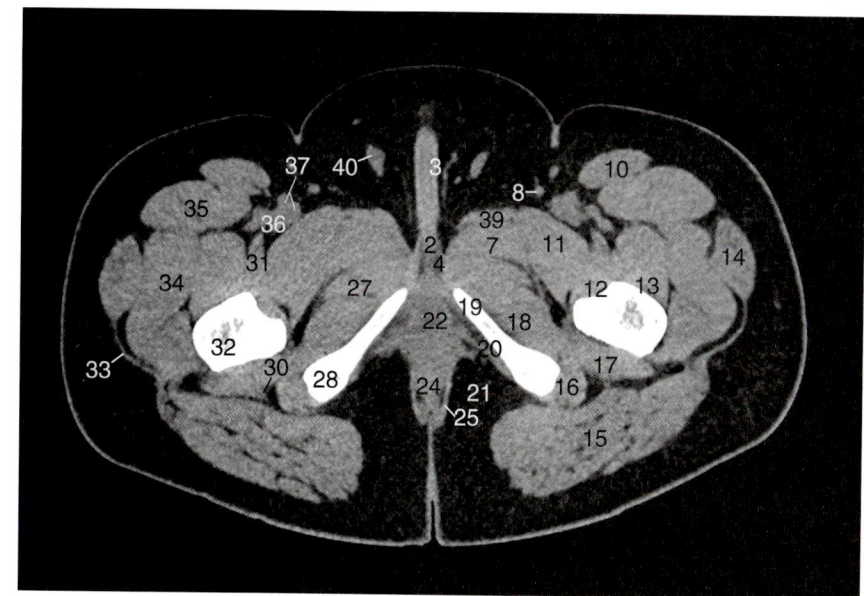
D. CT 平扫图像

1. 阴茎背浅静脉 superficial dorsal vein of penis
2. 尿道海绵体 cavernous body of urethra
3. 阴茎中隔 septum of penis
4. 阴茎脚 crus of penis
5. 输精管 ductus deferens
6. 鞘膜腔 cavity of tunica vaginaalis
7. 短收肌 adductor brevis
8. 大隐静脉 great saphenous vein
9. 股神经 femoral nerve
10. 缝匠肌 sartorius
11. 耻骨肌 pectineus
12. 髂股韧带 iliofemoral ligament
13. 股中间肌 vastus intermedius
14. 阔筋膜张肌 tensor fasciae latae
15. 臀大肌 gluteus maximus
16. 半膜肌肌腱 tendon of semimembranosus
17. 股方肌 quadratus femoris
18. 闭孔外肌 obturator externus
19. 坐骨支 ramus of ischium
20. 坐骨海绵体肌 ischiocavernosus
21. 坐骨肛门窝 ischioanal fossa
22. 会阴深横肌 deep transverse muscles of perineum
23. 尿道膜部 membranous portion of urethra
24. 肛管 anal canal
25. 肛门外括约肌 sphincter ani externus
26. 闭孔内肌 obturator internus
27. 大收肌 adductor magnus
28. 坐骨结节 ischial tuberosity
29. 股二头肌长头和半腱肌 long head of biceps femoris and semitendinosus
30. 坐骨神经 sciatic nerve
31. 髂腰肌 iliopsoas
32. 大转子 greater trochanter
33. 阔筋膜 fasciae lata
34. 股外侧肌 vastus lateralis
35. 股直肌 rectus femoris
36. 股深动脉 deep femoral artery
37. 股动、静脉 femoral artery and vein
38. 腹股沟浅淋巴结 superficial inguinal lymph nodes
39. 长收肌 adductor longus
40. 精索 spermatic cord
41. 肉膜 dartos coat
42. 阴茎海绵体白膜 albuginea of cavernous body of penis

关键结构：尿生殖膈，尿道膜部，肛门外括约肌。

此断面经过耻骨联合下缘。断面显示耻骨弓，耻骨弓由耻骨联合下缘、耻骨下支和坐骨支构成，此断面中耻骨下支与坐骨支成"八"形，其间的结构前份为尿生殖三角区，内有尿生殖膈，前列腺消失，可见会阴深横肌及尿道膜部。盆腔后份为肛门三角区，内有肛管通过，肛管周围为肛门外括约肌，可分浅、深两层。浅层肌束呈梭形，后端起自肛尾韧带，前端终于会阴中心腱；深层肌呈环形，环绕肛管下端。断面前部可见阴茎根、阴囊及其内的精索。在MRI上，与肛周呈高信号的脂肪组织相比，肛门括约肌呈等低信号，显示清晰，肛门内括约肌呈与直肠肌层直接延续的圆环形，厚约为 2.5 mm；肛门外括约肌在最低部呈两个分离的括号形，向上逐渐靠近变成圆环形，其前部厚约为 2.5 mm，侧壁厚约为 3.0 mm，后部厚约为 16.0 mm[16]。膜部为尿道穿过尿生殖膈的部分，长约为 1.5 cm；周围有属于横纹肌的尿道外括约肌环绕，该肌有控制排尿的作用。膜部位置比较固定，当骨盆骨折时，易损伤此部[56]。

男性盆部连续横断层 30（MH.6290）

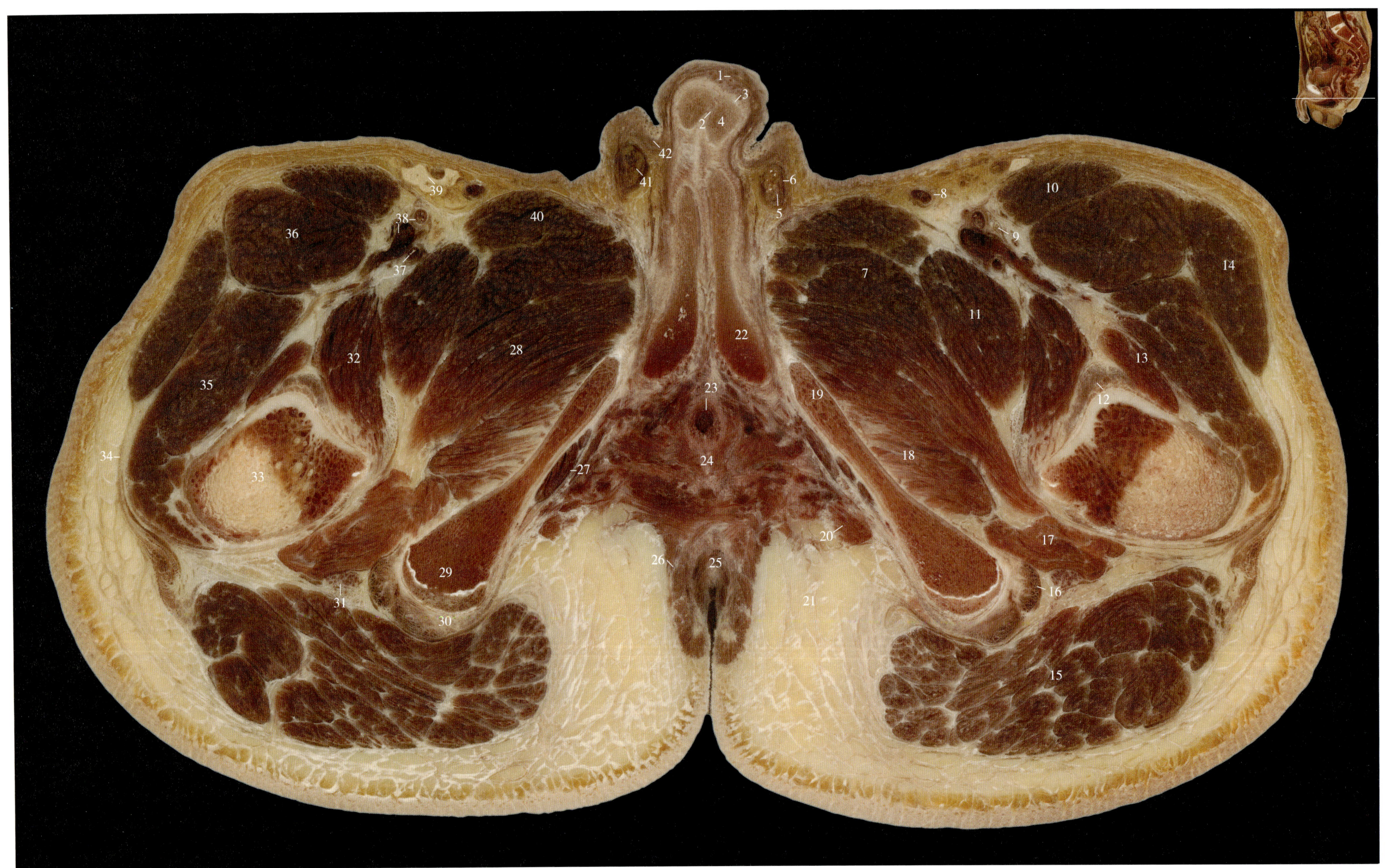

A. 断层标本图像

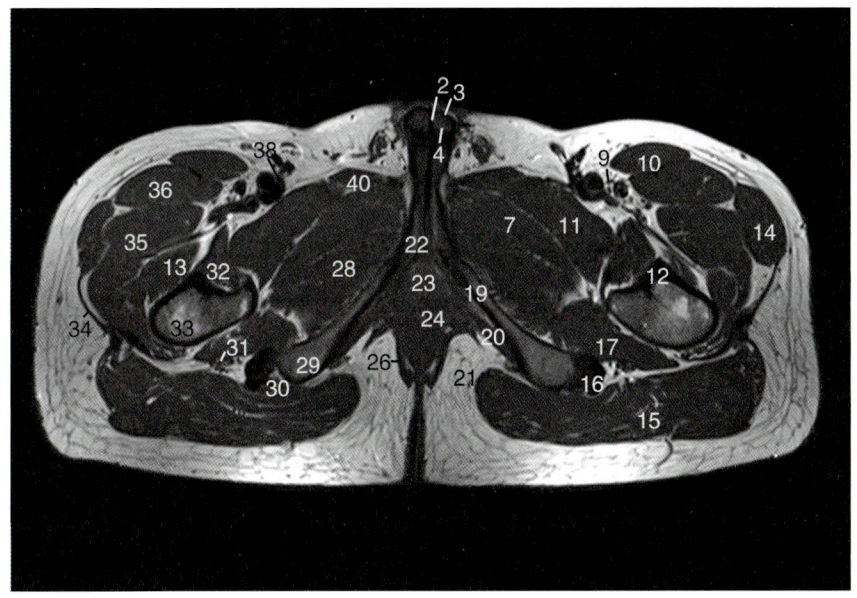
B. MR T1WI

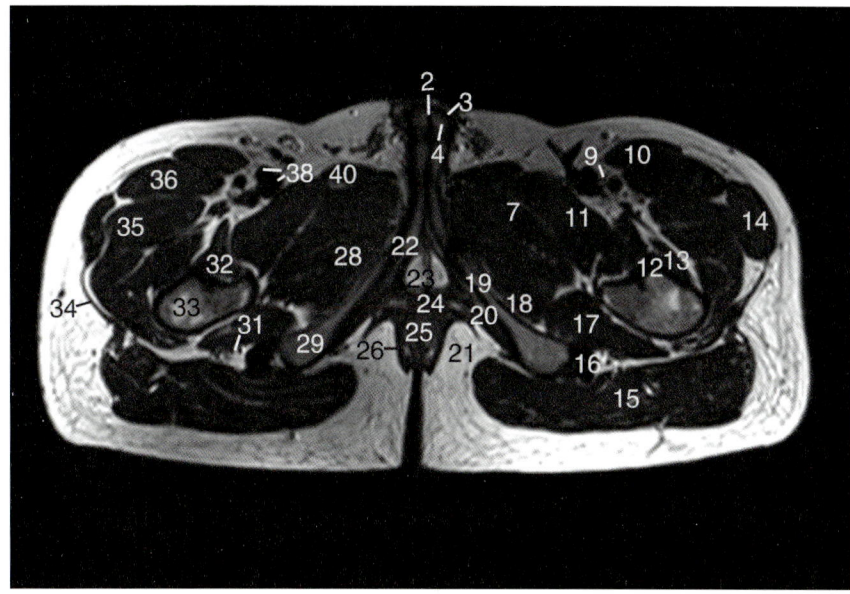
C. MR T2WI

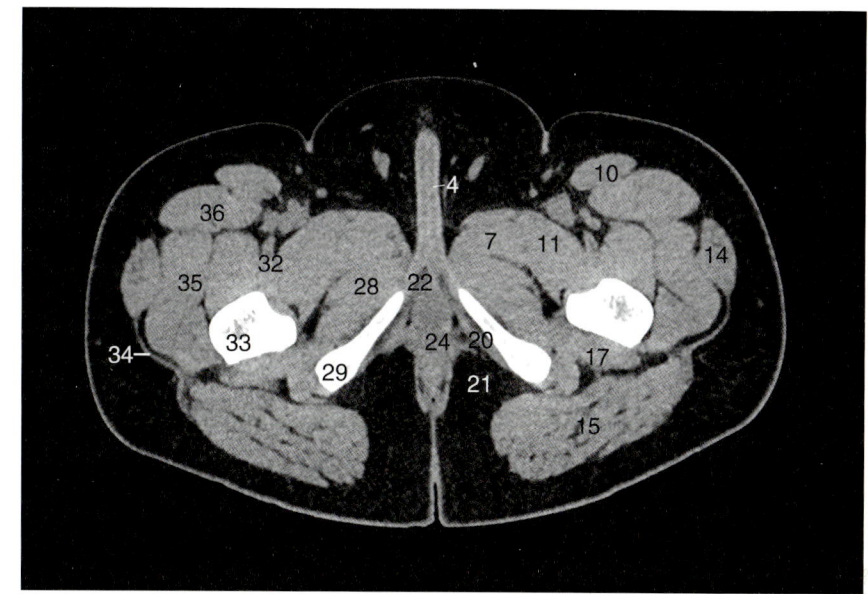
D. CT 平扫图像

1. 阴茎背深静脉 deep dorsal vein of penis
2. 阴茎中隔 septum penis
3. 阴茎海绵体白膜 albuginea of cavernous body of penis
4. 阴茎海绵体 cavernous body of penis
5. 输精管 ductus deferens
6. 鞘膜腔 cavity of tunica vaginaalis
7. 短收肌 adductor brevis
8. 大隐静脉 great saphenous vein
9. 股神经 femoral nerve
10. 缝匠肌 sartorius
11. 耻骨肌 pectineus
12. 髂股韧带 iliofemoral ligament
13. 股中间肌 vastus intermedius
14. 阔筋膜张肌 tensor fasciae latae
15. 臀大肌 gluteus maximus
16. 半膜肌肌腱 tendon of semimembranosus
17. 股方肌 quadratus femoris
18. 闭孔外肌 obturator externus
19. 坐骨支 ramus of ischium
20. 坐骨海绵体肌 ischiocavernosus
21. 坐骨肛门窝 ischioanal fossa
22. 阴茎脚 crus of penis
23. 尿道膜部 membranous portion of urethra
24. 尿生殖膈 urogenital diaphragm
25. 肛管 anal canal
26. 肛门外括约肌 sphincter ani externus
27. 闭孔内肌 obturator internus
28. 大收肌 adductor magnus
29. 坐骨结节 ischial tuberosity
30. 股二头肌长头和半腱肌 long head of biceps femoris and semitendinosus
31. 坐骨神经 sciatic nerve
32. 髂腰肌 iliopsoas
33. 大转子 greater trochanter
34. 阔筋膜 fasciae lata
35. 股外侧肌 vastus lateralis
36. 股直肌 rectus femoris
37. 股深动脉 deep femoral artery
38. 股动、静脉 femoral artery and vein
39. 腹股沟浅淋巴结 superficial inguinal lymph nodes
40. 长收肌 adductor longus
41. 附睾头 head of epididymis
42. 肉膜 dartos coat

关键结构：尿生殖膈，尿道膜部，阴茎。

此断面经过坐骨支层面。阴囊前端可见阴茎中隔分隔开两侧的阴茎海绵体，其周围有阴茎海绵体白膜围绕，两侧为精索和附睾头。耻骨下支与坐骨支呈"八"形，其内侧左侧的闭孔内肌将近消失。耻骨下支内侧可见阴茎脚，有尿道海绵体行于中线位置，阴茎脚、阴茎海绵体及尿道海绵体在MRI上均呈长T1、长T2信号。盆腔前份为尿生殖三角区，内有尿生殖膈，可见会阴横深肌及尿道膜部；会阴深横肌是一层扁肌，张于耻骨弓，后面的纤维起自坐骨支内侧面，行向内附于会阴中心腱，是会阴深隙的主要结构，收缩时可加强会阴中心腱的稳定性。会阴深隙中有阴茎背神经，与阴茎背动脉伴行，穿入会阴深间隙后，沿坐骨下支和耻骨下支前行，穿尿生殖膈下筋膜，经耻骨弓状韧带下方至阴茎背部。阴茎海绵体后端称阴茎脚，分别附于两侧的耻骨下支和坐骨支，被坐骨海绵体肌所覆盖，前端尖锐，嵌入阴茎头底面的凹陷内[41]。盆腔后份为肛门三角区，其内有肛管通过，肛管周围为肛门外括约肌，肛管两侧为坐骨肛门窝。该断面可见的大腿肌肉有：前群的缝匠肌、股四头肌，内侧群的耻骨肌、长收肌、短收肌、大收肌；后群的股二头肌、半腱肌、半膜肌；髋肌前群的髂腰肌即将止于股骨小转子。臀大肌下间隙内的坐骨神经及股三角内的股神经与股血管在标本上亦可显示。

男性盆部连续横断层 31（MH.6280）

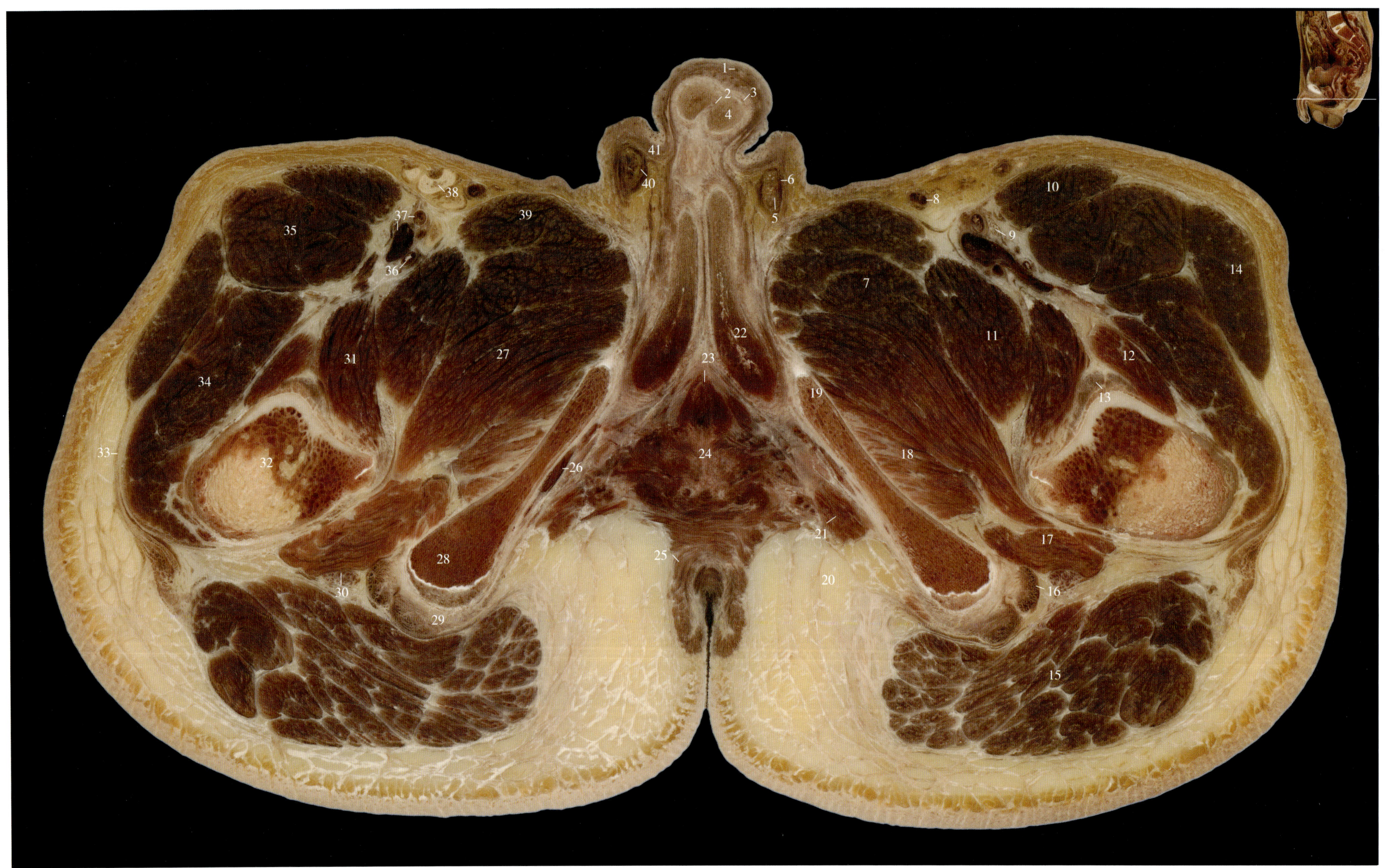

A. 断层标本图像

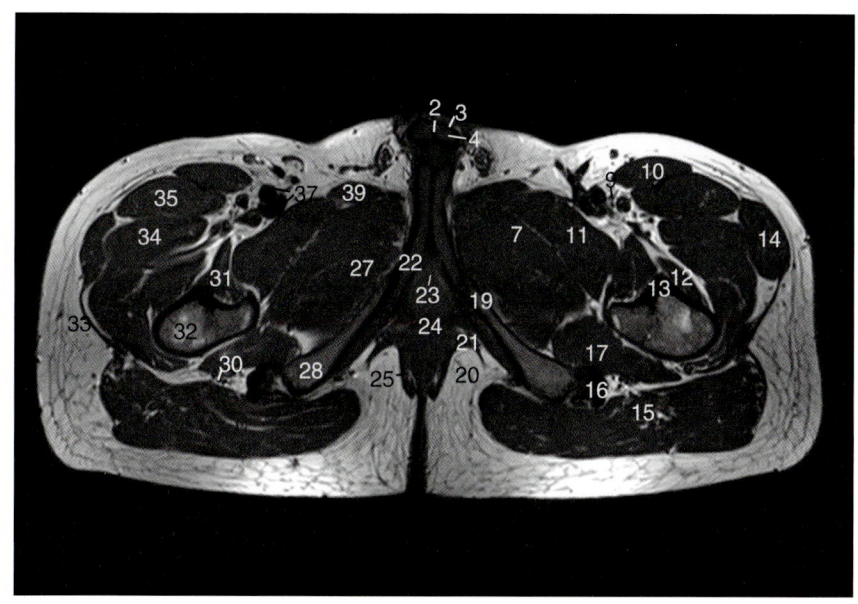

B. MR T1WI

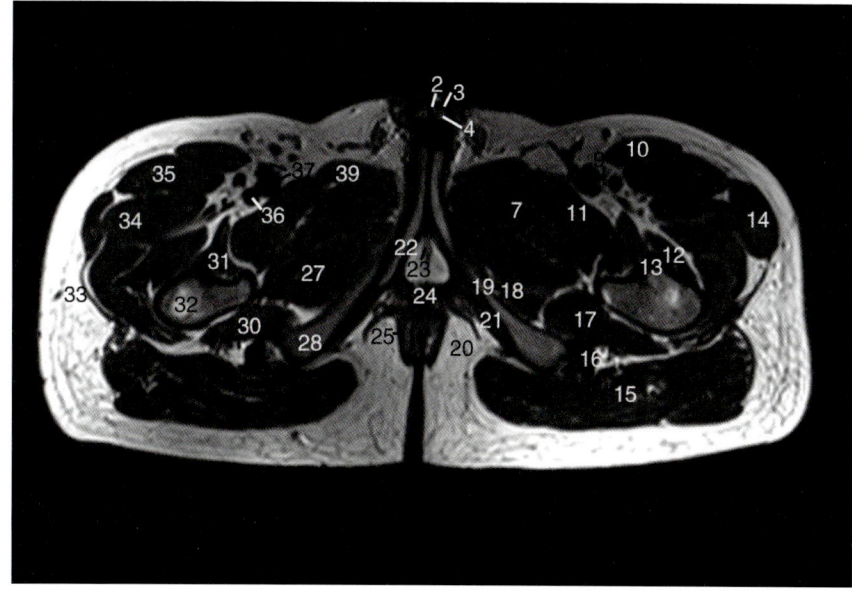

C. MR T2WI

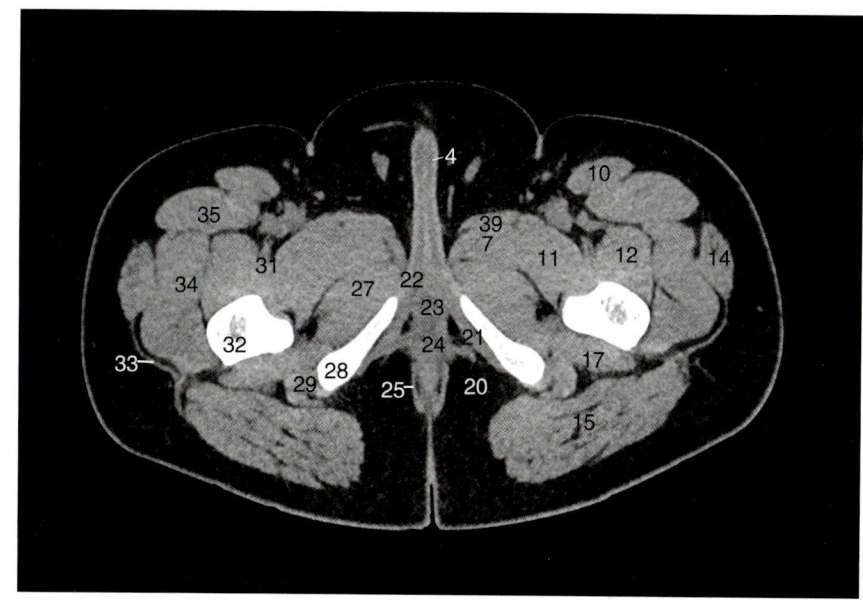

D. CT 平扫图像

1. 阴茎背深静脉 deep dorsal vein of penis
2. 阴茎中隔 septum penis
3. 阴茎海绵体白膜 albuginea of cavernous body of penis
4. 阴茎海绵体 cavernous body of penis
5. 输精管 ductus deferens
6. 鞘膜腔 cavity of tunica vaginaalis
7. 短收肌 adductor brevis
8. 大隐静脉 great saphenous vein
9. 股神经 femoral nerve
10. 缝匠肌 sartorius
11. 耻骨肌 pectineus
12. 股中间肌 vastus intermedius
13. 髂股韧带 iliofemoral ligament
14. 阔筋膜张肌 tensor fasciae latae
15. 臀大肌 gluteus maximus
16. 半膜肌肌腱 tendon of semimembranosus
17. 股方肌 quadratus femoris
18. 闭孔外肌 obturator externus
19. 坐骨支 ramus of ischium
20. 坐骨肛门窝 ischioanal fossa
21. 坐骨海绵体肌 ischiocavernosus
22. 阴茎脚 crus of penis
23. 尿道 urethra
24. 尿生殖膈 urogenital diaphragm
25. 肛门外括约肌 sphincter ani externus
26. 闭孔内肌 obturator internus
27. 大收肌 adductor magnus
28. 坐骨结节 ischial tuberosity
29. 股二头肌长头和半腱肌 long head of biceps femoris and semitendinosus
30. 坐骨神经 sciatic nerve
31. 髂腰肌 iliopsoas
32. 大转子 greater trochanter
33. 阔筋膜 fasciae lata
34. 股外侧肌 vastus lateralis
35. 股直肌 rectus femoris
36. 股深动脉 deep femoral artery
37. 股动、静脉 femoral artery and vein
38. 腹股沟浅淋巴结 superficial inguinal lymph nodes
39. 长收肌 adductor longus
40. 附睾头 head of epididymis
41. 肉膜 dartos coat

关键结构：尿生殖膈，尿道海绵体，阴茎。

此断面经过坐骨支层面。断面前部可见阴茎海绵体、尿道海绵体、阴囊及其内的精索和附睾头。双侧耻骨下支前内侧可见对称排列的阴茎海绵体的起始部阴茎脚，阴茎海绵体、尿道海绵体在T2WI上呈明显高信号；耻骨下支与坐骨支形成的耻骨弓呈"八"形，紧贴其内侧的闭孔内肌，在闭孔内肌内后侧可见坐骨海绵体肌；盆腔前份为尿生殖三角区，内有尿生殖膈，可见会阴深横肌及尿道膜部；后份为肛门三角区，其内有肛管通过，肛管周围为肛门外括约肌，肛管两侧为坐骨肛门窝。胚胎第4周时，在尿生殖窦膜的头侧间充质增生形成一个隆起，称生殖结节。在睾丸产生的雄激素作用下，生殖结节伸长形成阴茎[57]。阴茎主要由髂内动脉脏支阴部内动脉发出阴茎动脉进行血液供应。阴部神经（S2~S4）在会阴部分支阴茎背神经行于阴茎背侧，分布于阴茎的海绵体及皮肤。阴茎根固定在会阴浅隙内，阴茎体和头游离，呈圆柱状。阴茎体上面叫阴茎背，下面叫尿道面。尿道面正中有阴茎缝，与阴囊缝相接。阴茎由外到内依次为皮肤、阴茎浅筋膜、阴茎深筋膜、白膜构成[41]。白膜分别包裹3条海绵体，阴茎海绵体部略厚，尿道海绵体部较薄，左、右阴茎海绵体之间形成阴茎中隔[25]。

251

男性盆部连续横断层 32（MH.6270）

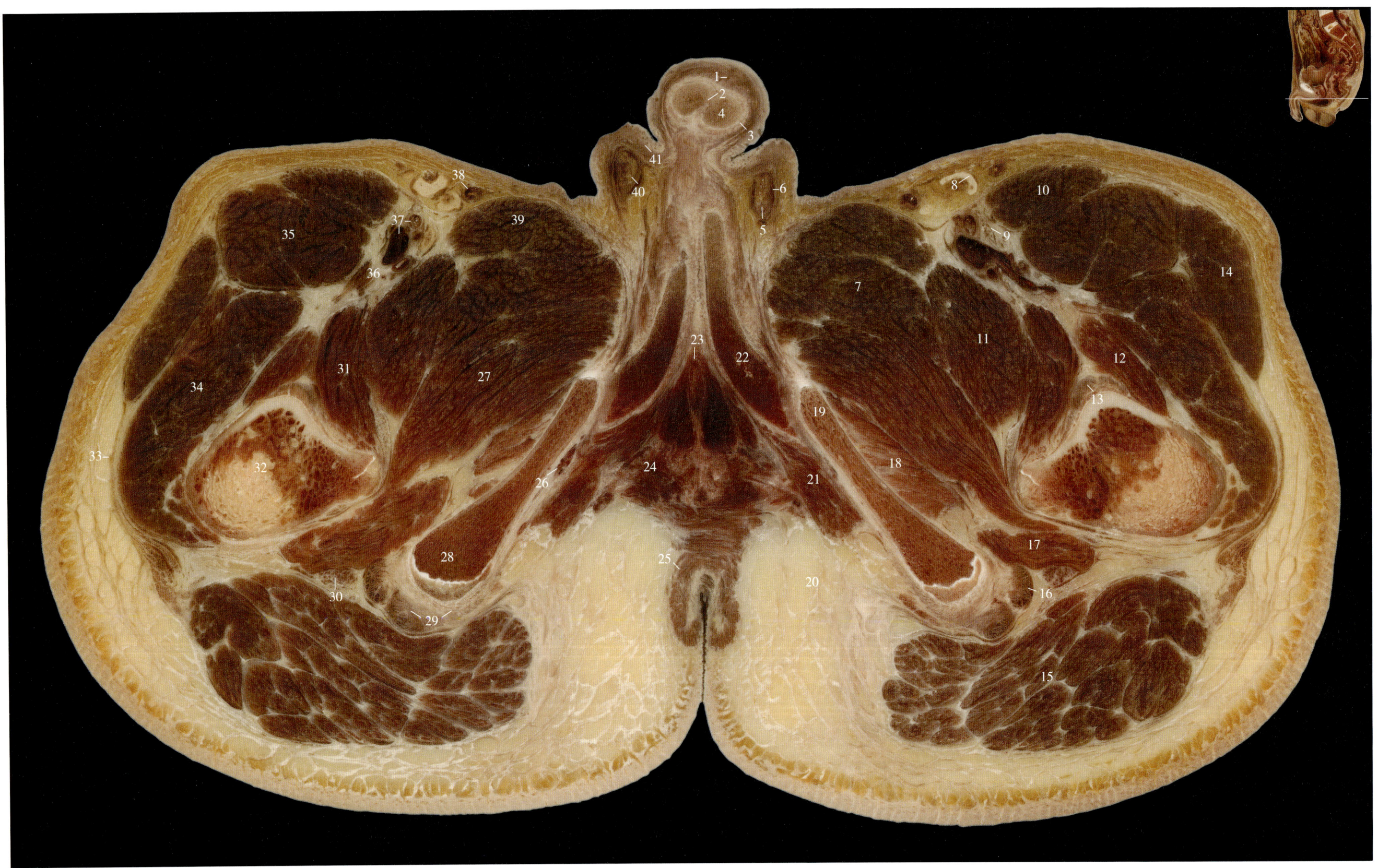

A. 断层标本图像

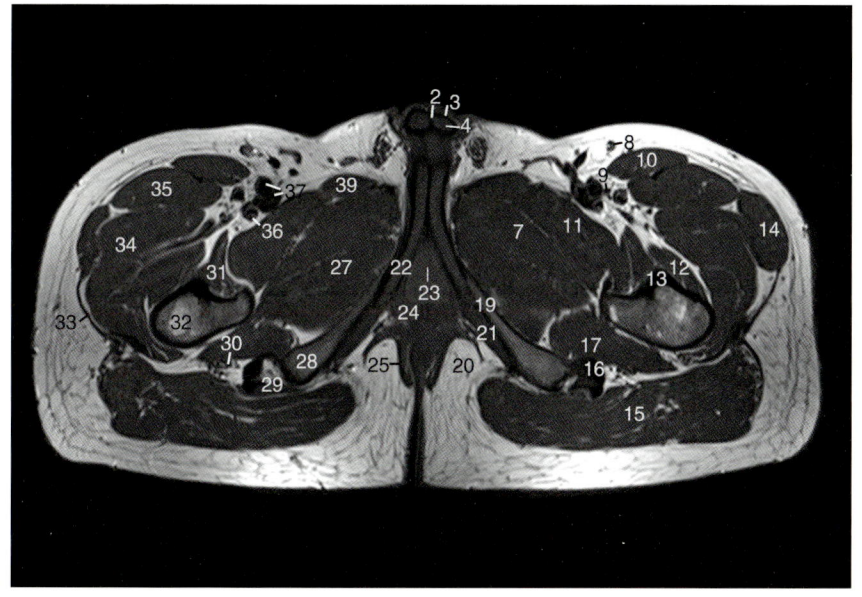

B. MR T1WI

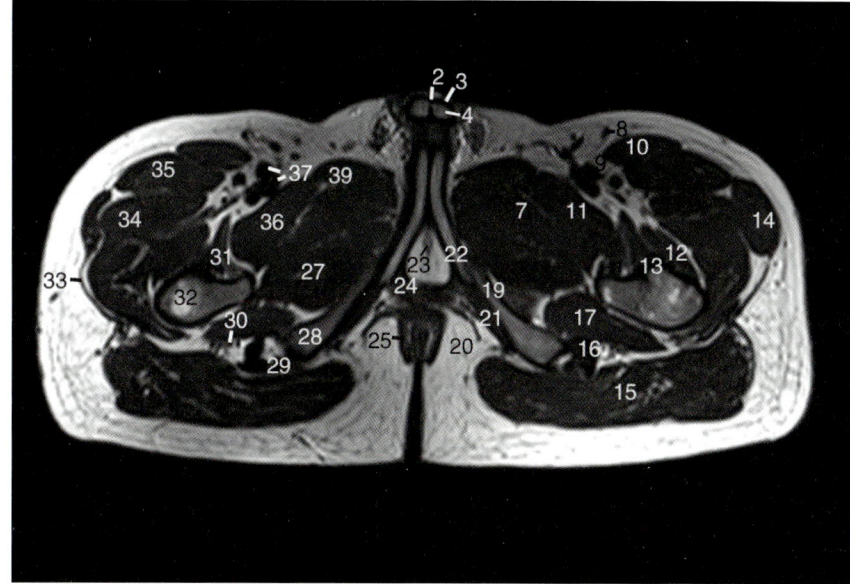

C. MR T2WI

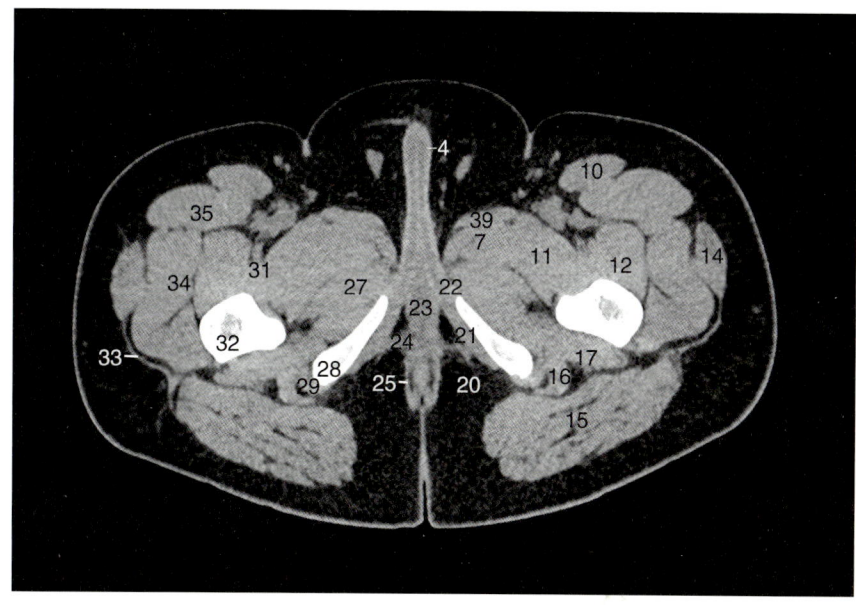

D. CT 平扫图像

1. 阴茎背深静脉 deep dorsal vein of penis
2. 阴茎中隔 septum penis
3. 阴茎海绵体白膜 albuginea of cavernous body of penis
4. 阴茎海绵体 cavernous body of penis
5. 输精管 ductus deferens
6. 鞘膜腔 cavity of tunica vaginaalis
7. 短收肌 adductor brevis
8. 腹股沟浅淋巴结 superficial inguinal lymph nodes
9. 股神经 femoral nerve
10. 缝匠肌 sartorius
11. 耻骨肌 pectineus
12. 股中间肌 vastus intermedius
13. 髂股韧带 iliofemoral ligament
14. 阔筋膜张肌 tensor fasciae latae
15. 臀大肌 gluteus maximus
16. 半膜肌肌腱 tendon of semimembranosus
17. 股方肌 quadratus femoris
18. 闭孔外肌 obturator externus
19. 坐骨支 ramus of ischium
20. 坐骨肛门窝 ischioanal fossa
21. 坐骨海绵体肌 ischiocavernosus
22. 阴茎脚 crus of penis
23. 尿道 urethra
24. 球海绵体肌 bulbocavernosus
25. 肛门外括约肌 sphincter ani externus
26. 闭孔内肌 obturator internus
27. 大收肌 adductor magnus
28. 坐骨结节 ischial tuberosity
29. 股二头肌长头和半腱肌 long head of biceps femoris and semitendinosus
30. 坐骨神经 sciatic nerve
31. 髂腰肌 iliopsoas
32. 大转子 greater trochanter
33. 阔筋膜 fasciae lata
34. 股外侧肌 vastus lateralis
35. 股直肌 rectus femoris
36. 股深动脉 deep femoral artery
37. 股动、静脉 femoral artery and vein
38. 大隐静脉 great saphenous vein
39. 长收肌 adductor longus
40. 附睾头 head of epididymis
41. 肉膜 dartos coat

关键结构：会阴浅横肌，坐骨海绵体肌，肛管。

　　此断面经过坐骨支层面。断面前部可见阴茎和阴囊，阴茎内可见阴茎海绵体，阴囊内可见附睾、鞘膜腔。尿道海绵体后端在正中线上，贴附于尿生殖膈下筋膜的下表面。尿道球的下表面有球海绵体肌覆盖。一对狭细的会阴浅横肌位于会阴浅隙的后份，起自坐骨结节的内前份，横行向内止于会阴中心腱。阴茎海绵体后端称阴茎脚，分别附于两侧的耻骨下支和坐骨支[41]。坐骨海绵体肌又名阴茎勃起肌，以肌肌腱和肌纤维起自坐骨结节内面和坐骨、耻骨支阴茎脚的附着部，肌向前内侧覆盖阴茎海绵体的游离面，以腱抵止于阴茎海绵体下面和外侧面的阴茎白膜，其中有一部分腱束抵达阴茎海绵体背面及两侧面，并相互交织。此肌收缩时可压迫阴茎海绵体而阻止静脉血回流，协助阴茎勃起[56]。断面中部两侧的骨性结构为坐骨支，其间主要内容为男性会阴浅隙结构—尿生殖三角浅层肌：会阴浅横肌、球海绵体肌和坐骨海绵体肌。位居中线的结构是尿道海绵体，其后方有球海绵体肌包绕。会阴深隙内的尿生殖三角深层肌（会阴深横肌和尿道括约肌）在此断面消失。尿生殖三角后部为肛管，肛管外有肛门外括约肌，肛管两侧为坐骨肛门窝。

男性盆部连续横断层 33（MH.6260）

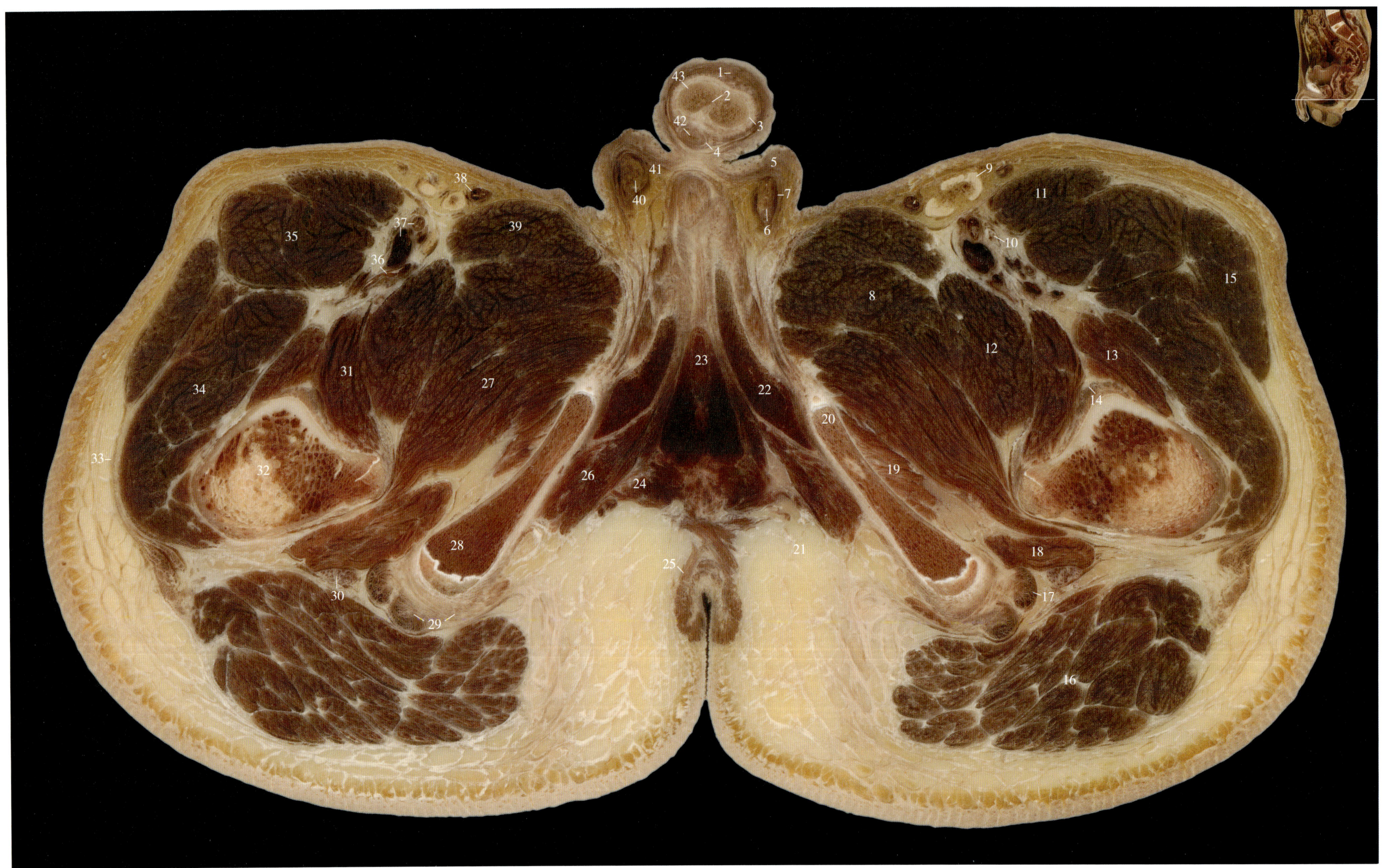

A. 断层标本图像

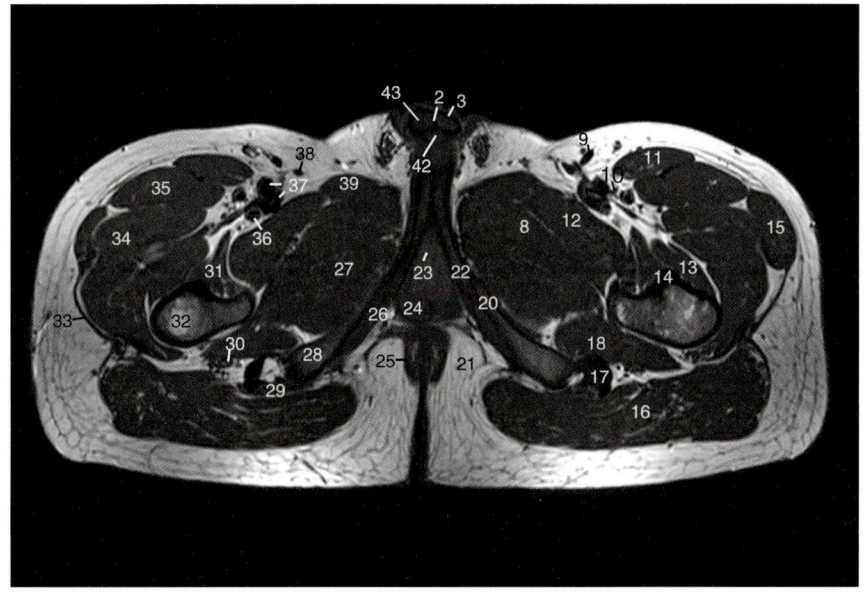
B. MR T1WI

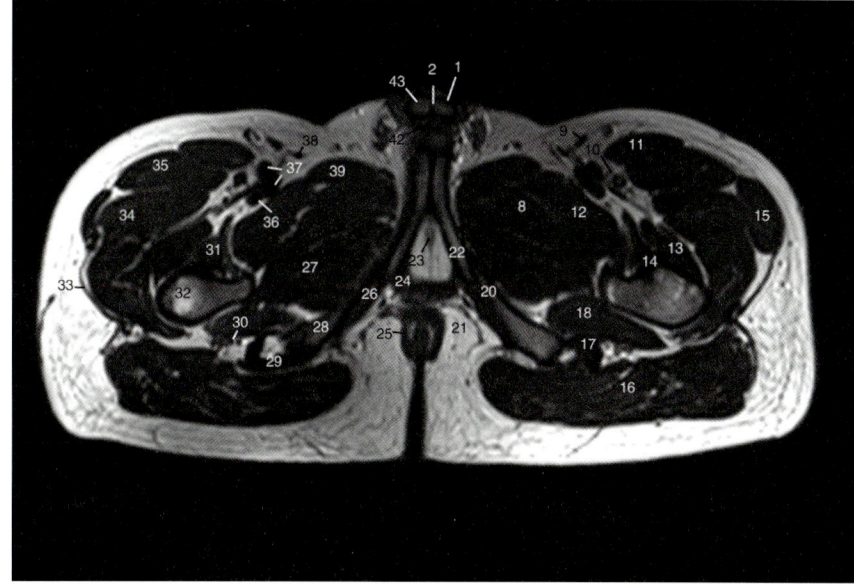
C. MR T2WI

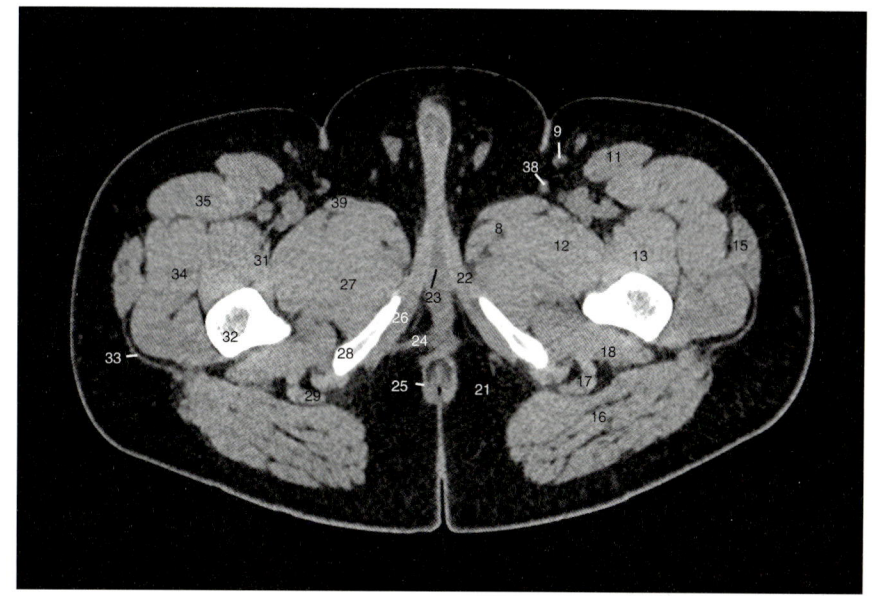
D. CT 平扫图像

1. 阴茎背深静脉 deep dorsal vein of penis
2. 阴茎中隔 septum penis
3. 阴茎海绵体白膜 albuginea of cavernous body of penis
4. 尿道海绵体白膜 albuginea of cavernous body of urethra
5. 阴囊 scrotum
6. 输精管 ductus deferens
7. 鞘膜腔 cavity of tunica vaginaalis
8. 短收肌 adductor brevis
9. 腹股沟浅淋巴结 superficial inguinal lymph nodes
10. 股神经 femoral nerve
11. 缝匠肌 sartorius
12. 耻骨肌 pectineus
13. 股中间肌 vastus intermedius
14. 髂股韧带 iliofemoral ligament
15. 阔筋膜张肌 tensor fasciae latae
16. 臀大肌 gluteus maximus
17. 半膜肌肌腱 tendon of semimembranosus
18. 股方肌 quadratus femoris
19. 闭孔外肌 obturator externus
20. 坐骨支 ramus of ischium
21. 坐骨肛门窝 ischioanal fossa
22. 阴茎脚 crus of penis
23. 尿道 urethra
24. 球海绵体肌 bulbocavernosus
25. 肛门外括约肌 sphincter ani externus
26. 坐骨海绵体肌 ischiocavernosus
27. 大收肌 adductor magnus
28. 坐骨结节 ischial tuberosity
29. 股二头肌长头和半腱肌 long head of biceps femoris and semitendinosus
30. 坐骨神经 sciatic nerve
31. 髂腰肌 iliopsoas
32. 大转子 greater trochanter
33. 阔筋膜 fasciae lata
34. 股外侧肌 vastus lateralis
35. 股直肌 rectus femoris
36. 股深动脉 deep femoral artery
37. 股动、静脉 femoral artery and vein
38. 大隐静脉 great saphenous vein
39. 长收肌 adductor longus
40. 附睾头 head of epididymis
41. 肉膜 dartos coat
42. 尿道海绵体 cavernous body of urethra
43. 阴茎海绵体 cavernous body of penis

关键结构：鞘膜腔，尿道海绵体，球海绵体肌。

此断面经过坐骨支层面。断面前部为阴茎和阴囊，于阴茎内可见阴茎海绵体、尿道海绵体，其周围分别有阴茎海绵体白膜和尿道海绵体白膜围绕；阴囊内可见附睾、鞘膜腔。断面中部两侧的骨性结构为坐骨支，其间位居中线的结构是尿道海绵体，其后方有球海绵体肌包绕。两侧阴茎脚及坐骨海绵体肌附于坐骨支内侧。断面后部为肛管，其外有肛门外括约肌，肛管两侧为坐骨肛门窝。睾丸鞘膜不包裹精索，可分脏层和壁层，脏层贴于睾丸和附睾的表面，在附睾后缘与壁层相移行，两层之间为鞘膜腔，内有少量浆液。临床上常见的有：先天性鞘膜积液，为腹膜鞘突未闭锁，积液可自鞘膜腔流入腹膜腔，腹膜腔内液体亦可流入鞘膜腔。这种交通性鞘膜积液可伴有先天性腹股沟斜疝。婴儿期鞘膜积液，为腹膜鞘突仅在腹股沟管腹环处闭锁，其余部分仍未闭锁成腔。精索鞘膜积液，系腹膜鞘突的精索部部分闭锁，另一部分未闭锁形成的；一般的睾丸鞘膜积液，是腹膜鞘突正常团锁，而由于外伤等原因引起的鞘膜积液，此种类型最常见[56]。

男性盆部连续横断层 34（MH.6250）

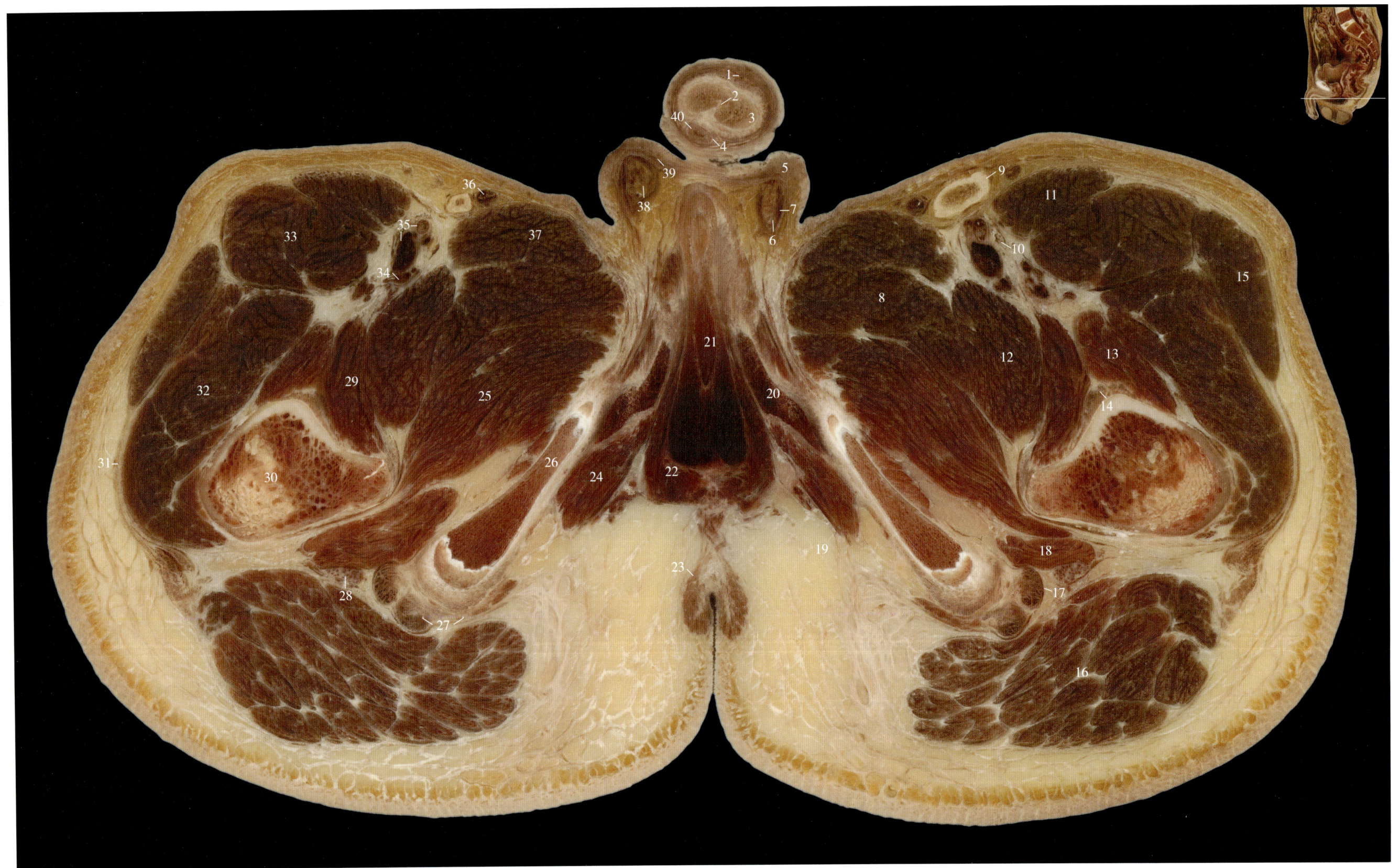

A. 断层标本图像

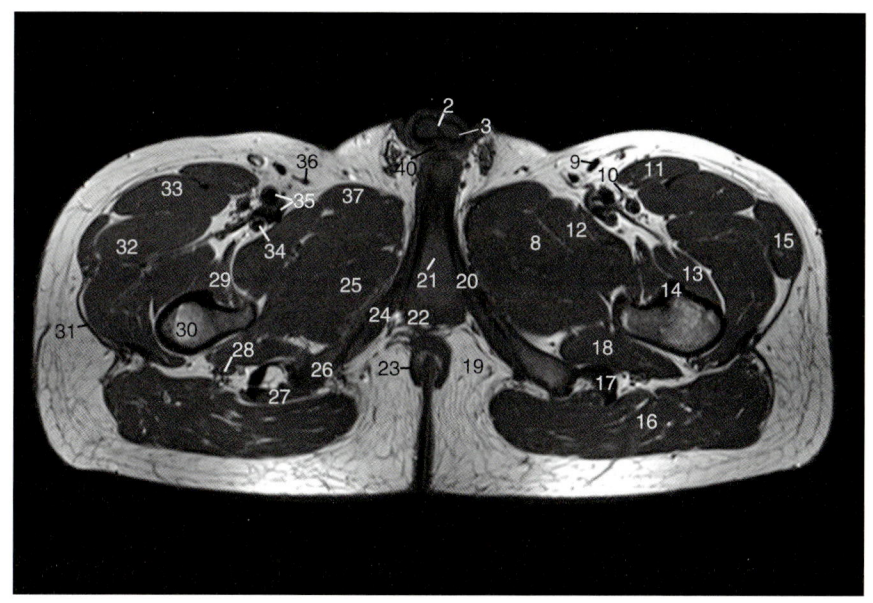
B. MR T1WI

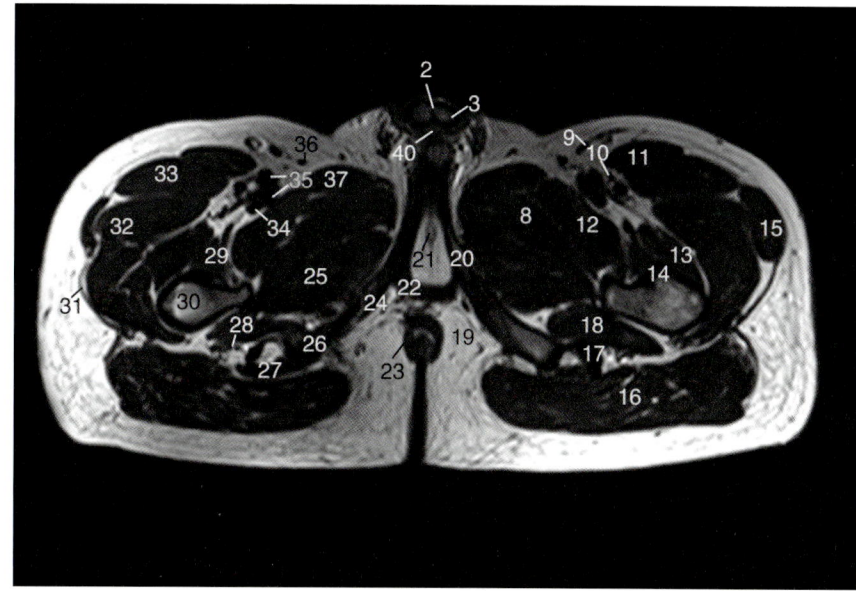
C. MR T2WI

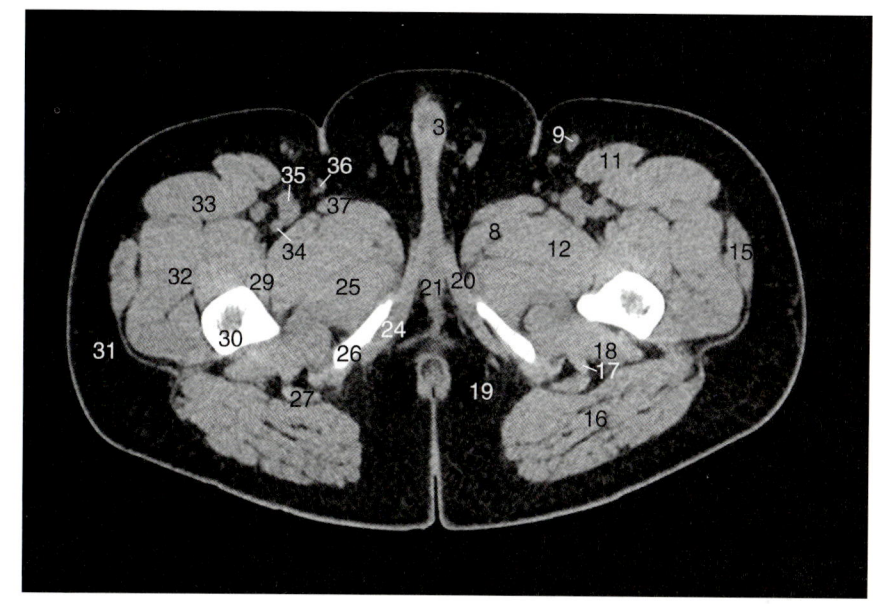
D. CT 平扫图像

1. 阴茎背深静脉 deep dorsal vein of penis
2. 阴茎中隔 septum penis
3. 阴茎海绵体 cavernous body of penis
4. 尿道海绵体白膜 albuginea of cavernous body of urethra
5. 阴囊 scrotum
6. 输精管 ductus deferens
7. 鞘膜腔 cavity of tunica vaginaalis
8. 短收肌 adductor brevis
9. 腹股沟浅淋巴结 superficial inguinal lymph nodes
10. 股神经 femoral nerve
11. 缝匠肌 sartorius
12. 耻骨肌 pectineus
13. 股中间肌 vastus intermedius
14. 髂股韧带 iliofemoral ligament
15. 阔筋膜张肌 tensor fasciae latae
16. 臀大肌 gluteus maximus
17. 半膜肌肌腱 tendon of semimembranosus
18. 股方肌 quadratus femoris
19. 坐骨肛门窝 ischioanal fossa
20. 阴茎脚 crus of penis
21. 尿道 urethra
22. 球海绵体肌 bulbocavernosus
23. 肛门外括约肌 sphincter ani externus
24. 坐骨海绵体肌 ischiocavernosus
25. 大收肌 adductor magnus
26. 坐骨支 ramus of ischium
27. 股二头肌长头和半腱肌 long head of biceps femoris and semitendinosus
28. 坐骨神经 sciatic nerve
29. 髂腰肌 iliopsoas
30. 大转子 greater trochanter
31. 阔筋膜 fasciae lata
32. 股外侧肌 vastus lateralis
33. 股直肌 rectus femoris
34. 股深动脉 deep femoral artery
35. 股动、静脉 femoral artery and vein
36. 大隐静脉 great saphenous vein
37. 长收肌 adductor longus
38. 附睾头 head of epididymis
39. 肉膜 dartos coat
40. 尿道海绵体 cavernous body of urethra

关键结构：附睾，球海绵体肌，会阴神经。

此断面为经过阴囊上份层面。断面前部为阴囊和近将分离的阴茎，于阴囊内可见附睾及其周围的鞘膜腔，阴茎海绵体、尿道海绵体的周围有白膜围绕。附睾呈新月形，紧贴睾丸的上端及后缘，主要由附睾管盘曲而成。附睾的主要功能是暂时储藏精子，并促使精子进一步成熟[41]。成人附睾的各径：头尾长度左侧为 4.50 cm ± 0.53 cm；右侧为 4.53 cm ± 0.53 cm。附睾头襞处宽度左侧为 0.86 cm ± 0.14 cm；右侧 0.85 cm ± 0.13 cm。附睾下襞处宽度左侧为 0.69 cm ± 0.12 cm；右侧为 0.70 cm ± 0.13 cm[16]。断面中部两侧的骨性结构为坐骨支，其间居中的结构是尿道海绵体，其后方膨大部分构成的尿道球，尿道海绵体后方及两侧被"U"形的球海绵体肌包绕。球海绵体肌两侧、坐骨支内侧分别见阴茎脚及坐骨海绵体肌。球海绵体肌为成对肌，由对称性的左、右两部肌包围尿道球，两侧肌借尿道球中隔相连接。球海绵体肌分为浅、中、深3层。浅层的肌纤维起自尿道球中隔，肌纤维行向前外侧；中层起自会阴中心腱，肌纤维近似矢状位向前；深层呈环形，环绕尿道球后部。3层肌纤维均抵止于阴茎海绵体侧面和背侧面的阴茎筋膜[1]。此肌收缩时可压迫尿道海绵体、尿道球、阴茎海绵体及阴茎背深静脉，以协助阴茎勃起，并可缩窄和缩短尿道，帮助排尿和射精。会阴神经伴行会阴动脉进入浅隙，发出阴囊后神经与动脉伴行，支配会阴浅横肌、球海绵体肌和坐骨海绵体肌。断面后部为肛门，其外有肛门外括约肌，两侧为坐骨肛门窝。

男性盆部连续横断层 35（MH.6240）

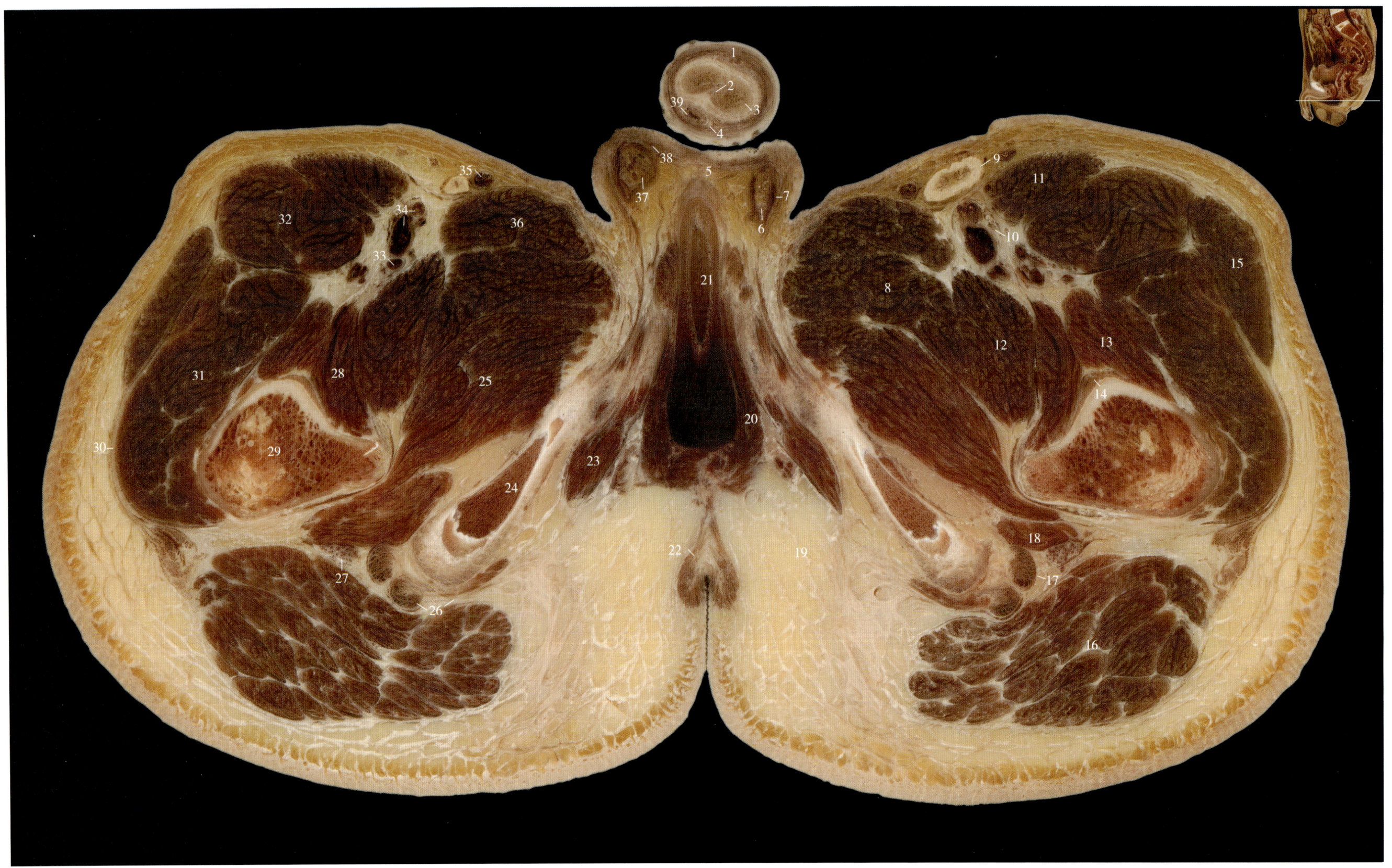

A. 断层标本图像

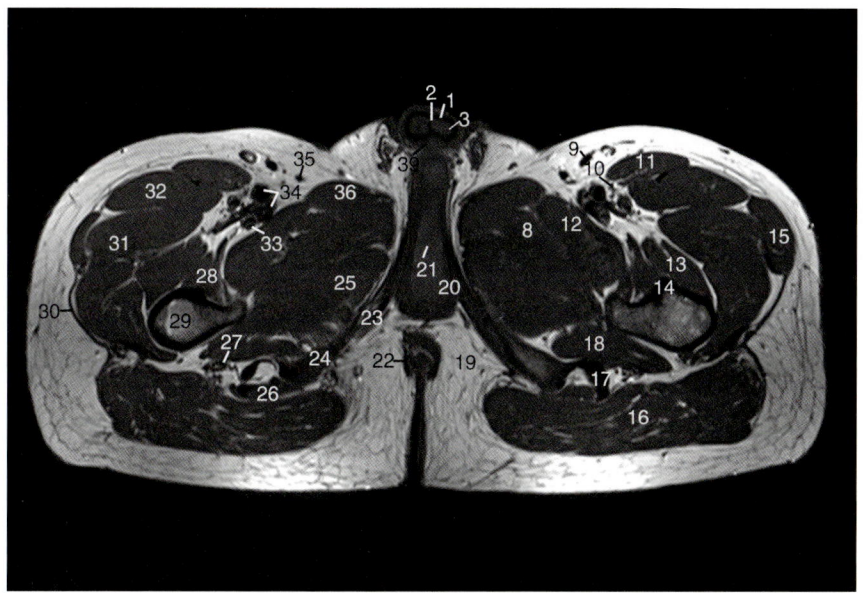

B. MR T1WI

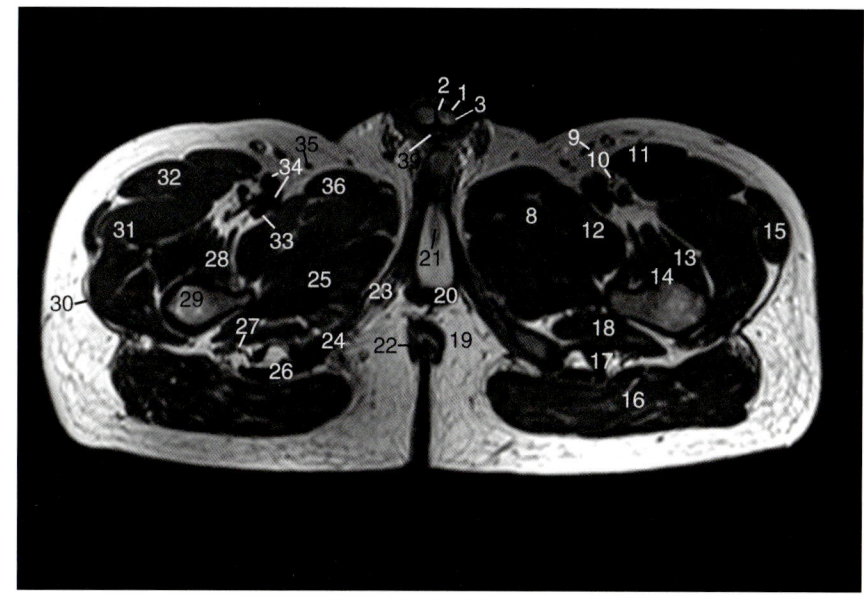

C. MR T2WI

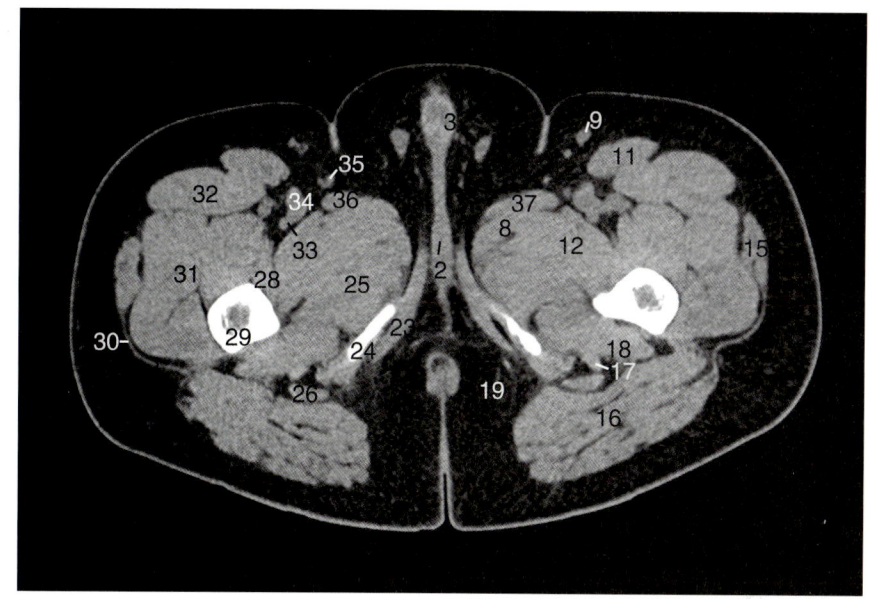

D. CT 平扫图像

关键结构：阴茎海绵体，尿道海绵体，腹股沟淋巴结，白膜。

此断面为经过阴囊上份层面。断面前部可见分离的阴茎头，其内可见阴茎海绵体白膜、尿道海绵体白膜分别包绕阴茎海绵体和尿道海绵体。阴囊内结构为附睾及鞘膜腔。断面中部居中线位置为尿道海绵体，其后方有呈"U"形的球海绵体肌包绕；两侧的骨性结构为坐骨支，其内侧为坐骨海绵体肌，二者间出现充填脂肪组织的一间隙，与断面后部的坐骨肛门窝内脂肪组织相延续。断面后部见肛门外括约肌围绕。在该断面股三角前方皮下见淋巴结影，股三角区淋巴结一般分为4群：①骶淋巴结，沿骶正中动脉排列，收纳盆后壁、直肠的部分淋巴；②髂内淋巴结，沿髂内动脉及其分支排列，收纳盆腔脏器、会阴和臀区的淋巴；③髂外淋巴结，沿髂外动脉排列，收纳腹股沟浅、深淋巴结的输出淋巴管及部分盆腔脏器和腹前壁的淋巴；④髂总淋巴结，沿髂总动脉排列，主要收纳上述3群淋巴结的输出淋巴管，然后注入腰淋巴结[55]。

1. 阴茎 penis
2. 阴茎中隔 septum penis
3. 阴茎海绵体 cavernous body of penis
4. 尿道海绵体白膜 albuginea of cavernous body of urethra
5. 阴囊 scrotum
6. 输精管 ductus deferens
7. 鞘膜腔 cavity of tunica vaginaalis
8. 短收肌 adductor brevis
9. 腹股沟浅淋巴结 superficial inguinal lymph nodes
10. 股神经 femoral nerve
11. 缝匠肌 sartorius
12. 耻骨肌 pectineus
13. 股中间肌 vastus intermedius
14. 髂股韧带 iliofemoral ligament
15. 阔筋膜张肌 tensor fasciae latae
16. 臀大肌 gluteus maximus
17. 半膜肌肌腱 tendon of semimembranosus
18. 股方肌 quadratus femoris
19. 坐骨肛门窝 ischioanal fossa
20. 球海绵体肌 bulbocavernosus
21. 尿道 urethra
22. 肛门外括约肌 sphincter ani externus
23. 坐骨海绵体肌 ischiocavernosus
24. 坐骨支 ramus of ischium
25. 大收肌 adductor magnus
26. 股二头肌长头和半腱肌 long head of biceps femoris and semitendinosus
27. 坐骨神经 sciatic nerve
28. 髂腰肌 iliopsoas
29. 大转子 greater trochanter
30. 阔筋膜 fasciae lata
31. 股外侧肌 vastus lateralis
32. 股直肌 rectus femoris
33. 股深动脉 deep femoral artery
34. 股动、静脉 femoral artery and vein
35. 大隐静脉 great saphenous vein
36. 长收肌 adductor longus
37. 附睾头 head of epididymis
38. 肉膜 dartos coat
39. 尿道海绵体 cavernous body of urethra

男性盆部连续横断层 36（MH.6230）

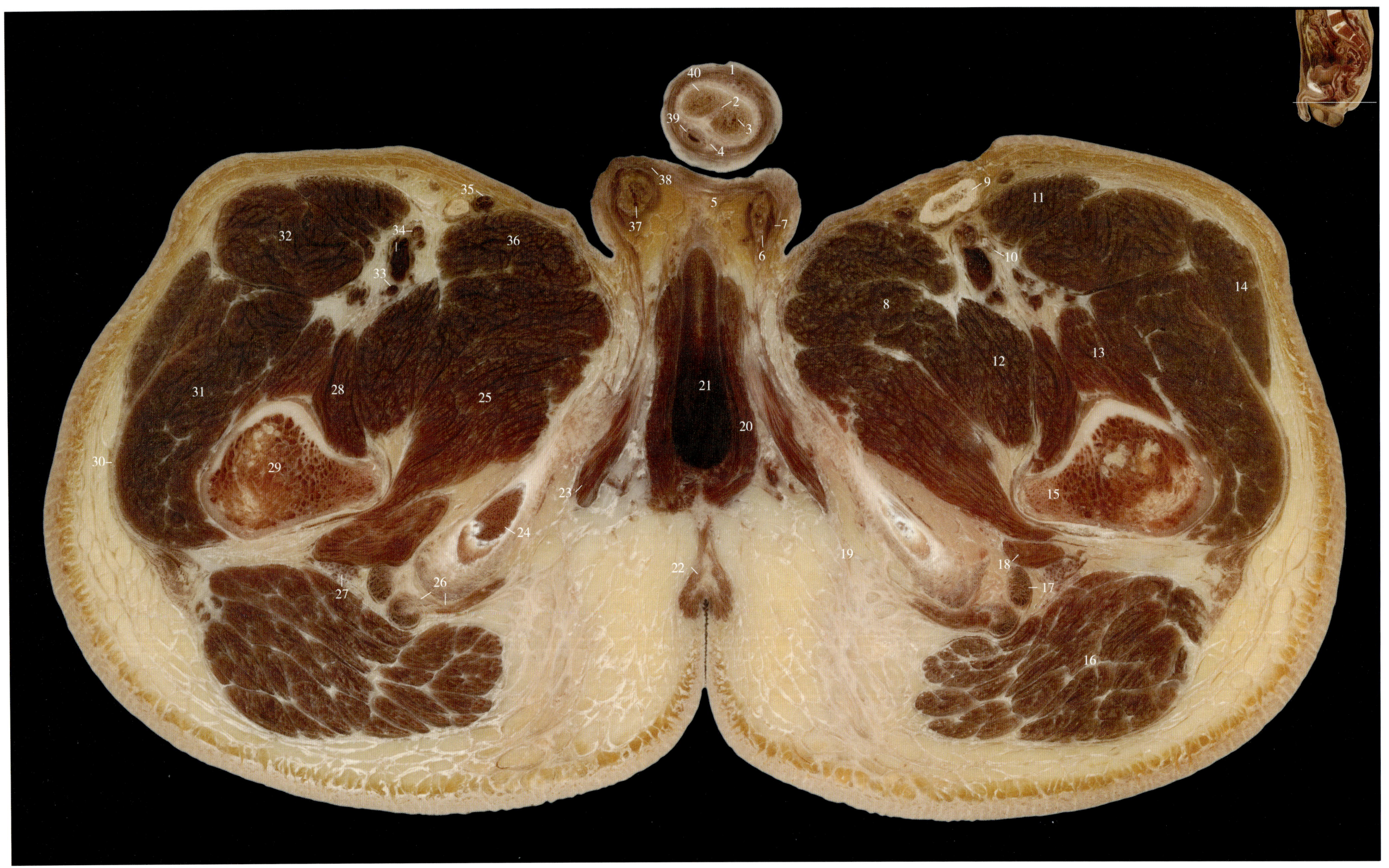

A. 断层标本图像

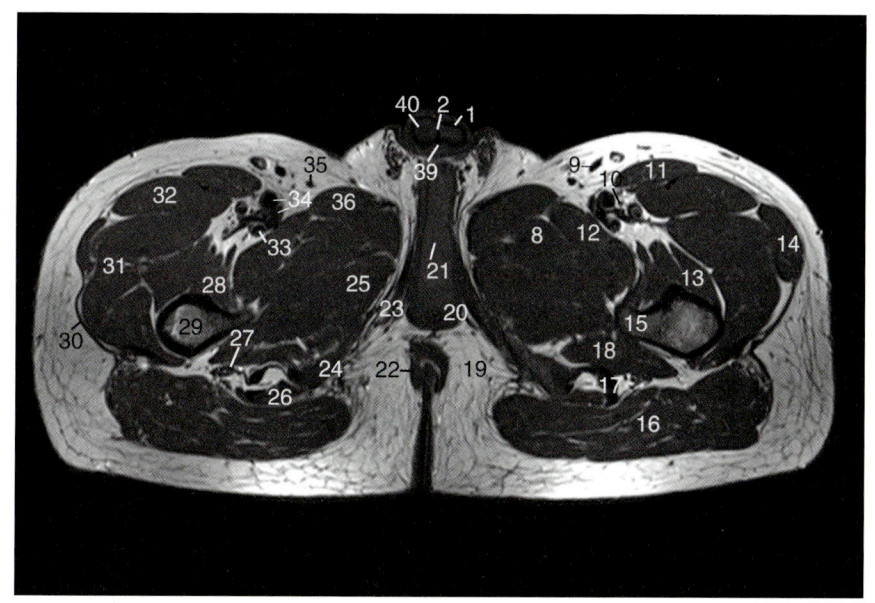
B. MR T1WI

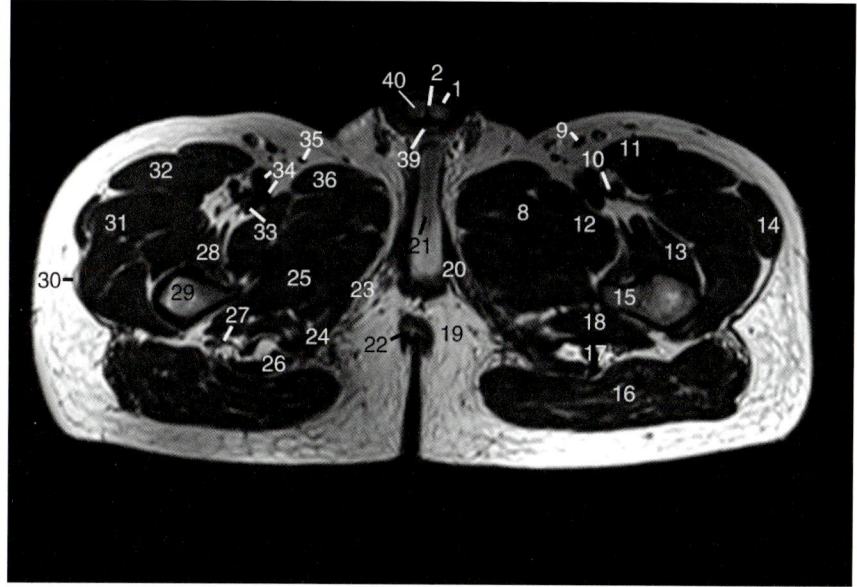
C. MR T2WI

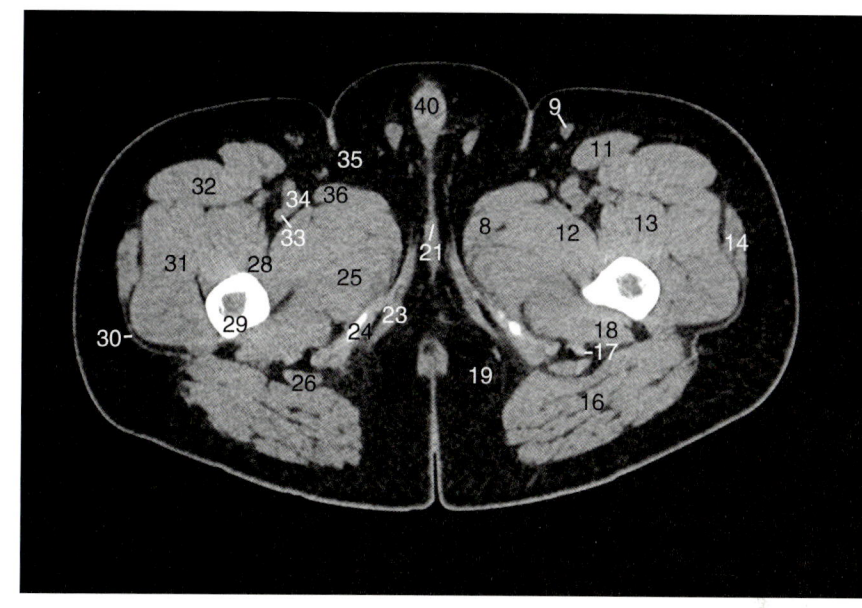
D. CT 平扫图像

关键结构：球海绵体肌，坐骨海绵体肌，腹股沟浅淋巴结。

  此断面为经过阴囊上份层面。断面左侧的坐骨支几近消失，其内侧为坐骨海绵体肌，尿道海绵体居中线位置，其外有呈"U"形的球海绵体肌包绕，与坐骨海绵体肌间存在一间隙，内有疏松结缔组织和静脉丛。断面前部可见分离的阴茎头，内为阴茎海绵体和尿道海绵体及周围的阴茎海绵体白膜和尿道海绵体白膜，阴囊内结构为附睾及鞘膜腔。断面后部为肛门，其外有肛门括约肌，两侧为坐骨肛门窝。该断面在腹股沟区可见腹股沟浅淋巴结。腹股沟浅淋巴结分上、下两群，上群6~7个，位于腹股沟下方与其平行，收集脐以下腹壁浅层、臀外生殖器、会阴及肛管下端的浅淋巴结管；下群4~5个，沿大隐静脉末段纵行排列，收集下肢浅淋巴管。腹股沟浅淋巴结的输出管注入沿股静脉排列的腹股沟深淋巴结或经股管注入髂外淋巴结[58]。

1. 阴茎 penis
2. 阴茎中隔 septum penis
3. 阴茎深动脉 deep artery of penis
4. 尿道海绵体白膜 albuginea of cavernous body of urethra
5. 阴囊 scrotum
6. 输精管 ductus deferens
7. 鞘膜腔 cavity of tunica vaginaalis
8. 短收肌 adductor brevis
9. 腹股沟浅淋巴结 superficial inguinal lymph nodes
10. 股神经 femoral nerve
11. 缝匠肌 sartorius
12. 耻骨肌 pectineus
13. 股中间肌 vastus intermedius
14. 阔筋膜张肌 tensor fasciae latae
15. 小转子 lesser trochanter
16. 臀大肌 gluteus maximus
17. 半膜肌肌腱 tendon of semimembranosus
18. 股方肌 quadratus femoris
19. 坐骨肛门窝 ischioanal fossa
20. 球海绵体肌 bulbocavernosus
21. 尿道 urethra
22. 肛门外括约肌 sphincter ani externus
23. 坐骨海绵体肌 ischiocavernosus
24. 坐骨支 ramus of ischium
25. 大收肌 adductor magnus
26. 股二头肌长头和半腱肌 long head of biceps femoris and semitendinosus
27. 坐骨神经 sciatic nerve
28. 髂腰肌 iliopsoas
29. 大转子 greater trochanter
30. 阔筋膜 fasciae lata
31. 股外侧肌 vastus lateralis
32. 股直肌 rectus femoris
33. 股深动脉 deep femoral artery
34. 股动、静脉 femoral artery and vein
35. 大隐静脉 great saphenous vein
36. 长收肌 adductor longus
37. 附睾头 head of epididymis
38. 肉膜 dartos coat
39. 尿道海绵体 cavernous body of urethra
40. 阴茎海绵体 cavernous body of penis

男性盆部连续横断层 37（MH.6220）

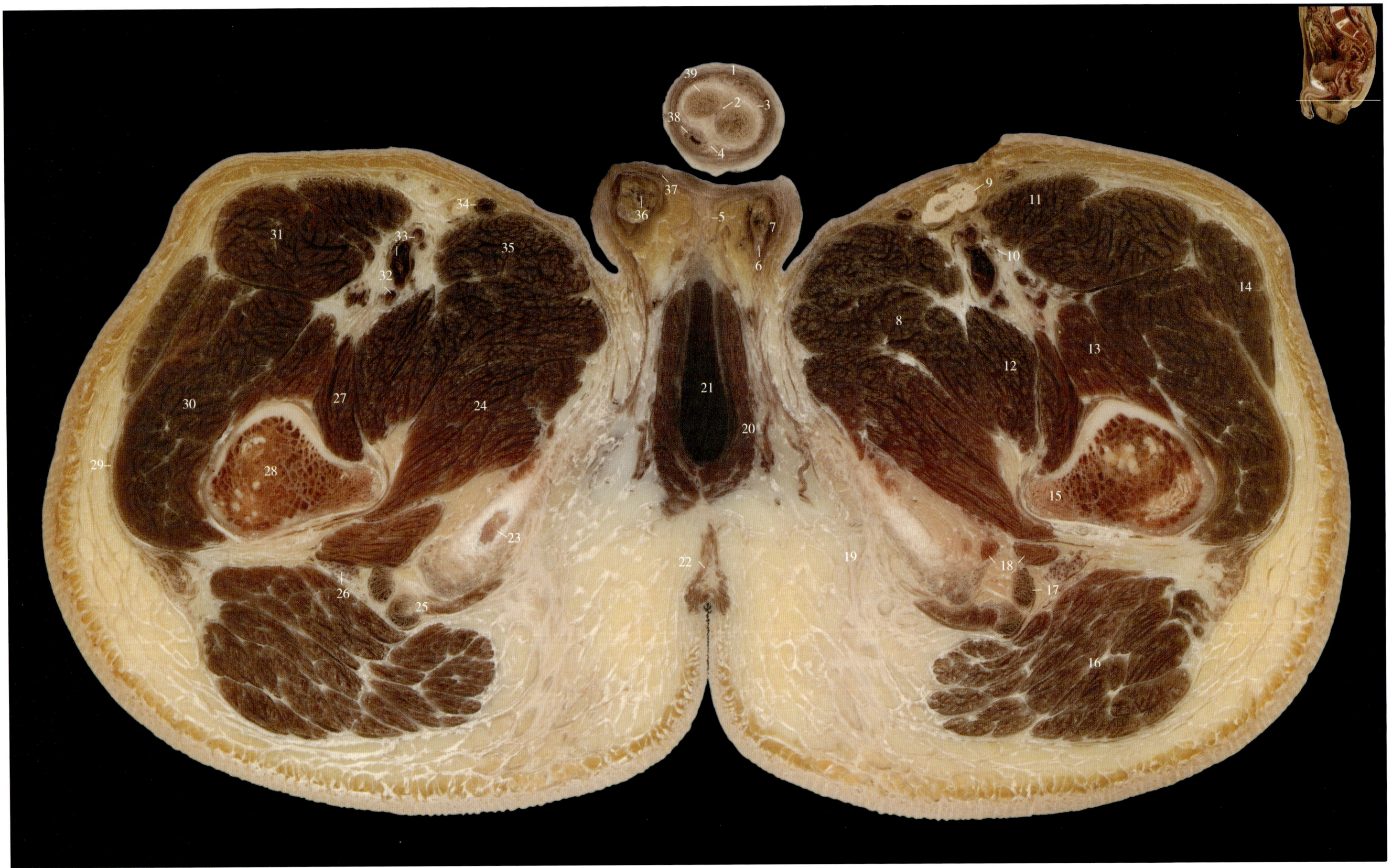

A. 断层标本图像

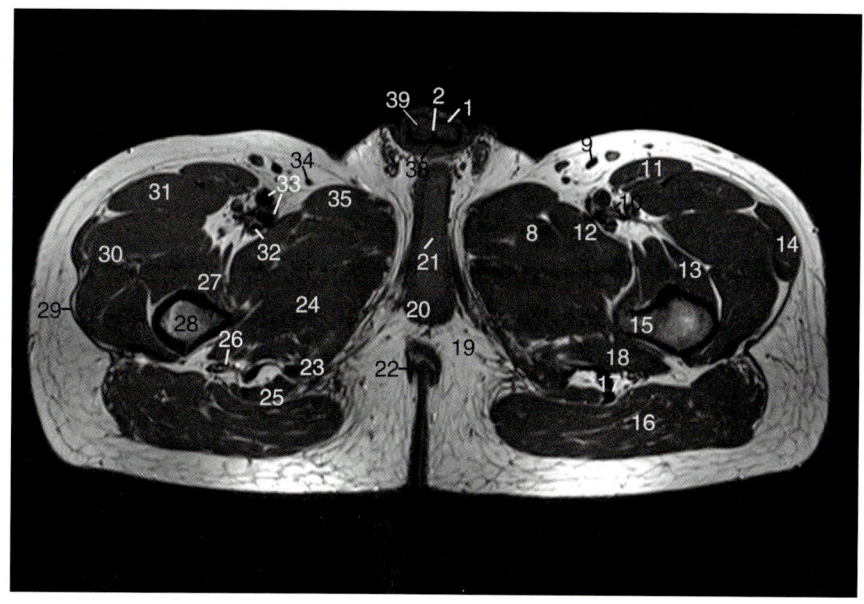
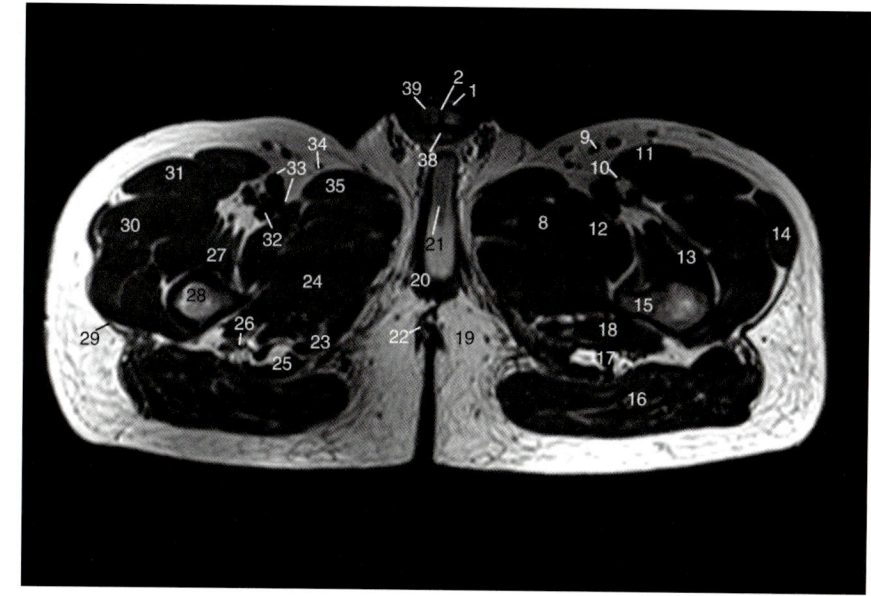
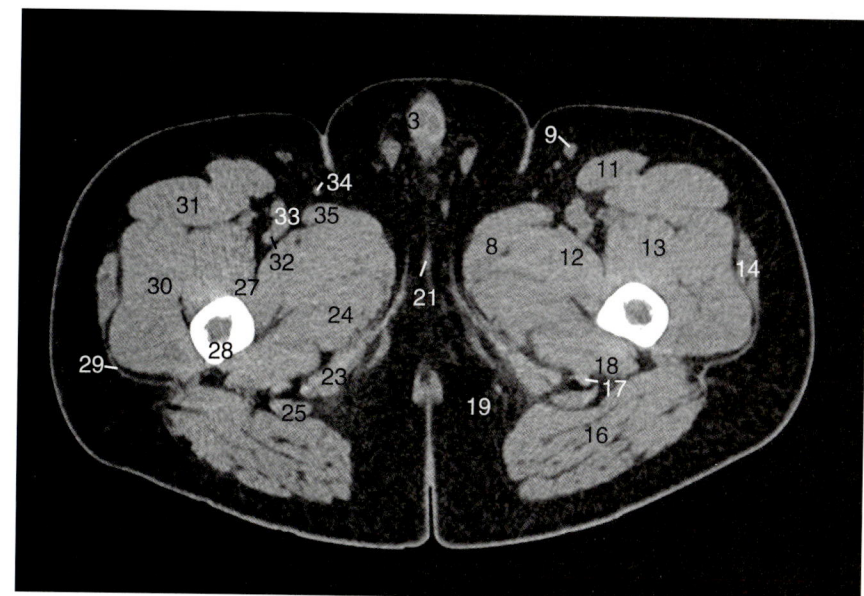

B. MR T1WI　　　　　C. MR T2WI　　　　　D. CT 平扫图像

1. 阴茎 penis
2. 阴茎中隔 septum penis
3. 阴茎海绵体白膜 albuginea of cavernous body of penis
4. 尿道海绵体白膜 albuginea of cavernous body of urethra
5. 阴囊中隔 septum of scrotum
6. 输精管 ductus deferens
7. 鞘膜腔 cavity of tunica vaginaalis
8. 短收肌 adductor brevis
9. 腹股沟浅淋巴结 superficial inguinal lymph nodes
10. 股神经 femoral nerve
11. 缝匠肌 sartorius
12. 耻骨肌 pectineus
13. 股中间肌 vastus intermedius
14. 阔筋膜张肌 tensor fasciae latae
15. 小转子 lesser trochanter
16. 臀大肌 gluteus maximus
17. 半膜肌肌腱 tendon of semimembranosus
18. 股方肌 quadratus femoris
19. 坐骨肛门窝 ischioanal fossa
20. 球海绵体肌 bulbocavernosus
21. 尿道 urethra
22. 肛门外括约肌 sphincter ani externus
23. 坐骨支 ramus of ischium
24. 大收肌 adductor magnus
25. 股二头肌长头和半腱肌 long head of biceps femoris and semitendinosus
26. 坐骨神经 sciatic nerve
27. 髂腰肌 iliopsoas
28. 大转子 greater trochanter
29. 阔筋膜 fasciae lata
30. 股外侧肌 vastus lateralis
31. 股直肌 rectus femoris
32. 股深动脉 deep femoral artery
33. 股动、静脉 femoral artery and vein
34. 大隐静脉 great saphenous vein
35. 长收肌 adductor longus
36. 附睾头 head of epididymis
37. 肉膜 dartos coat
38. 尿道海绵体 cavernous body of urethra
39. 阴茎海绵体 cavernous body of penis

关键结构：白膜，阴茎筋膜，阴囊。

此断面为经过阴囊上份层面。

左侧的坐骨支仅见皮质，坐骨海绵体肌仅右侧尚存细丝状的肌纤维，尿道海绵体居中线位置，其内有扩大的尿道球部，其外有呈"U"形的球海绵体肌包绕。断面前部可见分离的阴茎头，一对阴茎海绵体居前，尿道海绵体居后，周围均有白膜围绕。阴茎或尿道海绵体的白膜是由胶原纤维组织和弹性纤维组织组成的双层结构，该双层结构具有特殊性，其内环层为完整360°。环绕内层和并不完整的300°纵向外层。因为白膜由成熟的纤维组织形成，所以其在MRI上表现为T1WI、T2WI低信号。当阴茎损伤累及白膜时，表现为低信号的白膜不连续，可伴有散在高信号的血肿，需行外科修补术治疗[59]。阴囊内结构为附睾及鞘膜腔。断面后部为肛门括约肌，两侧为坐骨肛门窝，与臀部皮下脂肪相延续。左侧股鞘前方见淋巴结。阴茎的3个海绵体外面包裹有深、浅筋膜和皮肤。深筋膜在阴茎前端逐渐变薄而消失；在阴茎根处，深筋膜形成富含弹性纤维的阴茎悬韧带，将阴茎悬吊于耻骨联合前面[41]。阴茎深筋膜外面包有阴茎浅筋膜和皮肤，浅筋膜疏松无脂肪组织。阴茎的皮肤薄而柔软，向阴茎头延伸形成双层的皮肤皱襞，即阴茎包皮。阴囊皮肤较薄而多褶皱，皮下组织内缺乏脂肪而含有平滑肌纤维，特称肉膜。在阴囊的正中面上，肉膜向深部延伸为阴囊中隔，将阴囊分为左、右各半，分别容纳两侧的睾丸、附睾、输精管的起始段和它们周围的被膜。

男性盆部连续横断层 38（MH.6210）

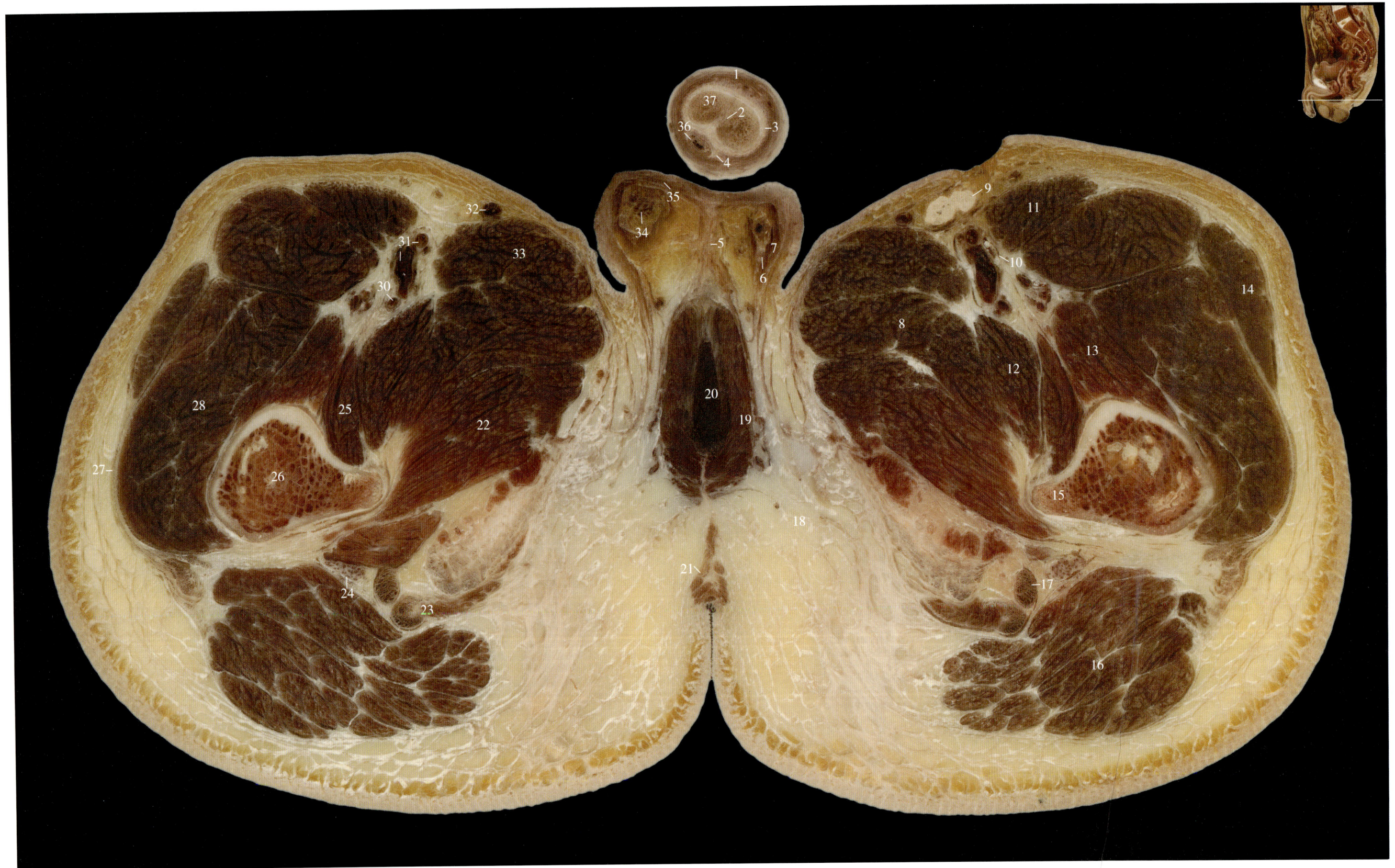

A. 断层标本图像

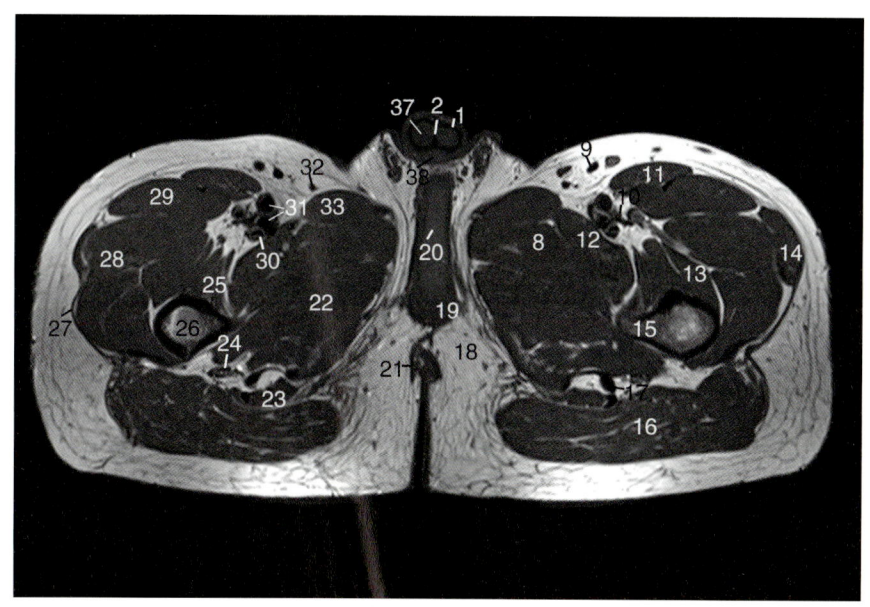
B. MR T1WI

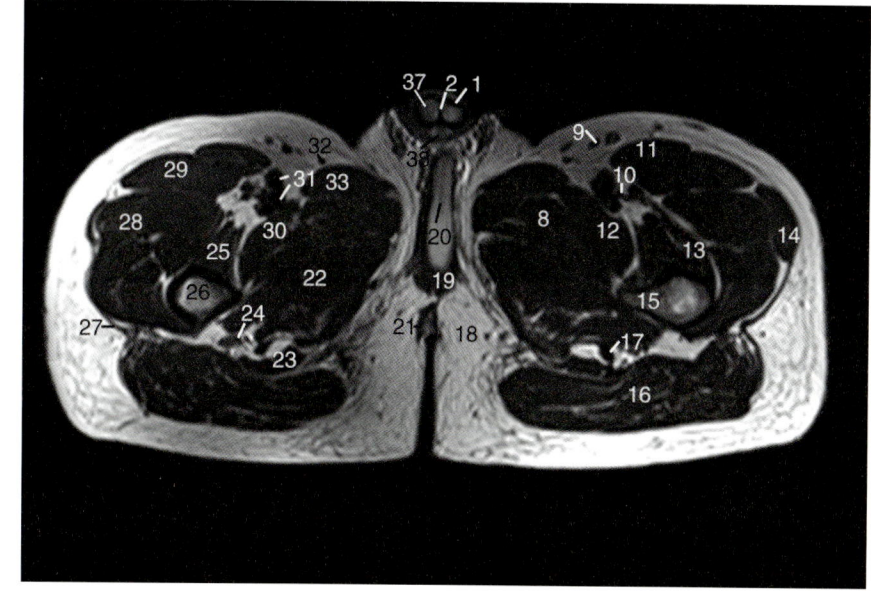
C. MR T2WI

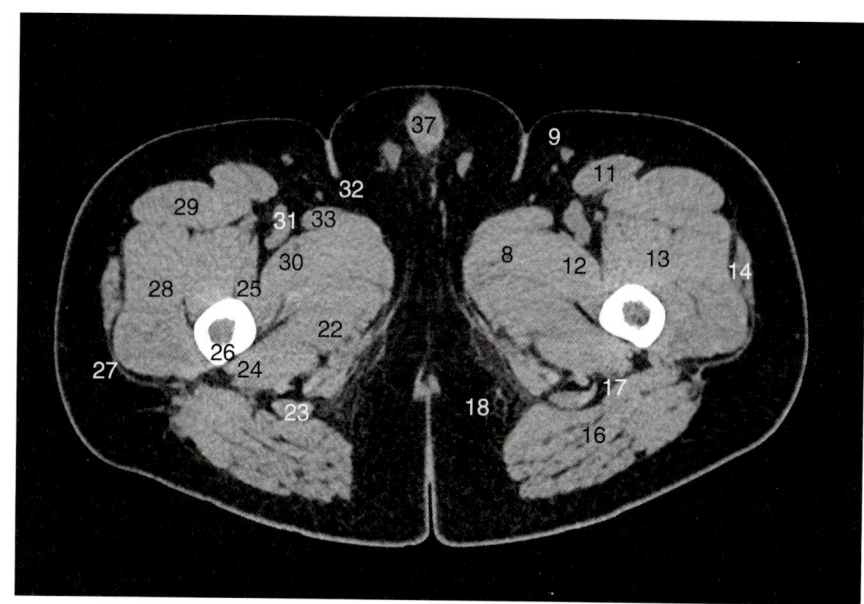
D. CT 平扫图像

关键结构：尿道球部，白膜，肛门外括约肌。

此断面为经过阴囊上份层面。双侧坐骨支、坐骨海绵体肌消失。断面前部可见分离的阴茎头，成对的阴茎海绵体居前，尿道海绵体居后，周围均有白膜围绕；阴囊内结构为附睾及鞘膜腔。断面中部可见尿道海绵体及尿道球部的内腔，其外有呈括弧状的球海绵体肌包绕。断面后部为肛门括约肌，两侧为坐骨肛门窝。来自腰大肌及髂肌的髂腰肌经过髋关节前方在此断面达其止点小转子前缘。尿道球部是男性尿道的三个膨大之一，为男性尿道海绵体后端的膨大部分，位于两侧阴茎脚之间，固定在尿生殖膈的下面。经过此部的尿道称为尿道球部，为尿道全长最宽的部分，并有尿道球腺开口于此[1]。发生骑跨伤时将尿道挤向耻骨联合下方，从而引起球部损伤。肛门外括约肌的深、浅两部，直肠纵行平滑肌和肛门内括约肌在肛管直肠移行处共同形成一肌性环，称为肛直肠环，有括约肛门的重要作用. 手术中如严重损伤此环，可引起大便失禁[52]。

1. 阴茎 penis
2. 阴茎中隔 septum penis
3. 阴茎海绵体白膜 albuginea of cavernous body of penis
4. 尿道海绵体白膜 albuginea of cavernous body of urethra
5. 阴囊中隔 septum of scrotum
6. 输精管 ductus deferens
7. 鞘膜腔 cavity of tunica vaginaalis
8. 短收肌 adductor brevis
9. 腹股沟浅淋巴结 superficial inguinal lymph rodes
10. 股神经 femoral nerve
11. 缝匠肌 sartorius
12. 耻骨肌 pectineus
13. 股中间肌 vastus intermedius
14. 阔筋膜张肌 tensor fasciae latae
15. 小转子 lesser trochanter
16. 臀大肌 gluteus maximus
17. 半膜肌肌腱 tendon of semimembranosus
18. 坐骨肛门窝 ischioanal fossa
19. 球海绵体肌 bulbocavernosus
20. 尿道 urethra
21. 肛门外括约肌 sphincter ani externus
22. 大收肌 adductor magnus
23. 股二头肌长头和半腱肌 long head of biceps femoris and semitendinosus
24. 坐骨神经 sciatic nerve
25. 髂腰肌 iliopsoas
26. 大转子 greater trochanter
27. 阔筋膜 fasciae lata
28. 股外侧肌 vastus lateralis
29. 股直肌 rectus femoris
30. 股深动脉 deep femoral artery
31. 股动、静脉 femoral artery and vein
32. 大隐静脉 great saphenous vein
33. 长收肌 adductor longus
34. 附睾头 head of epididymis
35. 肉膜 dartos coat
36. 尿道海绵体 cavernous body of urethra
37. 阴茎海绵体 cavernous body of penis

男性盆部连续横断层 39（MH.6200）

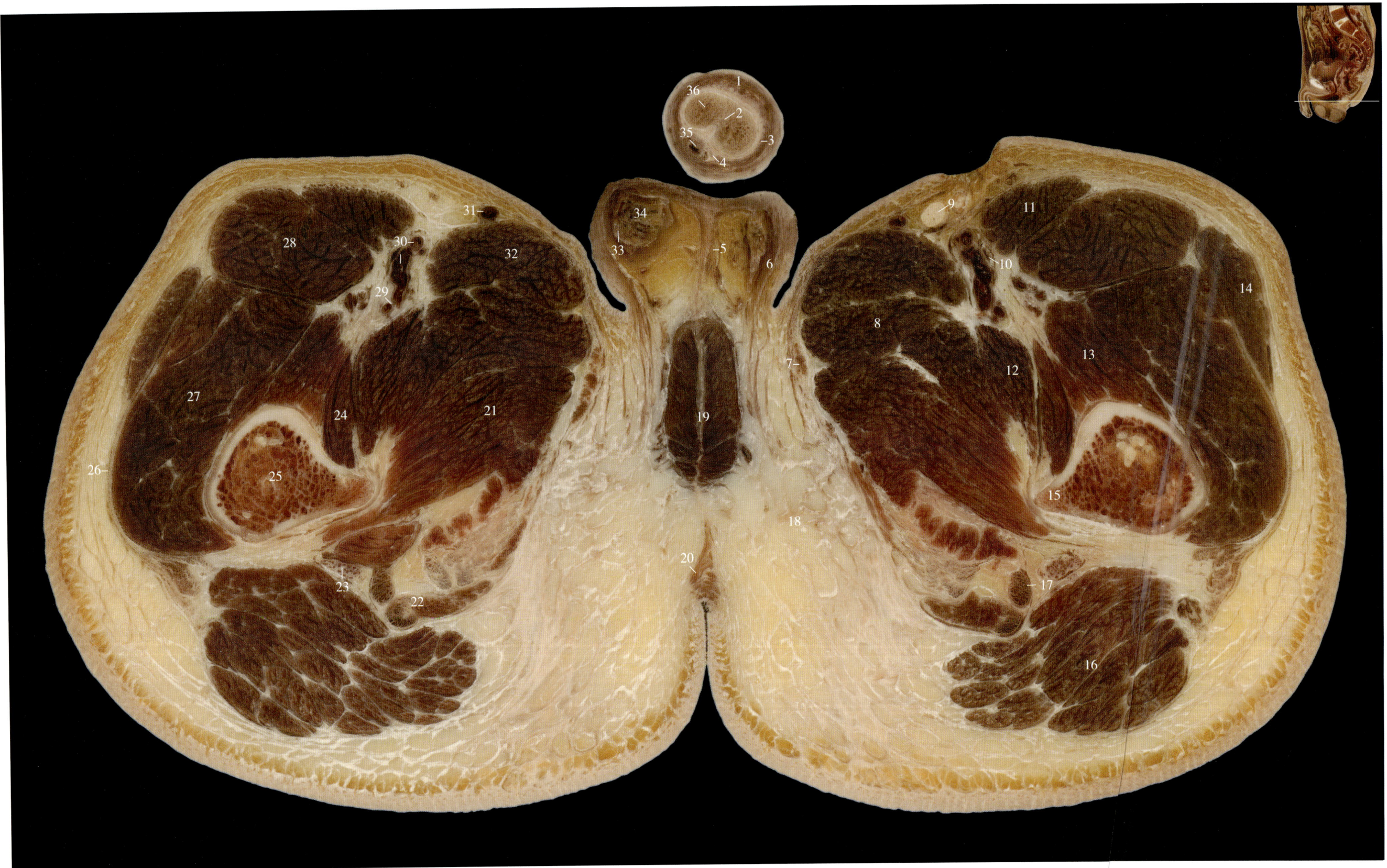

A. 断层标本图像

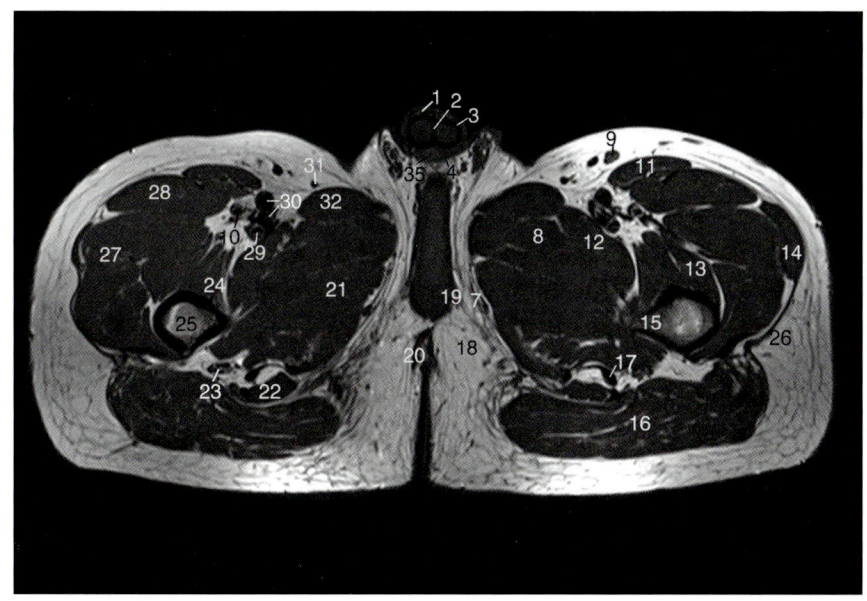

B. MR T1WI

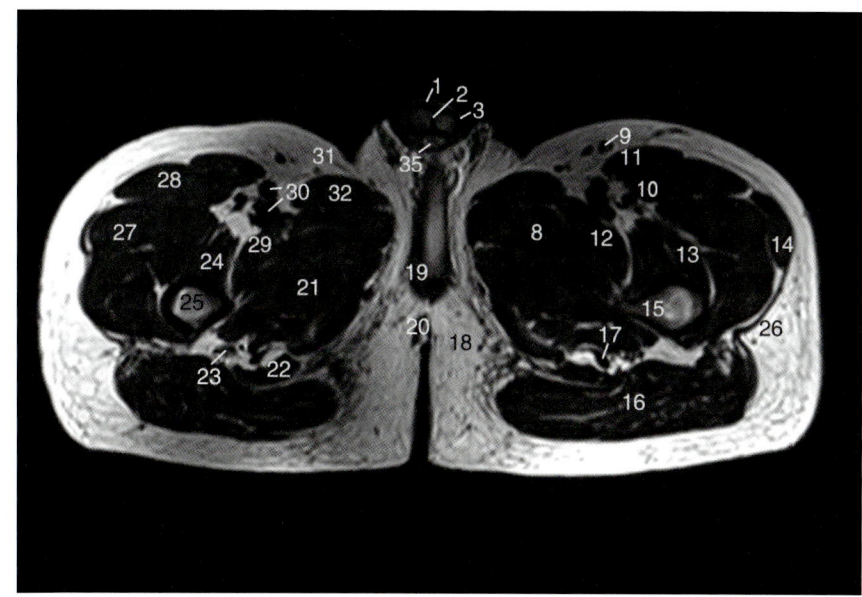

C. MR T2WI

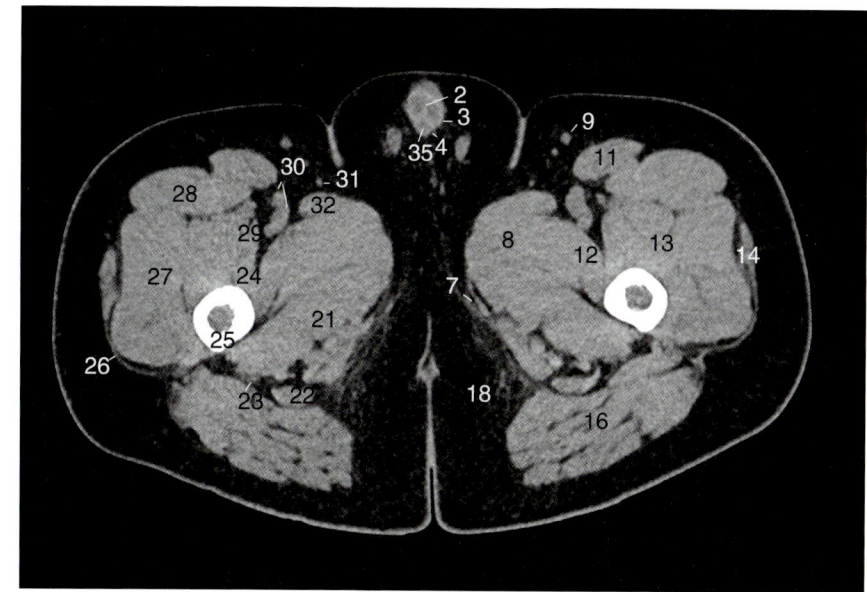

D. CT 平扫图像

关键结构：阴茎包皮，坐骨肛门窝，白膜。

此断面为经过阴囊上份层面。

断面前部可见分离的阴茎头，居前者为成对的阴茎海绵体，居后者为尿道海绵体，周围均有白膜围绕；阴囊内结构为附睾及鞘膜腔[52]。断面中部可见长条形的球海绵体肌。断面后部为肛门括约肌，两侧为坐骨肛门窝。股三角内见股神经位于股动脉外侧，股深动脉位于股动脉后方，股静脉位于股动脉内侧。阴茎的皮肤薄弱、柔软，富于伸展性。皮肤从阴茎颈开始游离向前延伸，形成双层皮肤皱襞，称阴茎包皮[41]。小儿时期包皮包被阴茎头，成年后阴茎头外露。如果成年后包皮仍包被阴茎头，称包皮过长，或包皮不能上翻露出阴茎头，称包茎。在这种情况下可行包皮环切手术。男性青少年和成人阴茎包皮状况：10~12岁包皮过长占71.8%，包茎占11.5%；13~16岁包皮过长占64.75%，包茎占5.57%；17~18岁包皮过长占40.45%，包茎占2.75%；18岁以上包皮过长占18.11%，包茎占0.98%[16]。

1. 阴茎包皮 prepuce of penis
2. 阴茎中隔 septum penis
3. 阴茎海绵体白膜 albuginea of cavernous body of penis
4. 尿道海绵体白膜 albuginea of cavernous body of urethra
5. 阴囊中隔 septum of scrotum
6. 鞘膜腔 cavity of tunica vaginaalis
7. 股薄肌 gracilis
8. 短收肌 adductor brevis
9. 腹股沟浅淋巴结 superficial inguinal lymph nodes
10. 股神经 femoral nerve
11. 缝匠肌 sartorius
12. 耻骨肌 pectineus
13. 股中间肌 vastus intermedius
14. 阔筋膜张肌 tensor fasciae latae
15. 小转子 lesser trochanter
16. 臀大肌 gluteus maximus
17. 半膜肌肌腱 tendon of semimembranosus
18. 坐骨肛门窝 ischioanal fossa
19. 球海绵体肌 bulbocavernosus
20. 肛门外括约肌 sphincter ani externus
21. 大收肌 adductor magnus
22. 股二头肌长头和半腱肌 long head of biceps femoris and semitendinosus
23. 坐骨神经 sciatic nerve
24. 髂腰肌 iliopsoas
25. 大转子 greater trochanter
26. 阔筋膜 fasciae lata
27. 股外侧肌 vastus lateralis
28. 股直肌 rectus femoris
29. 股深动脉 deep femoral artery
30. 股动、静脉 femoral artery and vein
31. 大隐静脉 great saphenous vein
32. 长收肌 adductor longus
33. 输精管 ductus deferens
34. 附睾头 head of epididymis
35. 尿道海绵体 cavernous body of urethra
36. 阴茎深动脉 deep artery of penis

男性盆部连续横断层 40（MH.6190）

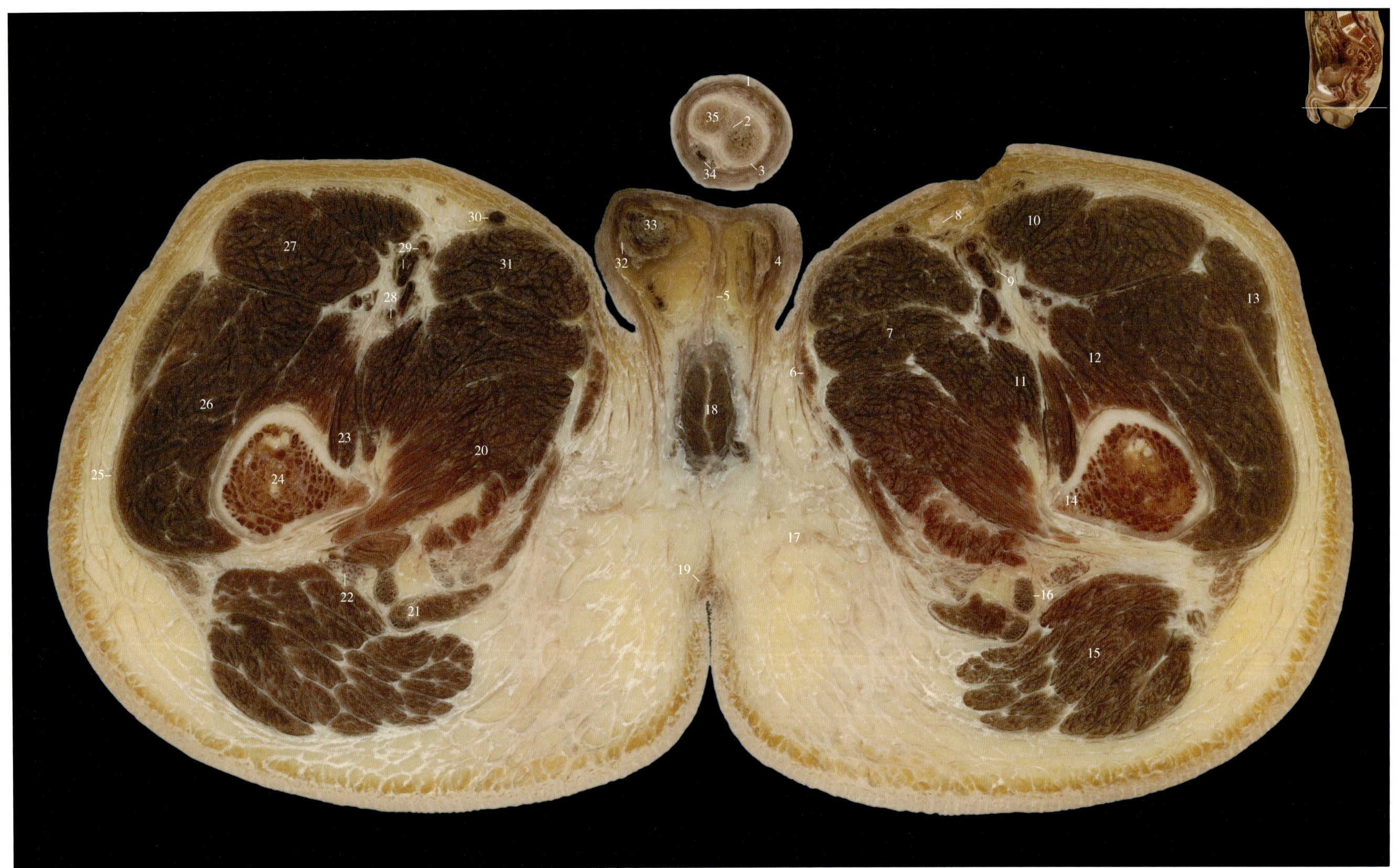

A. 断层标本图像

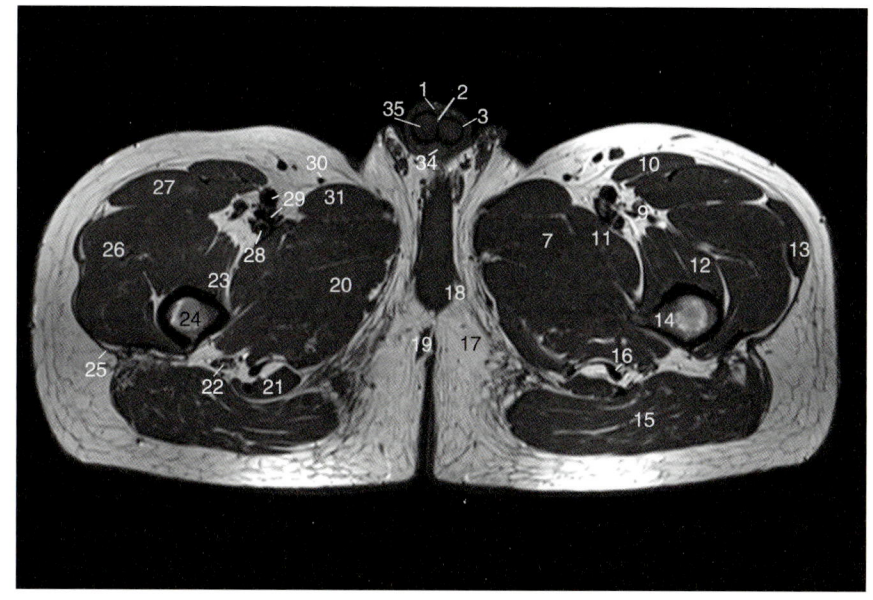
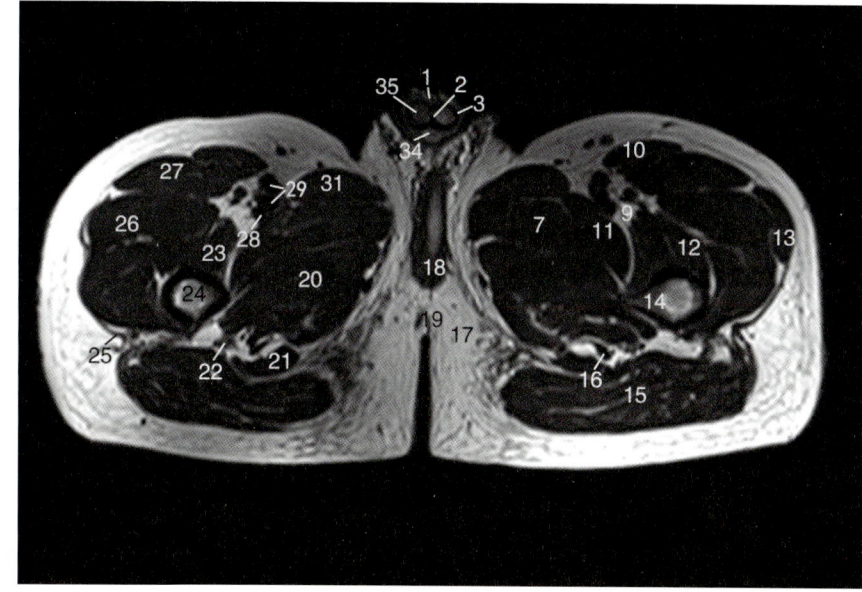
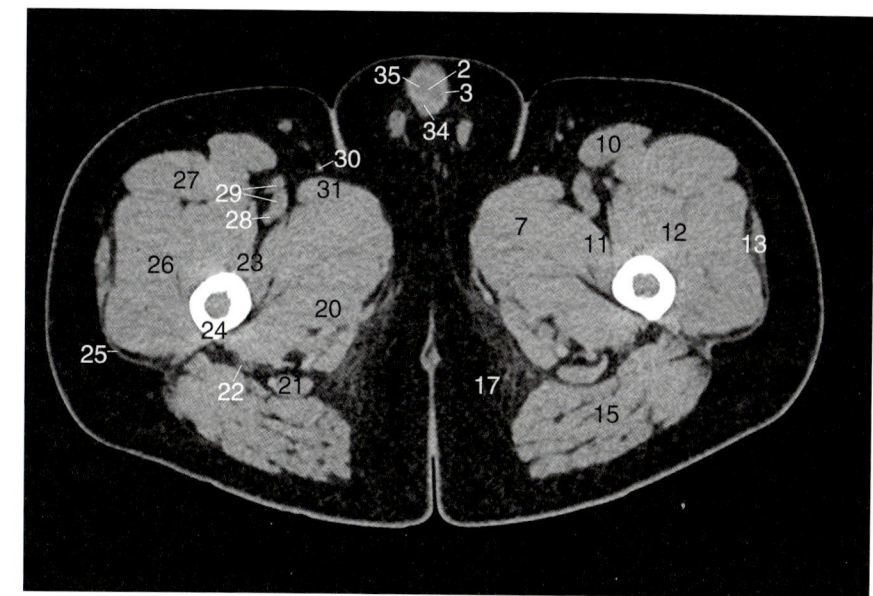

B. MR T1WI 　　　　　　　　C. MR T2WI　　　　　　　　D. CT 平扫图像

1. 阴茎包皮 prepuce of penis
2. 阴茎中隔 septum penis
3. 阴茎海绵体白膜 albuginea of cavernous body of penis
4. 鞘膜腔 cavity of tunica vaginaalis
5. 阴囊中隔 septum of scrotum
6. 股薄肌 gracilis
7. 短收肌 adductor brevis
8. 腹股沟浅淋巴结 superficial inguinal lymph nodes
9. 股神经 femoral nerve
10. 缝匠肌 sartorius
11. 耻骨肌 pectineus
12. 股中间肌 vastus intermedius
13. 阔筋膜张肌 tensor fasciae latae
14. 小转子 lesser trochanter
15. 臀大肌 gluteus maximus
16. 半膜肌肌腱 tendon of semimembranosus
17. 坐骨肛门窝 ischioanal fossa
18. 球海绵体肌 bulbocavernosus
19. 肛门外括约肌 sphincter ani externus
20. 大收肌 adductor magnus
21. 股二头肌长头和半腱肌 long head of biceps femoris and semitendinosus
22. 坐骨神经 sciatic nerve
23. 髂腰肌 iliopsoas
24. 大转子 greater trochanter
25. 阔筋膜 fasciae lata
26. 股外侧肌 vastus lateralis
27. 股直肌 rectus femoris
28. 股深动脉 deep femoral artery
29. 股动、静脉 femoral artery and vein
30. 大隐静脉 great saphenous vein
31. 长收肌 adductor longus
32. 输精管 ductus deferens
33. 附睾头 head of epididymis
34. 尿道海绵体 cavernous body of urethra
35. 阴茎海绵体 cavernous body of penis

关键结构：尿生殖区，肛门三角区，坐骨神经。

　　此断面为经过附睾上份层面。尿生殖三角区已近皮下组织，球海绵体肌即将消失。肛门三角区内的肛门及肛门括约肌几乎消失。断面前部可见分离的阴茎头，居前的是一对阴茎海绵体，居后的为尿道海绵体，周围均有白膜围绕；阴囊内结构为附睾及鞘膜腔。断面两侧为大腿结构，以股骨为中心，其周围分别是股内侧肌群、股外侧肌群和股后肌群。股骨后方的臀大肌体积变小，其前方与股后肌群间隙内见坐骨神经。股三角已达尖部。尿生殖三角又称尿生殖区，区内有生殖器官，并有尿道（女性还有阴道）通过。由浅入深为皮肤、浅筋膜、深层肌和海绵体、尿生殖膈。其中，坐骨海绵体肌覆盖阴茎脚的浅面，可助阴茎勃起；球海绵体肌在男性包绕尿道球，收缩时可助排尿和射精，在女性此肌覆盖前庭球，收缩时可助缩小阴道口[60]。尿生殖膈位于盆膈前份下方，封闭盆膈裂孔，男性有尿道通过，女性有尿道和阴道通过。尿生殖膈由深层肌和其上、下的两层筋膜构成。肛门三角区内有肛管及坐骨肛门窝等，窝内充满脂肪组织，并有阴部内血管及阴部神经沿窝外侧壁通过。在坐骨结节下缘上方2.5 cm处，闭孔筋膜包绕上述血管、神经，形成阴部管[12, 41]。

男性盆部连续横断层 41（MH.6180）

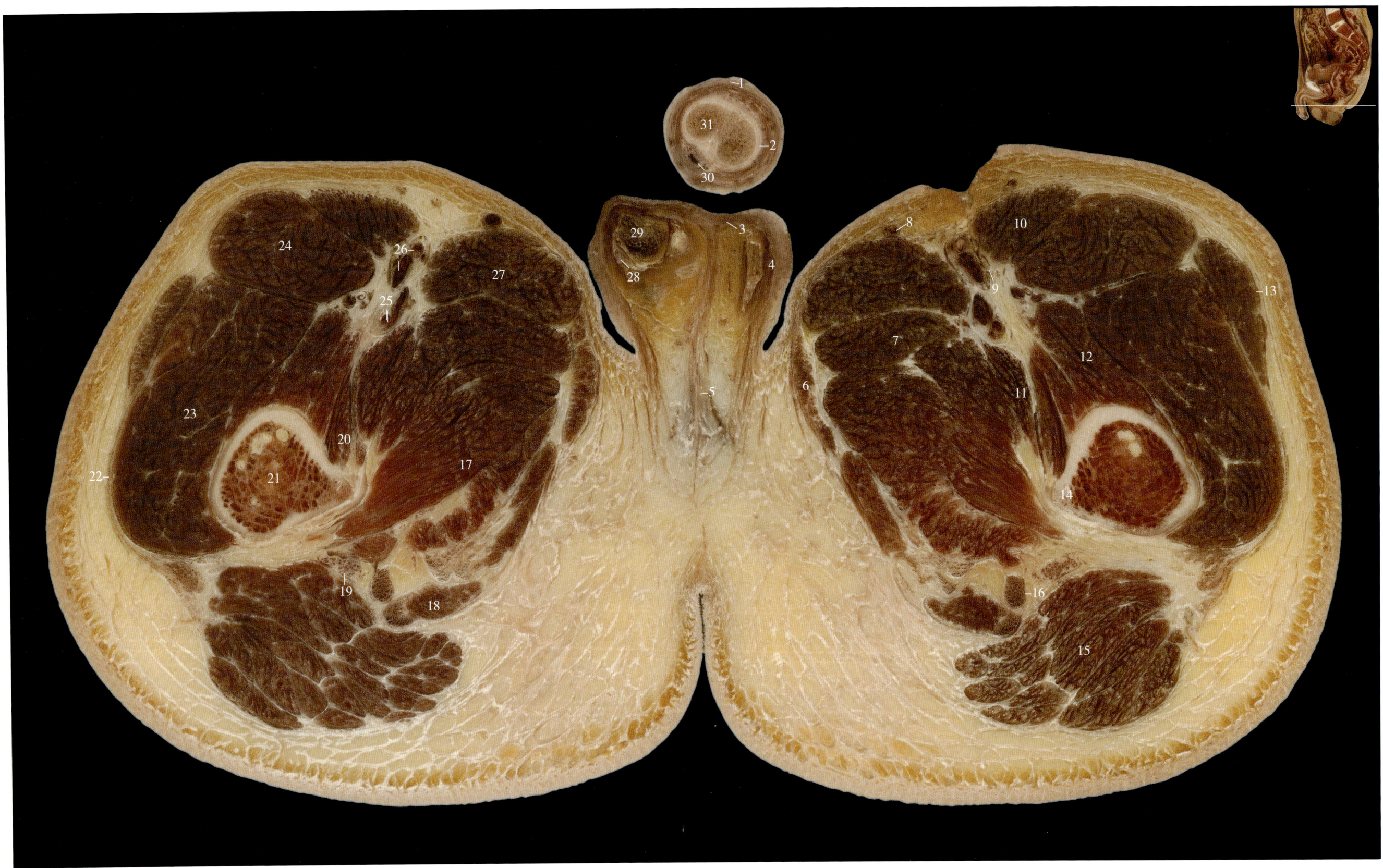

A. 断层标本图像

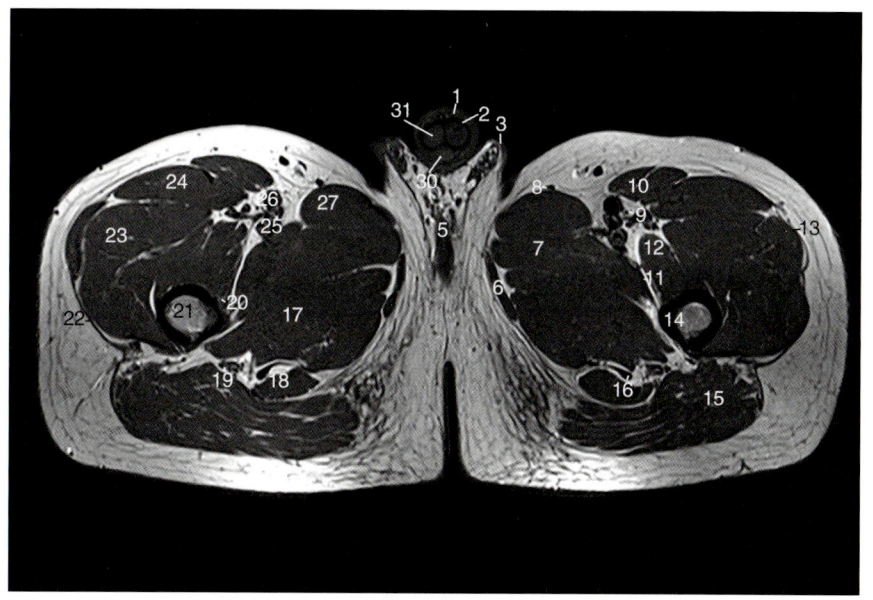

B. MR T1WI

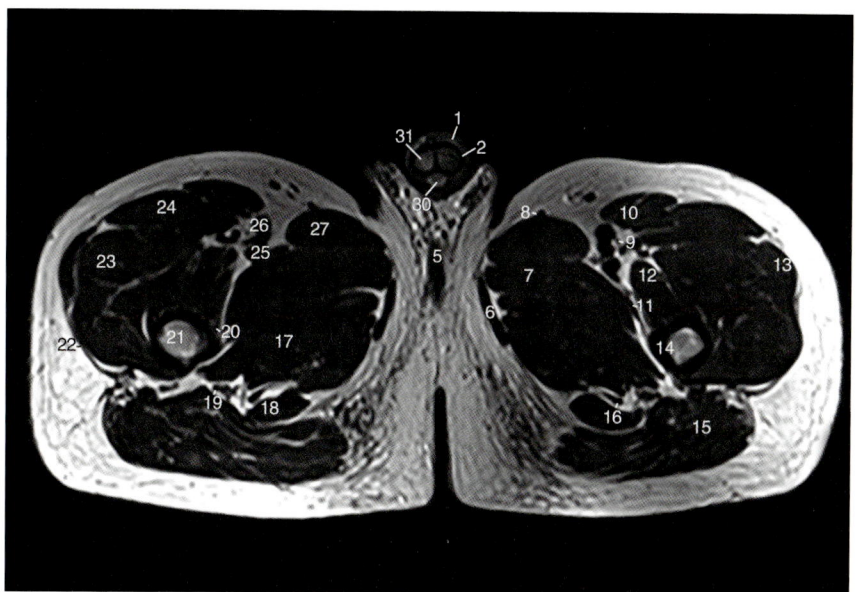

C. MR T2WI

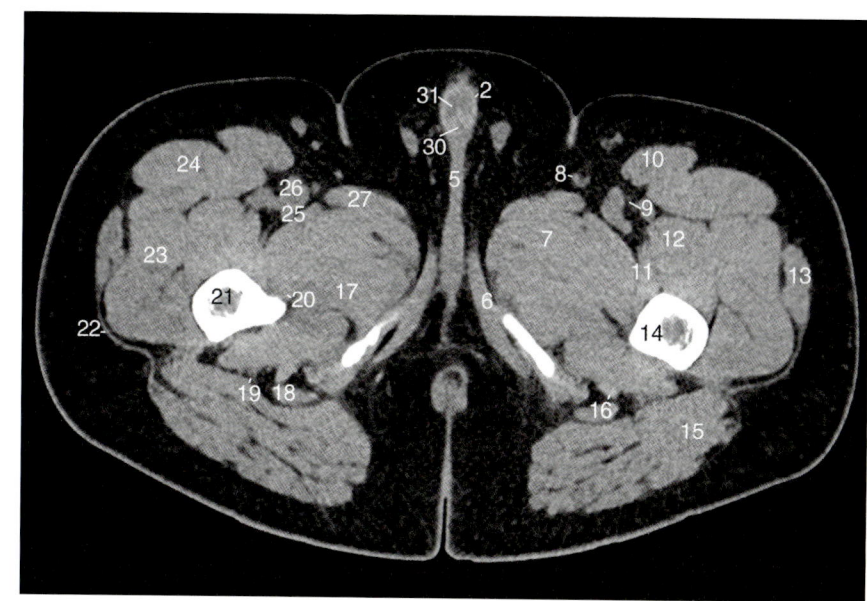

D. CT 平扫图像

1. 阴茎包皮 prepuce of penis
2. 阴茎海绵体白膜 albuginea of cavernous body of penis
3. 肉膜 dartos coat
4. 鞘膜腔 cavity of tunica vaginaalis
5. 阴囊中隔 septum of scrotum
6. 股薄肌 gracilis
7. 短收肌 adductor brevis
8. 大隐静脉 great saphenous vein
9. 股神经 femoral nerve
10. 缝匠肌 sartorius
11. 耻骨肌 pectineus
12. 股中间肌 vastus intermedius
13. 阔筋膜张肌 tensor fasciae latae
14. 小转子 lesser trochanter
15. 臀大肌 gluteus maximus
16. 半膜肌肌腱 tendon of semimembranosus
17. 大收肌 adductor magnus
18. 股二头肌长头和半腱肌 long head of biceps femoris and semitendinosus
19. 坐骨神经 sciatic nerve
20. 髂腰肌 iliopsoas
21. 股骨 femur
22. 阔筋膜 fasciae lata
23. 股外侧肌 vastus lateralis
24. 股直肌 rectus femoris
25. 股深动脉 deep femoral artery
26. 股动、静脉 femoral artery and vein
27. 长收肌 adductor longus
28. 输精管 ductus deferens
29. 附睾 epididymis
30. 尿道海绵体 cavernous body of urethra
31. 阴茎海绵体 cavernous body of penis

关键结构：尿道海绵体，阴囊，附睾。

此断面为经过阴囊上份层面。断面中部尿生殖三角区已近皮下组织，球海绵体肌消失。肛门三角区内肛门及肛门括约肌消失。断面前部可见阴茎，居阴茎前部的是一对阴茎海绵体，居后的为尿道及尿道海绵体，海绵体周围有白膜围绕。海绵体在T1WI上呈等信号，与大腿肌肉信号类似，T2WI上呈高信号，明显高于肌肉信号。包绕海绵体的白膜在T1WI及T2WI上均呈明显低信号。CT平扫图像上，阴茎及阴囊均呈软组织密度，不能区分其内的结构[61]。阴囊内结构为附睾、鞘膜腔。肉膜为阴囊的浅筋膜，与皮肤组成阴囊壁，并在正中线上向深部发出阴囊中隔，将阴囊分为左、右两腔，分别容纳两侧的睾丸、附睾及精索等[41]。附睾在T2WI上呈不均一中等信号，强度低于睾丸。

男性盆部连续横断层 42 (MH.6170)

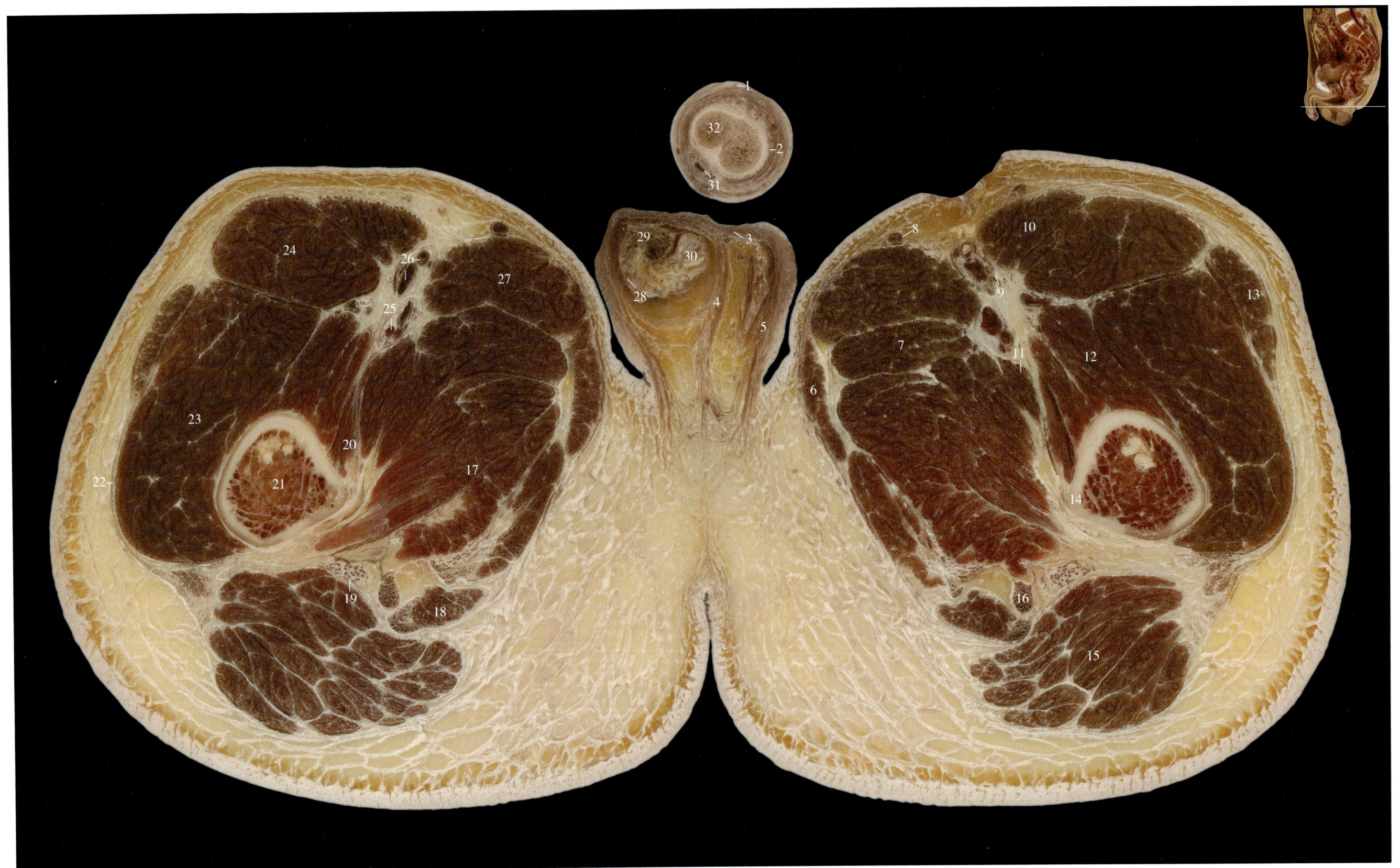

A. 断层标本图像

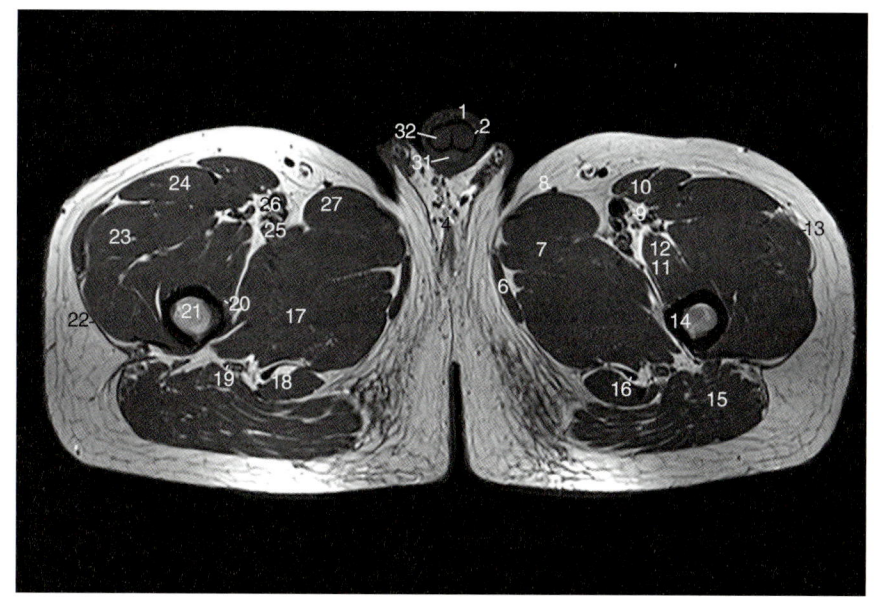

B. MR T1WI

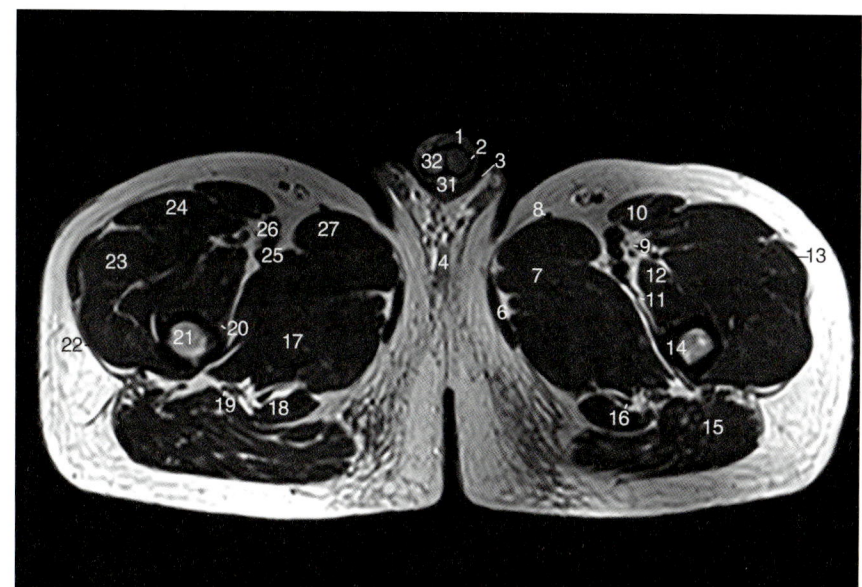

C. MR T2WI

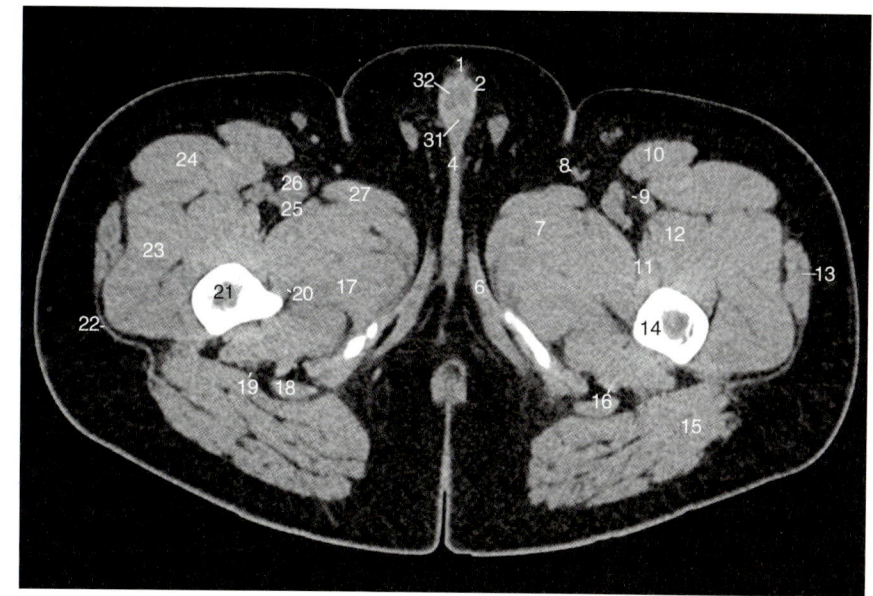

D. CT 平扫图像

1. 阴茎包皮 prepuce of penis
2. 阴茎海绵体白膜 albuginea of cavernous body of penis
3. 肉膜 dartos coat
4. 阴囊中隔 septum of scrotum
5. 鞘膜腔 cavity of tunica vaginaalis
6. 股薄肌 gracilis
7. 短收肌 adductor brevis
8. 大隐静脉 great saphenous vein
9. 股神经 femoral nerve
10. 缝匠肌 sartorius
11. 耻骨肌 pectineus
12. 股中间肌 vastus intermedius
13. 阔筋膜张肌 tensor fasciae latae
14. 小转子 lesser trochanter
15. 臀大肌 gluteus maximus
16. 半膜肌肌腱 tendon of semimembranosus
17. 大收肌 adductor magnus
18. 股二头肌长头和半腱肌 long head of biceps femoris and semitendinosus
19. 坐骨神经 sciatic nerve
20. 髂腰肌 iliopsoas
21. 股骨 femur
22. 阔筋膜 fasciae lata
23. 股外侧肌 vastus lateralis
24. 股直肌 rectus femoris
25. 股深动脉 deep femoral artery
26. 股动、静脉 femoral artery and vein
27. 长收肌 adductor longus
28. 输精管 ductus deferens
29. 附睾 epididymis
30. 睾丸 testis
31. 尿道 urethra
32. 阴茎海绵体 cavernous body of penis

关键结构：尿道海绵体，阴茎海绵体，阴部内动脉。

此断面为经过睾丸上份层面。断面前部为阴茎头，阴茎海绵体居阴茎前份、成对，尿道海绵体居后，周围均有白膜围绕。右侧阴囊内结构为附睾、睾丸及鞘膜腔。临床上将尿道海绵体部称为前尿道。前尿道损伤多见于会阴部骑跨伤所致的球部尿道损伤。如仅尿道海绵体部有破裂，阴茎深筋膜完好，渗出尿液可被局限在阴茎范围；如阴茎深筋膜也破裂，尿液可随阴茎浅筋膜蔓延到阴囊和腹前壁[62]。尿生殖区的血供来自阴部内动脉。阴部内动脉沿坐骨肛门窝侧壁前行至尿生殖膈后缘，分成会阴动脉和阴茎动脉。会阴动脉入会阴浅隙，并分支至阴囊。阴茎动脉入会阴深隙，分成阴茎背动脉和阴茎深动脉两终支，前者行于阴茎背面，后者穿入阴茎海绵体[25]。大腿肌群：断面两侧为股骨和大腿肌群，臀大肌前面可见大腿后肌群，起于坐骨结节跨髋、膝止于胫腓骨的半腱肌、半膜肌和股二头肌。股骨前外侧可见大腿前外侧群的股四头肌、缝匠肌、阔筋膜张肌；内侧群可见耻骨肌、长收肌、短收肌、大收肌和最内侧的股薄肌。另外，在股骨小转子前可见髂腰肌止于小转子，臀大肌深面可见坐骨神经，长收肌与缝匠肌间脂肪间隙内见股神经及股血管。

男性盆部连续横断层 43（MH.6160）

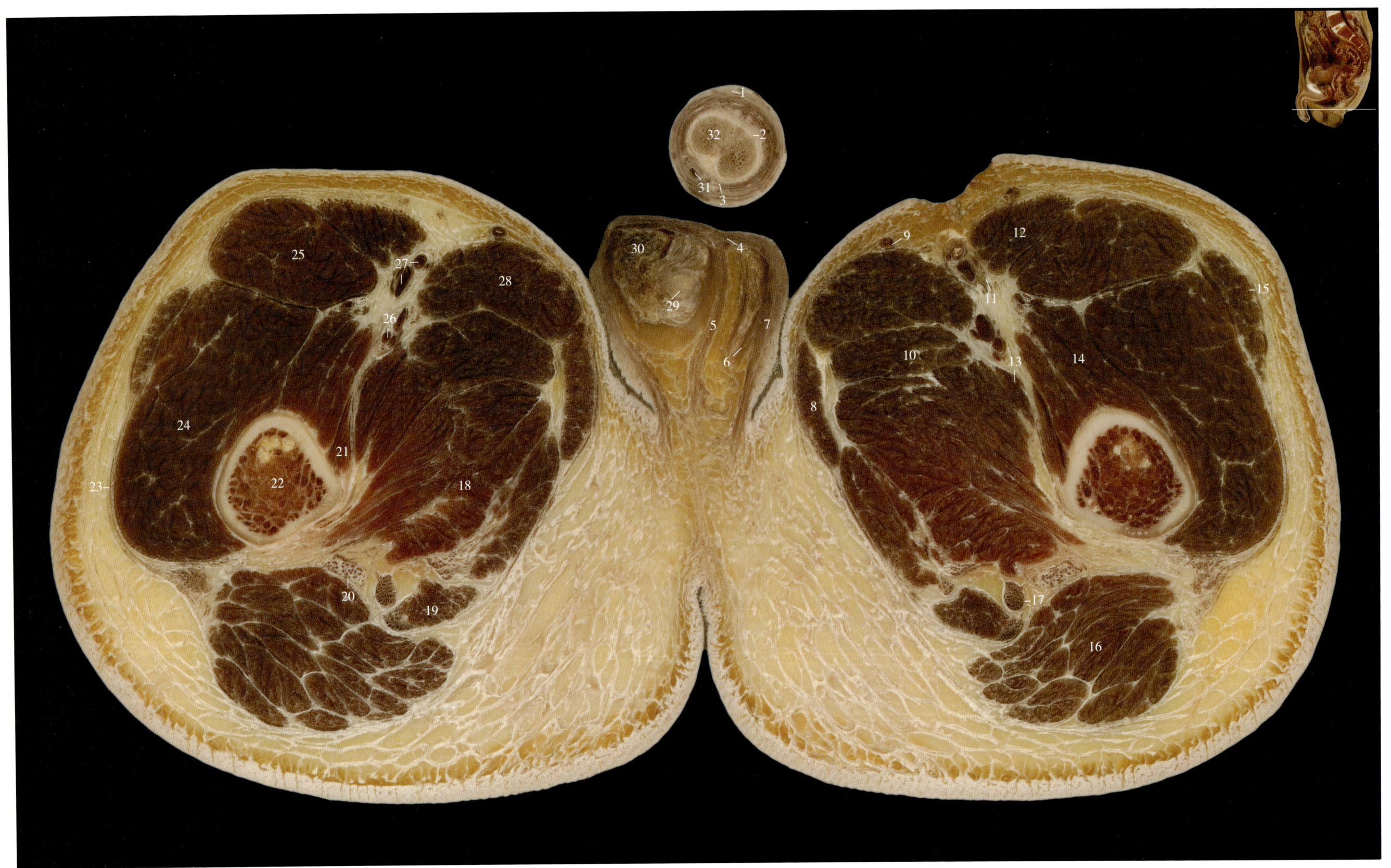

A. 断层标本图像

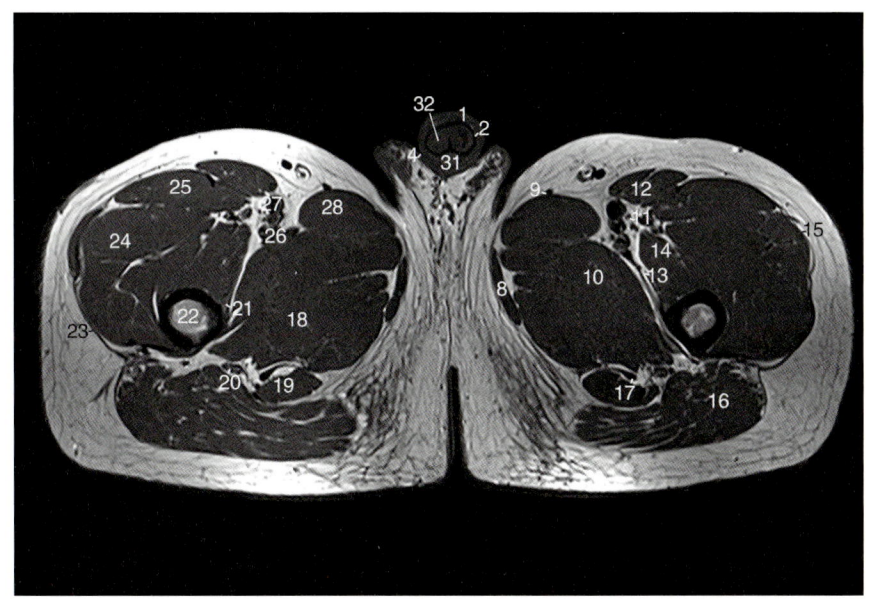

B. MR T1WI

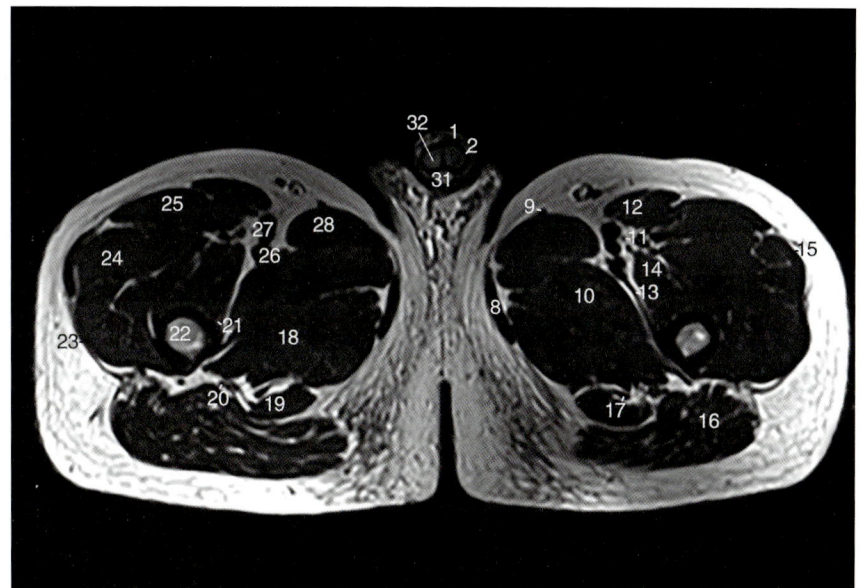

C. MR T2WI

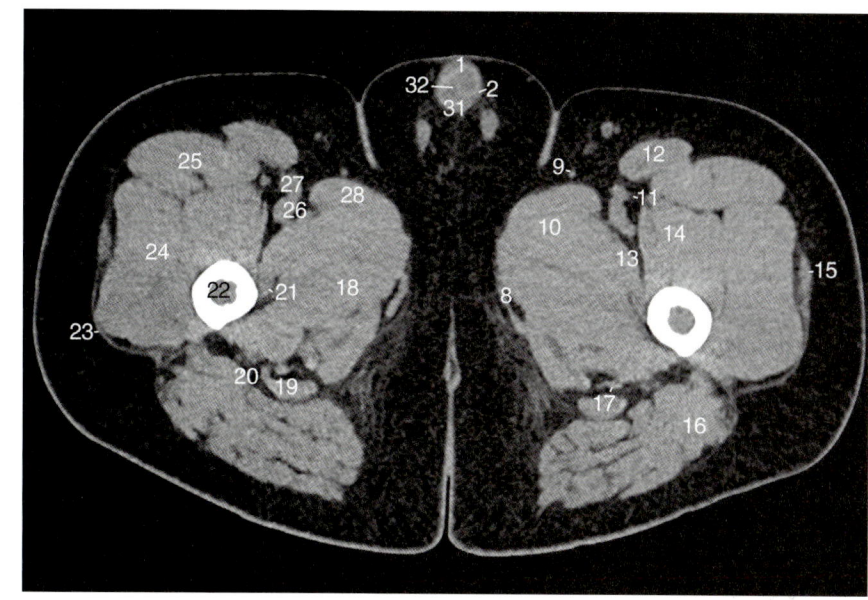

D. CT 平扫图像

关键结构：阴茎深筋膜，阴茎背神经，睾丸。

1. 阴茎包皮 prepuce of penis
2. 阴茎海绵体白膜 albuginea of cavernous body of penis
3. 阴茎深筋膜 deep fascia of penis
4. 肉膜 dartos coat
5. 阴囊中隔 septum of scrotum
6. 输精管 ductus deferens
7. 鞘膜腔 cavity of tunica vaginaalis
8. 股薄肌 gracilis
9. 大隐静脉 great saphenous vein
10. 短收肌 adductor brevis
11. 股神经 femoral nerve
12. 缝匠肌 sartorius
13. 耻骨肌 pectineus
14. 股中间肌 vastus intermedius
15. 阔筋膜张肌 tensor fasciae latae
16. 臀大肌 gluteus maximus
17. 半膜肌 semimembranosus
18. 大收肌 adductor magnus
19. 股二头肌长头和半腱肌 long head of biceps femoris and semitendinosus
20. 坐骨神经 sciatic nerve
21. 髂腰肌 iliopsoas
22. 股骨 femur
23. 阔筋膜 fasciae lata
24. 股外侧肌 vastus lateralis
25. 股直肌 rectus femoris
26. 股深动脉 deep femoral artery
27. 股动、静脉 femoral artery and vein
28. 长收肌 adductor longus
29. 睾丸 testis
30. 附睾 epididymis
31. 尿道 urethra
32. 阴茎海绵体 cavernous body of penis

此断面为经过睾丸上份层面。断面前部可见分离的阴茎头、阴茎包皮，阴茎海绵体居前、成对，尿道海绵体居后，周围均有白膜围绕。阴茎深筋膜又称 Buck 筋膜，包裹阴茎的 3 条海绵体，前端始于冠状沟，后续于腹白线。深筋膜在阴茎前端逐渐变薄而消失；在阴茎根处，深筋膜形成富含弹性纤维的阴茎悬韧带，将阴茎悬吊于耻骨联合前面[25]，此筋膜深面与白膜之间有阴茎背深静脉（正中）和阴茎背动脉和阴茎背神经（两侧）。包皮切除术或阴茎手术时，可在阴茎根背面两侧施行阴茎背神经阻滞麻醉[62]。阴囊由中隔分成左、右两部分，右侧内的结构为附睾、睾丸及鞘膜腔，左侧睾丸位置一般比右侧要低 1 cm 左右[16]。该断面在左侧阴囊内尚未出现睾丸及附睾，仅见输精管。

男性盆部连续横断层 44（MH.6150）

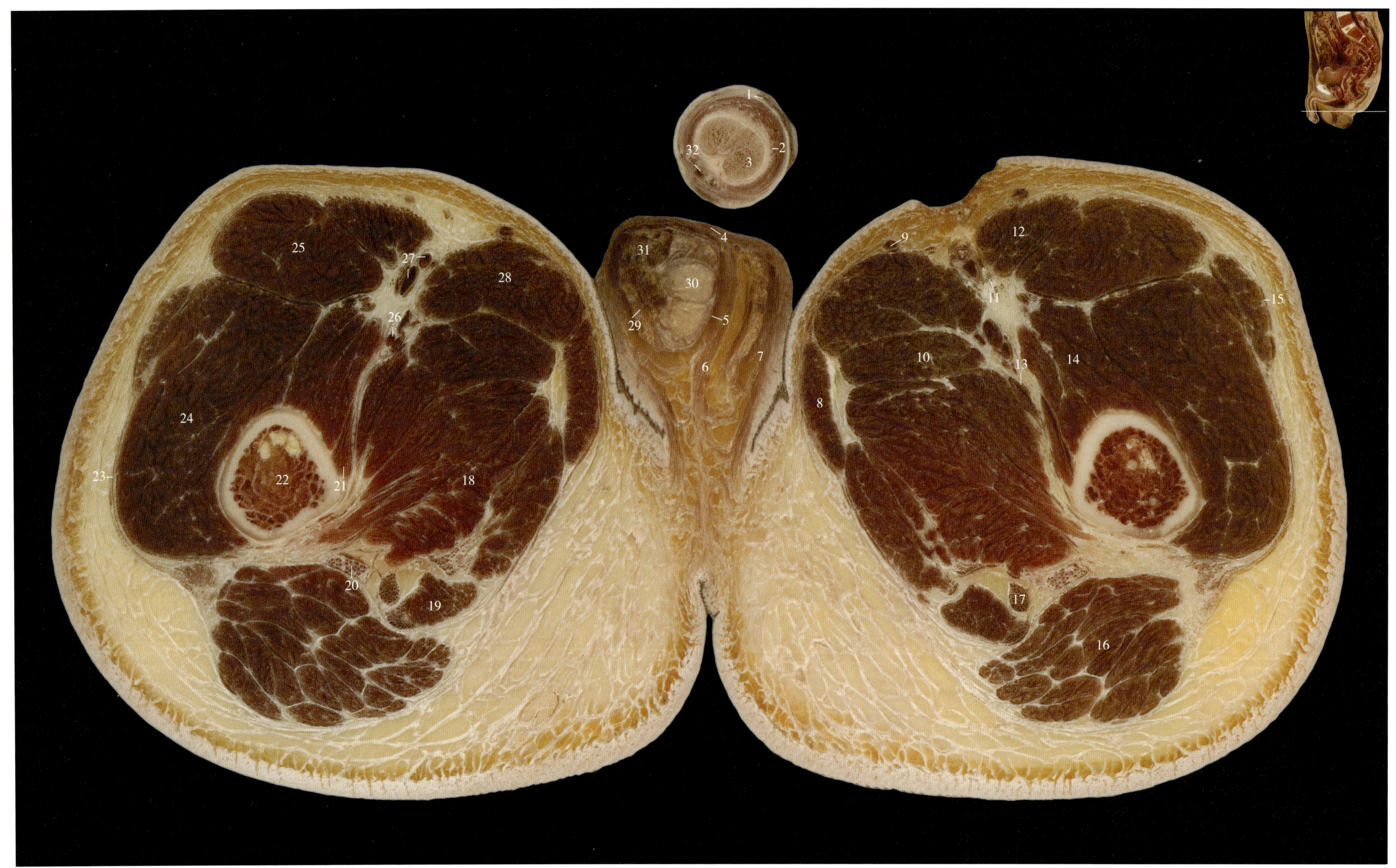

A. 断层标本图像

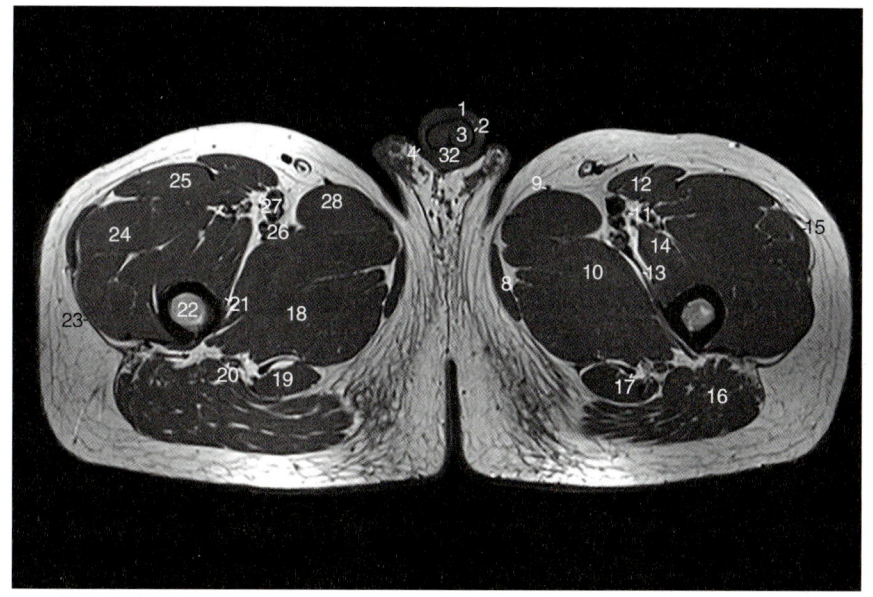
B. MR T1WI

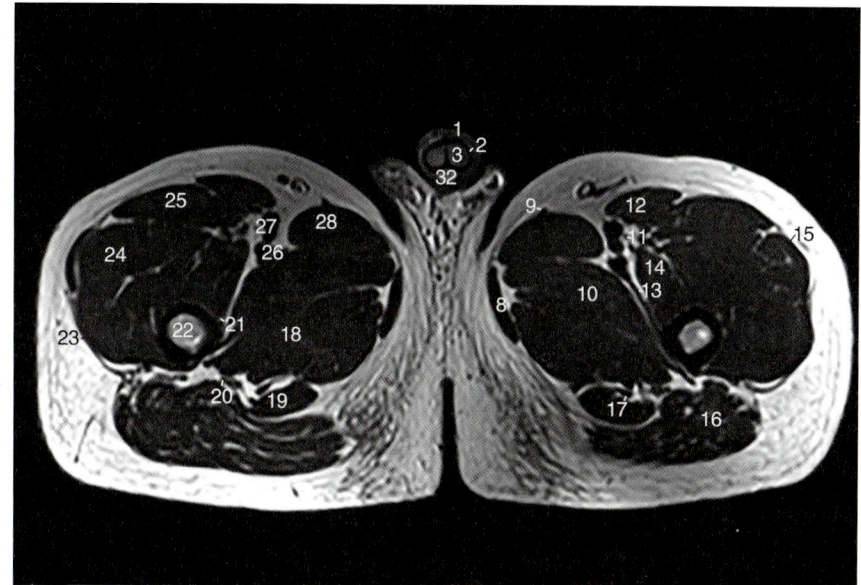
C. MR T2WI

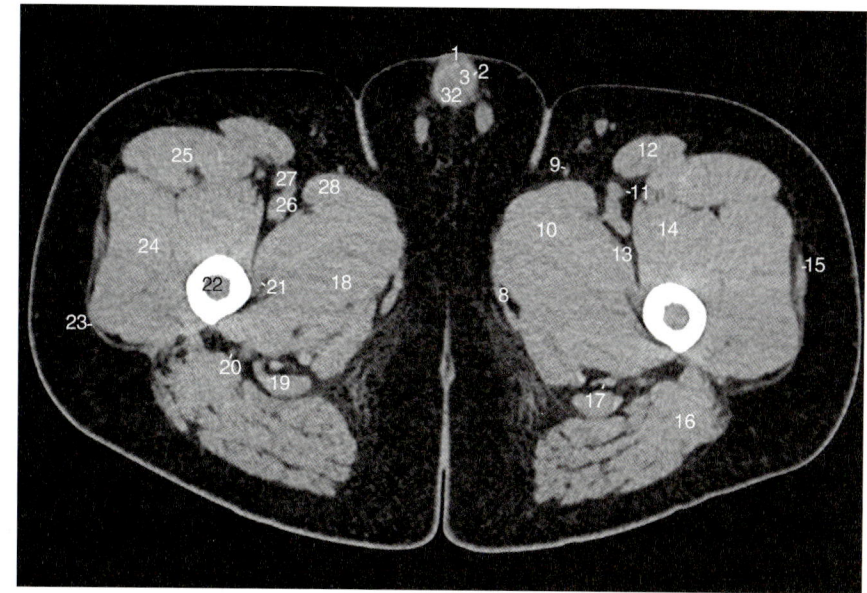
D. CT 平扫图像

1. 阴茎包皮 prepuce of penis
2. 阴茎海绵体白膜 albuginea of cavernous body of penis
3. 阴茎海绵体 cavernous body of penis
4. 肉膜 dartos coat
5. 提睾肌 cremaster
6. 阴囊中隔 septum of scrotum
7. 鞘膜腔 cavity of tunica vaginaalis
8. 股薄肌 gracilis
9. 大隐静脉 great saphenous vein
10. 短收肌 adductor brevis
11. 股神经 femoral nerve
12. 缝匠肌 sartorius
13. 耻骨肌 pectineus
14. 股中间肌 vastus intermedius
15. 阔筋膜张肌 tensor fasciae latae
16. 臀大肌 gluteus maximus
17. 半膜肌 semimembranosus
18. 大收肌 adductor magnus
19. 股二头肌长头和半腱肌 long head of biceps femoris and semitendinosus
20. 坐骨神经 sciatic nerve
21. 髂腰肌 iliopsoas
22. 股骨 femur
23. 阔筋膜 fasciae lata
24. 股外侧肌 vastus lateralis
25. 股直肌 rectus femoris
26. 股深动脉 deep femoral artery
27. 股动、静脉 femoral artery and vein
28. 长收肌 adductor longus
29. 输精管 ductus deferens
30. 睾丸 testis
31. 附睾 epididymis
32. 尿道 urethra

关键结构：阴囊，提睾肌，鞘膜腔。

此断面为经过睾丸上份层面。断面前部可见分离的阴茎头，内见成对的阴茎海绵体，周围有白膜围绕。阴囊由中隔分成左右两部分，右侧阴囊内的结构为附睾、睾丸及鞘膜腔，睾丸切面较上一断面增大，左侧睾丸及附睾尚未出现。阴囊的浅筋膜为肉膜，肉膜深面由外侧向内侧依次为精索外筋膜、提睾肌、精索内筋膜和睾丸鞘膜。提睾肌来自腹内斜肌和腹横肌的肌纤维束[57]。鞘膜腔为脏层睾丸鞘膜与壁层睾丸鞘膜之间的腔隙，内有少量浆液，呈长 T1 信号和长 T2 信号。睾丸鞘膜积液时表现为液体包绕睾丸。阴囊为阴茎根部下垂的皮肤囊袋，内有睾丸、附睾和输精管起始部。阴囊壁由皮肤和肉膜组成，是腹壁皮肤及浅筋膜的延续。肉膜含有平滑肌纤维，该平滑肌随外界温度变化可产生反射性舒缩活动，以调节阴囊内的温度，有利于精子的发育和生存[41]。

男性盆部连续横断层 45（MH.6140）

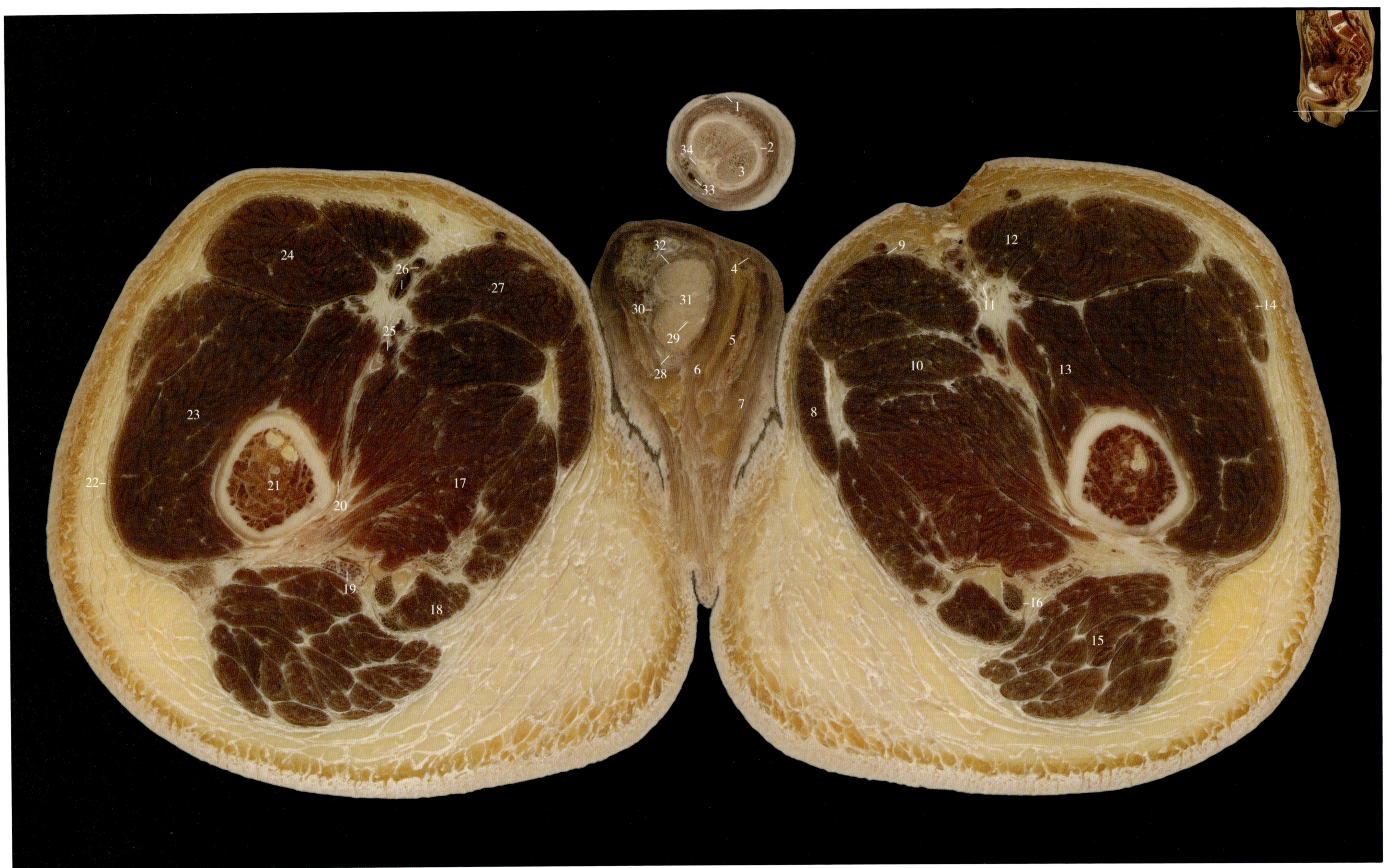

A. 断层标本图像

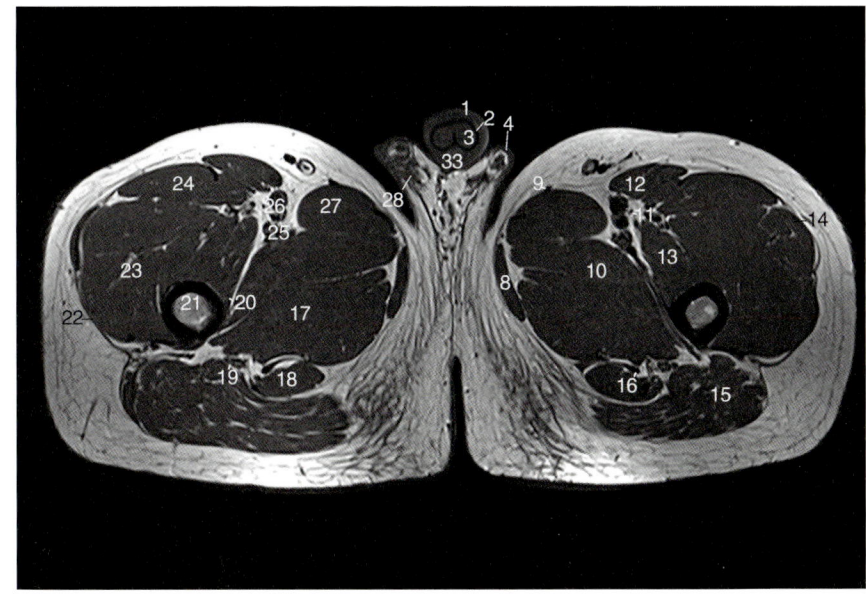
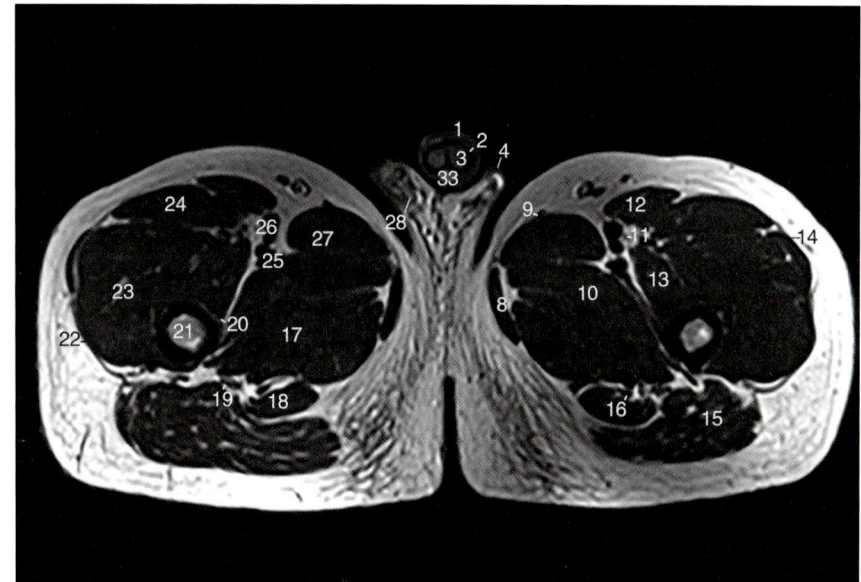
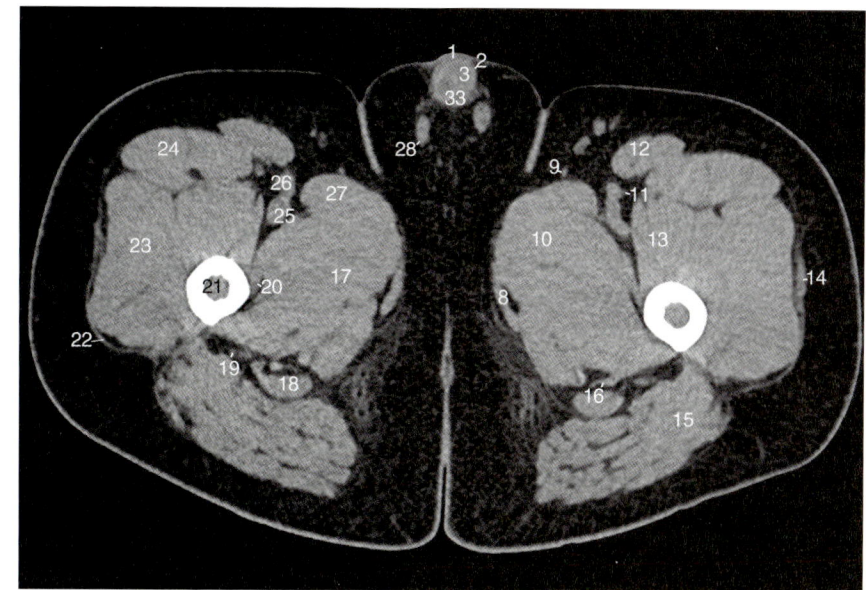

B. MR T1WI　　　　　　　　　　　　C. MR T2WI　　　　　　　　　　　　D. CT 平扫图像

1. 阴茎包皮 prepuce of penis
2. 阴茎海绵体白膜 albuginea of cavernous body of penis
3. 阴茎海绵体 cavernous body of penis
4. 肉膜 dartos coat
5. 提睾肌 cremaster
6. 阴囊中隔 septum of scrotum
7. 鞘膜腔 cavity of tunica vaginaalis
8. 股薄肌 gracilis
9. 大隐静脉 great saphenous vein
10. 短收肌 adductor brevis
11. 股神经 femoral nerve
12. 缝匠肌 sartorius
13. 股中间肌 vastus intermedius
14. 阔筋膜张肌 tensor fasciae latae
15. 臀大肌 gluteus maximus
16. 半膜肌 semimembranosus
17. 大收肌 adductor magnus
18. 股二头肌长头和半腱肌 long head of biceps femoris and semitendinosus
19. 坐骨神经 sciatic nerve
20. 髂腰肌 iliopsoas
21. 股骨 femur
22. 阔筋膜 fasciae lata
23. 股外侧肌 vastus lateralis
24. 股直肌 rectus femoris
25. 股深动脉 deep femoral artery
26. 股动、静脉 femoral artery and vein
27. 长收肌 adductor longus
28. 附睾 epididymis
29. 睾丸小隔 septula testis
30. 睾丸网 rete testis
31. 睾丸 testis
32. 白膜 tunica albuginea
33. 尿道 urethra
34. 阴茎深筋膜 deep fascia of penis

关键结构：附睾，坐骨神经，睾丸。

　　此断面为经过睾丸上份层面。断面前部可见分离的阴茎头，阴茎海绵体成对，周围均有白膜围绕；断面中会阴部的结构主要为皮下组织，其前方可见阴囊，其内为附睾、睾丸及鞘膜腔，附睾体部位于睾丸的背侧。附睾分为头、体、尾三部，头部由输出小管盘曲而成连接着睾丸的曲细精管，紧贴睾丸的上端；输出小管的末端连接一条附睾管，附睾管长 4~5 cm，盘曲构成体部和尾部，紧贴睾丸的后缘，管的末端急转向上直接延续成为输精管，进入精索。附睾管除贮存精子外还能分泌附睾液，助于精子的成熟[12, 52, 57]。在臀大肌下间隙可见粗大的坐骨神经，主干宽度可达 1.5~2 cm，由于是软组织密度，紧贴臀大肌，CT 不易显示；磁共振周围神经成像（MRN）可明确显示，主要采用两种序列：第一是 T2WI 或者重 T2WI；第二则是反映水分子扩散特性的 DWI（扩散加权成像）及 DTI（扩散张量成像）。坐骨神经经梨状肌下孔在臀大肌深面向下行，依次横过上孖肌、闭孔内肌、下孖肌及股方肌的后方并支配这些肌肉，经股骨大转子和坐骨结节之间，下降至股骨背侧[41]。

男性盆部连续横断层 46（MH.6130）

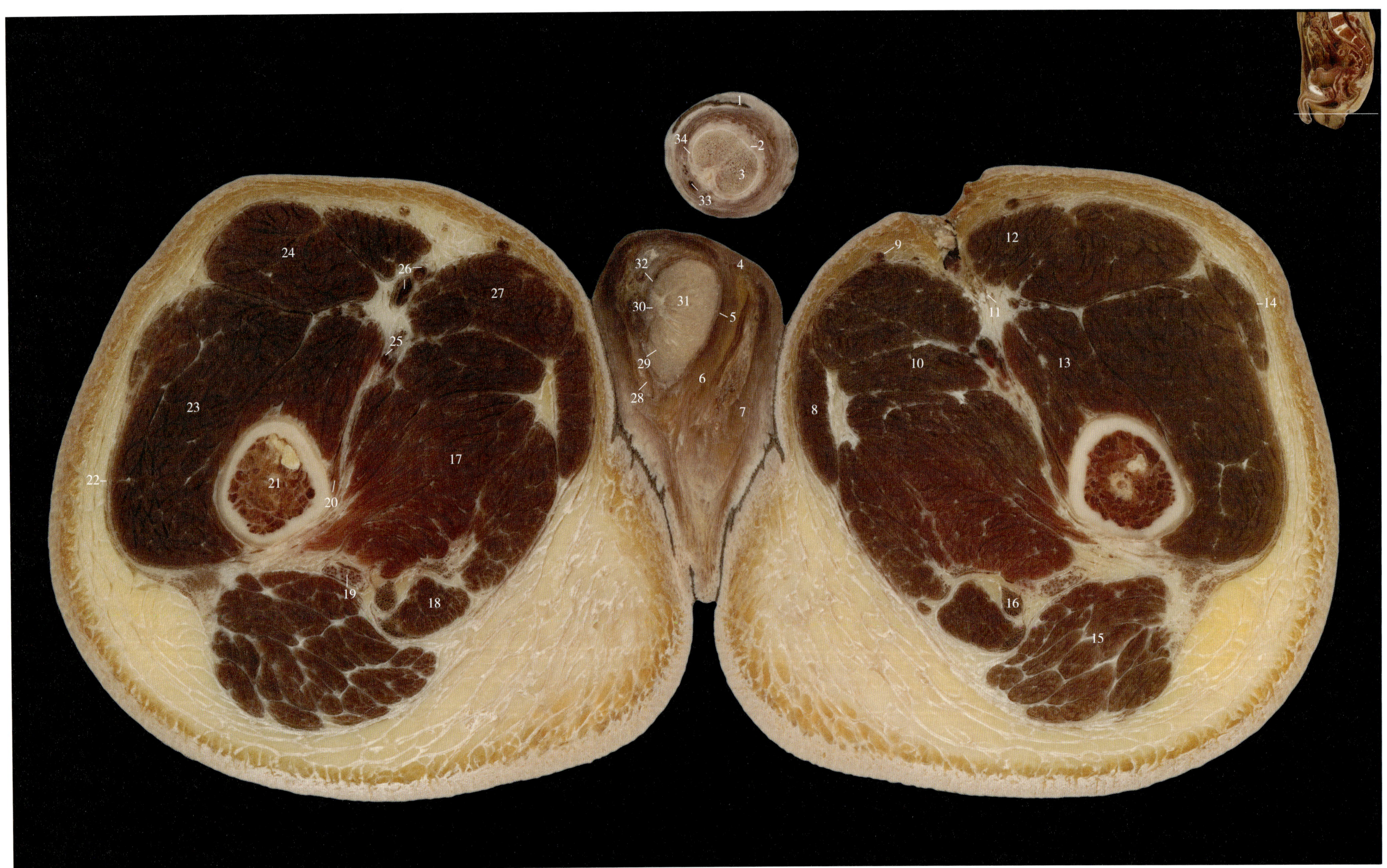

A. 断层标本图像

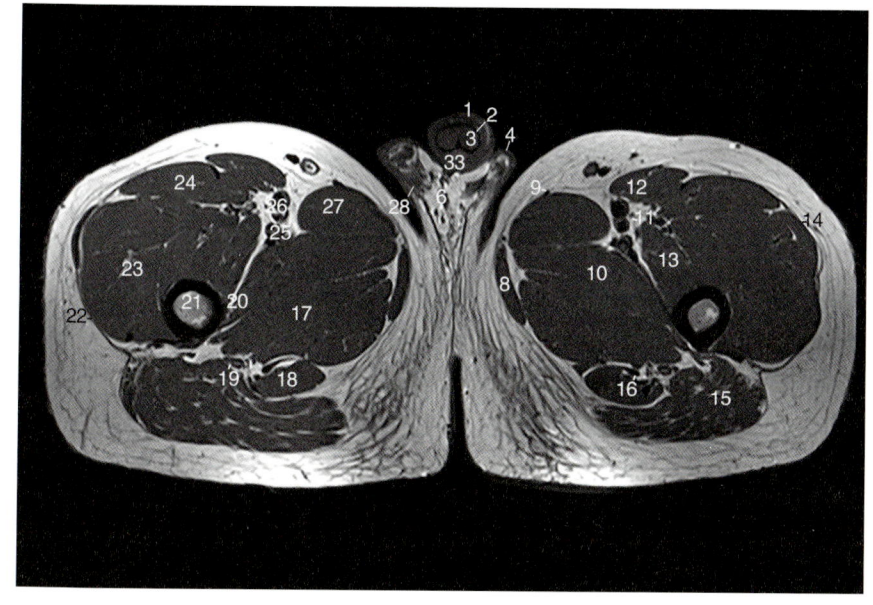

B. MR T1WI

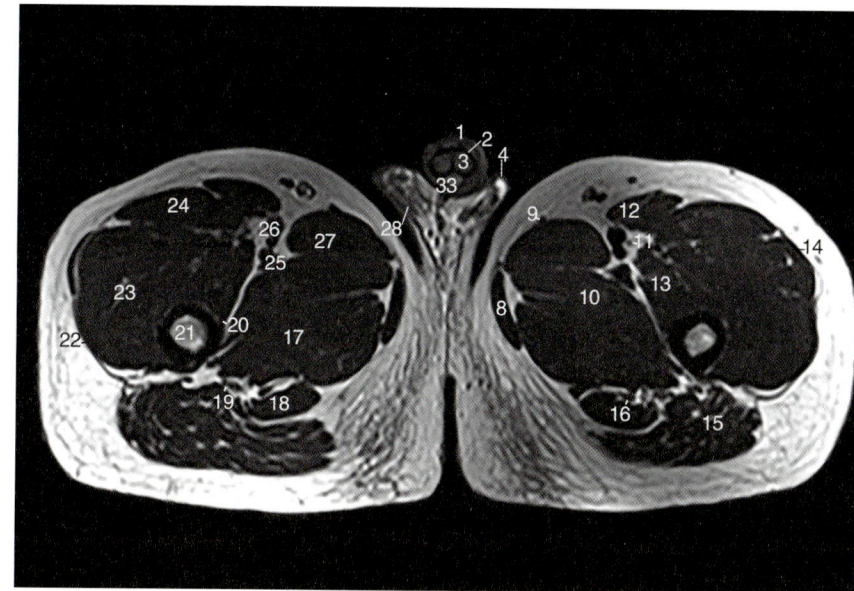

C. MR T2WI

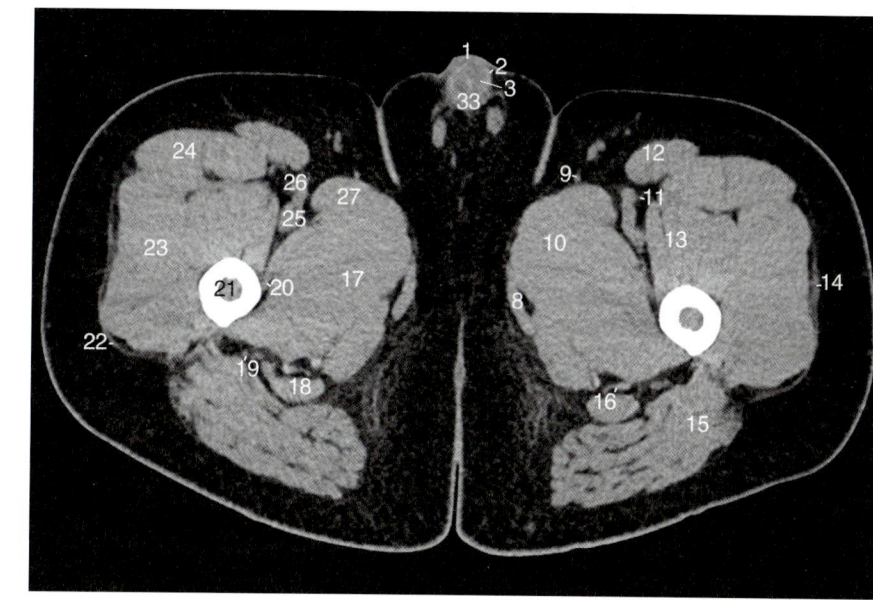

D. CT 平扫图像

1. 阴茎包皮 prepuce of penis
2. 阴茎海绵体白膜 albuginea of cavernous body of penis
3. 阴茎海绵体 cavernous body of penis
4. 肉膜 dartos coat
5. 提睾肌 cremaster
6. 阴囊中隔 septum of scrotum
7. 鞘膜腔 cavity of tunica vaginaalis
8. 股薄肌 gracilis
9. 大隐静脉 great saphenous vein
10. 短收肌 adductor brevis
11. 股神经 femoral nerve
12. 缝匠肌 sartorius
13. 股中间肌 vastus intermedius
14. 阔筋膜张肌 tensor fasciae latae
15. 臀大肌 gluteus maximus
16. 半膜肌 semimembranosus
17. 大收肌 adductor magnus
18. 股二头肌长头和半腱肌 long head of biceps femoris and semitendinosus
19. 坐骨神经 sciatic nerve
20. 髂腰肌 iliopsoas
21. 股骨 femur
22. 阔筋膜 fasciae lata
23. 股外侧肌 vastus lateralis
24. 股直肌 rectus femoris
25. 股深动脉 deep femoral artery
26. 股动、静脉 femoral artery and vein
27. 长收肌 adductor longus
28. 附睾 epididymis
29. 睾丸小隔 septula testis
30. 睾丸网 rete testis
31. 睾丸 testis
32. 白膜 tunica albuginea
33. 尿道 urethra
34. 阴茎深筋膜 deep fascia of penis

关键结构：阴茎，尿道，阴茎海绵体。

此断面经过阴囊下份。断面前部见分离的阴茎头，从外侧向内侧可见包皮、浅筋膜、深筋膜包绕尿道和阴茎海绵体，尿道及阴茎海绵体周围有白膜包绕，并在两个阴茎海绵体间形成间隔，中国男性尿道的长度：全长为 171.81 mm ± 27.14 mm，其中前尿道长为 138.81 mm ± 32.03 mm，后尿道长为 33.05 mm ± 4.96 mm[16]。阴茎分为阴茎根、阴茎体及阴茎头三部分，阴茎根位于会阴部尿生殖三角内，由阴茎海绵体左右侧脚及尿道球组成，附于耻骨弓边缘及尿生殖膈下筋膜上，是阴茎的固定部；中部为阴茎体，呈圆柱形，悬于耻骨联合前下方，为阴茎的可动部；阴茎头也称龟头，为阴茎前端的膨大部，尖端有尿道外口；阴茎头底部的游离缘明显隆起，称阴茎头冠，下方浅沟为冠状沟，其前上面为阴茎背，后下面为阴茎尿道面。阴茎的被膜有皮肤、浅筋膜、深筋膜及白膜。浅筋膜为阴茎的皮下组织，疏松无脂肪，内有阴茎背浅血管和淋巴管，向四周分别移行于阴囊肉膜、会阴浅筋膜（colles筋膜）及腹前外侧壁的浅筋膜深层（scarpa筋膜）。阴茎深筋膜即 Buck 筋膜，近端至阴茎根部向上续于腹白线，在阴茎根部形成阴茎悬韧带，将阴茎悬吊于耻骨联合前面和白线，远端至龟头底部与阴茎海绵体紧密愈着。

男性盆部连续横断层 47（MH.6120）

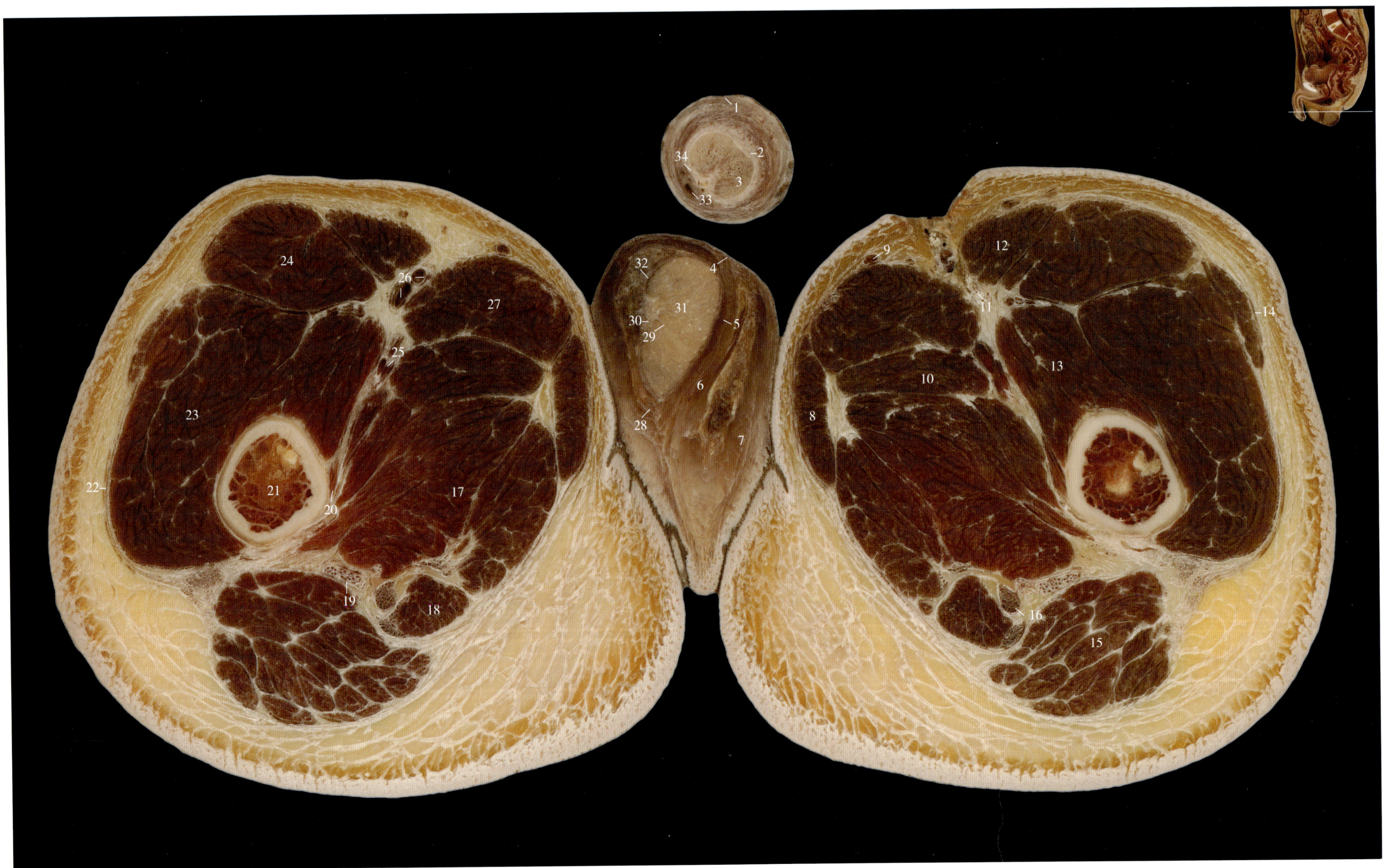

A. 断层标本图像

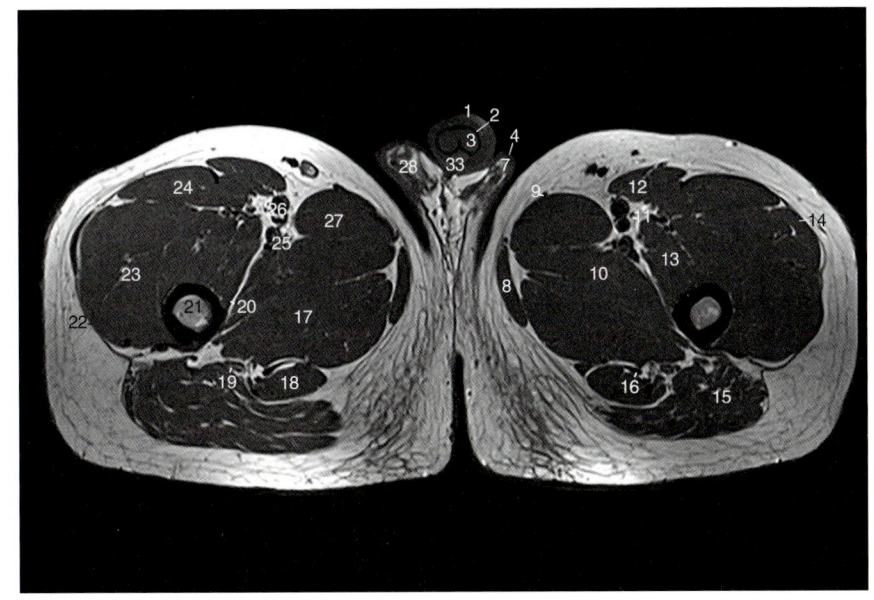

B. MR T1WI

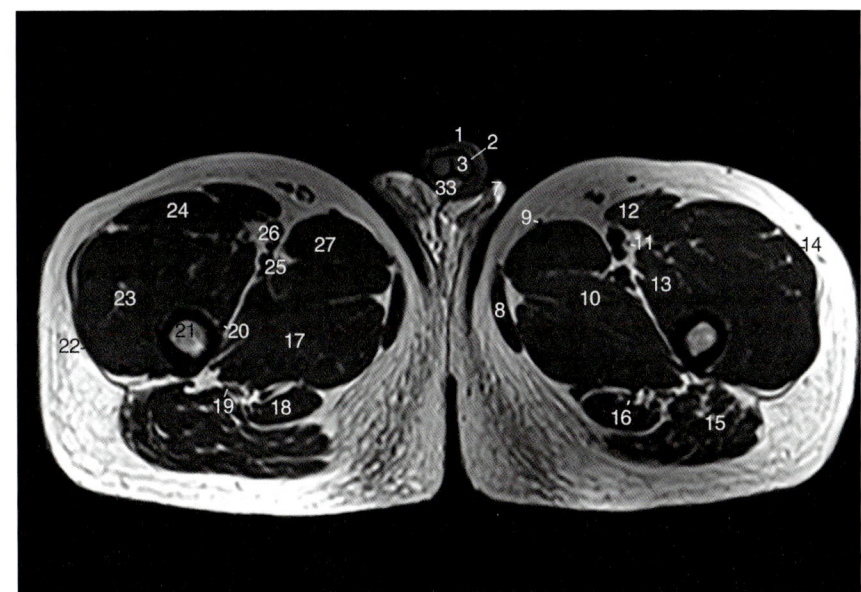

C. MR T2WI

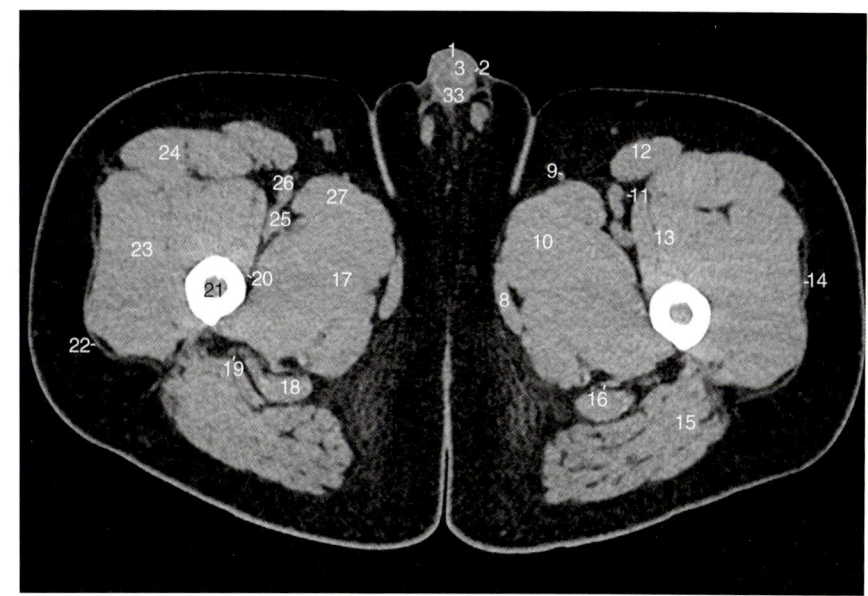

D. CT 平扫图像

关键结构：睾丸网，睾丸白膜，阴茎海绵体。

  此断面经过阴囊下份。断面前部可见分离的阴茎头，成对的阴茎海绵体周围有白膜围绕，之间见白膜形成的分隔，尿道位于阴茎断面的后部。阴茎海绵体白膜为双层结构，导静脉穿行其间，外层在勃起时对导静脉具有压迫作用。不同部位的白膜强度和厚度有明显差异，最脆弱的区域是腹侧沟处，此处外层阙如，因此许多假体植入后由此突出。断面的中份、两股之间为阴囊，阴囊是由两个位于早期阴茎两侧的阴囊组织与尿道背侧的中间基质成分共同发育而成[63]，阴囊内结构为附睾、睾丸及鞘膜腔。睾丸周边为睾丸白膜，在T2WI上呈短低信号薄环。睾丸白膜是睾丸表面的一层厚的致密结缔组织膜，在后缘增厚进入睾丸形成睾丸纵隔，睾丸小隔由纵隔发出，呈扇形伸入睾丸实质并与白膜相连，将实质分为100~200个睾丸小叶。睾丸网由小叶内的生精小管汇合呈精直小管进入睾丸纵隔交织形成。睾丸网发出12~15条睾丸输出小管经睾丸后缘上部进入附睾。睾丸的主要功能是产生精子和分泌雄性激素。睾丸和附睾淋巴引流系统由4~8个集合淋巴管组成。这些淋巴伴行于精索血管，穿过输尿管，然后从肾静脉与主动脉分叉处汇入腰丛淋巴结。在右侧，淋巴管汇入腔静脉后和前淋巴结；在左侧，流入主动脉后、主动脉前和腰丛中间淋巴结。有些淋巴管在到达膀胱腹膜后离开精索血管，侧向弯曲并汇入髂外淋巴结。

1. 阴茎包皮 prepuce of penis
2. 阴茎海绵体白膜 albuginea of cavernous body of penis
3. 阴茎海绵体 cavernous body of penis
4. 肉膜 dartos coat
5. 提睾肌 cremaster
6. 阴囊中隔 septum of scrotum
7. 鞘膜腔 cavity of tunica vaginaalis
8. 股薄肌 gracilis
9. 大隐静脉 great saphenous vein
10. 短收肌 adductor brevis
11. 股神经 femoral nerve
12. 缝匠肌 sartorius
13. 股中间肌 vastus intermedius
14. 阔筋膜张肌 tensor fasciae latae
15. 臀大肌 gluteus maximus
16. 半膜肌 semimembranosus
17. 大收肌 adductor magnus
18. 股二头肌长头和半腱肌 long head of biceps femoris and semitendinosus
19. 坐骨神经 sciatic nerve
20. 髂腰肌 iliopsoas
21. 股骨 femur
22. 阔筋膜 fasciae lata
23. 股外侧肌 vastus lateralis
24. 股直肌 rectus femoris
25. 股深动脉 deep femoral artery
26. 股动、静脉 femoral artery and vein
27. 长收肌 adductor longus
28. 附睾 epididymis
29. 睾丸小隔 septula testis
30. 睾丸网 rete testis
31. 睾丸 testis
32. 白膜 tunica albuginea
33. 尿道 urethra
34. 阴茎深筋膜 deep fascia of penis

283

男性盆部连续横断层 48（MH.6110）

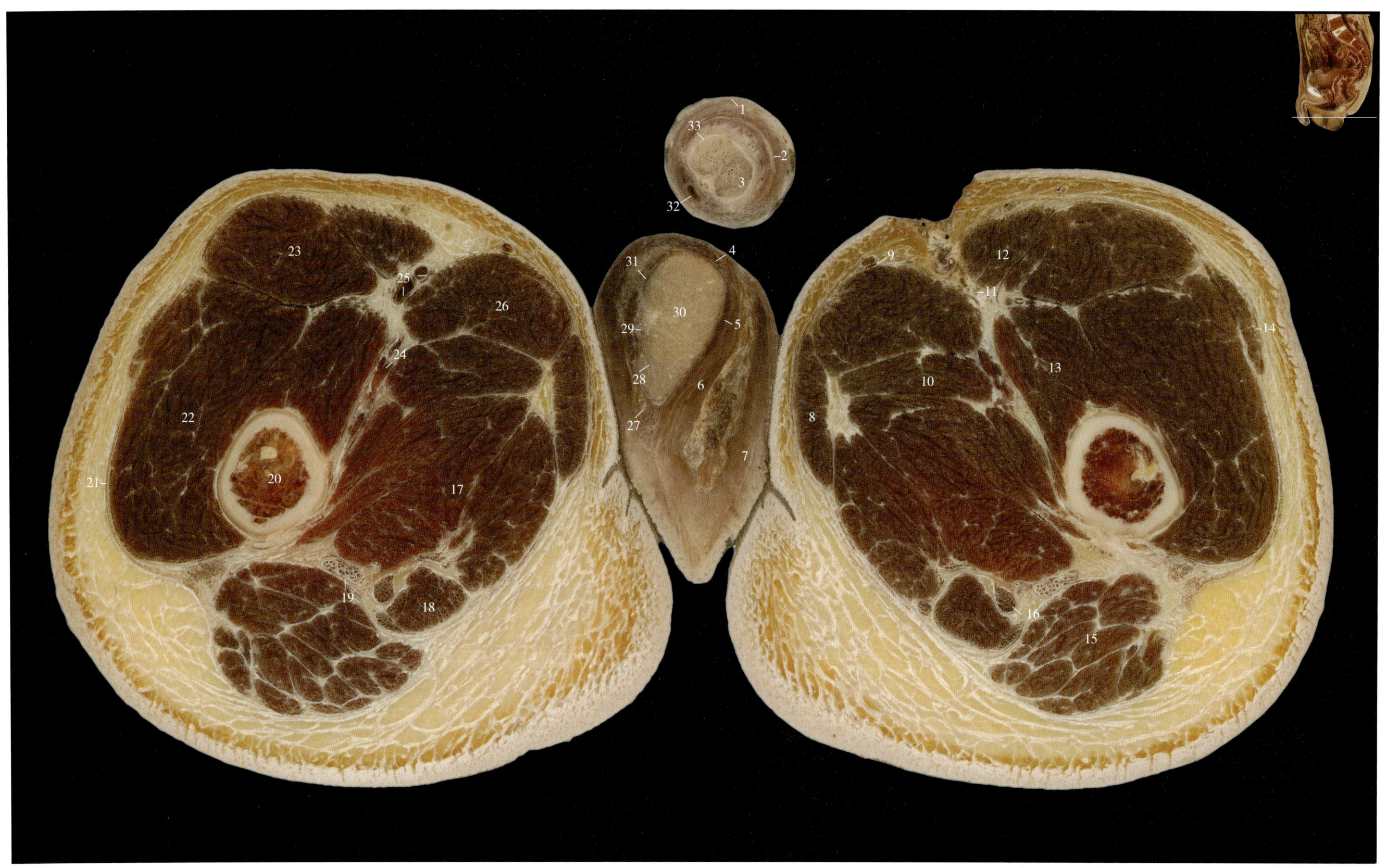

A. 断层标本图像

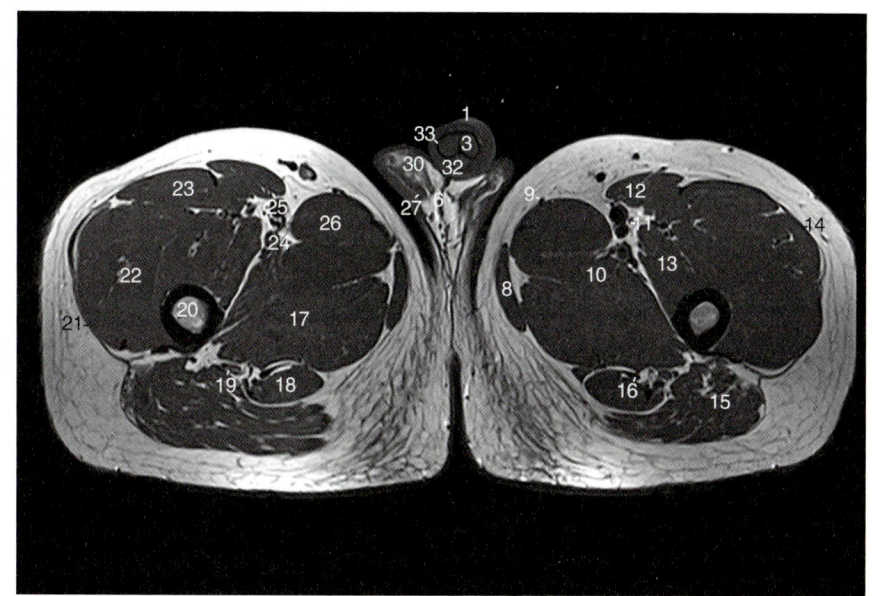
B. MR T1WI

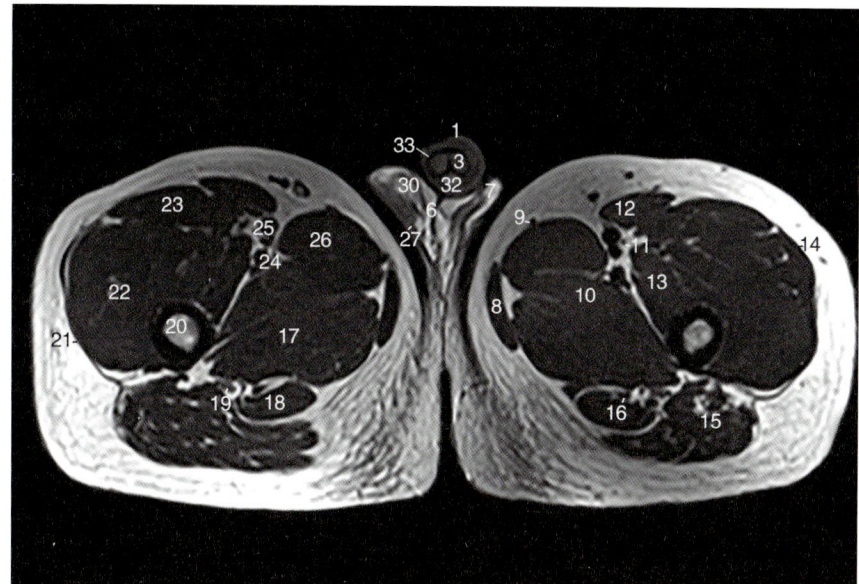
C. MR T2WI

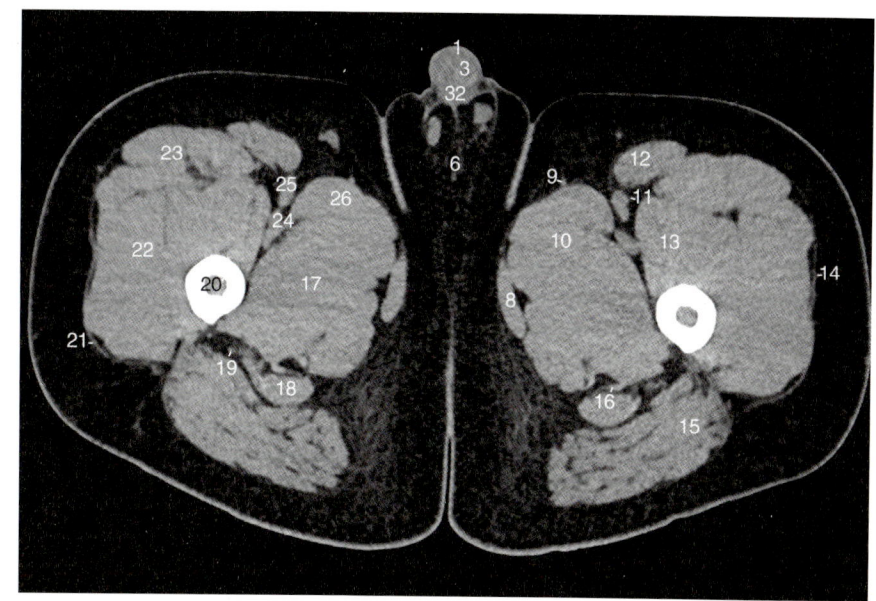
D. CT 平扫图像

关键结构：睾丸，睾丸小隔，睾丸网。

此断面经过右侧睾丸上份。断面前部见阴茎头，成对的阴茎海绵体周围有白膜围绕，之间见白膜形成的分隔，尿道位于阴茎断面的后部。断面的中份、两股之间为阴囊，阴囊内结构为附睾、睾丸及鞘膜腔。该断面左侧睾丸体积较上一断面变大，其外缘处可见睾丸小隔和睾丸网；附睾在睾丸背侧；睾丸内侧见提睾肌，阴囊中隔把阴囊分成左右两侧，该断面左侧睾丸及附睾尚未出现。膀胱、阴道上段、直肠、睾丸的胚胎发生来自腰部，睾丸动脉起自腹主动脉，伴随精索降至阴囊，分布于睾丸和附睾。它的痛觉传入按规律应是沿睾丸动脉的交感神经丛经腹腔丛传入下胸和上腰段脊髓。但现在知道睾丸的交感神经也来自盆丛，沿输精管到睾丸，其内也有痛觉传入纤维，并且可能以其为主，所以慢性睾丸痛可以通过封闭盆丛而缓解。又由于睾丸的传出和传入神经在盆丛左右相通，因此一侧睾丸的肿痛或静脉曲张可影响对侧睾丸的功能[31]。睾丸和附睾的静脉汇合成蔓状静脉丛，经精索进入盆腔后汇合为睾丸静脉，左侧以直角汇入左肾静脉，右侧以锐角汇入下腔静脉[25]。

1. 阴茎包皮 prepuce of penis
2. 尿道海绵体白膜 albuginea of cavernous body of urethra
3. 阴茎海绵体 cavernous body of penis
4. 肉膜 dartos coat
5. 提睾肌 cremaster
6. 阴囊中隔 septum of scrotum
7. 鞘膜腔 cavity of tunica vaginaalis
8. 股薄肌 gracilis
9. 大隐静脉 great saphenous vein
10. 短收肌 adductor brevis
11. 股神经 femoral nerve
12. 缝匠肌 sartorius
13. 股中间肌 vastus intermedius
14. 阔筋膜张肌 tensor fasciae latae
15. 臀大肌 gluteus maximus
16. 半膜肌 semimembranosus
17. 大收肌 adductor magnus
18. 股二头肌长头和半腱肌 long head of biceps femoris and semitendinosus
19. 坐骨神经 sciatic nerve
20. 股骨 femur
21. 阔筋膜 fasciae lata
22. 股外侧肌 vastus lateralis
23. 股直肌 rectus femoris
24. 股深动脉 deep femoral artery
25. 股动、静脉 femoral artery and vein
26. 长收肌 adductor longus
27. 附睾 epididymis
28. 睾丸小隔 septula testis
29. 睾丸网 rete testis
30. 睾丸 testis
31. 白膜 tunica albuginea
32. 尿道 urethra
33. 阴茎海绵体白膜 albuginea of cavernous body of penis

男性盆部连续横断层 49（MH.6100）

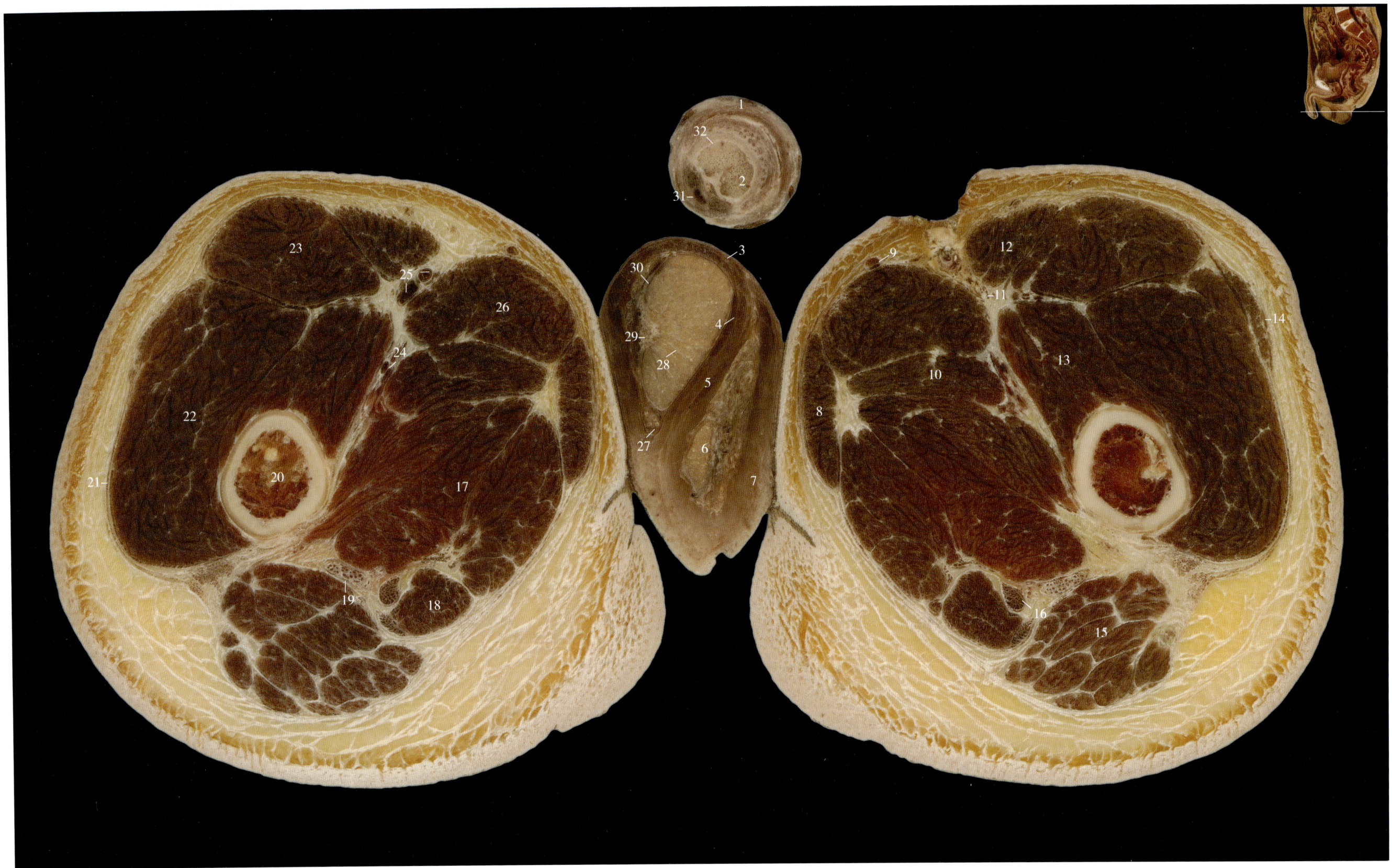

A. 断层标本图像

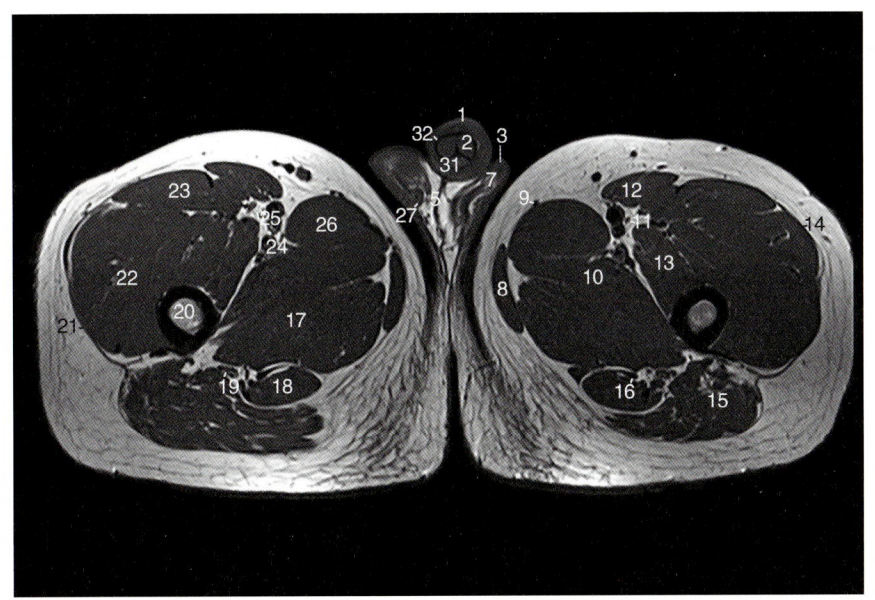
B. MR T1WI

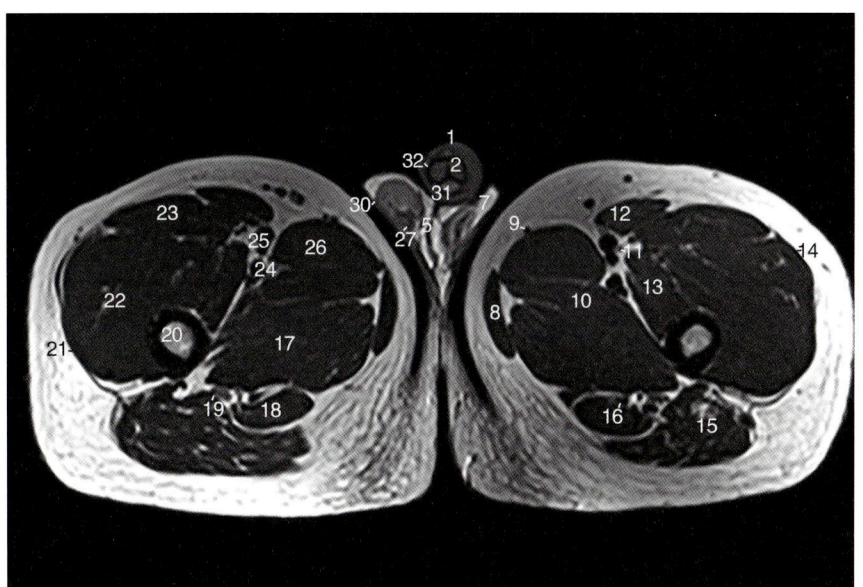
C. MR T2WI

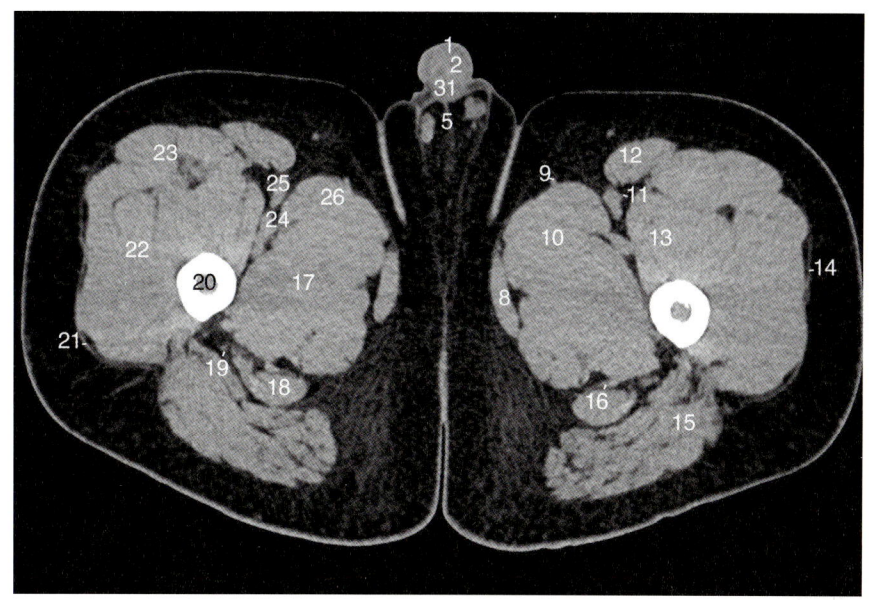
D. CT 平扫图像

1. 阴茎包皮 prepuce of penis
2. 阴茎海绵体 cavernous body of penis
3. 肉膜 dartos coat
4. 提睾肌 cremaster
5. 阴囊中隔 septum of scrotum
6. 睾丸 testis
7. 鞘膜腔 cavity of tunica vaginaalis
8. 股薄肌 gracilis
9. 大隐静脉 great saphenous vein
10. 短收肌 adductor brevis
11. 股神经 femoral nerve
12. 缝匠肌 sartorius
13. 股中间肌 vastus intermedius
14. 阔筋膜张肌 tensor fasciae latae
15. 臀大肌 gluteus maximus
16. 半膜肌 semimembranosus
17. 大收肌 adductor magnus
18. 股二头肌长头和半腱肌 long head of biceps femoris and semitendinosus
19. 坐骨神经 sciatic nerve
20. 股骨 femur
21. 阔筋膜 fasciae lata
22. 股外侧肌 vastus lateralis
23. 股直肌 rectus femoris
24. 股深动脉 deep femoral artery
25. 股动、静脉 femoral artery and vein
26. 长收肌 adductor longus
27. 附睾 epididymis
28. 睾丸小隔 septula testis
29. 睾丸网 rete testis
30. 白膜 tunica albuginea
31. 尿道 urethra
32. 阴茎海绵体白膜 albuginea of cavernous body of penis

关键结构：睾丸鞘膜，睾丸，阴茎海绵体。

　　此断面经过左侧睾丸上端。断面前部可见分离的阴茎头，阴茎从外侧向内侧可见包皮、浅筋膜、深筋膜包绕尿道和阴茎海绵体，尿道及阴茎海绵体周围还有白膜包绕，白膜在两个阴茎海绵体间形成间隔。尿道位于阴茎后方的尿道面。右侧阴囊内结构为附睾、睾丸、提睾肌及鞘膜腔；左侧阴囊内出现睾丸及附睾结构。正常睾丸呈卵圆形结构，T1WI上信号强度低于脂肪而高于水，T2WI上则高于脂肪低于水。一般左侧睾丸略低于右侧睾丸。睾丸呈卵圆形，左右各一，重为20~30g，纵径为4.3~5.1 cm，宽为2.6~3.1 cm，厚为2~3 cm。睾丸在胚胎发育期为腹膜后器官，在出生时睾丸已经腹股沟管下降至阴囊内[16]。在下降过程中把前后两层腹膜作为被覆睾丸的包膜，这两层包膜称为睾丸鞘膜，其间的空隙积存少量液体，称为睾丸鞘膜囊。睾丸内层鞘膜与睾丸的固有膜构成致密厚实的白膜，T2WI上呈明显低信号薄环。断面两侧为股骨和大腿的3个肌群，即前群、后群和内侧群。另外，臀大肌深面可见坐骨神经，长收肌与缝匠肌间脂肪间隙内可见股神经、股动脉及股静脉，股中间肌与短收肌间隙内可见股深动脉。

男性盆部连续横断层 50（MH.6090）

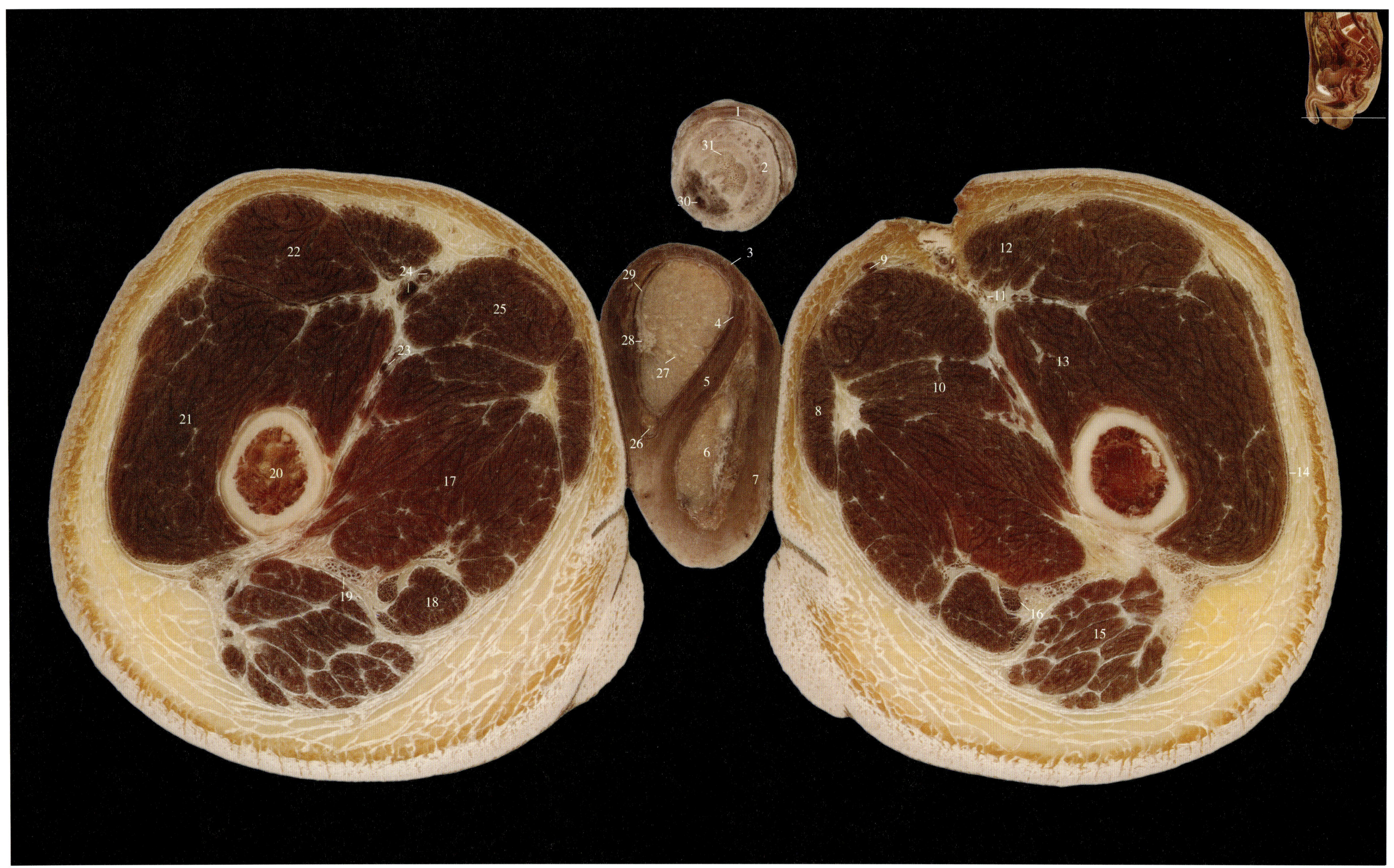

A. 断层标本图像

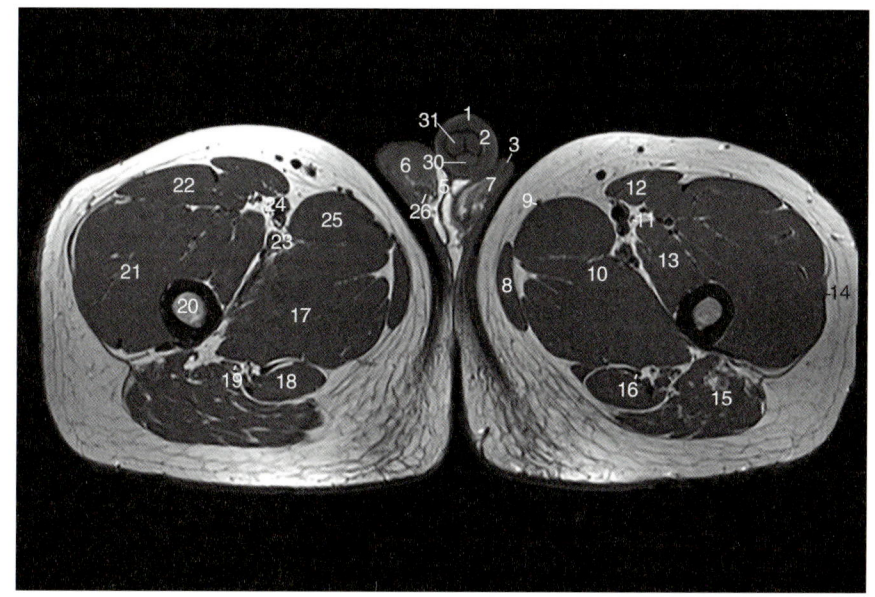

B. MR T1WI

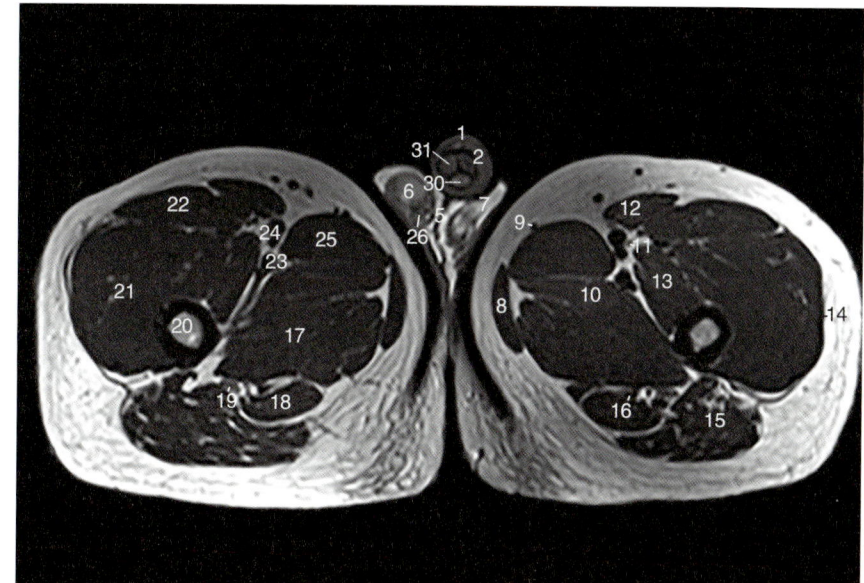

C. MR T2WI

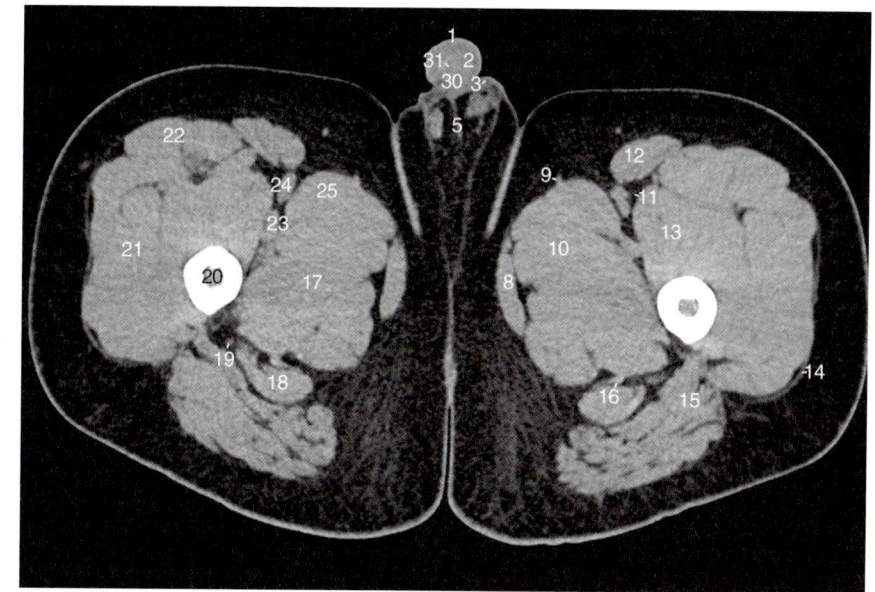

D. CT 平扫图像

1. 阴茎包皮 prepuce of penis
2. 阴茎头 glans penis
3. 肉膜 dartos coat
4. 提睾肌 cremaster
5. 阴囊中隔 septum of scrotum
6. 睾丸 testis
7. 鞘膜腔 cavity of tunica vaginaalis
8. 股薄肌 gracilis
9. 大隐静脉 great saphenous vein
10. 短收肌 adductor brevis
11. 股神经 femoral nerve
12. 缝匠肌 sartorius
13. 股中间肌 vastus intermedius
14. 阔筋膜 fasciae lata
15. 臀大肌 gluteus maximus
16. 半膜肌 semimembranosus
17. 大收肌 adductor magnus
18. 股二头肌长头和半腱肌 long head of biceps femoris and semitendinosus
19. 坐骨神经 sciatic nerve
20. 股骨 femur
21. 股外侧肌 vastus lateralis
22. 股直肌 rectus femoris
23. 股深动脉 deep femoral artery
24. 股动、静脉 femoral artery and vein
25. 长收肌 adductor longus
26. 附睾 epididymis
27. 睾丸小隔 septula testis
28. 睾丸网 rete testis
29. 白膜 tunica albuginea
30. 尿道 urethra
31. 阴茎海绵体 cavernous body of penis

关键结构：附睾静脉，附睾，睾丸。

此断面经过左侧睾丸上份。

断面前部可见分离的阴茎头及阴茎包皮。阴茎海绵体较上一断面略变小，周围有白膜围绕其后方的尿道；右侧阴囊内结构为附睾、睾丸、提睾肌及鞘膜腔；左侧阴囊内睾丸面积较上一断面变大。T2WI上，因睾丸、阴茎海绵体及尿道海绵体含水丰富，呈高信号，白膜呈环形低信号。睾丸动脉起自腹主动脉，伴随精索降至阴囊，分布于睾丸和附睾。睾丸和附睾的静脉汇合成蔓状静脉丛，经精索进入盆腔后汇合为睾丸静脉，左侧以直角汇入左肾静脉，右侧以锐角汇入下腔静脉。生殖股神经在腹股沟韧带上方分为生殖支和股支，生殖支于腹股沟管深环进入该管，随管内结构分布于提睾肌和阴囊。在此断面，双侧大腿肌肉大致对称，事实上，肌肉体积在分析个人身体表现和疾病或年龄相关的肌肉形态学改变中至关重要，但是，很少有准确的参考数据。有学者利用MRI对健康青年志愿者双侧大腿肌肉群进行体积的研究发现，优势侧的臀大肌、臀小肌、闭孔内肌、股薄肌、腘肌、缝匠肌、股内侧肌、短收肌、大收肌、耻骨肌、半膜肌和下肢深后肌群肌肉体积均大于非优势侧[60]。

男性盆部连续横断层 51（MH.6080）

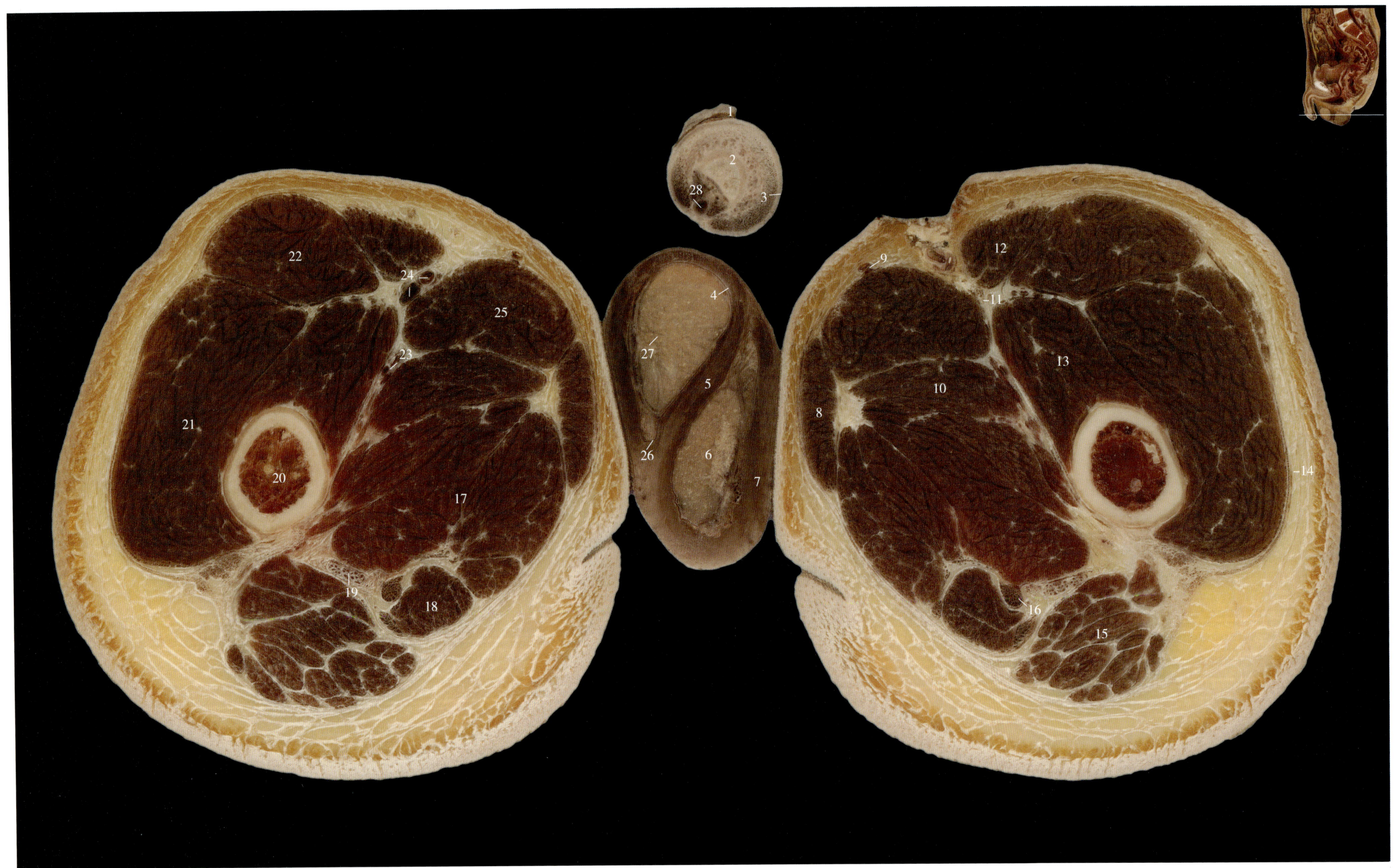

A. 断层标本图像

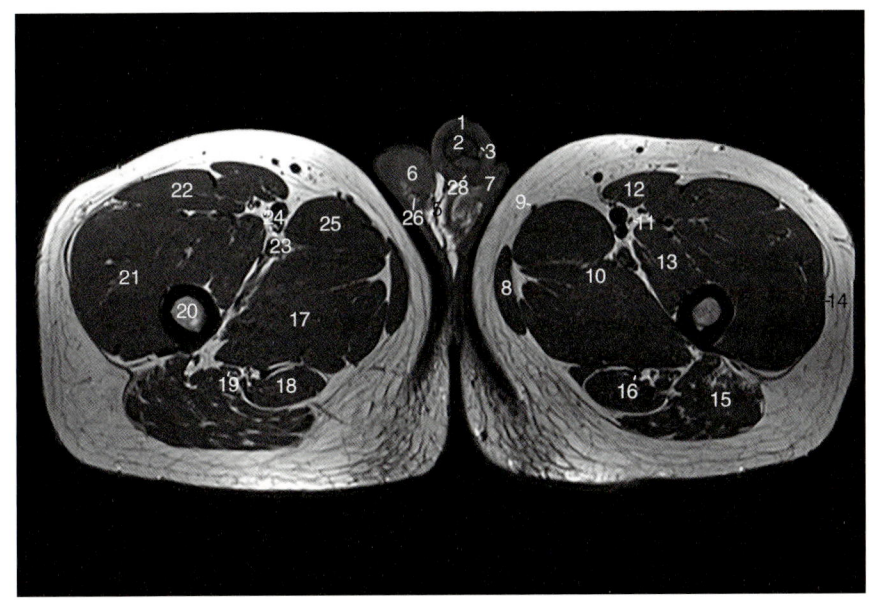

B. MR T1WI

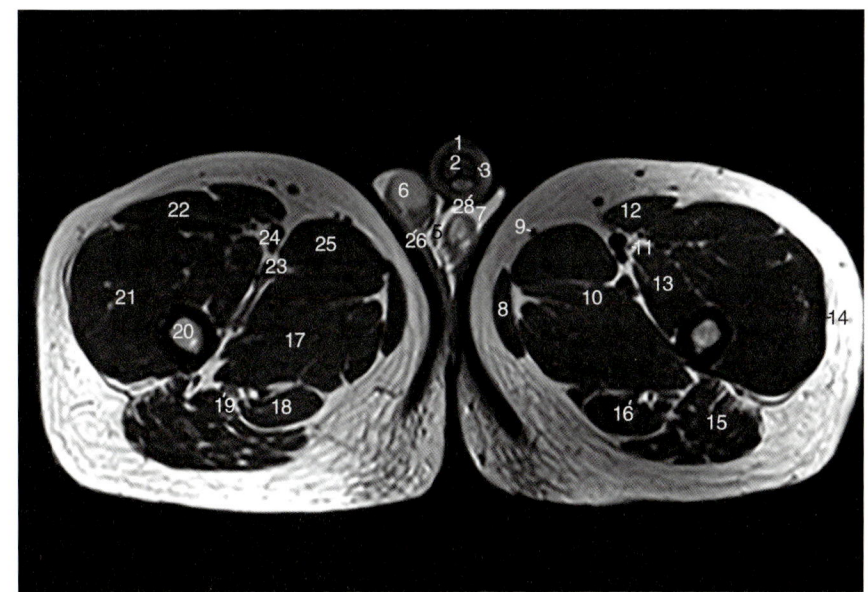

C. MR T2WI

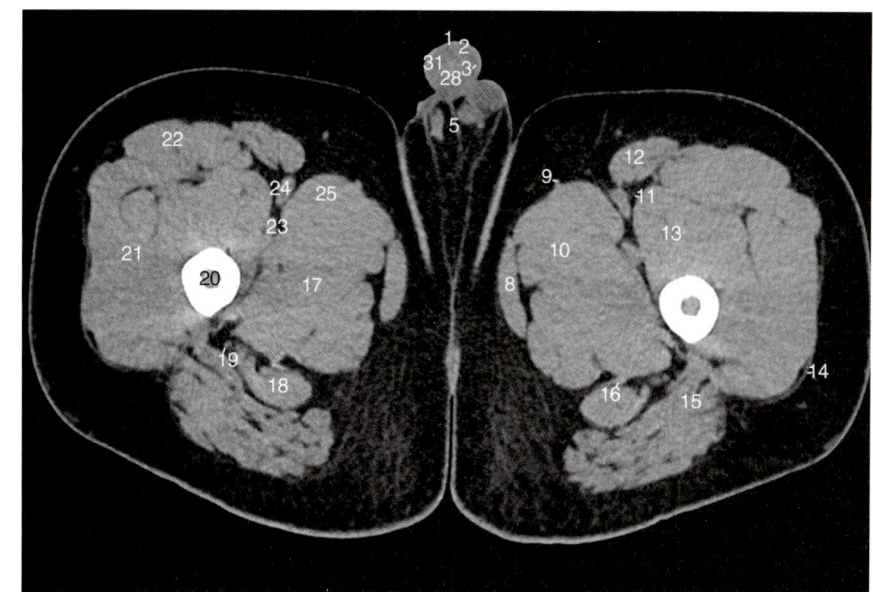

D. CT 平扫图像

1. 阴茎包皮 prepuce of penis
2. 阴茎头 glans penis
3. 尿道海绵体白膜 albuginea of cavernous body of urethra
4. 提睾肌 cremaster
5. 阴囊中隔 septum of scrotum
6. 睾丸 testis
7. 鞘膜腔 cavity of tunica vaginaalis
8. 股薄肌 gracilis
9. 大隐静脉 great saphenous vein
10. 短收肌 adductor brevis
11. 股神经 femoral nerve
12. 缝匠肌 sartorius
13. 股中间肌 vastus intermedius
14. 阔筋膜 fasciae lata
15. 臀大肌 gluteus maximus
16. 半膜肌 semimembranosus
17. 大收肌 adductor magnus
18. 股二头肌长头和半腱肌 long head of biceps femoris and semitendinosus
19. 坐骨神经 sciatic nerve
20. 股骨 femur
21. 股外侧肌 vastus lateralis
22. 股直肌 rectus femoris
23. 股深动脉 deep femoral artery
24. 股动、静脉 femoral artery and vein
25. 长收肌 adductor longus
26. 附睾 epididymis
27. 睾丸小隔 septula testis
28. 尿道舟状窝 navicular fossa of urethra

关键结构：附睾，睾丸，提睾肌。

此断面经过左侧睾丸上份。

断面前部可见分离的阴茎头，阴茎头内的尿道扩大成尿道舟状窝，为男性尿道三个膨大之一。双侧阴囊内结构均为附睾、睾丸、提睾肌及鞘膜腔，中国成人男性附睾的各径：头尾长度左侧为 4.50 cm ± 0.53 cm；右侧为 4.53 cm ± 0.53 cm。附睾头端宽度左侧为 0.86 cm ± 0.14 cm；右侧为 0.85 cm ± 0.13 cm。附睾下端宽度左侧为 0.69 cm ± 0.12 cm；右侧为 0.70 cm ± 0.13 cm[16]；左侧阴囊内睾丸面积较上一断面变大。阴茎结构在磁共振 T2WI 上，层次结构清晰，阴茎海绵体及尿道海绵体含水丰富，呈高信号，白膜呈环形低信号，阴茎病变时结构失常、信号异常，并可明确识别淋巴结转移；阴茎癌侵犯阴茎海绵体时，T2WI 上病变相对于阴茎体呈低信号，III 期病灶扩散至腹股沟淋巴结、IV 期累及深部盆腔淋巴结。当腹股沟淋巴结短径超过 7 mm、盆腔淋巴结短径超过 6 mm 时，即考虑淋巴结转移[3]。阴囊和阴茎的皮肤淋巴管和会阴淋巴管彼此吻合。包皮的内表面和外表面的淋巴管向背侧汇聚，与皮肤的淋巴管汇合，形成数个集合淋巴管回流到耻骨区，沿着股管并汇入腹股沟浅淋巴结。阴茎头的丰富的淋巴管汇聚到系带，在那里与尿道的淋巴管吻合，沿着阴茎筋膜下紧靠背深静脉，通常穿过股管并汇入同侧浅表的腹股沟淋巴结。也有少量的淋巴流入内侧腔隙或引流至腹股沟深部淋巴结。海绵体也可能表现出相同的淋巴引流。

男性盆部连续横断层 52（MH.6070）

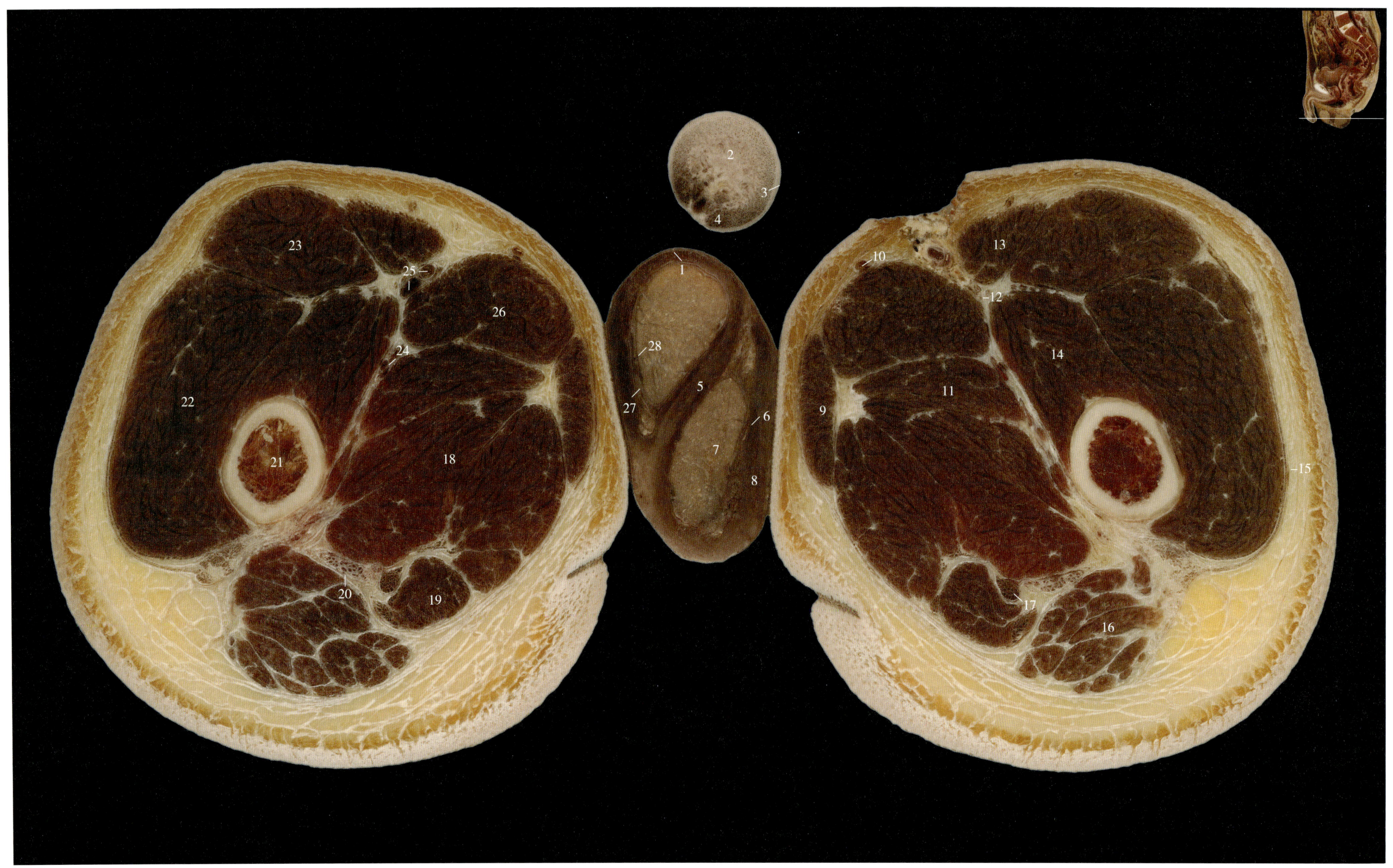

A. 断层标本图像

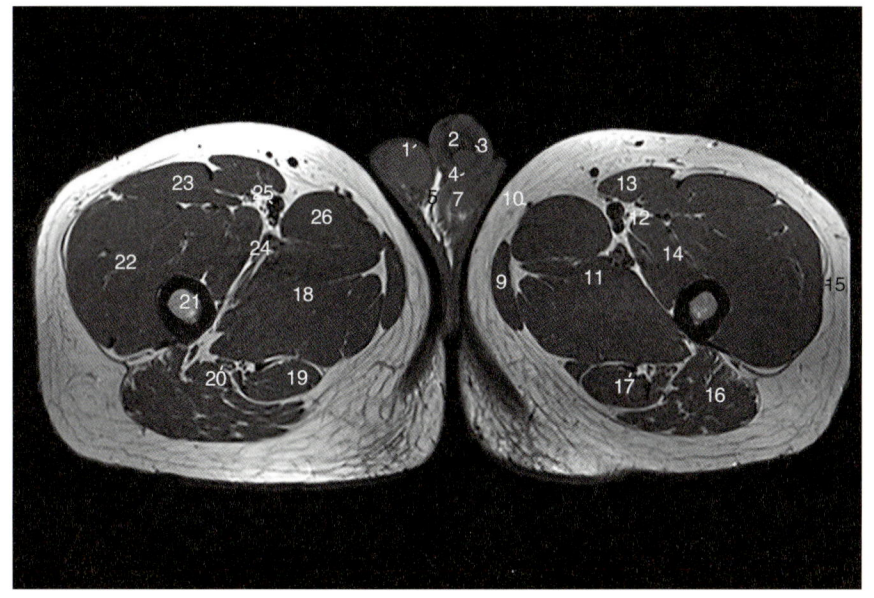

B. MR T1WI

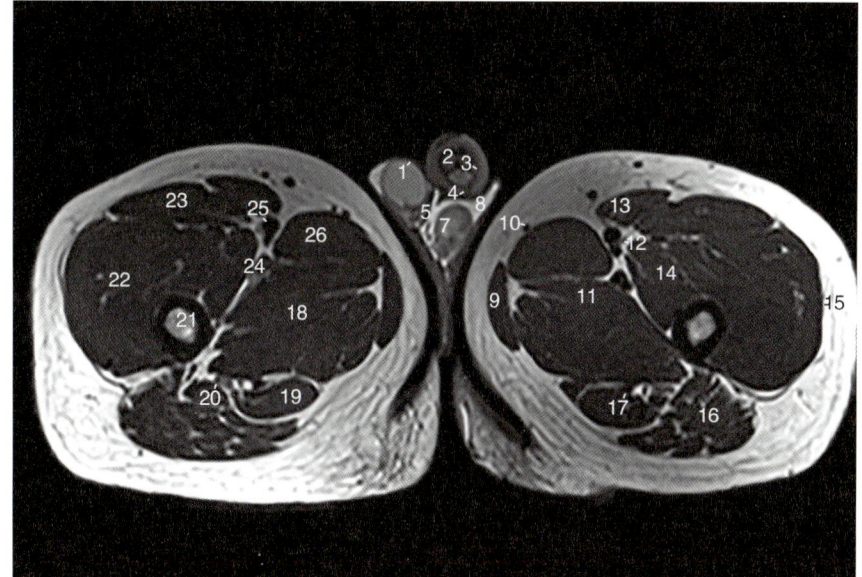

C. MR T2WI

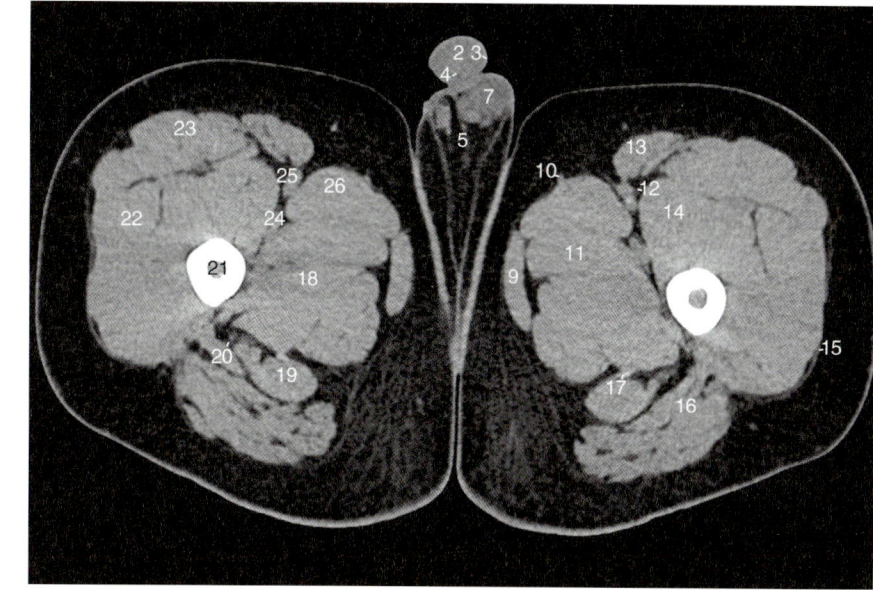

D. CT 平扫图像

关键结构：阴囊，睾丸，鞘膜腔。

此断面经过右侧睾丸下份。断面前部可见分离的阴茎头，在阴茎头处的尿道扩大成尿道舟状窝。断面中部、两股之间为阴囊，阴囊内结构可见睾丸及鞘膜腔，右侧睾丸已达下份。阴囊壁由皮肤和肉膜组成。阴囊的皮肤薄而柔软，有少量阴毛，色素沉着明显。肉膜为浅筋膜，与腹前外侧壁的 Scarpa 筋膜和会阴部的 Colles 筋膜相延续，肉膜内含有平滑肌纤维，可随外界温度的变化而舒缩，以调节阴囊内的温度，利于精子的发育和生存；阴囊肉膜深面由外侧向内侧依次为精索外筋膜、提睾肌、精索内筋膜和睾丸鞘膜。T2WI 上，阴茎海绵体断面明显缩小，信号减低，左侧睾丸出现，呈高信号，白膜呈环形低信号。

1. 肉膜 dartos coat
2. 阴茎头 glans penis
3. 尿道海绵体白膜 albuginea of cavernous body of urethra
4. 尿道舟状窝 navicular fossa of urethra
5. 阴囊中隔 septum of scrotum
6. 提睾肌 cremaster
7. 睾丸 testis
8. 鞘膜腔 cavity of tunica vaginaalis
9. 股薄肌 gracilis
10. 大隐静脉 great saphenous vein
11. 短收肌 adductor brevis
12. 股神经 femoral nerve
13. 缝匠肌 sartorius
14. 股中间肌 vastus intermedius
15. 阔筋膜 fasciae lata
16. 臀大肌 gluteus maximus
17. 半膜肌 semimembranosus
18. 大收肌 adductor magnus
19. 股二头肌长头和半腱肌 long head of biceps femoris and semitendinosus
20. 坐骨神经 sciatic nerve
21. 股骨 femur
22. 股外侧肌 vastus lateralis
23. 股直肌 rectus femoris
24. 股深动脉 deep femoral artery
25. 股动、静脉 femoral artery and vein
26. 长收肌 adductor longus
27. 精索外筋膜 external spermatic fascia
28. 精索内筋膜 internal spermatic fascia

男性盆部连续横断层 53（MH.6060）

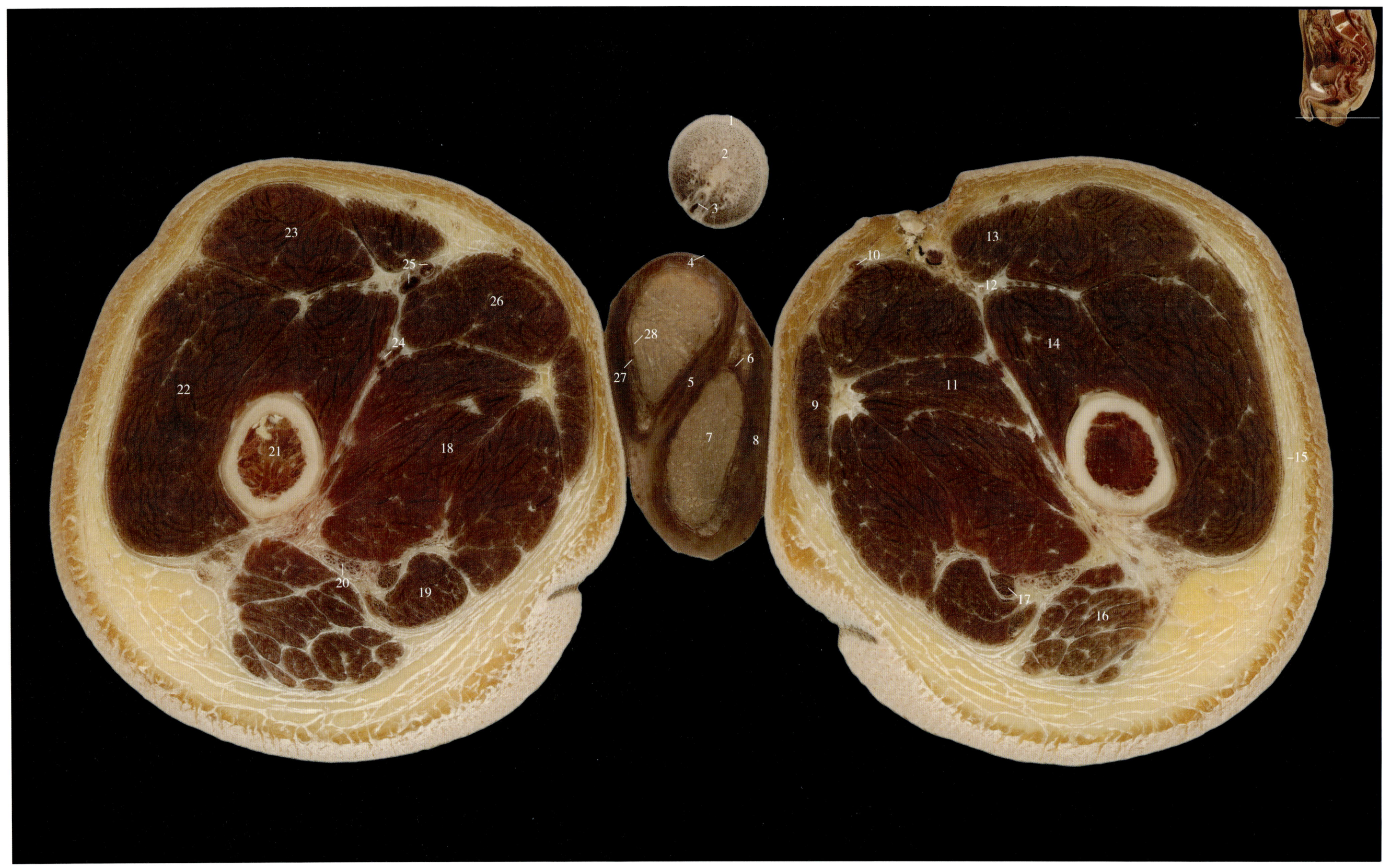

A. 断层标本图像

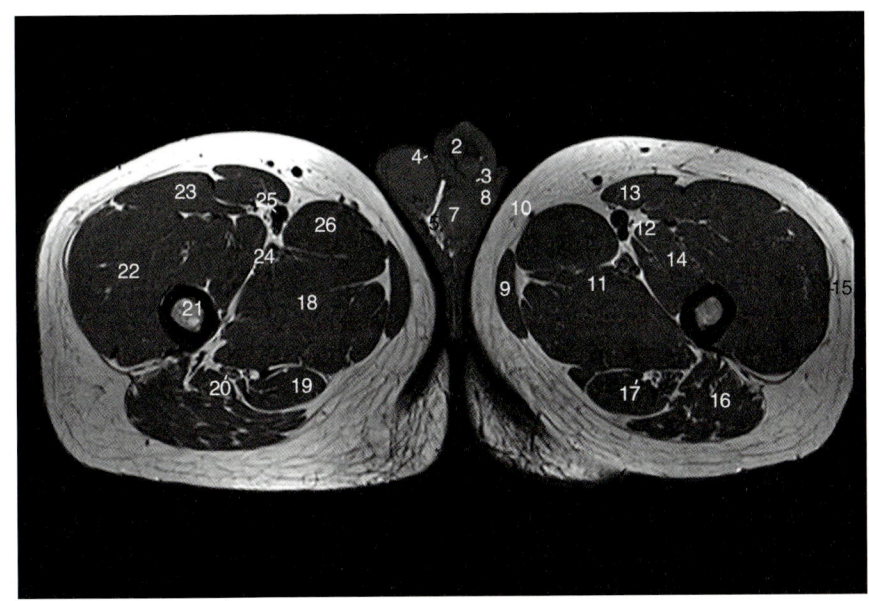
B. MR T1WI

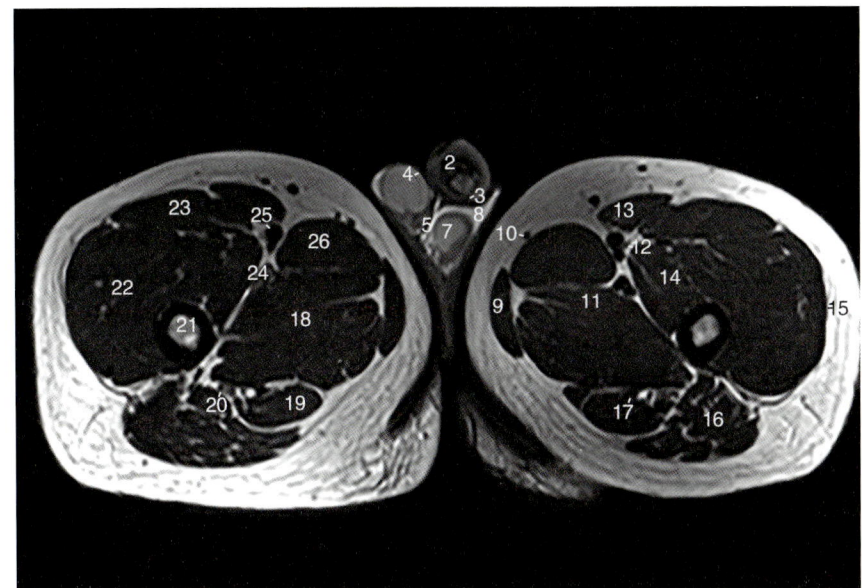
C. MR T2WI

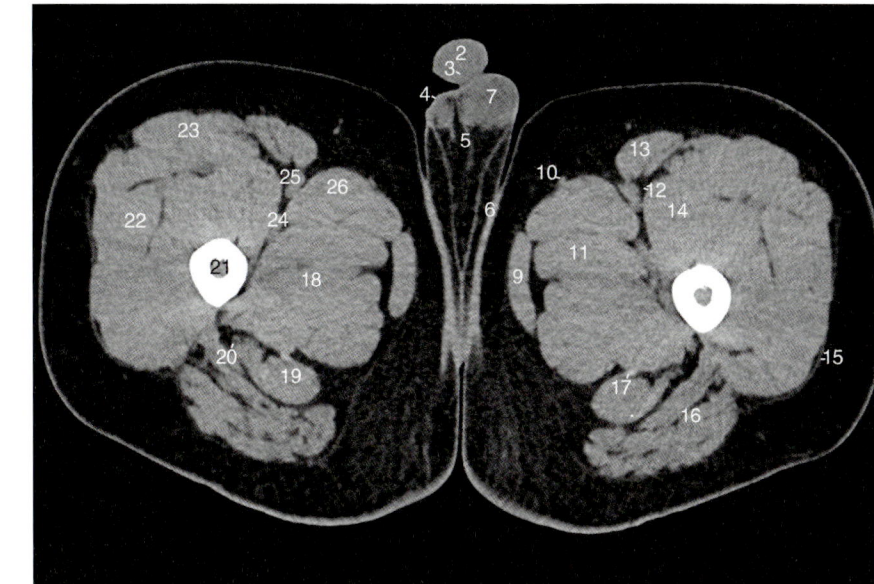
D. CT 平扫图像

关键结构：睾丸，睾丸白膜，鞘膜腔。

1. 尿道海绵体白膜 albuginea of cavernous body of urethra
2. 阴茎头 glans penis
3. 尿道 urethra
4. 肉膜 dartos coat
5. 阴囊中隔 septum of scrotum
6. 提睾肌 cremaster
7. 睾丸 testis
8. 鞘膜腔 cavity of tunica vaginaalis
9. 股薄肌 gracilis
10. 大隐静脉 great saphenous vein
11. 短收肌 adductor brevis
12. 股神经 femoral nerve
13. 缝匠肌 sartorius
14. 股中间肌 vastus intermedius
15. 阔筋膜 fasciae lata
16. 臀大肌 gluteus maximus
17. 半膜肌 semimembranosus
18. 大收肌 adductor magnus
19. 股二头肌长头和半腱肌 long head of biceps femoris and semitendinosus
20. 坐骨神经 sciatic nerve
21. 股骨 femur
22. 股外侧肌 vastus lateralis
23. 股直肌 rectus femoris
24. 股深动脉 deep femoral artery
25. 股动、静脉 femoral artery and vein
26. 长收肌 adductor longus
27. 精索外筋膜 external spermatic fascia
28. 精索内筋膜 internal spermatic fascia

此断面经过左侧睾丸中份。断面前部可见分离的阴茎头，阴茎头断面的后缘见尿道。阴囊内结构为睾丸及鞘膜腔，左侧睾丸断面增大，已达中份，右侧睾丸断面变小，达下份；阴囊肉膜深面由外侧向内侧依次为精索外筋膜、提睾肌、精索内筋膜和睾丸鞘膜。T2WI上，阴茎海绵体断面进一步缩小，信号减低，尿道海绵体呈高信号，左侧睾丸断面增大，呈高信号，白膜呈低信号。睾丸发生于腹腔后壁，以后随胚体的发育逐渐下移，降至阴囊。正常者于孕 28~36 周睾丸进入阴囊；如发育受阻，睾丸可停留在腹膜后间隙或腹股沟管内，也可能伴有睾丸结构的异常。若出生后 3~5 个月内睾丸仍未降至阴囊，即为隐睾症。隐睾的出现率约为 0.48%，早产儿发病率高达 30%[64]。其中单侧隐睾 80.00%，左、右侧之比约为 1:1.5，双侧隐睾 20.00%。其中腹股沟管型占 81.43%，腹腔型占 14.76%，皮下环型占 3.81%。先天性单侧睾丸阙如占隐睾占 5.4%，其中左、右侧之比约为 3:1[16]。在超声检查中，阴囊内不能探及睾丸，可于同侧腹股沟探及未降睾丸。声像图表现为较正常睾丸稍小的卵圆形实质性结构，形态与正常侧睾丸相似，轮廓清晰，边界光整，内部回声分布与正常睾丸无异，呈均匀分布的细小点状实性低回声结构，但隐睾无正常睾丸的可压缩性及其周围的液性暗区。隐睾的睾丸常萎缩并可钙化。CDFI 表现为隐睾症的睾丸内部的血流信号较少。

男性盆部连续横断层 54（MH.6050）

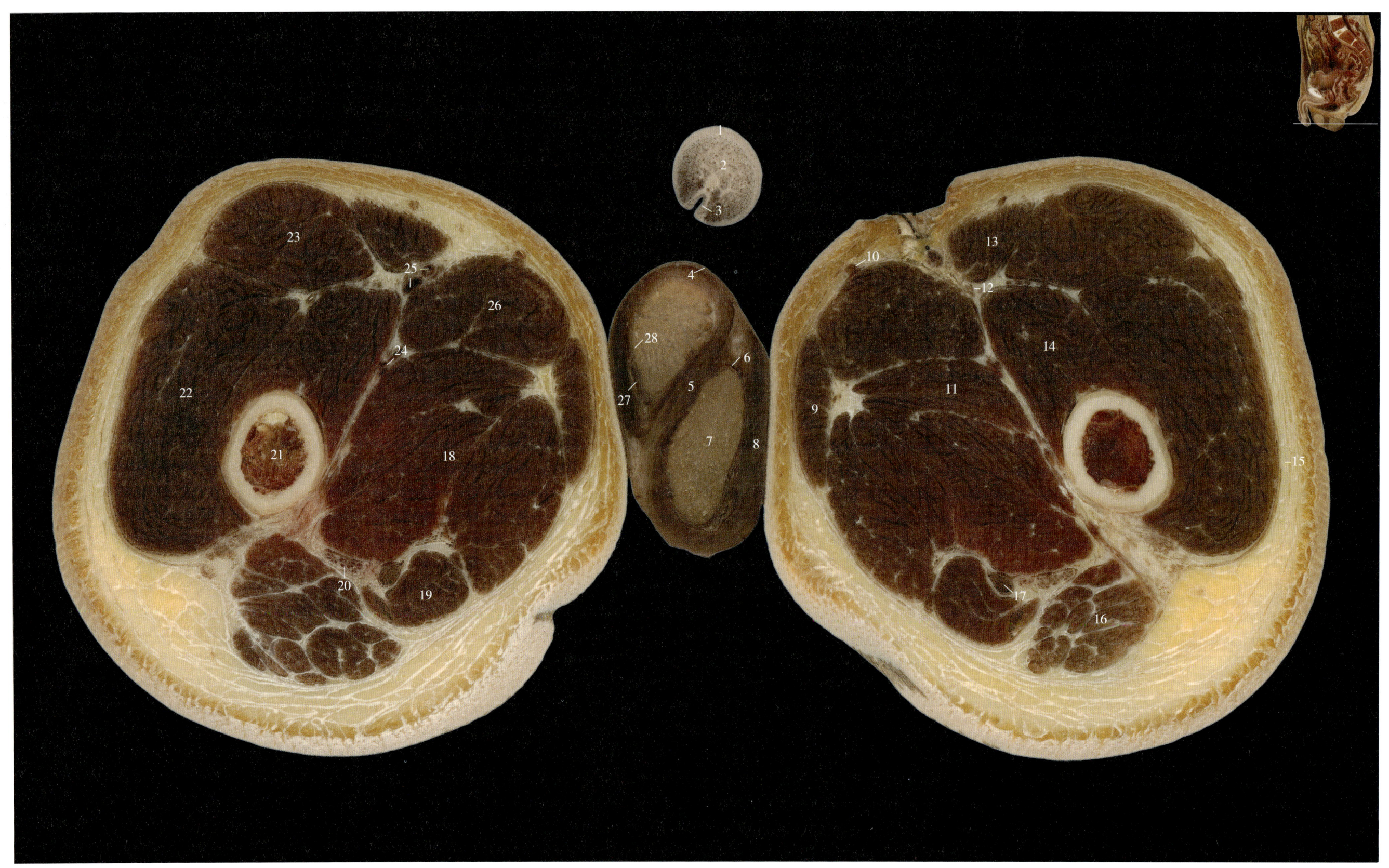

A. 断层标本图像

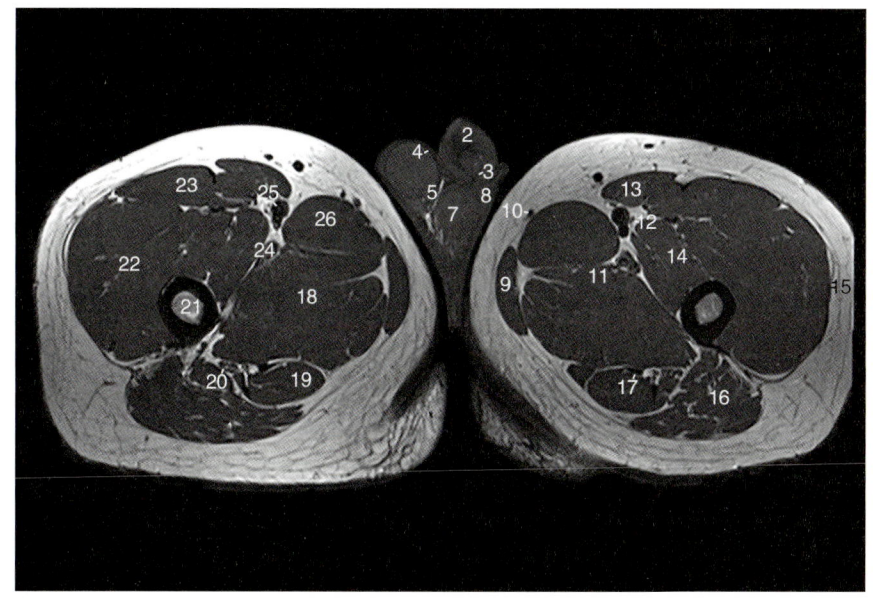

B. MR T1WI

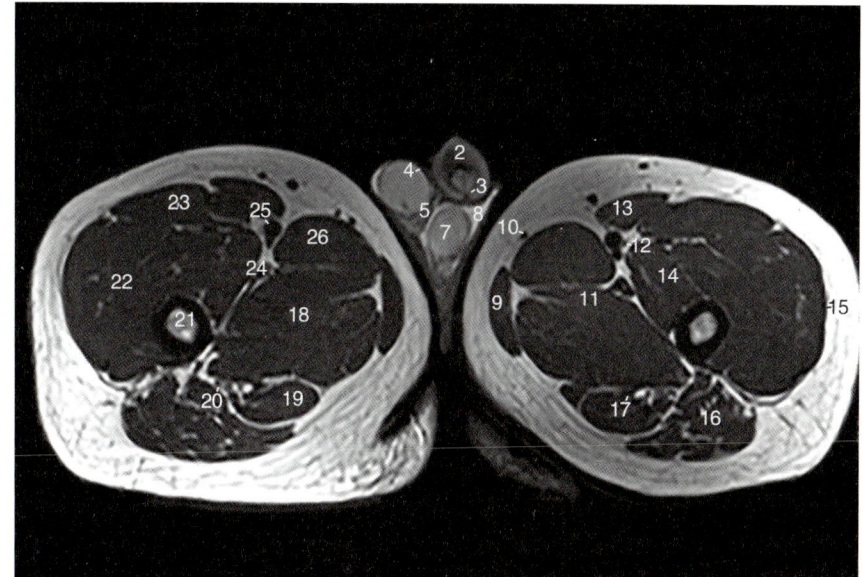

C. MR T2WI

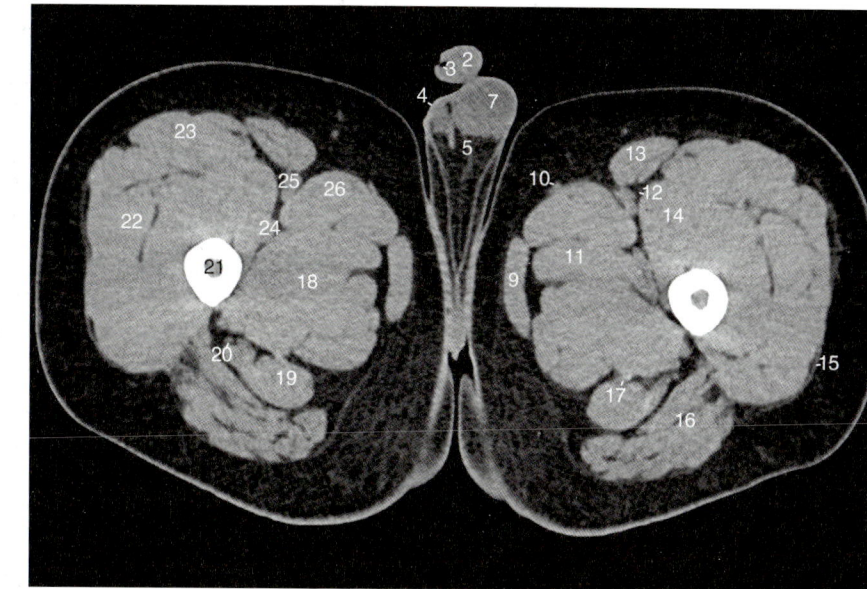

D. CT 平扫图像

关键结构：尿道，阴囊肉膜，睾丸。

　　此断面经过左侧睾丸中份。断面前部可见分离的阴茎头。男性尿道止于阴茎头的尿道外口，尿道外口呈矢状裂隙。断面中部为阴囊，阴囊内结构为睾丸及鞘膜腔；阴囊肉膜深面由外侧向内侧依次为精索外筋膜、提睾肌、精索内筋膜和睾丸鞘膜。T2WI 上，阴茎海绵体仅有很小断面，尿道海绵体断面缩小，呈高信号，双侧睾丸断面呈高信号，鞘膜腔内液体呈现明显高信号，白膜呈低信号。男性尿道有排精和排尿功能，起自膀胱的尿道内口止于阴茎头的尿道外口。成人尿道管径平均为 5~7 mm，长为 16~22 cm；分前列腺部、膜部和海绵体部三部分[31]。尿道有 3 个狭窄、3 个膨大和 2 个弯曲。3 个狭窄分别是尿道内口、尿道膜部和尿道外口，其中外口最窄，呈矢状裂隙。尿道结石易嵌顿在这些狭窄部位。

1. 尿道海绵体白膜 albuginea of cavernous body of urethra
2. 阴茎头 glans penis
3. 尿道外口 external orifice of urethra
4. 肉膜 dartos coat
5. 阴囊中隔 septum of scrotum
6. 提睾肌 cremaster
7. 睾丸 testis
8. 鞘膜腔 cavity of tunica vaginaalis
9. 股薄肌 gracilis
10. 大隐静脉 great saphenous vein
11. 短收肌 adductor brevis
12. 股神经 femoral nerve
13. 缝匠肌 sartorius
14. 股中间肌 vastus intermedius
15. 阔筋膜 fasciae lata
16. 臀大肌 gluteus maximus
17. 半膜肌 semimembranosus
18. 大收肌 adductor magnus
19. 股二头肌长头和半腱肌 long head of biceps femoris and semitendinosus
20. 坐骨神经 sciatic nerve
21. 股骨 femur
22. 股外侧肌 vastus lateralis
23. 股直肌 rectus femoris
24. 股深动脉 deep femoral artery
25. 股动、静脉 femoral artery and vein
26. 长收肌 adductor longus
27. 精索外筋膜 external spermatic fascia
28. 精索内筋膜 internal spermatic fascia

男性盆部连续横断层 55（MH.6040）

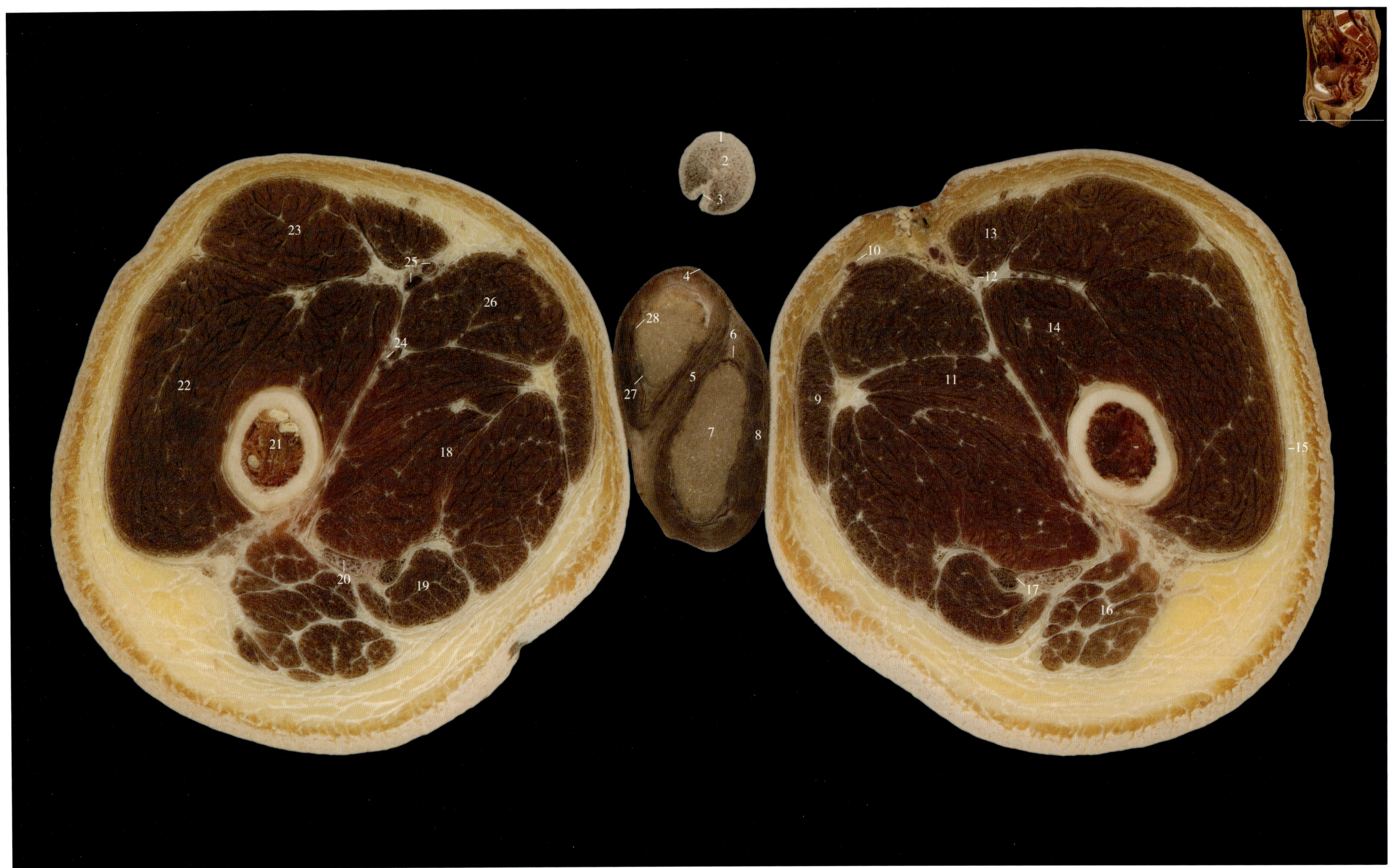

A. 断层标本图像

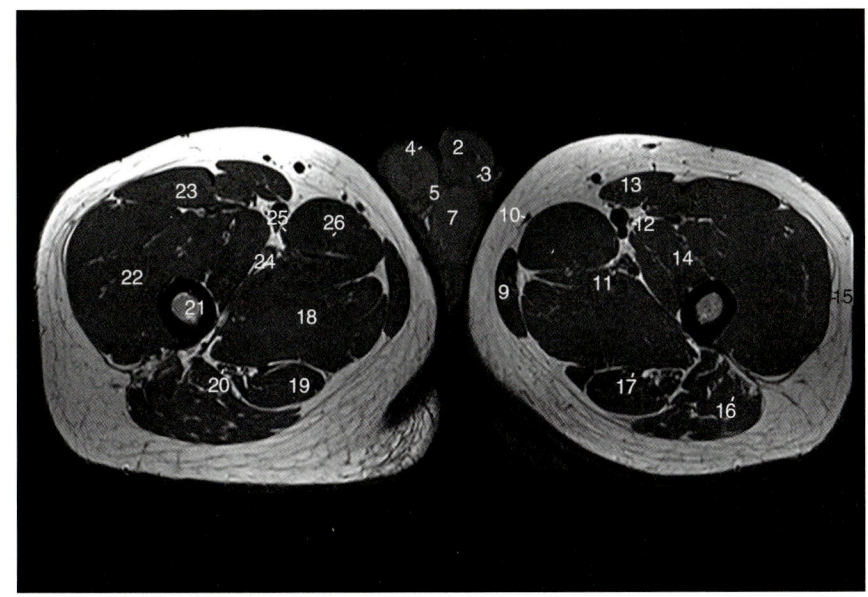
B. MR T1WI

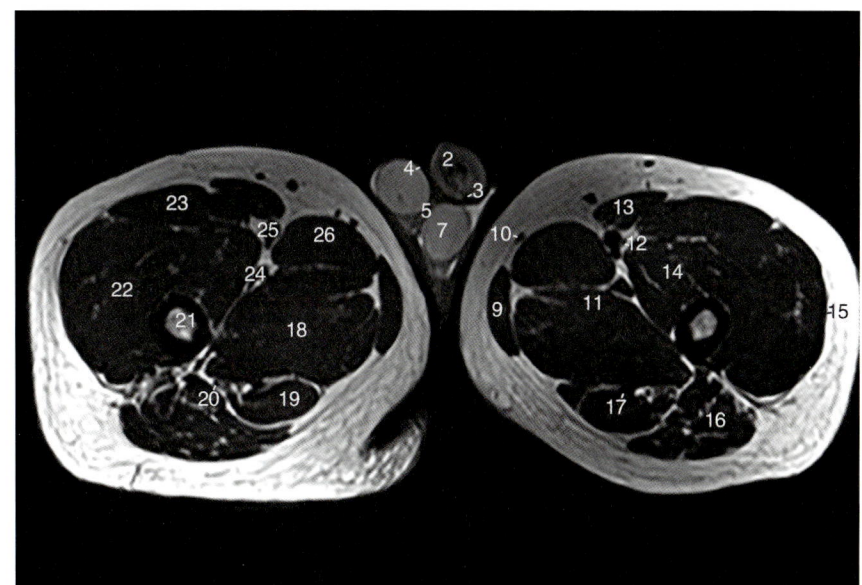
C. MR T2WI

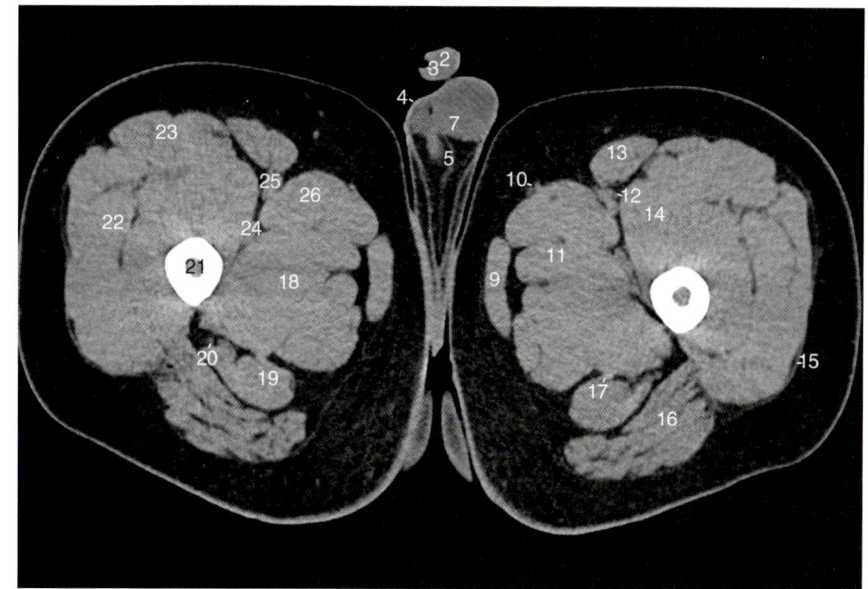
D. CT 平扫图像

关键结构：阴囊，精索筋膜，睾丸鞘膜。

此断面经过右侧睾丸下份。

断面前部可见分离的阴茎头。阴茎头的尿道外口呈矢状裂隙。阴囊内结构为睾丸及鞘膜腔，右侧睾丸断面较上一断面变小；阴囊肉膜深面由外侧向内侧依次为精索外筋膜、提睾肌、精索内筋膜和睾丸鞘膜。T2WI 上，阴茎海绵体几近消失，尿道海绵体断面缩小，呈高信号，双侧睾丸断面呈椭圆形高信号，鞘膜腔内液体呈现明显高信号，白膜呈低信号。阴囊深面见包被精索的被膜，由外侧向内侧有：①精索外筋膜为腹外斜肌肌腱膜的延续；②提睾肌来自腹内斜肌和腹横肌的肌纤维束，排列稀疏呈袢状，可反射性提起睾丸；③精索内筋膜为腹横筋膜的延续，较薄弱[25]。精索静脉曲张，即蔓状静脉丛扩张和迂曲，多发生于左侧，在 MRI 表现为多个直径>2 mm 的浆液性管状结构[64]。发病时，因静脉回流受阻，睾丸功能受影响，严重时可引起不育。

1. 尿道海绵体白膜 albuginea of cavernous body of urethra
2. 阴茎头 glans penis
3. 尿道外口 external orifice of urethra
4. 肉膜 dartos coat
5. 阴囊中隔 septum of scrotum
6. 提睾肌 cremaster
7. 睾丸 testis
8. 鞘膜腔 cavity of tunica vaginaalis
9. 股薄肌 gracilis
10. 大隐静脉 great saphenous vein
11. 短收肌 adductor brevis
12. 股神经 femoral nerve
13. 缝匠肌 sartorius
14. 股中间肌 vastus intermedius
15. 阔筋膜 fasciae lata
16. 臀大肌 gluteus maximus
17. 半膜肌 semimembranosus
18. 大收肌 adductor magnus
19. 股二头肌长头和半腱肌 long head of biceps femoris and semitendinosus
20. 坐骨神经 sciatic nerve
21. 股骨 femur
22. 股外侧肌 vastus lateralis
23. 股直肌 rectus femoris
24. 股深动脉 deep femoral artery
25. 股动、静脉 femoral artery and vein
26. 长收肌 adductor longus
27. 精索外筋膜 external spermatic fascia
28. 精索内筋膜 internal spermatic fascia

男性盆部连续横断层 56（MH.6030）

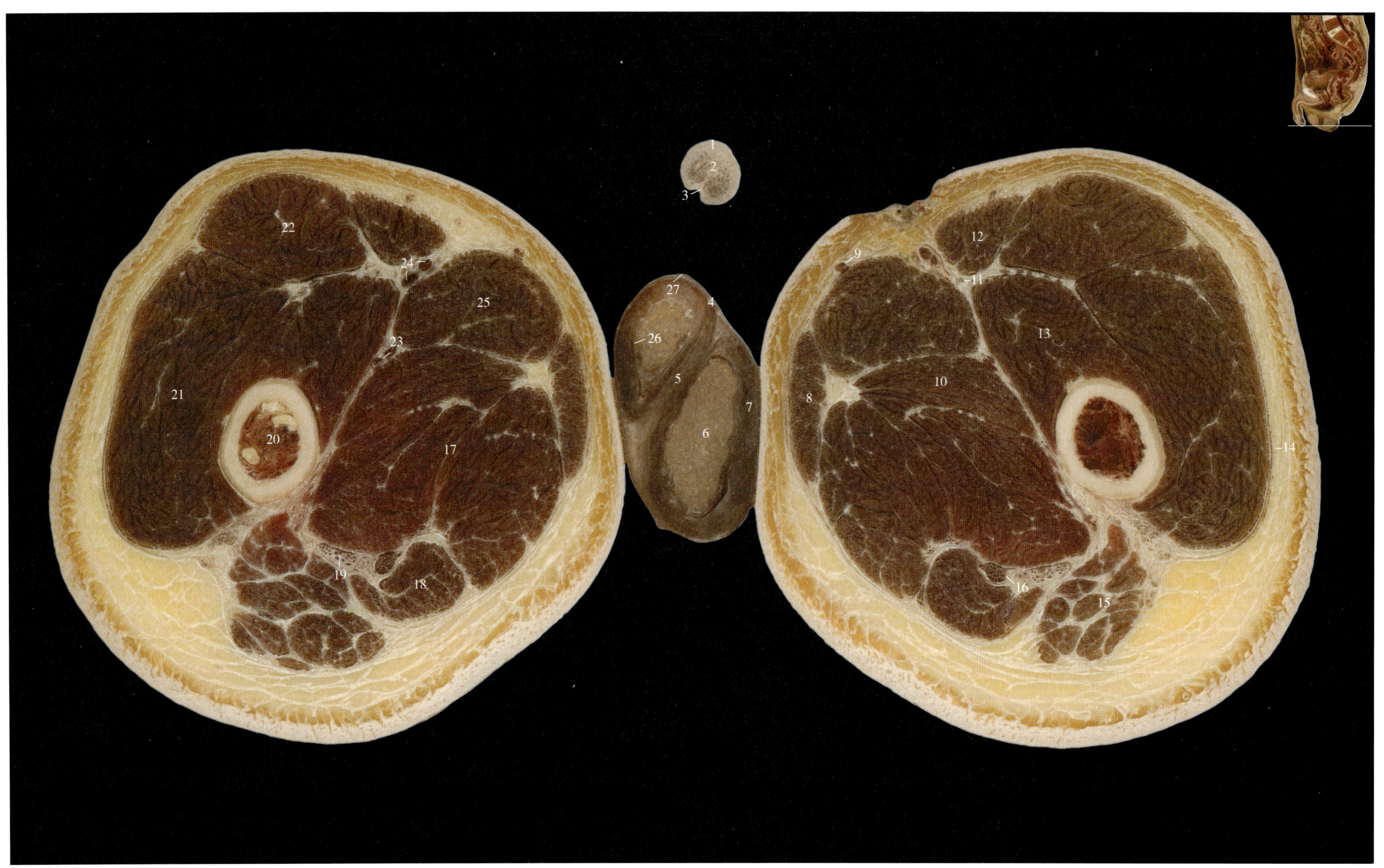

A. 断层标本图像

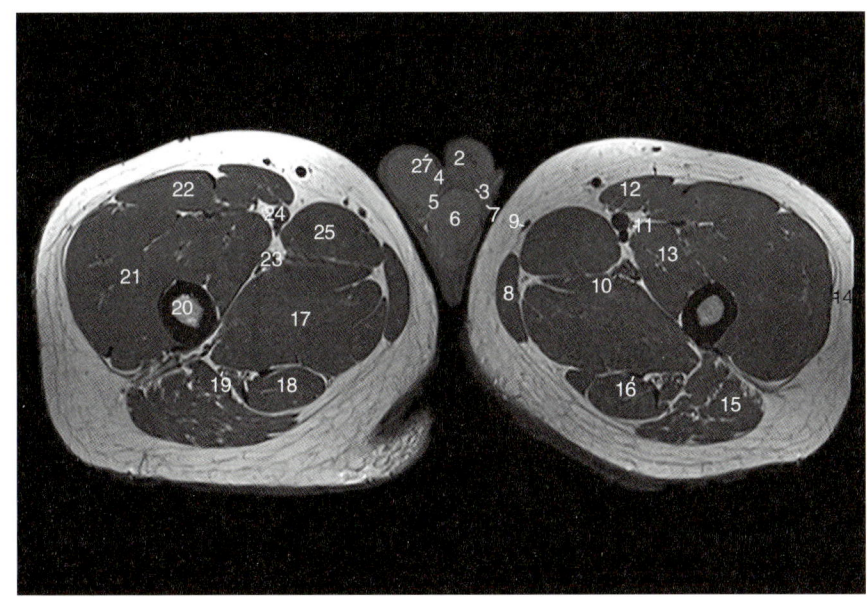
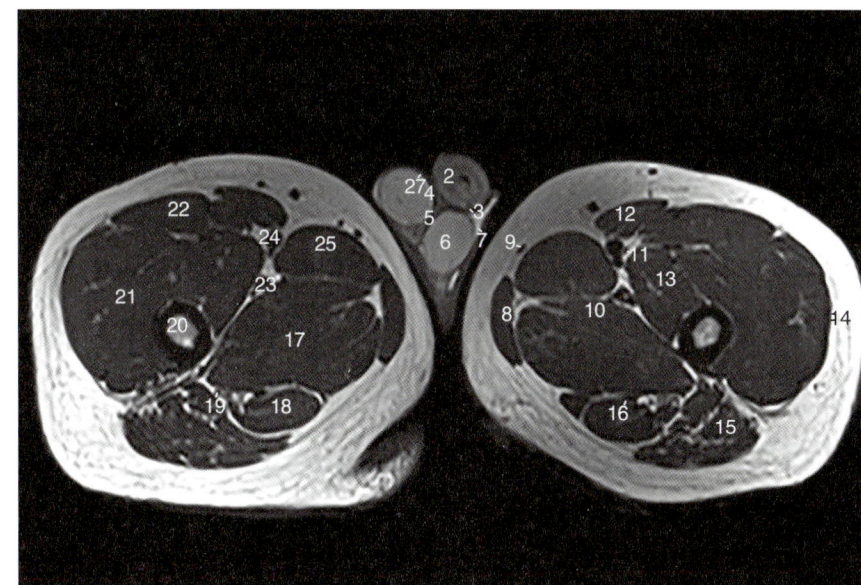
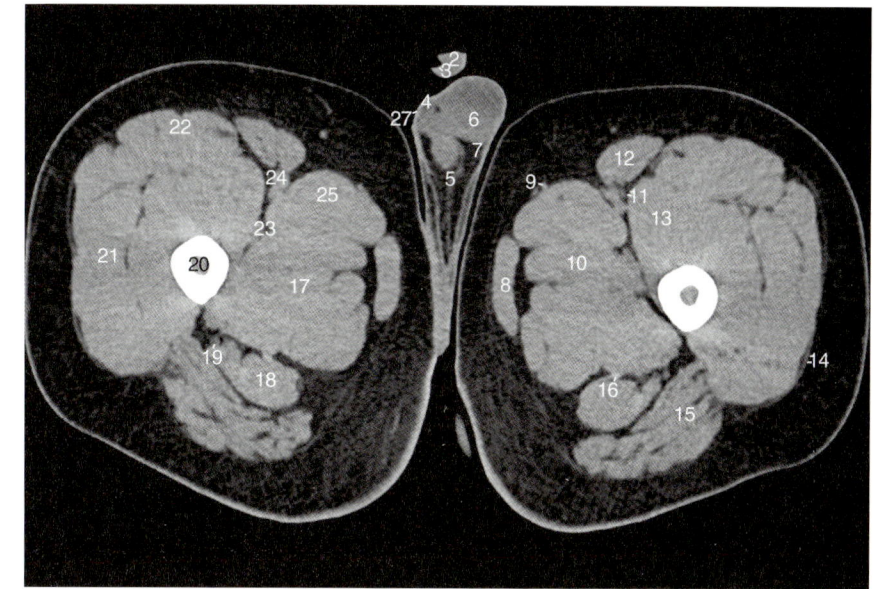

B. MR T1WI   C. MR T2WI   D. CT 平扫图像

关键结构：鞘膜腔，包皮系带，睾丸。

此断面经过左侧睾丸下份。

断面前部可见分离的阴茎头、尿道外口、阴茎包皮。与阴茎头腹侧中线处连有一条皮肤皱褶，称包皮系带。做包皮环切术时勿损伤该韧带，以免影响阴茎的勃起。阴囊内结构为睾丸下份及鞘膜腔。T2WI 上，双侧睾丸断面呈椭圆形高信号，鞘膜腔内液体呈现明显高信号，白膜呈低信号。睾丸鞘膜来源于腹膜，分为壁层和脏层，壁腹膜紧贴于精索内筋膜内面，脏腹膜包贴睾丸和附睾表面。脏、壁两层在睾丸后缘处互相反折移行，二者之间的腔隙即为鞘膜腔，内有少量浆液。若腹膜鞘突上部闭锁不全或鞘膜腔感染发炎时，可出现鞘膜积液，鞘突在不同的部位闭合不全，可形成睾丸鞘膜积液、精索鞘膜积液、睾丸精索鞘膜积液（婴儿型）和交通性鞘膜积液（先天性）。在男性中，尿道海绵体部分淋巴管汇入阴茎海绵体的区域淋巴。前列腺的淋巴管与前列腺共享区域淋巴结。至于尿道膜部，可以分为 3 个主要的淋巴管：第 1 个伴行阴部内动脉汇入臀下淋巴结。第 2 个位于耻骨联合之后，汇入腔隙内淋巴结。第 3 个位于前列腺的前面，与膀胱的传出淋巴管汇合在一起，后者流入髂外淋巴结内侧链的中上淋巴结[55]。

1. 尿道海绵体白膜 albuginea of cavernous body of urethra
2. 阴茎头 glans penis
3. 包皮系带 frenulum of prepuce
4. 阴囊 scrotum
5. 阴囊中隔 septum of scrotum
6. 睾丸 testis
7. 鞘膜腔 cavity of tunica vaginaalis
8. 股薄肌 gracilis
9. 大隐静脉 great saphenous vein
10. 短收肌 adductor brevis
11. 股神经 femoral nerve
12. 缝匠肌 sartorius
13. 股中间肌 vastus intermedius
14. 阔筋膜 fasciae lata
15. 臀大肌 gluteus maximus
16. 半膜肌 semimembranosus
17. 大收肌 adductor magnus
18. 股二头肌长头和半腱肌 long head of biceps femoris and semitendinosus
19. 坐骨神经 sciatic nerve
20. 股骨 femur
21. 股外侧肌 vastus lateralis
22. 股直肌 rectus femoris
23. 股深动脉 deep femoral artery
24. 股动、静脉 femoral artery and vein
25. 长收肌 adductor longus
26. 提睾肌 cremaster
27. 肉膜 dartos coat

男性盆部连续横断层 57（MH.6020）

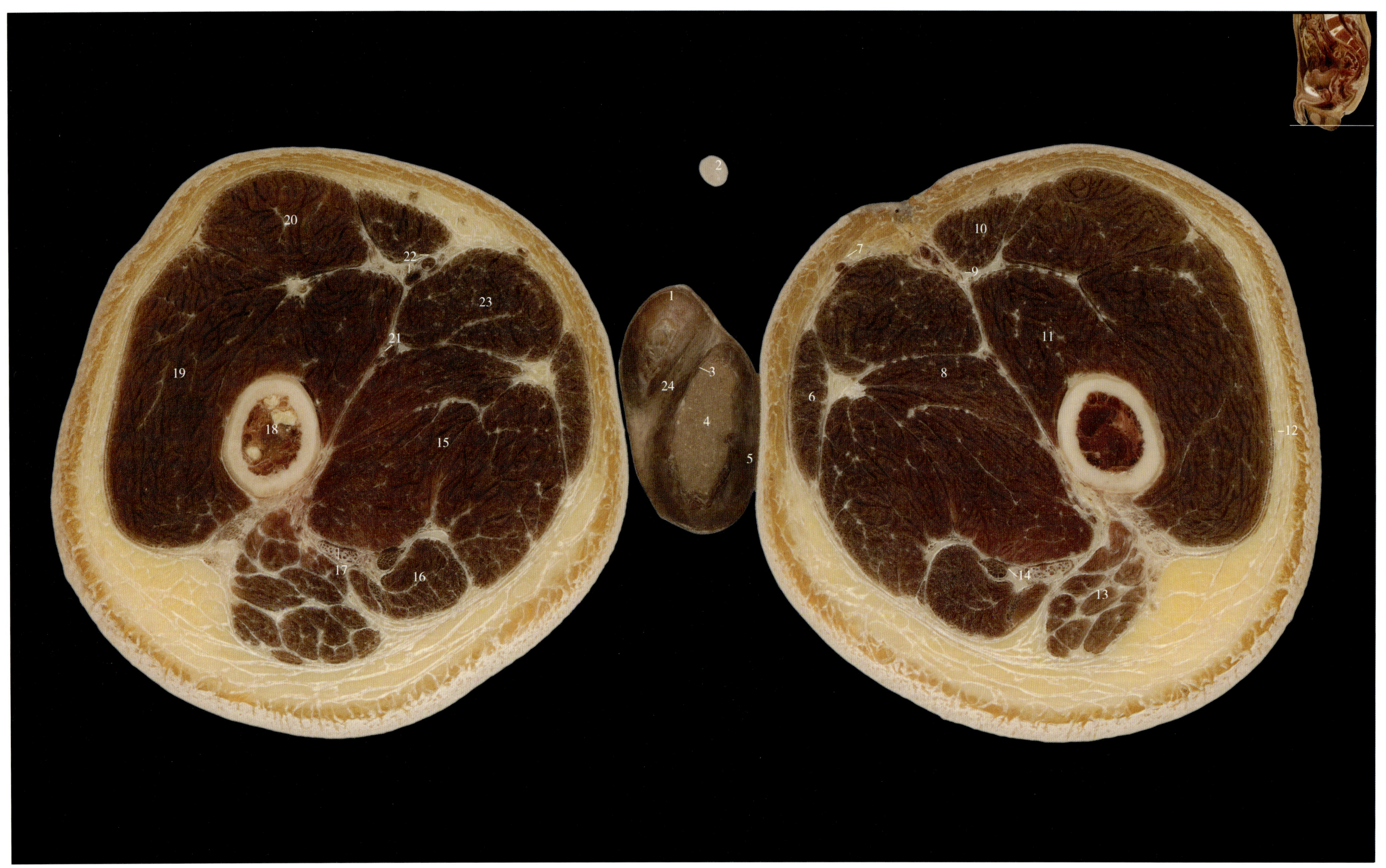

A. 断层标本图像

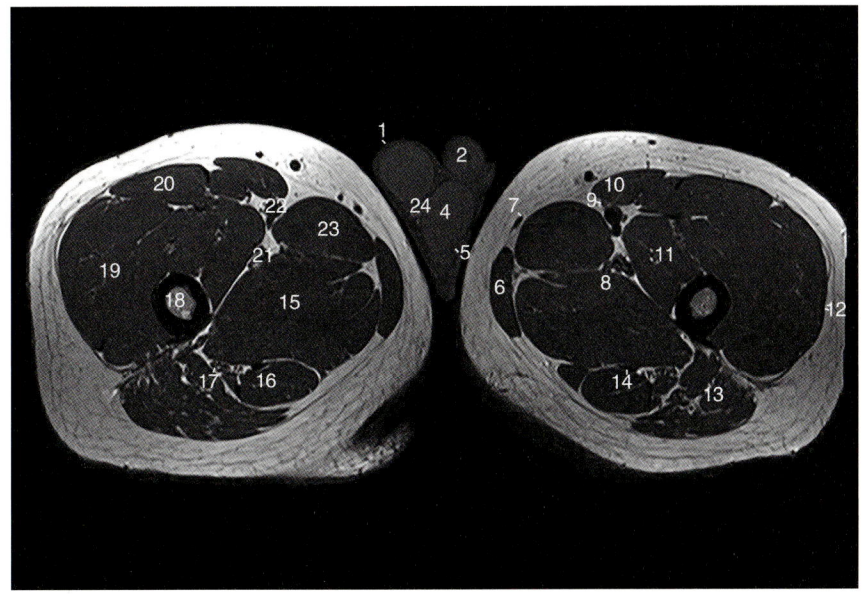
B. MR T1WI

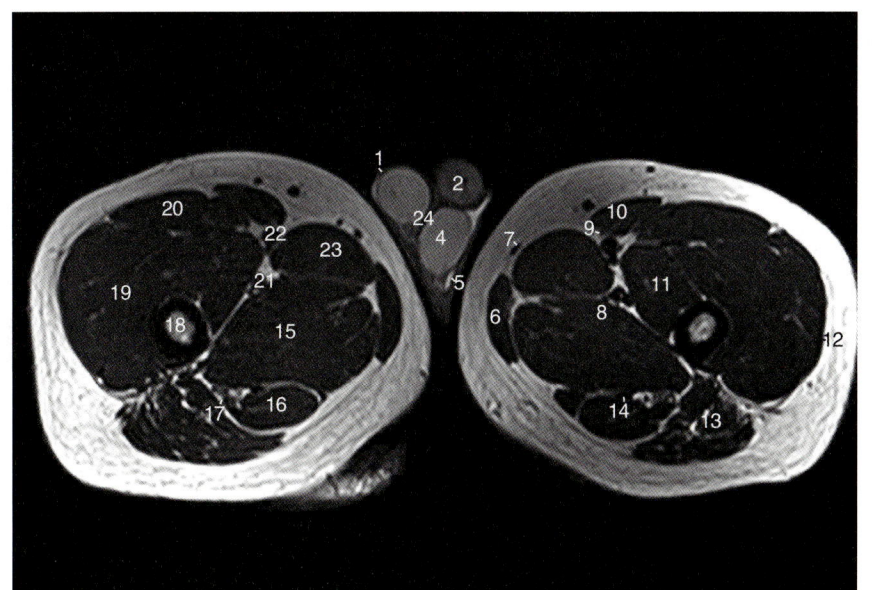
C. MR T2WI

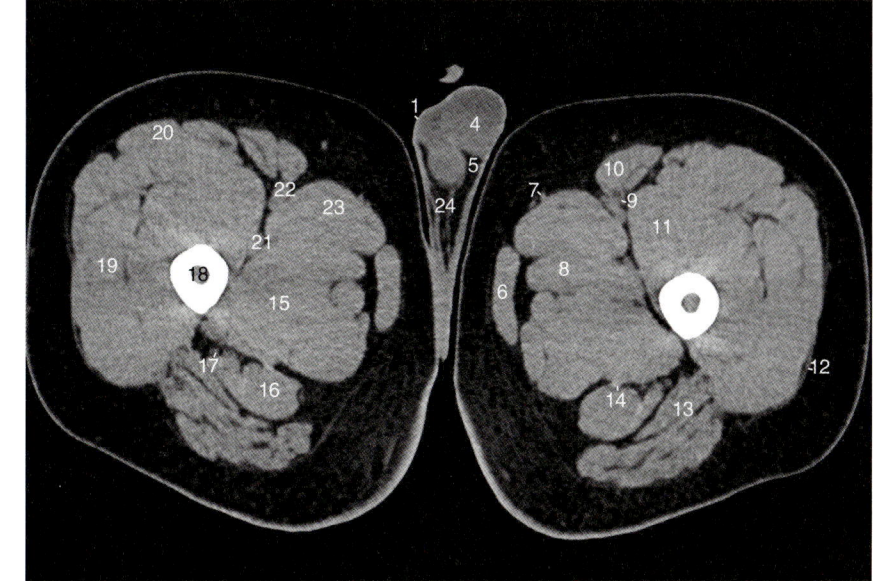
D. CT 平扫图像

1. 肉膜 dartos coat
2. 阴茎头 glans penis
3. 提睾肌 cremaster
4. 睾丸 testis
5. 鞘膜腔 cavity of tunica vaginaalis
6. 股薄肌 gracilis
7. 大隐静脉 great saphenous vein
8. 短收肌 adductor brevis
9. 股神经 femoral nerve
10. 缝匠肌 sartorius
11. 股中间肌 vastus intermedius
12. 阔筋膜 fasciae lata
13. 臀大肌 gluteus maximus
14. 半膜肌 semimembranosus
15. 大收肌 adductor magnus
16. 股二头肌长头和半腱肌 long head of biceps femoris and semitendinosus
17. 坐骨神经 sciatic nerve
18. 股骨 femur
19. 股外侧肌 vastus lateralis
20. 股直肌 rectus femoris
21. 股深动脉 deep femoral artery
22. 股动、静脉 femoral artery and vein
23. 长收肌 adductor longus
24. 阴囊中隔 septum of scrotum

关键结构：睾丸，阴囊，鞘膜腔。

此断面经过右侧睾丸下端。

断面前部可见分离的阴茎头及阴茎包皮。断面中心显示阴囊下份，其内可见睾丸及鞘膜腔，右侧睾丸已达下端，左侧睾丸达下份。T2WI 上，双侧睾丸断面呈椭圆形高信号，鞘膜腔内液体呈现明显高信号。临床上，睾丸损伤常见，主要影像学检查方法依赖于超声检查，表现为患侧睾丸肿大，内部回声不均，包膜可不完整，血肿时可见无回声区或高回声区，CDFI 在暗区内无血流显像。睾丸破裂 MRI 表现为形态失常，白膜中断，睾丸实质呈混杂信号，鞘膜内积血或混合破碎睾丸组织，T1WI 和 T2WI 均为混杂信号；睾丸挫伤出血急性期 MRI 表现为等信号或稍高信号，T2WI 表现为以低信号为主的混杂信号；白膜下血肿 MRI 表现为白膜下环形 T1WI 高信号，T2WI 低信号[64]。断面侧部为股骨和大腿的 3 个肌群。臀大肌断面变小，其深面仍可见坐骨神经，长收肌与缝匠肌间隙内见股神经及股动脉及股静脉，股中间肌与短收肌及长收肌间隙内见股深动脉，长收肌表面皮下浅筋膜内见大隐静脉。

参考文献

［1］ 刘树伟.断层解剖学.3 版.北京：高等教育出版社,2017.

［2］ Steinke H,Hammer N,Slowik V,et al. Novel insights into the sacroiliac joint ligaments. Spine (Phila Pa 1976),2010,35(3):257-263.

［3］ 赖剑强,王钢.骶髂关节周围韧带的解剖及磁共振成像研究进展.中华创伤杂志,2015,31(09):856-858.

［4］ 徐克,龚启勇,韩萍.医学影像诊断学.8 版.北京：人民卫生出版社,2018.

［5］ Susan Standring.格氏解剖学.41 版.丁自海,刘树伟,译.济南：山东科学技术出版社,2017.

［6］ Cheng L,Zhao H,Zhang FX. Iliac vein compression syndrome in an asymptomatic patient population: a prospective study.Chin Med J (Engl),2017,130(11):1269-1275.

［7］ 刘竞艳,万业达.卵巢动脉的影像学研究进展及临床意义.国际医学放射学杂志,2013,36(01):29-33.

［8］ 刘凤永,王茂强,王志军,等.卵巢动脉的血管造影解剖及其临床意义.解剖学杂志,2007(06):783-786.

［9］ Baraliakos X,Haibel H,Listing J,et al.Continuous long-term anti-TNF therapy does not lead to an increase in the rate of new bone formation over 8 years in patients with ankylosing spondylitis. Ann Rheum Dis,2014,73(4):710-715.

［10］ Biancheri R,Mancardi MM,Celle ME,et al.Cranial nerve and cauda equina contrast enhancement in Cockayne syndrome. Neurology,2014,83(17):1581.

［11］ 潘国平,王国平,华群,等.马尾神经冗余征 100 例 MRI 诊断及鉴别诊断分析.解剖学报,2018,25(21):44-45.

［12］ 丁文龙,刘学政.系统解剖学.9版.北京：人民卫生出版社,2018.

［13］ Jian N,Tian MM,Xiao LX,et al.Normal development of sacrococcygeal centrum ossification centers in the fetal spine: a postmortem magnetic resonance imaging study. Neuroradiology,2018,60(8):821-833.

［14］ Jackson LA, Ramirez DMO,Carrick KS, et al.Gross and Histologic Anatomy of the pelvic ureter: clinical applications to pelvic surgery. Obstet Gynecol,2019, 133(5): 896-904.

［15］ 马建军,徐连本,杨培学,等．臀大肌相关解剖学研究.齐齐哈尔医学院学报,2004(10):1121-1122.

［16］ 中国解剖学会体质调查委员会.中国人解剖学数值.北京：人民卫生出版社,2002.

［17］ 汪忠镐,舒畅.血管外科临床解剖学（钟世镇现代临床解剖学全集）.济南：山东科学技术出版社,2020.

［18］ Park IJ,Choi GS,Lim KH,et al. Metastasis to the sigmoid or sigmoid mesenteric lymph nodes from rectal cancer. Ann Surg,2009,249(6):960-964.

［19］ Huang JJ,Ruaan MK,Lan RR,et al. Acute pyogenic iliopsoas abscess in Taiwan: clinical features,diagnosis,treatments and outcome . J Infect,2000,40(3):248-255.

［20］ Muavha DA,L Ras,S Jeffery. Laparoscopic surgical anatomy for pelvic floor surgery. Best Pract Res Clin Obstet Gynaecol,2019,54: 89-102.

［21］ 郎景和,张晓东.妇产科临床解剖学.2 版.济南：山东科学技术出版社,2020.

［22］ 崔慧先,李瑞锡.局部解剖学.9版.北京：人民卫生出版社,2018.

［23］ Harisinghani MG. Atlas of lymph node anatomy. Berlin: Springer New York Heidelberg Dordrecht London,2013: 91-102.

［24］ 基思·L·莫尔,阿瑟·F·达利.临床应用解剖学.4 版.李云庆,译.郑州：河南科学技术出版社,2006.

［25］ 丁文龙,王海杰.系统解剖学.3版.北京：人民卫生出版社,2015.

［26］ 艾里·克豪里.骨骼肌肉 MRI/CT 断层解剖.3 版.韩洪宾,余家阔,王福生,译.北京：北京大学医学出版社,2009: 228.

［27］ 靳安民,汪华侨.骨科临床解剖学.2 版.济南：山东科学技术出版社,2020.

［28］ Richter E,Feyerabend T. Normal Lymph Node Topography CT Atlas. Berlin:Springer-Verlag Berlin Heidelberg,2004.

［29］ 吕维富,张爱武,周春泽,等.子宫动脉的三维 DSA 表现及其最佳显示体位探讨.介入放射学杂志,2011,20(11): 853-856.

［30］ 张朝佑.人体解剖学.3 版.北京：人民卫生出版社,2009.

［31］ 苏泽轩,邱剑光.泌尿外科临床解剖学.2 版.济南：山东科学技术出版社,2020.

［32］ Sora MC,Jilavu R,Matusz P. Computer aided three-dimensional reconstruction and modeling of the pelvis,by using plastinated cross sections,as a powerful tool for morphological investigations. Surg Radiol Anat,2012,34(8): 731-736.

［33］ Shin DS,Jang HG,Hwang SB,et al. Two-dimensional sectioned images and three-dimensional surface models for learning the anatomy of the female pelvis. Anat Sci Educ,2013,6(5): 316-323.

［34］ Zijta FM, Lakeman MM, Froeling M, et al.Evaluation of the female pelvic floor in pelvic organ prolapse using 3.0-Tesla diffusion tensor imaging and fibre tractography. European Radiology,2012,22(12): 2806-2813.

［35］ MA Gatellier,EJD Gautier, O Mayeur, et al.Complete 3 dimensional reconstruction of parturient pelvic floor.J Gynecol Obstet Hum Reprod,2020,49(1): 9-10

［36］ Elroy P Weledji, D Eyongeta, E Ngounou. The anatomy of urination: What every physician should know. Clin Anat,2019,32(1): 60-67.

［37］ 张逸仲.实时三维超声结合高频超声对正常成年女性尿道长度与相关因素的影像学研究.现代医用影像学,2016,25(03): 462-465.

［38］ Hennigan HJ,DuBose TJ. Sonography of the normal female urethra. AJR Am J Roentgenol,1985,145(4): 839-841.

［39］ Erden A.MRI of anal canal:normal anatomy,imaging protocol,and perianal fistulas: Par 1.Abdom Radiol (NY),2018,43(6):1334-1352.

［40］ Moore KL. The developing human. 10th edition. Canada: Elsevier,2017.

［41］ 王怀经,应大君.局部解剖学.3 版.北京：高等教育出版社,2014.

［42］Ramirez M,Ingrand P,Richer JP,et al. What is the pelvic lymph node normal size? Determination from normal MRI examinations. Surg Radiol Anat,2016,38(4): 425-431.

［43］刘吉华, 杨本涛, 徐爱德. 正常成人髋臼断面角的CT测量. 中华放射学杂志,1999(05): 3-5.

［44］中休医学会男科学分会编写组. 精索静脉曲张诊断与治疗中国专家共识. 中华男科学杂志,2015,21(11):1035-1042.

［45］Temel T. Prostate MRI essentials l a practical guide for radiologists. Berlin Springer,2020.

［46］黄晓芹. 组织学与胚胎学.3版. 上海: 上海科技教育出版社,2018.

［47］Eckart R,Thomas F. Normal lymph node topography CT atlas. Berlin Springer,2004.

［48］郭光文, 王序. 人体解剖彩色图谱.2版. 北京: 人民卫生出版社,2018.

［49］金征宇. 医学影像学.2版. 北京: 人民卫生出版社,2010.

［50］汪亚晴, 刘永寿, 马维义. 临床实用解剖图谱—盆部及会阴部分册. 北京: 世界图书出版公司北京公司,2000.

［51］王世栋, 邓雪飞, 王娜, 等. 前列腺周围筋膜及其毗邻结构的三维断层解剖研究. 中国临床解剖学杂志,2010,28(6):643-646.

［52］Khaled ME. Cross-Sectional Imaging of the abdomen and pelvis:a practical algorithmic approach. New York: Springer,2015.

［53］Michelle D Bardis ,Roozbeh Houshyar ,Peter D Chang ,et al. Applications of Artificial Intelligence to Prostate Multiparametric MRI (mpMRI): Current and Emerging Trends. Cancers (Basel),2020,12(5):1204.

［54］Armando Stabile,Francesco Giganti,Andrew B Rosenkrantz,et al.Multiparametric MRI for prostate cancer diagnosis: current status and future directions. Nat Rev Urol,2020,17(1):41-61.

［55］王云祥. 实用淋巴系统解剖学. 北京: 人民卫生出版社,1984.

［56］韩永坚. 临床解剖学丛书—腹、盆部分册. 北京: 人民卫生出版社,1992.

［57］李和, 李继承. 组织学与胚胎学.3版. 北京: 人民卫生出版社,2015.

［58］Bontumasi N,Jacobson JA,Caoili E,et al. Inguinal lymph nodes: size,number,and other characteristics in asymptomatic patients by CT. Surg Radiol Anat,2014,36(10): 1051-1055.

［59］张龙江, 祁吉. 阴茎的MRI检查及应用. 国外医学·临床放射学分册,2005,28(3):167-169.

［60］Lube J,Cotofana S,Bechmann I,et al. Reference data on muscle volumes of healthy human pelvis and lower extremity muscles: an in vivo magnetic resonance imaging feasibility study. Surg Radiol Anat,2016,38(1): 97-106.

［61］王海屹, 袁静, 伍兵. 男性与女性盆腔MRI诊断学. 郑州: 河南科学技术出版社,2019.

［62］Jean-Michel Dubernard J, Claude Abbou, Léon Dorn, 等. 泌尿外科手术学. 闵志廉, 译. 北京: 人民卫生出版社,2007.

［63］van der Putte SC. The devlopment of the perineum in the human. A comprehensive histological study with a special reference to the role of the stromal components. Adv Anat Embryol Cell Biol,2005,177: 23-118.

［64］Riccardo M,Roberto PM. MRI of the female and male pelvis. Berlin Springer, 2014.

索 引

B

白膜 tunica albuginea 279~289
半腱肌 semitendinosus 157~187,275~303
半膜肌 semimembranosus 159~167,275~303
半膜肌肌腱 tendon of semimembranosus 157,169~187,227~273
膀胱 urinary bladder 13~137,191~231
膀胱颈 neck of bladder 133~139
膀胱静脉丛 vesical venous plexus 127~145,191~209
膀胱前间隙 prevesical space 197~215
膀胱阴道隔 vesicovaginal septum 135,173
膀胱肿瘤 bladder tumor 141,217
包皮过长 redundant prepuce 267
包皮系带 frenulum of prepuce 301
闭孔动、静脉 obturator artery and vein 83~117,121,129~133,137~141
闭孔动、静脉和神经 obturator artery, vein and nerve 123
闭孔动脉 obturator artery 127
闭孔静脉 obturator vein 135,143
闭孔淋巴结 glandulae foraminis obturatorii 201
闭孔膜 obturator membrane 137,139,141,143
闭孔内肌 obturator internus 65,75~149,191~253
闭孔内肌肌腱 tendon of obturator internus 111
闭孔神经 obturator nerve 47~55,83~103,191~193
闭孔外肌 obturator externus 129~157,217~255
闭孔血管、神经 obturator vessels and nerve 119
闭孔血管 obturator blood vessels 193
闭孔血管和神经 obturator blood vessels and nerve 195~213

C

长收肌 adductor longus 143~187,229~303
长收肌肌腱 tendon of adductor longus 141
肠系膜及肠系膜动、静脉 mesentery and mesenteric artery and vein 63~67
耻骨 pubis 87
耻骨弓状韧带 arcuate pubic ligament 151,229~245
耻骨后间隙 retropubic space 137~145,233~237
耻骨肌 pectineus 113~149,153~277
耻骨联合 pubic symphysis 127~149,219~245
耻骨上韧带 superior public ligament 205~217
耻骨上支 superior ramus of pubis 119~141,205~227
耻骨体 body of pubis 89~121,191~203
耻骨体 body of pubis 107~111
耻骨下支 inferior ramus of pubis 143~159,229~245

D

大便失禁 fecal incontinence 159
大收肌 adductor magnus 149~187,233~303
大阴唇 greater lip of pudendum 169~187
大隐静脉 great saphenous vein 133~187,221~303
大转子 greater trochanter 201~227,247~269
骶骨侧部 lateral part of sacrum 3
骶管 sacral canal 19~41
骶结节韧带 sacrotuberous ligament 115~121
骶髂骨间韧带 interosseous sacroiliac ligaments 3
骶髂关节 sacroiliac joint 15~49
骶髂关节炎 sacroiliitis 17
骶前间隙 presacral space 201
第1骶神经 1st sacral nerve 3~59
第1骶椎 1st sacral vertebra 5~23
第2骶神经 2nd sacral nerve 19~61
第2骶椎 2nd sacral vertebra 25~39
第3骶神经 3rd sacral nerve 21~65
第4骶神经 4th sacral nerve 43~47,55~61,67~71
第5骶椎 5th sacral vertebra 71~79
短收肌 adductor brevis 139~187,229~303

F

缝匠肌 sartorius 79~187,191~303
附睾 epididymis 271~291
附睾头 head of epididymis 249~269
腹壁下动、静脉 inferior epigastric artery and vein 85~99
腹股沟浅淋巴结 superficial inguinal lymph nodes 89~117,123~127,151~155,165~269
腹股沟深淋巴结 deep inguinal lymph node 89~105
腹横肌 transversus abdominis 3~69
腹内斜肌 obliquus internus abdominis 3~93
腹直肌 rectus abdominis 3~125,191~219
腹直肌鞘 sheath of rectus abdominis 101~113

G

肛管 anal canal 127~161,231~249
肛门 anus 169~167
肛门外括约肌 sphincter ani externus 159~179,225~269
肛提肌 levator ani 97~165,191~245
睾丸 testis 273~303
睾丸网 rete testis 279~289
睾丸小隔 septula testis 279~291
宫颈管囊肿 cervical duct cyst 103
宫颈黏膜 cervical mucosa 81,95~103
股薄肌 gracilis 169~187,267~303
股动、静脉 femoral artery and vein 195~213,221~303

股动脉 femoral artery　　　123~193,215~219
股二头肌、半腱肌和半膜肌总腱 tendons of biceps femoris,
　　semitendinous and semimembranousus　　123~155
股二头肌长头 long head of biceps femoris　　159~187
股二头肌长头和半腱肌 long head of biceps femoris and
　　semitendinosus　　229~303
股二头肌长头肌肌腱 tendon of long head of biceps femoris　　157
股方肌 quadratus femoris　　119~169,221~263
股骨 femur　　135~141,275~303
股骨大转子 greater trochanter　　103~131
股骨颈 neck of femur　　111~133,207~245
股骨颈疝窝　fossil of femoral neck hernia　　215
股骨体 shaft of femur　　151~157,161
股骨体与小转子 shaft and lesser trochanter of femur　　145~149
股骨头 femoral head　　65,87~121,191~227
股骨头韧带 ligament of head of femur　　97~121，191~211
股骨小转子 femur,lesser trochanter　　151~161
股静脉 femoral vein　　123~187,191~193,215~219
股内侧肌间隔 medial femoral intermuscular septum　　177~187
股深动脉 deep femoral artery　　121~187,231~303
股深静脉 deep femoral vein　　167~187
股神经 femoral nerve　　3~55,59~67,71~167,191~303
股外侧肌 vastus lateralis　　127~187,217~303
股外侧肌间隔 lateral femoral intermuscular septum　　171~187
股直肌 rectus femoris　　99~187,191~303
股中间肌 vastus intermedius　　155~187,239~303
骨折 fracture　　81,87,111,119,137,149

H

回肠 ileum　　3~121,191~195
会阴深横肌 deep transverse muscles of perineum　　243~247

J

降结肠 descending colon　　3~31
精囊 seminal vesicle　　191~227
精索 spermatic cord　　191~247
精索静脉 varicocele　　195,299
精索内筋膜 internal spermatic fascia　　293~299
精索外筋膜 external sepermatic fascia　　293~299

K

空肠 jejunum　　3~53
髋关节 hip joint　　191~201
髋臼 acetabulum　　85
髋臼唇 acetabular labrum　　195~215
髋臼窝 acetabular fossa　　95
阔筋膜 fasciae latae　　117~187,195~303
阔筋膜张肌 tensor fasciae latae　　79~287

L

L5-S1 椎间盘 L5-S1 intervertebral disc　　3~11
阑尾 vermiform appendix　　15~39
梨状肌 piriformis　　49~57,61~95,191
梨状肌肌腱 tendon of piriformis　　89~95

M

马尾 cauda equina　　3~17
马尾综合征　cauda equina syndrome　　19
盲肠 cecum　　3~27

N

尿道 urethra　　141~177,223~225,251~265,273~289,295
尿道海绵体 cavernous body of urethra　　247，255~271
尿道海绵体白膜 albuginea of cavernous body of urethra　　255~267,
　　285,291~301
尿道嵴 urethral ridge　　239~241
尿道膜部 membranous portion of urethra　　243~249
尿道内口 internal urethra orifice　　221
尿道前列腺部 prostatic portion of urethra　　227~237
尿道外口 external orifice of urethra　　179~183,297~299
尿道舟状窝 navicular fossa of urethra　　291~293
尿生殖膈 urogenital diaphragm　　249~251

Q

髂股韧带 iliofemoral ligament　　79~147,191~259
髂骨体 body of ilium　　71~83
髂骨翼 ala of ilium　　3~69
髂肌 iliacus　　3~43

髂静脉压迫综合征　iliac vein compression syndrome　　13
髂内静脉属支 tributary of internal iliac vein　　51
髂前上棘 anterior superior iliac spine　　49~51
髂外淋巴结 external iliac lymph nodes　　51~53
髂腰肌 iliopsoas　　45~175,191~283
髂腰肌肌腱 iliopsoas tendon　　123~129,133,137~149,153~161
前列腺 prostate　　203,207~241
前列腺肥大　prostatic hyperplasia　　231
前列腺静脉丛 prostatic venous plexus　　239~243
前庭球 bulb of vestibule　　155~165
鞘膜积液　hydrocele of tunica vaginalis　　255,277,301
鞘膜腔 cavity of tunica vaginaalis　　247~303
球海绵体肌 bulbocavernosus　　253~269

R

肉膜 dartos coat　　245~265,271~289,293~303

S

S1-2 骶椎间盘 S1-2 intervertebral disc　　19
S1-2 椎间盘 S1-2 intervertebral disc　　21~29
S2-3 椎间盘 S2-3 intervertebral disc　　39~45
S3-4 椎间盘 S3-4 intervertebral disc　　53~57
S4-5 椎间盘 S4-5 intervertebral disc　　71
上孖肌 gemellus superior　　97~109,203~209
上孖肌肌腱 tendon of gemellus superior　　97
射精管 ejaculatory　　229~239
输精管 ductus deferens　　191~209,217~221,239~277
输精管壶腹 ampulla of ductus deferens　　211~215
输尿管 ureter　　197~203
输尿管壁内部 intramural part of ureter　　123~125
竖脊肌 erector spinae　　3~53

T

提睾肌 cremaster　　277~303
臀大肌 gluteus maximus　　3~187,191~303
臀上静脉 superior gluteal vein　　49
臀上静脉属支 tributary of superior gluteal vein　　53
臀下动、静脉 inferior gluteal artery and vein　　123~129,137~145,159,
　　163,171~179
臀下动、静脉和神经 inferior gluteal artery，vein and nerve　　131

臀下动脉 inferior gluteal artery　　　133~135,147~157,161~169, 181~183
臀小肌 gluteus minimuss　　37~113,191~197
臀中肌 gluteus medius　　3~141,191~223
臀中肌肌腱 tendon of gluteus medius　　89~101
外阴疼痛综合征 vulva pain syndrome　　187
尾骨 coccyx　　81~119,191~211
尾骨肌 coccygeus　　191~205

X

下孖肌 gemellus inferior　　113~121,211~219
先天性腹股沟斜疝　congenital indirect inguinal hernia　　169,255
小阴唇 lesser lip of pudendum　　179~187
小转子 lesser trochanter　　261~273
悬韧带 suspensory ligament　　221~233
旋股内侧动、静脉 medial femoral circumflex artery andvein　　141~143,151~157
旋股内侧动脉 medial femoral circumflex artery　　131~139,145~149,155,159~167
旋股外侧动、静脉 lateral femoral circumflex artery and vein　　151~167
旋股外侧动脉 lateral femoral circumflex artery　　157~165,169
旋股外侧动脉降支 descending branch of lateral femoral circumflex artery　　171~183
旋股外侧动脉升支 ascending branch of lateral femoral circumflex artery　　135~137,141~149
旋股外侧静脉降支 descending tributaries of lateral femoral circumflex vein　　179,185~187,175~177,181~183
旋股外侧血管升支 lateral femoral circumflex vessel ascending branch　　139
旋股外动脉降支 descending branch of lateral femoral circumflex artery　　185~187
血栓　thrombus　　11
腰大肌 psoas major　　3~43
腰骶干 lumbosacral trunk　　3~59

Y

乙状结肠 sigmoid colon　　33~97
乙状结肠扭转　volvulus of sigmoid colon　　87
乙状结肠系膜 sigmoid mesocolon　　55,61
异位妊娠　ectopic gestation　　73

阴部内动、静脉 internal pudendal artery and vein　　123~139,143~145,153
阴部内动、静脉和阴部神经 internal pudendal artery and vein & pudendal nerve　　141
阴部内静脉 internal pudendal vein　　147~151,155~167
阴部内血管和阴部神经 internal pudendal blood vessels and pudendal nerve　　203~213
阴部神经 pudendal nerve　　215~235
阴道 vagina　　65,81,121~171
阴道静脉丛 vaginaal venous plexus　　123~179
阴道口 vaginaal orifice　　173~175
阴道前庭 vaginaal vestibule　　177
阴道穹后部 posterior part of fornix of vaginaa　　117~119
阴蒂 clitoris　　161~183
阴蒂海绵体 cavernous body of clitoris　　173~177
阴蒂脚 clitoral crura　　161~167
阴阜 mons pubis　　127~149
阴茎 penis　　259~265
阴茎包皮 prepuce of penis　　267~291
阴茎背浅静脉 superficial dorsal vein of penis　　243~247
阴茎背深静脉 deep dorsal vein of penis　　249~257
阴茎海绵体 cavernous body of penis　　237~245,249~265,269~289
阴茎海绵体白膜 albuginea of cavernous body of penis　　247~255,263~287
阴茎脚 crus of penis　　247~257
阴茎深动脉 deep artery of penis　　261,267,275,279~283
阴茎头 glans penis　　289~303
阴茎中隔 septum of penis　　245~269
阴囊 scrotum　　255~261,301
阴囊中隔 septum of scrotum　　263~303
隐睾症　cryptorchism　　295
硬脊膜 spinal dura mater　　5
右股动脉 right femoral artery　　85~121
右股静脉 right femoral vein　　85~121
右卵巢 right ovary　　15~33,47~59,65
右卵巢动、静脉 right ovarian artery and vein　　3~49,63~69
右髂内动脉 right internal iliac artery　　3~47
右髂内动脉分支 branches of right internal iliac artery　　49
右髂内静脉 right internal iliac vein　　13~29,33~49
右髂内静脉属支 right tributary of internal iliac vein　　31~81
右髂外动脉 right external iliac artery　　3~83
右髂外静脉 right external iliac vein　　13~83
右髂外淋巴结 right external iliac lymph nodes　　71

右髂总静脉 right common iliac vein　　3~11
右输卵管 right uterine tube　　47~73
右输尿管 right ureter　　5~19,25,31~33,107~121
右臀上动、静脉 right superior gluteal artery and vein　　57~65,69
右臀上动、静脉分支 branches of right superior gluteal artery and vein　　69~71
右臀上动脉 right superior gluteal artery　　51~55
右臀上静脉 right superior gluteal vein　　51~55,67
右臀下动、静脉 right inferior gluteal artery and vein　　71~105
右臀下动脉 right inferior gluteal artery　　51~61
右臀下静脉 right inferior gluteal vein　　51~61
右阴部内动、静脉 right internal pudendal artery and vein　　107~121

Z

直肠 rectum　　61~125,191~229
直肠癌　rectal carcinoma　　67,219
直肠膀胱陷凹 rectovesical pouch　　191~205
直肠系膜 mesorectum　　87~89,105~113
直肠系膜筋膜 mesorectal fascia　　87~89
直肠肿瘤　rectal tumor　　67,205
椎间盘突出症　disc herniation　　3
子宫底 fundus of uterus　　31~37,51,57~81
子宫动、静脉 uterine artery and vein　　85~87,91,99~107
子宫动脉 uterine artery　　89
子宫肌层 myometrium of uterus　　65,81
子宫结合带 uterine junction zone　　65,81
子宫颈 neck of uterus　　81,89~119
子宫颈管 canal of cervix of uterus　　89~119
子宫阔韧带 broad ligament of uterus　　91~97
子宫阔韧带前叶 anterior layer of cardinal ligament of uterus　　85~89
子宫内膜 endometrium　　41~61,65,69~93
子宫腔 cavity of uterus　　55~87
子宫体 body of uterus　　39~87
子宫阴道静脉丛 uterovaginaal venous plexus　　95~121
子宫圆韧带 round ligament of uterus　　73~79
左股动脉 left femoral artery　　85~121
左股静脉 left femoral vein　　85~121
左卵巢 left ovary　　15~41,57~83
左卵巢动、静脉 left ovarian artery and vein　　3~11,69~71
左髂内动脉 left internal iliac artery　　3~29,33~49
左髂内动脉分支 branch of left internal iliac artery　　31
左髂内静脉 left internal iliac vein　　19~29,33~49

左髂内静脉属支 tributary of left internal iliac vein　31
左髂外动脉 left external iliac artery　3~61,69~83
左髂外动脉 left external iliac artery　63~67
左髂外静脉 left external iliac vein　19~83
左髂外淋巴结 left external iliac lymph nodes　73~83
左髂总静脉 left common iliac vein　3~17
左输卵管 left uterine tube　57~65,73~83
左输尿管 left ureter　5~7,13~19,45~55,59~121
左臀上动、静脉 left superior gluteal artery and vein　61~63
左臀上动脉 left superior gluteal artery　51~59
左臀上静脉 left superior gluteal vein　51~59
左臀下动、静脉 left inferior gluteal artery and vein　57~113
左阴部内动、静脉 left internal pudental artery and vein　115~121
坐股韧带 ischiofemoral ligament　109~121,199~219
坐骨 ischium　65,125
坐骨肛门窝 ischioanal fossa　65,105~113,123~145,149,151,207~269
坐骨海绵体肌 ischiocavernosus　99~109,157~159,191~211,247~261
坐骨结节 ischial tuberosity　127~157,213~255
坐骨神经 sciatic nerve　61~303
坐骨神经滋养静脉 veins of sciatic nerve　185~187
坐骨体 body of ischium　85~123,191~203
坐骨支 ramus of ischium　159~161,247~263